Essential Nursing Care for
Children and
Young People

Essential Nursing Care for Children and Young People

Theory, Policy and Practice

Chris Thurston

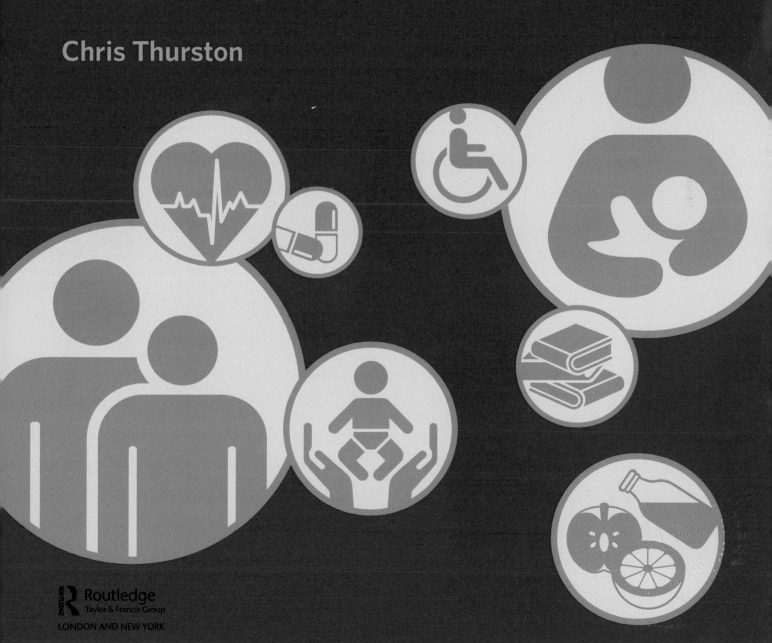

Routledge
Taylor & Francis Group

LONDON AND NEW YORK

First published 2013
by Routledge
2 Park Square, Milton Park, Abingdon, Oxon OX14 4RN

and by Routledge
711 Third Avenue, New York, NY 10017

Routledge is an imprint of the Taylor & Francis Group, an informa business

British Library Cataloguing in Publication Data
A catalogue record for this book is available from the British Library

Library of Congress Cataloging in Publication Data
[CIP data]

ISBN: 978-0-273-75239-4

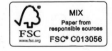

Printed and bound in Great Britain by
TJ International Ltd, Padstow, Cornwall

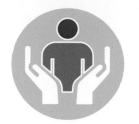
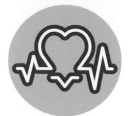
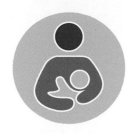
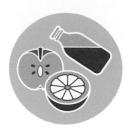
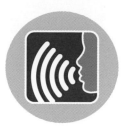

BRIEF CONTENTS

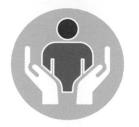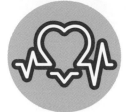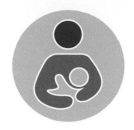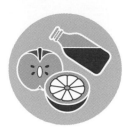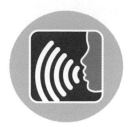

CONTENTS

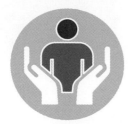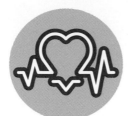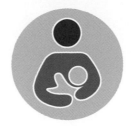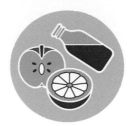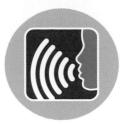

PREFACE

INTRODUCTION

As the nature of children's nurses is progressive both in relation to the developing child and young person, so is their illness and the child branch nursing student; this book offers an exciting and appropriate format to guide the student or child care professional through the process of caring for children and young people in a variety of settings and with an array of needs and conditions. The focus is on the appropriate management of children, young people and their families to ensure a child centred approach using specific conditions within case studies. The book is packed with information and key terms, using the child or young person's voice and case studies; there are interactive exercises, bullet point summaries of complex issues and guidance. With a case study pertinent to each chapter and interactive exercises, this encourages reflection on the key points.

RATIONALE

The changing context of children and young people's health and well-being and the evolving health services they require means that every health practitioner working with the child, young person and their families has to develop the capacity to undertake assessments and interventions in a wide variety of settings while acknowledging the frequently changing environment that the families live in. This needs to be understood in the context of nursing care, family requirements and the needs and wishes of the children and young people. The book explores the challenges of working with children and young people who have a variety of health care needs both in hospital and the community and from infancy to young adulthood.

THE AIM OF THE BOOK

The aim of this book is to develop practitioners 'Fit for Purpose', 'Fit for Practice' and 'Fit for Award' (Nursing and Midwifery Council (NMC) 2004), and therefore the focus of learning in this book is exploring the underpinning theory that will inform developing practice. The learning strategy that underpins the book aims to ensure a student centred and inquiring approach which develops creative problem solving abilities and integrates and utilises research evidence in practice, encouraging the reader to learn from examples to ensure that care given to children, young people and their families is of a consistent high quality and seamless in delivery. Therefore, both an inter-professional and an inquiry-based learning approach have been combined to facilitate this approach. The text will offer resources to fulfil the NMC requirement for the minimum award for pre-registration nursing programmes in the UK.

WHO SHOULD USE THIS BOOK?

This book is focused on the needs of the pre-register child branch nursing student undertaking the modernised pathways leading to registration as a nurse in the field of child nursing. This text offers focused insight with flexible boundaries between the generic and field specific child branch components. Also explored is community and public health practice. The text will therefore fit within a 'typical' programme structure for pre-reg students on nursing degrees on the whole. The package will enhance the student and lecturer experience by focusing on and exploring the main issues which challenge children's nurses and the children and families they care for including emergency care, long-term conditions and the transitions between the community and the hospital and transferring to adult services. The book will also offer supportive text for the period after registration relating to objectives and nature of assessed outcomes. There is a need to provide student nurses with an accessible, practice-oriented book to help guide their work in the developing context of empowering children and young people and their families as users of health services. This book will be packed with information case studies, interactive exercises and bullet points.

This book is also aimed at nursing professionals who work with children and young people and their families in a variety of health care settings in hospital and the community including Student Children's Nurses and Children's Nurses, Learning Disabilities Student Nurses, School Nurses and Community Children's Nurses. The book may also be relevant to students on foundation degrees in health and social care, youth workers and practitioners embarking on NVQ and child care courses.

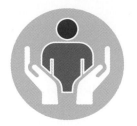 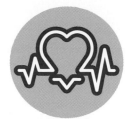 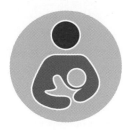 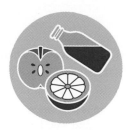 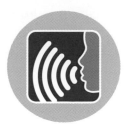

CHAPTER SUMMARIES

CHAPTER 1
Foundations of Children and Young People's Nursing
Sue Collier

On completion of this chapter the reader will be able to:

- Explore historical perspectives of children's nursing in order to understand the origins of professional values.
- Critically explain the impact of policy and guidelines on children and young people's nursing and 'why children and young people's nurses do what they do'.
- Appraise frameworks of care and their appropriateness when caring for children and young people.
- Critically explore the concept of the family and the principles of family-centred care and partnership when caring for children and young people.
- Critically explore the impact of communication leading to a therapeutic relationship with the child or young person and their family.
- Explore the development of the self as a developing children and young people's nurse.

This chapter seeks to place children and young person's nursing into the context of contemporary health care during the twenty-first century, providing key information related to the professional values and the foundations of children and young people's nursing. The children and young people's nurse will be required to follow the guiding professional principles and underpinning theories; assess, plan and implement care; discern when care is not progressing appropriately and to build a therapeutic relationship with the child, young person, parents or carers. This requires effective communication, team work and decision-making (see chapter on long-term care). In order to understand 'why we do what we do in children's and young people's nursing it is important to understand where the discipline has arisen.'

CHAPTER 2
Using Developmental Theories to Enhance Holistic Care
Steve Bilham

On completion of this chapter the reader will be able to:

- Describe the factors that may result in variations in the growth and development of children and young people.
- Reflect upon the role of the family in the development of children and young people.
- Explore the theories of play in relation to the growth and development of children and young people and discuss their value in practice.
- Have knowledge of physical growth and maturation of children and young people in the assessment and planning of care.
- Use theories of child development and play to reflect on the care that respects the child and young person's ability and developing autonomy.

This chapter will explore the social construction of childhood, alongside basic genetics, and variations in growth and development. Examination will also include assessment of physical and developmental growth to include discussion of developmental milestones. Important developmental theories will be discussed including Piaget, Freud, Vygotsky, Erikson, Bronfenbrenner, Skinner and Watson, from birth to adolescence. Attachment theories will also acknowledge Bowlby, while language development will include Chomsky, Brunner and developmental theorists. Alongside this moral development the chapter will reflect upon Piaget, Kohlberg, Berryman and Gilligan. A child's temperament and the value of an understanding of normative play will also be highlighted.

CHAPTER 3
Health Promotion Needs of Children and Young People
Hilary Collins

On completion of this chapter the reader will be able to:

- Identify issues in child health promotion and understand the role of the children's nurse in addressing these.
- Describe the legislation and/or policies and research which influence the health trends and targets for children and young people.
- Understand the children's nurse's role in enabling the care of children, young people with long-term health needs and their families.
- Reflect upon the role of the children's nurse as part of an inter-professional team when promoting health and well-being of children and young people.

- Identify approaches to health promotion that are appropriate to children and young people and consider their relevance and effectiveness.

This chapter aims to raise awareness of the multiplicity of factors that may impact the health and well-being of children in contemporary society and evaluate the role of the health professional as a health promoter. The emphasis on holistic care, health care legislation and policy and other developments has encouraged health professionals to examine practice to use research and to approach change in a dynamic way. If children and young people's nurses are proactive as well as responsive to children, young people and their families/carers, successful health improvement outcomes can be achieved

CHAPTER 4
Cultural Aspects for Children and Young People
Steve Bilham

On completion of this chapter the reader will be able to:

- Reflect upon society's views of the role and position of the child and young person and the implications for practice.
- Reflect upon how personal beliefs and cultural practices impact upon the delivery of holistic care to children and young people and their families.
- Explore how children's nurses can offer culturally appropriate nursing care.

An understanding of culture helps to equip the health professional with beliefs and values that give individuals a sense of identity, self-worth and belonging, as well as providing the rules for behaviour. This enables the child or young person to physically survive and provide for the welfare and support of its members a particular culture and therefore its health care system, including the values, beliefs and practices that group members possess about health promotion and illness prevention. Culture can also help establish the cause, detection and treatment of illness. As a result, concepts of health, illness and care are integral parts of general cultural values, beliefs and practices. By the professional recognizing their own cultural biases, you can learn about or remove unintentional influences. This awareness process must involve examination of one's own prejudices and biases towards diverse groups, as well as an in-depth exploration of one's own cultural background.

CHAPTER 5
Safeguarding Children and Young People
Steven Walker

On completion of this chapter the reader will be able to:

- Describe risk and resilience factors in children and young people.
- Identify the signs, symptoms and effects of abuse.
- Understand how the inter-professional team can use protocols and policies related to children and young people at risk.

- To reflect upon issues of confidentiality in regards to safeguarding children and young people.

Each child is unique and therefore blanket policies and procedures will not support every child, rather a focused approach is required that acknowledges the rights of the child to have holistic and optimum growth and for the reader to be able to assess if abuse has occurred. Children therefore need to feel safe to communicate with professionals, which may lead to issues of confidentiality for the carers working with the child. In order to achieve a balance between family support and safeguarding individual children, the readers need to consider the factors involved in the investigation and intervention in child abuse.

CHAPTER 6
Caring for Children in a Variety of Settings
Sharon Clarke

On completion of this chapter the reader will be able to:

- Identify issues in child health and explain the role of the children's nurse in a variety of settings.
- Explain the children's nurse's role in enabling the care of children, young people with long-term health needs and their families.
- Discuss the role of the children's nurse as part of an inter-professional team when promoting the health and well-being of children and young people in the community setting.
- Identify approaches to health care that are appropriate to children and young people and consider their relevance and effectiveness.

The vast majority of contacts with the health service for children are with primary health care teams. Primary care, through Children's Clinical Networks, Primary Care Trusts and Children's Trusts, has a key role in improving the health and well-being of the children in their local area and addressing health inequalities, both through local strategic partnerships and through work with individual children, young people, families and communities. In a typical year, pre-school children will see their general practitioner about six times while school-aged children will visit two or three times. Most consultations in primary care are for minor illnesses that can be effectively dealt with by the general practitioner, practice nurse or health visitor, together with the family. This chapter aims to provide a resource for workers in a variety of contexts in voluntary or statutory agencies. It will analyse local Children's Clinical Networks by taking a 'journey' approach in identifying the local network, assessment, diagnosis and treatment and specifically addressing access points. It will focus on the relationships between the different parts of the local service. Finally, consideration will be given to the provision of a comprehensive and integrated service, highlighting good practice.

CHAPTER 7
Caring for Children and Young People in the Medical Setting
Carolyn Seeman

On completion of this chapter the reader will be able to:

- Consider the importance of a holistic approach to care through collaboration with the family and MDT.
- Explore the more common interventions of care required for children in a medical setting.
- Understand the appropriate practice required for IV sites and IV infusion.
- Investigate the importance of skin integrity and monitoring.
- Reflect upon the pain management required for a child with medical needs.
- Explore the rationale for evidence-based infection control.

At times it can feel daunting when entering the children's acute medical ward following handover, due to the variety, complexity and sometimes unpredictability of the work that lies ahead. The essence of children's medical nursing is that of holism, considering that the children are usually admitted unexpectedly, have suddenly fallen ill and a trip to the doctors or the emergency department has meant a referral to the children's ward. Children and young people usually arrive with significant others, parents, siblings, grandparents or carers. Most children in today's society live busy, full and active lives and in confining them to hospital there is a danger of shrinking their world considerably. It is recognised that where possible children and young people should be in hospital for the shortest stay possible (DoH 2004) and only if absolutely necessary.

CHAPTER 8
Caring for Children and Young People in the Surgical Setting
Chris Thurston

On completion of this chapter the reader will be able to:

- Explore why accidents and injuries may occur in children and young people.
- Reflect upon assessment with children, young people and families when challenges to LOC and pain are present.
- Plan and implement surgical care for orthopaedic conditions.
- Investigate legal and professional themes around consent to surgical treatment.
- Discuss the effectiveness of surgical nursing care interventions for peri-operative orthopaedic care management.

This chapter will discuss the occurrence of accidents and injuries and the effects of surgery on the child or young person, highlighting how good assessment and planning are vital in helping professionals to develop individualised planning, resulting in optimum quality of care and swift post-operative recovery. The approach will acknowledge the challenges faced by staff in surgical settings and encourage the reader to develop suitable strategies to aid in delivery of peri-operative care. The specific needs and care required for general and orthopaedic surgery will also be highlighted.

CHAPTER 9
Neonatal Nursing Care
Jacki (Oughton) Dopran and Sue Collier

On completion of this chapter the reader will be able to:

- Critically explore the political drivers and professional values which impact on the ethos of neonatal nursing.
- Critically explore the environmental, developmental, social and cultural factors relating to the delivery of holistic and family centred care to the infant and their family when special and/or transitional care are required.
- Critically reflect upon nursing and medical interventions required for the appropriate management of the infant needing special and/or transitional care.
- Critically explore the delivery of evidence-based holistic care to the neonate and their family when special and/or transitional care is needed.

The neonatal unit is a very different environment from any other unit or ward, and the new parents may not have been expecting their new baby to be born early or to require neonatal services. Parents and their families can be experiencing a range of emotions and are possibly just trying to cope with this new and unexpected event. During the past two decades, neonatal care has changed dramatically, which has led to new developments in technology, improved understanding through research and changes to the organisation of neonatal care nationally. This adds further mystification to the care of the preterm baby and potentially adds to the stresses the parents are already experiencing.

CHAPTER 10
Emergency Care of Children and Young People
Carolyn Seeman and Joanne Outridge

On completion of this chapter the reader will be able to:

- Discuss the use of a structured approach to assessing children and young people with emergency care needs.
- Outline the appropriate interventions in managing the care needs of the deteriorating child or young person.
- Identify key individuals involved in the care of the child or young person who presents with emergency care needs, recognising the importance of communication throughout the patient's journey.
- Analyse the impact that acute/stressful situations may have on the family of a child or young person who is receiving emergency care.

For many health care professionals, children are often perceived as being more challenging to manage in an emergency due to the very nature of being a child (Davies 2011). However once these challenges are faced and understood, it becomes clear that a systematic approach to assessment, timely intervention and good communication with appropriate professionals will assist all those caring for children to deliver effective care and management for patients who are deteriorating or who need immediate intervention. The assessment processes will be discussed in more detail further on. This chapter aims to equip nurses with the essential tools that are required to enable safe and sound assessments and initiate interventions to care for these sick children. The aim is to explore some of the objectives using a case study approach, following the journey of a child assisting identification of the factors to consider when caring for any child who may deteriorate.

CHAPTER 11
The Challenges of Sexual Exploration for Young People
Susan Walker

On completion of this chapter the reader will be able to:

- Talk about the main methods of contraception available in the UK.
- Describe and explain how each method of contraception works, what may make it fail, how often it may fail and the risks and benefits associated with it.
- Talk about the most common sexually transmitted diseases affecting young people in the UK and how these can be prevented.
- Understand the law regarding sexual practice and young people.
- Understand the social, cultural and political contexts in which young people explore their sexuality.
- Reflect upon the ethical and professional challenges of caring for young people as they mature and explore their sexuality.
- Apply this knowledge in a non-judgemental and ethical manner which respects the diverse views and experiences of young people and their families.

The issue of young people and sexual behaviour is a complex one. It cannot simply be addressed within a biological context but involves social, ethical, cultural, religious and legal aspects. A health professional working with young people will inevitably encounter the issue of sexuality and must be equipped to deal with the subject compassionately and knowledgeably. Sexual desire, sexual behaviour, specific sexual practices and sexual orientation are highly charged areas of human existence, which arouse strong emotions. This is particularly the case where young people are concerned because the gradual transition from childhood to adulthood is not clearly defined in mainstream twenty-first century culture in the UK.

CHAPTER 12
Mental Health and the Challenges of Mental Ill Health
Steven Walker and Dave Hawkes

On completion of this chapter the reader will be able to:

- Explore the impact and implications of policy and legislation on the services delivered to children and adolescents for mental health.
- Evaluate the collaboration at the personal, organisational and societal level in providing child and adolescent mental health services.
- Analyse the evidence base for health promotion in child and adolescent mental health services.
- Reflect upon the appropriate approaches when communicating with a child in distress.
- Review the evidence base for care or service delivery to children and adolescents for those with mental health problems and/or disorders.
- Understand and explore the therapeutic interventions used with children who have mental health issues.
- Explore the overview of family and system therapies for children and young people.

The chapter aspires to provide a foundation of theoretical ideas and practical guidance that will offer support and create the basis for informed, reflective, confident practice. For a minority of young people, the issues for mental health become more challenging, and they will require further support to resolve the problems that arise; this will also be explored. While there is a real need for mental health nurses specialising in children and young people's mental health, it is not the role of this chapter to explore this specialist training rather, it is important in any setting where children and young people are to offer guidance on how to assess, offer simple interventions which cause no harm to the child or young person and refer to the appropriate services, including Child And Family Consultation (CAFC) or Child And Adolescent Health Services (CAMHS).

CHAPTER 13
The Challenges for Children and Young People with Learning Disability from Black Asian Minority Ethnic (BAME) Background
Rena Williams

On completion of this chapter the reader will be able to:

- Explore the term learning disabilities and have an understanding of the categories of learning disabilities.
- Have an awareness of the impact that a child with severe learning disabilities has on the family unit.
- Analyse some of the dynamics faced with providing support to families from BAME backgrounds.
- Plan a package of health and social care based on holistic and multicultural needs.
- Analyse and evaluate your skills in providing family friendly care support within diverse communities.

A key factor to effective LD care is inter-professional and inter-agency team work with an approach; this person centered approach to the young person and family will endeavour to diminish the expert power that can often act as a barrier towards families as well as encourage engagement, mutual learning, peer support and partnership working. Such working practice will have more therapeutic effect for the family and young person as opposed to a prescriptive model of care. The health practitioner should be working alongside a theme of family focus and well-being, which is also paramount to the delivery of effective care for people with LD as the family more often takes on the full time caring role, which can lead to family burn out, resentment and breakdown, all of which have physiological and psychological pitfalls.

CHAPTER 14
Children and Young People with Life-Limiting Conditions
Sharon Clarke

On completion of this chapter the reader will be able to:

- Analyse the needs of children, young people and their families requiring respite and palliative care.
- Review the evidence base for care or service delivery to children and young people and their families with respite and palliative care needs.
- Critically appraise the effectiveness of personal, organisational and societal collaboration in providing respite and palliative care for children and young people and their families.
- Critically reflect upon the impact that cultural, psychological, social and spiritual perceptions of death and dying can have upon the delivery of palliative care to children, young people and their families.

This chapter is intended for professionals working with children and young people and/or their families who require palliative care. The purpose of this chapter is to develop knowledge and understanding of the needs of children and young people who require palliative care and the evidence-based interventions and strategies that might be used to better enable the care of such individuals. Consideration will also be given to the needs of the child and young person's family, carers and society and how these might be most effectively met. Finally, this chapter will identify good practices in how children's needs require health, education and social services to work together.

CHAPTER 15
Preparation for Professional Practice
Sue Collier

On completion of this chapter the reader will be able to:

- Critically explore political drivers to protect patients and promote health and well-being.
- Assess the mechanisms and processes which are utilised in monitoring, evaluating and improving standards of care delivered.
- Critically reflect upon team working in terms of leadership qualities, management skills, communication skills and evidence-based practice.

- Critically evaluate the concepts of professional/inter-professional collaboration and issues around accountability and responsibility in managing the delivery of care.
- Explore how organisational systems facilitate the quality of care delivery and safeguard quality.
- Be able to understand the key skills required to lead a team of nurses and to effectively manage the care of a group of patients.

Current policy statements emphasise the need for clinical governance and interprofessional collaboration to reflect the necessity for risk assessment, risk management, research and evidence-based practice, in the provision of healthcare. Leading, managing or co-ordinating care for a group of children and young people can be a rewarding experience, yet it requires practice and a range of honed skills. Preparing to extend those experiences to include overseeing an entire ward requires a 'fluency' with the skills, knowledge and understanding of the key concepts on which the organisation operates and a contemporary knowledge of key professional issues. This chapter will enable the reader to consider aspects of organisation and management of care and understanding of the organisational processes that influence the delivery of care.

CHAPTER 16
Transferring to Adult Services for Young People with Long-Term Conditions
Chris Thurston

On completion of this chapter the reader will be able to:

- Explore transitional processes in relation to young people as they become adults.
- Understand the challenges in the lives of young people with a lifelong or life limiting illness.
- Critically analyse the issues affecting young people with long-term health conditions.
- Explore the development of services, during and after transferring to adult services.
- Critically evaluate provision for young people with long-term health conditions.

This chapter will discuss how to improve the practice of health professionals in understanding the transitional experiences of young people with long-term conditions. While the young people have lifelong conditions, they also have commonalities with their peers who are unaffected.

Reading this chapter will enable the understanding of the physical, psychological and social support required when transferring to adult services for a young person with long-term health needs. The changing context of young people's lives and the services they require mean that every health practitioner working with young people has to develop the capacity to undertake assessments and interventions in a wide variety of settings. Such activity needs to be understood in the context of statutory duties, agency requirements and the needs and wishes of the young people. Young people already feel disempowered by society, and this is before they have any further challenges in their lives. To start the transition into adulthood for Jenny (from the case study in the chapter) with her health needs, transferring into adult services issues may arise as she is required to adapt to adult health care. An exploration of the definition of transition and its importance will offer explanations of the journey from child to young adult, when transitioning with a long-term illness. This includes an acknowledgement of the effects of physical and human development on the young person and also the attributes of the young person with long-term illness, including the debilitating effect the condition has on the young person and their body. There will also be a focused exploration of themes related to transition including youth culture, comparative youth and the biographical perspective of youth.

CHAPTER 17
Research with Children and Young People
Tina Moules and Darren Sharpe

On completion of this chapter the reader will be able to:

- Discuss different approaches, techniques and methods for researching with children and young people.
- Search for and interpret information from a variety of sources.
- Understand the ethical issues involved in carrying out research with children and young people.
- Explain the importance of disseminating the findings of research into the practice arena.
- Understand the requirement for developing the capacity for conceptual, critical and independent thinking.

This chapter starts by giving an overview of how the involvement of children and young people has changed over recent years and the different level at which they can and are involved. It then goes through the research process, specifically focusing on issues related to doing research with children. The chapter concentrates on non-therapeutic research with children and young people. This type of research aims only to gain new knowledge and so is unlikely to benefit the participants. Therapeutic research, sometimes referred to as clinical research, on the other hand aims to benefit a particular group of patients by improving available treatment. Find out more about this type of research with children and young people in the following readings:

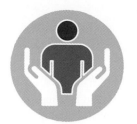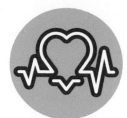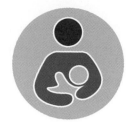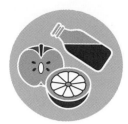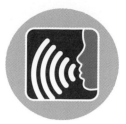

AUTHORS

Chris Thurston

Director of Teaching and Learning, Anglia Ruskin University (ARU)

RN, RSCN, Dip N, BSc [Hon's] in Health Studies [Nursing]. MA Sociology and Health Studies, MA Teaching and Learning in Higher and Further education. NMC Nurse Tutor, PhD, Fellow of The Academy Higher Education, panel member for the NMC.

Chris worked with children and families on the children's ward, which had children who had a variety of challenges including issues around long-term conditions and child protection. She then started working within the university's teaching modules with child branch nursing students on pre-registration programmes and also multi-professional groups about issues surrounding safeguarding children. In 2010 she completed a PhD describing young people with CF, their feelings, emotions and memories around their life story and their health care experiences including transition. The young people have been encouraged through taped interviews to reflect upon their life and transitions they have experienced. Her present role is to support fellow academics in teaching and assessing health, social care and educational students.

Publications

Thurston, C. (2006) Child abuse: Recognition of Causes and Types of Abuse, Advanced Practice. *Practice Nurse* 26 May, Part 29e.

Thurston, C. (2006) Child protection: Primary Prevention and Early Intervention, Advanced Practice. *Practice Nurse,* 9 June, Part 29f.

Thurston, C. and Bird, M. (2009) *Pre-Registration Nursing, Common Foundation Programme.* Pearson Custom Publication: Harlow, UK.

Thurston, C. and Church, J. (2001) Involving Children and Families in Decision Making about Health, (Ed.) P. Foley et al. *Children in Society.* The Open University/Palgrave, Basingstoke.

Walker, S. and Thurston, C. (2006) *Safeguarding Children and Young People, a Guide to Integrated Practice.* Russell House publishing Ltd: Lyme Regis.

Steven Walker

MSc, CQSW, Dip FT

Steven is a registered social worker and UKCP Psychotherapist and programme leader for Child and Adolescent Mental Health in the Faculty of Health and Social Care, Anglia Ruskin University. He qualified in 1985 at the London School of Economics and Political Science and worked in London and Essex in child protection and child and adolescent mental health services. Steven has published over 50 scholarly articles in national and international journals as well as eight textbooks. His recent research has included an evaluation of a young person's mental health and an investigation into the emotional and mental health needs of young ex-soldiers.

Susan Walker

Senior Lecturer, ARU

MB BCh DFFP BA (Hons) MPhil PhD

Dr Susan Walker is a senior lecturer in sexual health at ARU. She qualified in medicine from Queen's University, Belfast, in 1990 and worked as a GP until 2008, during which time she developed a particular interest in the sociological and cultural influences upon sexual and reproductive health. She undertook a BA in Women's Studies and Sociology at Anglia Ruskin University in 2005 and completed a PhD in 'The Effect of Body Image upon Contraceptive Outcomes' at Cambridge University in 2010. Her area of special interest is the intersection of gender, culture and health.

Dave Hawkes

Senior Lecturer, ARU

Dave is a Senior Lecturer in Mental Health at ARU. He is a mental health nurse and has an MA in Mental Health and teaches on solution focused therapy. He has undertaken research with a study on exploring the impact of the miracle question in solution focused therapy. Dave also runs modules on Solution Focused Brief Therapy in Clinical Practice, which is designed to enable practitioners in a variety of clinical settings to use Solution Focused Brief Therapy (SFBT) skills in their day-to-day work. It explores the development and application of SFBT, the philosophical and research base that underpins the model and the implications of the approach on partnership and collaboration with people seeking help for a variety of difficulties in a variety of settings.

Publications

Hawkes, D. (2007) Book review of 'Humanising Psychiatry and Mental Health Care: The Challenge of the Person-centred

Approach'. *Health and Social Care in the Community*, 15(5), 505–506.

Hingley, D. and Hawkes, D. (2007) Recovery intelligence and 'Groundhog Day' effect in mental health care. *Mental Health Nursing*, 1 July.

Rena Williams

Senior Lecturer, ARU

Masters Level, Mentorship Preparation, BSC Hons Specialist Practitioner – Community Learning Disabilities, Project 2000. Registered Nurse (Mental Handicap/learning disability)

Starting as Community Auxiliary Nurse, Rena qualified as a learning disabilities nurse and became in time a school nurse for children with special needs. She has also used her experience and knowledge to be a management board member of Anika Patrice Project, a voluntary organisation for people with a learning difficulty with family and carers who come from the African, Caribbean and Asian communities. Rena was a Health Facilitator at Barking and Dagenham PCT in London/Essex, during which time she undertook an Evaluation of Health Facilitation.

Sharon Clarke

Senior Lecturer, ARU

RGN, RSCN, BSc [Hons] in Child Health Nursing. Postgraduate Diploma in Community Specialist Practice. Postgraduate Diploma in Teaching and Learning in Higher and Further Education.

Sharon has worked for twenty years within the NHS as a children's nurse in a variety of settings. Initially she worked with children and families on children's wards followed by a number of years working within paediatric intensive care units before moving to community children's nursing. In 2006 Sharon started working within the university teaching modules with child branch nursing students on pre-registration programmes. Presently Sharon facilitates child branch groups and supervises undergraduate projects, alongside teaching and running modules. Sharon has been involved in the design and provision of programmes of education and training, including educational audits, to evaluate the quality and outcomes of professional education and training. Currently, Sharon is completing her MA research in developing educational resources to support the continuous professional development of professionals caring for children with life limiting and life threatening conditions. Throughout her career Sharon has embodied lifelong learning and fully endorses that there is a need for an unequivocal commitment to continued investment in nursing, midwifery and health visiting education with the aim of improving the quality of care provided for patients and clients, their families and the wider community by nurses. Amid the enormous changes continuing to take place in health care provision, Sharon believes that education must be accessible, relevant and flexible in order to prepare knowledgeable, flexible and competent practitioners capable of meeting the varied health care needs of local communities.

Sue Collier

Senior Lecturer/Admissions Tutor (Child branch), ARU

MSc Professional Nursing Practice: Child Health Nursing Practice; English National Board Higher Award in Nursing; BSc. Professional Nursing Practice; Registered General Nurse; Post Graduate Diploma in Teaching and Learning; Registered Sick Children's Nurse; National Nursery Examinations Board;

Starting working in local authority day nurseries, Sue qualified as a nursery nurse and worked as a Nursery Officer with well children under five years and in the neonatal unit setting. Inspired by caring for vulnerable children and their families in the neonatal setting, Sue furthered her career by qualifying as a Registered Nurse and then a Registered Sick Children's Nurse. Sue has worked as a Senior Sister in the neonatal setting, Children's Services Co-ordinator, Matron and Named Nurse for Safeguarding Children and Young People.

Carolyn Seeman

NNEB, RGN, RSCN, BSc, PGDip HE

Over the last 16 years Carolyn has worked as a Children's Nurse primarily in a District General Hospital. Her experience has included nursing sick children in a medical, surgical and community setting. Within the practice setting she held the role of Clinical Facilitator for Acute Care within the Trust, and this role was a key factor in forming her interest in High Dependency care. Since entering Higher Education as a Lecturer in Children's Nursing, she has continued to develop this through the modules she delivers. She is currently undertaking a Masters in Teaching and Learning, which she hopes to complete in the next year.

Steve Bilham

RGN

Steve qualified as a Registered General Nurse in 1986 and moved quickly into working with children, young people and their families. After a number of years working in hospital, he moved to working in the community, qualifying as a Health Visitor in 1991. With a strong and long lasting interest in promoting all aspects of good health, he has worked in a number of settings, both urban and rural, interspersed with a period of time teaching in higher education. In 2010 Steve moved from the academic setting to continue working in practice. His current role sees him working in the East End of London. His research and academic interests include how children develop within all societies and how people perceive the world we live in.

Darren Sharpe

Postdoctoral Research Fellow Childhood and Youth Research Institute

Darren is a sociologist and specialises in the involvement of children, young people and vulnerable adults in social policy research. His work focuses primarily on (i) the theoretical development and practices of active youth participation/citizenship,

(ii) social innovation and e-inclusion and (iii) young people's mental health and well-being. Prior to his appointment at Anglia Ruskin University, Darren was the Development Officer at the National Youth Agency think tank. Darren also lectured at Nottingham Trent University and Loughborough University in the social sciences. He has taught and developed modules on Qualitative Research Methods, Social Structure, Race, Culture and Society and Criminal Justice Research. At Loughborough University he was a Research Associate in the Young Carers Research Group.

Joanne Outteridge

MSc Child Health Nursing, Postgraduate Diploma Higher Education, Postgraduate Diploma Health Care Ethics, Bachelor of Nursing, RN (Child), ENB 415 (Children's Intensive Care Nursing), Registered Nurse Teacher.

After qualifying as a children's nurse Joanne worked at Guy's and St Thomas' NHS Foundation Trust before moving to St Bartholomew School of Nursing and Midwifery, City University, as a Lecturer in Children's Nursing. Joanne moved to Anglia Ruskin University in 2004 where she continues to teach on pre-reg and CPD courses. She is course leader for the Graduate Certificate in Paediatric Intensive Care and Graduate Certificate in Special and Intensive Care of the Newborn; she is also actively involved with the Paediatric Intensive Care Society Educator's Group.

Tina Moules

PhD Health and Social Care, MSc Behavioural Biology, Cert. Ed, RN, RN(Child), Clinical Teacher, Registered Nurse Tutor.

After qualifying as a children's nurse and working as a charge nurse at Great Ormond Street Children's Hospital, Tina moved into lecturing in Children's Nursing. Tina moved to Anglia Ruskin University in 1994 as Head of Division, Childhood Studies and undertook a variety of roles including Head of Department, Advanced Practice and Research and until 2011 Director of Research. She has also has been a reviewer for the *Journal of Clinical Nursing*; *Journal of Child Health Care*, and an active member of a number of research groups including Royal College of Nursing (RCN) Research Society, Association of Child Health Nurse Researchers (ACHNR-UK), ReACH Network (Research in Adolescent and Child Health), East of England Nursing Research network and Researching Children Network (International Network).

Publications

Mantle, G., Moules, T. and Johnson, K. (2007) Whose Wishes and Feelings? Children's Autonomy and Parental Influence in Family Court Enquiries. *British Journal of Social Work*, 37(5), 785–805.

Moules, T. (2009) 'They wouldn't know how it feels…': characteristics of quality care from young people's perspectives: a participatory research project. *Journal of Child Health Care*, 13(4), 322–332.

Moules, T. and O'Brien, N. (2007) So Round the Spiral Again: a Reflective Participatory Research Project with Children and Young People. *Educational Action Research*, 15(3), 385–402.

Moules, T. and Ramsay, J. (2008) *The Textbook of Children's and Young People's Nursing*, 2nd edn. London: Blackwell.

O'Brien, N. and Moules. T. (2007) The child's perspective and Service delivery, in D. DeBell (ed.) *Public Health Practice and the School-age Population*. London: Hodder Arnold. Ch. 11. (An RCN Accredited book).

Jacki (Dopran) Oughton, MA in Law and Ethics, RGN, RM, 904,998. She has worked in neonatal nursing for the past 26 years, the last 12 being focused in education and management. Jackie's management experience is in level 2 and 3 services and across a neonatal network along with clinical interest for patient safety and risk management. Her current role is Senior Nurse NICU at the Homerton Hospital and Lead Nurse for North East London Perinatal Network. She has also has worked on the National Patients Safety agency website in regard to care bundles.

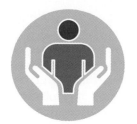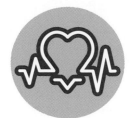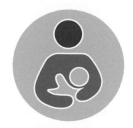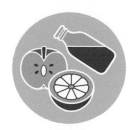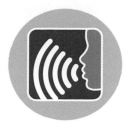

ACKNOWLEDGEMENTS

We would all like to thank the many children, families and students that we have had the pleasure to work with over the years who inspired us to create this essential children's nursing book. Whether in the capacity of children's nurses, researchers or nurse lecturers, also thanks go to lecturer colleagues Julie Teatheredge and Sally Goldspink who gave valuable insight into the mental health chapter.

PUBLISHER'S ACKNOWLEDGEMENTS

We are grateful to the following for permission to reproduce copyright material:

Cartoons

Cartoon 17.0 from Hospitalized children's views of the good nurse, *Nursing Ethics*, 16, pp. 543–60 (Brady, M. 2009), Sage Journals. © 2009 Sage Publications. Reprinted by permission of Sage Publications.

Figures

Figure 1.4 from *Politics UK*, 4th ed., p. 530 (Jones, B. 2001), Pearson Education Limited. © 2001 Pearson Education Limited; Figure 1.5 from Family centred care: a concept analysis, *Journal of Advanced Nursing*, 29, pp. 1178–1187 (Hutchfield, K. 1999), Blackwell Science; Figure 1.8 from *Children's and young people's nursing in practice: A problem-based learning approach*, Palgrave Macmillan (Coleman, V., Smith, L. and Bradshaw, M. 2007); Figure 3.5 from Health promotion: the Tannahill model revisited, *Public Health*, 122, pp. 1387–91 (Tannahill, A. 2008); Figure 7.5 from NICE Guidelines (2007) National Institute for Health and Clinical Excellence; Figure 8.8 from The development of the Glamorgan paediatric pressure ulcer risk assessment scale, *Journal of Wound Care*, 18, pp. 17–21 (Willock, J., Baharestani, M. and Anthony, D. 2009); Figure 9.6 from Extravasation of neonates revisited, http://www.nrls.npsa.nhs.uk/resources/type/signals/?entryid45=66756, © 2011 Crown; Figure 9.7 from Parer, J., Glob. libr. women's med. (IBSN: 1756-2228) 2008; DOI 10.3843/GLOWM.10194, http://www.glowm.com/index.html?p=glowm.cml/section_view&articleid=194, The Foundation for the Global Library of Women's Medicine Ltd; Figure 9.8 from http://catalog.nucleusinc.com/imagescooked/7021W.jpg, Nucleus Medical Media, Inc.; Figure 9.29 from Neonatal Jaundice CG9, http://guidance.nice.org.uk/CG98/Guidance/pdf/English, National Institute for Health and Clinical Excellence; Figure 10.6 from Guidelines, medical information and reports, http://www.resus.org.uk/pages/mediMain.htm, Resuscitation Council (UK); Figure 14.1 from Breaking bad news to parents: The children's nurses role, *International Journal of Palliative Nursing*, 12, pp. 115–120 (Price, P., McNeilly, P. and Surgenor, M. 2006), MA Healthcare Ltd.; Figure 14.2 from *Square Table: Local Learning and Evaluation Report*, Children's Hospices UK and ACT (2011). © 2011 Children's Hospices UK and Association for Children with Life Threatening or Terminal Conditions and their Families, ACT, the publisher/authors for the various publications is now called Together for Short Lives. The new organisation was launched in October 2011 following the merger of two children's palliative care charities, ACT and Children's Hospices UK. For more information see www.togetherforshortlives.org.uk; Figure 14.3 from *Children's Palliative Care in Africa*, Oxford University Press (Amery, J. 2009). © 2009 Oxford University Press; Figure 14.4 from *A framework for the development of integrated multi-agency care pathways for children with life-threatening and life-limiting conditions*, Children's Hospices UK and ACT (2004). © 2004 Children's Hospices UK and Association for Children with Life Threatening or Terminal Conditions and their Families, ACT, the publisher/authors for the various publications is now called Together for Short Lives. The new organisation was launched in October 2011 following the merger of two children's palliative care charities, ACT and Children's Hospices UK. For more information see www.togetherforshortlives.org.uk; Figure 14.5 from *Right People, Right Place, Right Time*, 1st ed., Association for Children with Life Threatening or Terminal Conditions (2009). © 2009 Children's Hospices UK and Association for Children with Life Threatening or Terminal Conditions, ACT, the publisher/authors of the various publications is now called Together for Short Lives. The new organisation was launched in October 2011 following the merger for two children's palliative care charities, ACT and Children's Hospices UK. For more information see www.togetherforshortlives.org.uk; Figure 14.6 from The Mercer model of paediatric palliative care, *European Journal Of Palliative Care*, 12, pp. 22–25 (Brown, E. and Mercer, A. 2005), Hayward Publishing; Figure 14.8 from *Palliative care services for children and young people in England: an independent review for the Secretary of State for Health*, Department of Health, UK (Craft, A. and Killen S. 2007). © 2007 Department of Health, UK; Figure 14.9 from Symptoms in children/young people with progressive malignant disease: United Kingdom Children's Cancer Study Group/Paediatric Oncology Nurses Forum survey, *Pediatrics*, 117, pp. 1179–86 (Goldman, A., Hewitt, M., Collins, G.S., Childs, M. and Hain, R. 2006), American Academy of Pediatrics. © 2006 AAP. Reproduced with permission from the AAP; Figure 14.11 from Symptom care flowcharts: a case study, *Paediatric Nursing*, 19, pp. 14–17 (Willis, E. 2007), RCN Publishing; Figure 14.12 from Hospital nurses' views of the signs and symptoms that herald the onset of the dying phase in oncology patients, *International Journal of Palliative Nursing* 18, pp. 143–49 (van der Werff, G., Paans, W. and Nieweg, R. 2012), MA Healthcare Ltd.; Figure 15.8 from *Leadership and Nursing Management*, 2nd ed., W.B. Saunders (Huber, D. 2000) Elsevier Health Sciences; Figure 17.3 from *Involving service users in health and social care research*, Routledge (Lowes, L. and Hulatt, I. 2005); Figure 17.4 from Gaining children's perspectives: A multiple method approach to explore environmental influences on healthy eating and physical activity, *Health & Place*, 15, pp. 614–21 (Pearce, A., Kirk, C., Cummins, S., Collins, M., Elliman, D., Connolly, A.M. and Law, C. 2009), Elsevier Health Sciences.

Tables

Table 7.3 from *The recognition and assessment of acute pain in children*, Royal College of Nursing (2009), pp. 6–7; Table 7.5 from National Institute of Health and Clinical Excellence; Table 7.8 from *Developing practical skills for nursing children and young people*, Hodder Arnold (Glasper, A., Aylott, M. and Battrick, C. 2010); Tables 9.1 and 9.2 from *Standards for hospitals providing neonatal intensive and high dependency care*, 2nd ed., British Association of Perinatal Medicine (2001); Table 14.1 from *Right People, Right Place, Right Time*, 1st ed., Association for Children with Life threatening or Terminal Conditions (ACT) (2009). © 2009 Association for Children with Life threatening or Terminal Conditions (ACT), ACT, the publisher/authors of the various publications is now called Together for Short Lives. The new organisation was launched in October 2011 following the merger for two children's palliative care charities, ACT and Children's Hospices UK. For more information see www.togetherforshortlives.org.uk; Table 14.3 from *A framework for the development of integrated multi-agency care pathways for children with life-threatening and life-limiting conditions,* Children's Hospices UK and ACT (2004). © 2004 Children's Hospices UK and Association for Children with Life Threatening or Terminal Conditions, ACT, the publisher/authors for the various publications is now called Together for Short Lives. The new organisation was launched in October 2011 following the merger for two children's palliative care charities, ACT and Children's Hospices UK. For more information see www.togetherforshortlives.org.uk; Table 14.4 adapted from Pediatric palliative care, *New England Journal of Medicine*, p. 350 (Himelstein, P., Hilden, M., Boldt, M. and Weissman, D. 2004); Table 14.5 from *Square Table: Local Learning and Evaluation Report*, Children's Hospices UK and Association for Children with Life threatening or Terminal Conditions (ACT) (2011). © 2011 Association for Children with Life threatening or Terminal Conditions (ACT), ACT, the publisher/authors of the various publications is now called Together for Short Lives. The new organisation was launched in October 2011 following the merger for two children's palliative care charities, ACT and Children's Hospices UK. For more information see www.togetherforshortlives.org.uk; Table 14.8 from *Withholding or withdrawing life sustaining treatment in children: A framework for practice*, 2nd ed., Royal College of Paediatrics and Child Health (RCPCH) London (2004); Table 15.5 from *Safeguarding children and young people: A guide to integrated practice*, Russell House Publishing Ltd. (Walker, S. and Thurston, C. 2006). © 2006 Walker, S. and Thurston, C.; Table 16.1 adapted from Transition to adult services for children and young people with palliative care needs: A systematic review, *Archives of Disease in Childhood*, p. 96 (Doug, M., Adi, Y., Williams, J., Paul, M., Kelly, D., Petchey, R. and Carter, Y.H. 2011), BMJ Publishing Group; Table 16.4 adapted from *Risk society: Towards a new modernity*, Sage Publications (Beck, U. 1992) © 1992 Sage Publications. Reproduced by permission of Sage Publications.

Text

Activity 9.1 from New Born Life Support, http://www.resus.org.uk/pages/nls.pdf, Resuscitation Council UK; Box 10. from 'Boy of 11 dies of asthma attack at school after teacher was "too busy to call him an ambulance"', *Daily Mail*, 18/03/2010 (Hull, L.), © 2010 Solo Syndication; Box 14 from *Square Table: Local Learning and Evaluation Report*, Children's Hospices UK and ACT (2011). © 2011 Children's Hospices UK and Association for Children with Life Threatening or Terminal Conditions, ACT, the publisher/authors for the various publications is now called Together for Short Lives. The new organisation was launched in October 2011 following the merger for two children's palliative care charities, ACT and Children's Hospices UK. For more information see www.togetherforshortlives.org.uk; Activity 14.1 from *A framework for the development of integrated multi-agency care pathways for children with life-threatening and life-limiting conditions*, Children's Hospices UK and ACT (2004). © 2004 Children's Hospices UK and Association for Children with Life-Threatening or Terminal Conditions (ACT), ACT, the publisher/authors for the various publications is now called Together for Short Lives. The new organisation was launched in October 2011 following the merger for two children's palliative care charities, ACT and Children's Hospices UK. For more information see www.togetherforshortlives.org.uk; Box 15.4 from Family centred care: A concept analysis, *Journal of Advanced Nursing*, 29, pp. 1178–87 (Hutchfield, K. 1999). © 1999 John Wiley & Sons Ltd.

Photographs

The publisher would like to thank the following for their kind permission to reproduce their photographs:

(Key: b-bottom; c-centre; l-left; r-right; t-top)

Alamy Images: Able Images 91b, Anna Omelchencko 215, Bubbles 91, James Davies 24; Mandy Godbehear 91cl, Megan

Maloy 91tr, Paul Hakimata, Young Woolff Photography 433; **Bridgeman Art Library Ltd:** National Museum, Oslo, Norway 345; **Corbis:** Bettmann 4; **Getty Images:** AFP 48, David Aaron Troy 209, Time & Life Images 50; **Harlow Healthcare**, www.healthforallchildren.co.uk 43; **Mary Evans Picture Library:** 85, 86; **Rex Features:** Daily Mail 121; **Science Photo Library Ltd:** A J Photo 27, Adam Gault 26, Garry Watson 122, Gusto Images 181, RIA Novosti 52, Scott Camazine; **Seca:** 43; **Shutterstock.com:** Lanych 91bl, Spotmatik, Studio1One 91tl

All other images © Pearson Education

In some instances we have been unable to trace the owners of copyright material, and we would appreciate any information that would enable us to do so.

CHAPTER 1
Foundations of Children and Young People's Nursing

Sue Collier

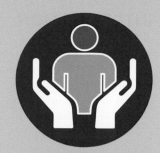

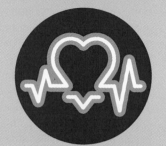

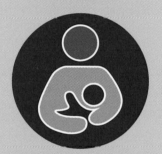

LEARNING OUTCOMES

On completion of this chapter, the reader will be able to:

- Explore historical perspectives of children's nursing in order to understand the origins of professional values.
- Critically explain the impact of policy and guidelines on children and young people's nursing and 'why children and young people's nurses do what they do.'
- Appraise frameworks of care and their appropriateness when caring for children and young people.
- Critically explore the concept of the family and the principles of family-centred care and partnership when caring for children and young people.
- Critically explore the impact of communication leading to a therapeutic relationship with the child or young person and their family.
- Explore the development of the self as a developing children and young people's nurse.

TALKING POINT

'Just over a quarter (26 per cent) of households with dependent children are single parent families, and there are 2 million single parents in Britain today. This figure has remained consistent since the mid-1990s.'
Office for National Statistics (2012)

'Children's nurses have always had to be creative to gain the cooperation of children.'
Crawford (2011)

'Between April 2006 and March 2007, the total hospital admissions due to asthma reached 80,595 which cost the NHS an estimated £61 million.'
Asthma UK (2011)

INTRODUCTION

This chapter seeks to place children and young people's nursing into the context of contemporary healthcare during the 21st century, providing key information related to the professional values and the foundations of children and young people's nursing. The children and young people's nurse will be required to follow the guiding professional principles; to understand the underpinning theories; to assess, plan and implement care; to discern when care is not progressing appropriately and to build a therapeutic relationship with the child, young person, parents or carers. This requires effective communication, teamwork and decision making (see Chapter 15). In order to understand *why we do what we do in children's and young people's nursing it is important to understand where the discipline has arisen.*

As healthcare practitioners, children's nurses are in a pivotal position to build a therapeutic relationship with the child, young person and their families. Effective communication and active listening are key to effective nursing care and documentation. The children and young people's nurse is required to integrate professional values and directives into the evidence based care of children and young people. The Nursing and Midwifery Council (2008) domains of nursing have been integrated into this chapter to demonstrate the correlation with children's nursing practice.

This case study will involve Rhys and his family to illustrate the issues children and young people face during they journey with asthma through healthcare. While the asthma journey through healthcare is relatively commonplace, the impact it has on each child or young person will differ, requiring individualised nursing assessments. Children and young people do not exist in isolation and have parents and carers who may wish to have a role in supporting and encouraging their offspring. The ethos of children's nursing is working in family centred care and partnership with parents and carers. There are many perspectives to children's nursing, including legal and ethical perspectives, professional, interprofessional practice and external partnerships. Children's nursing must comply with key government policies and guidance.

HISTORICAL PERSPECTIVES OF CHILDREN AND YOUNG PEOPLE'S NURSING

If the historical perspectives of children's nursing are explored in conjunction with the society of the day, it will allow some insight as to why some initiatives were successful while others clearly failed. Although contemporary society has changed, some of the issues have similarities with the past. Jolley (2011) has undertaken research into the history of children's nursing giving valuable insight into the origins of children's nursing, frequently explaining how external influences have helped to shape children's nursing. Ramsay (2008) points out that children's nursing is a comparatively recent specialism, traceable only to the 18th and 19th century yet Jolley (2011) identifies that all healthcare professions have existed for substantial periods of time. According to Lumsden (2010) professions have developed in 'silos' rather than in an integrated way. This means that each of the healthcare professions has established its 'professional identity', which shapes and influences service development and service issues (Figure 1.1). It may have been due to prevailing issues in society and political drivers at the time, as to whether children required a child-focused nurse to provide care. Jolley (2011) highlights that in order to understand what shapes the standards of care and the standards of the professional children's nurse in contemporary nursing it is essential to consider the historical perspectives. Lumsden (2010) reports that during the 19th century the professionals had expertise in a specific area and were autonomous practitioners, but were both predominantly male and also unregulated, and compares this to a contemporary professional who works for an organisation in which there is professional regulation and should no longer be predominately led by males or upper classes. There is a tendency in contemporary children's nursing for a predominantly female workforce.

An insight to the way in which children were treated in society can be traced back to Thomas Coram in 1739. Coram

---

CASE STUDY 1.1

Rhys Jones is a 4-year-old boy, who lives with his mother, Amanda, step-father, Huw, and 2-year-old sister, Bethan. Amanda is 7 months pregnant with Rhys's half-sibling. Rhys has been diagnosed with asthma and takes preventative medication. Amanda is torn between caring for both her children. Amanda's mum, Marge, lives 30 miles away and does not drive. Rhys visits his biological father, Anthony, and his stepmother, Ellen, every other weekend. Ellen has a little boy, Ben, aged 6, from a previous relationship.

Rhys has been admitted to hospital with acute exacerbation of asthma. Due to Rhys's respiratory status, an intravenous fluid regime has been prescribed. Rhys has also been prescribed nebulisers and oral prednisolone to aid his recovery.

During the night Rhys said he had a bad dream and wet the bed. The practice supervisor discovered this at the ward handover and asks Paige, the student nurse, to attend to Rhys's hygiene needs. On her way to collect the equipment, another nurse stops Paige and asks her to give her a hand. Paige tries to explain that her practice supervisor has asked her to care for Rhys. The other nurse says 'He does not need any help, his mum is with him and can manage on her own.'

Paige feels uncomfortable as this is not apparent from the initial care assessment from the previous day. Rhys's mother is heavily pregnant and is unable to fully participate in direct care. Amanda also thought she would not be allowed to stay with Rhys and needs to make arrangements for Bethan's care.

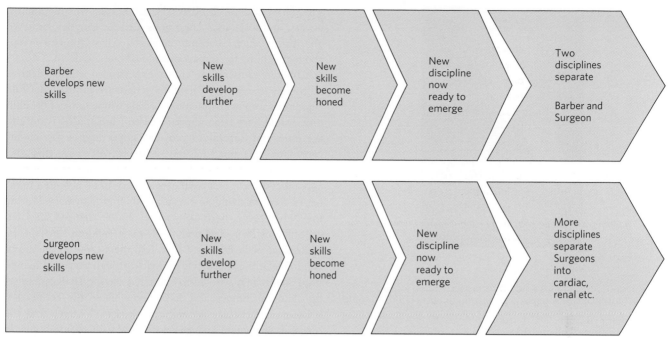

By the same processes nursing, midwifery, physiotherapy and occupational therapy have developed

Figure 1.1 Developing as a discipline

spent a great deal of time exploring the world as a sea captain. Ramsay (2008) provides information that, at the end of his sea-faring days, Coram returned to London and was clearly moved by the plight of children. Coram found dying children in the streets and corpses on dung heaps. In an attempt to provide care for the growing number of babies abandoned on London's streets (often illegitimate children of the poor or working class), Coram proffered the idea of a foundling hospital for unwanted children, for which he was given a Royal Charter. Funding for the foundling hospital from the Anglican Church was rejected. The reasons for this are not entirely clear but could have some relationship to church values about families and views on illegitimacy and relationships outside marriage. Through perseverance and charitable funding, he was able to establish a hospital but quickly became overwhelmed with admissions. Coram was concerned with protecting children and providing them with an education. Clearly, Coram was a man of influence whose work occurred approximately 100 years before the Public Health Act of 1848. Makins (1999) identified that William Hogarth donated paintings and Handel conducted the oratorio, *The Messiah*, at a concert to benefit funds for the foundlings.

Loudon (1979) undertook some research on George Armstrong and identified that he opened the first dispensary for children established in 1769. The dispensary for the infant poor survived for a shorter period of time than the general dispensaries. In contemporary terms, dispensaries would equate to the present day outpatient setting. It was largely funded by George Armstrong's own funds and collapsed soon after he died in 1789. A children's dispensary was established in 1816 by Dr John Bunnell Davis, who set out to treat children and train parents. The dispensary became known as the Royal Universal Dispensary,

but this too declined after Davis' death in 1834. Dr Charles West worked at the Waterloo Road Dispensary for approximately 10 years and was interested in opening inpatient facilities but became frustrated due to slow bureaucratic responses before resigning in 1850. It is understood that Charles West also worked at L'Hôpital des Enfant Malades in Paris, which was the world's first children's hospital, opening in 1802. These experiences have influenced his beliefs and values in caring for sick children within an institution designed for them. According to Jolley (2010), Charles West provided the 'blueprint' for hospitals for children across the United Kingdom.

In 1850 Charles West began negotiations relating to what would become Great Ormond Street Hospital (Loudon 1979) and succeeded in opening the Hospital for Sick Children in 1852. Glasper and Charles-Edwards (2002) identify that Charles Dickens was a benefactor to Great Ormond Street Hospital and a close friend of Charles West. Jolley (2010) adds that Queen Victoria was also a supporter. Media reports were limited and the literature was often used to record or inform readers of social issues. According to Ramsay (2008), Charles Dickens and Charles Kingsley both gave insight to poor child care practices within society at the time and that societal attitudes began to change.

A further contemporary of Charles West was Florence Nightingale who authored *Notes on Nursing* in 1859. Florence Nightingale had clear ideas on hygiene standards and nursing issues, and was able to articulate clear documentation. To the present day, these remain key elements of nursing in general. Florence Nightingale was influential in society but disagreed with the idea of a children's hospital, yet she portrayed nursing as a 'motherly' occupation (Jolley 2007; Jolley and Shields

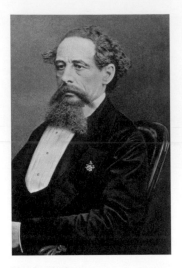

Charles Dickens

2009). Florence Nightingale was of the belief that children could be cared for in adult wards. She had concerns about recruiting sufficient nurses (Jolley 2010).

Catherine Wood was appointed as a 'lady visitor' to Great Ormond Street Hospital during the late 1850s and later joined as a ward superintendent. Wood is also credited with setting up her institution for children with hip diseases at Queen Square and subsequently acted as matron at Cromwell House, which was a convalescent home in Highgate, from 1869 to 1878. Wood returned to Great Ormond Street as lady superintendent (matron). Wood identified that children's nurses should act in a motherly fashion and show love. Wood authored two publications, *Handbook of nursing* and *The training of nurses for sick children* (Ramsay 2008). Jolley (2011) identifies that at this time children's nurses were portrayed as hard working, dedicated people, who served God and his children. These values are congruent with an era where there was social class division and the lower classes 'went into service'.

Ramsay (2008, page 614) highlights that from the mid-1850s and for almost a century, the involvement of parents in the care of children in hospital was considered to be superfluous and suggests that this may be due to the 'military philosophy of the Nightingale training'. Ramsay (2008) reports that this may have been the case due to maintaining of ward routines or anxieties about the spread of contamination or the possible distress felt by parents and their children because of the frequency of visiting. Lindsay (2011) has a different point of view, suggesting there is evidence that demonstrates mothers being able to stay with their children in hospital during the earlier part of the 19th century, but parents were excluded towards the end of the 19th century. The understanding of historical events is reliant on access to historical records; however, developments in children's nursing may well have been 'patchy'. It could be that some organisations were visionary about children's needs and some were slower to consider children's needs.

Eminent writers of the era identified the plight of children in society through novels such as *Oliver Twist*, *David Copperfield*

and *Martin Chuzzlewit*, all by Charles Dickens, who highlighted poverty and unsanitary conditions. Charles Kingsley authored *The Water Babies*, recording the plight of boy chimney sweeps and highlighting the impact of child labour and death.

Children in the 19th century experienced varying degrees of poverty in a society where no welfare system existed. Child labour was seen as acceptable in society where some of the children would have been apprenticed to learn trades. For some, the Industrial Revolution provided opportunities for income generation and financial independence. Although this may seem an action for liberation from poverty, for some trades or apprenticeships, it was a dangerous place to be in with a number of workers dying as a result of their employment. During the 19th century the Industrial Revolution changed lifestyles, expectations of society and the lives of children through the beginnings of healthcare. Social reformers came to the aid of children offering alternative lifestyles through varying schemes. Lord Shaftesbury worked to end child slavery, Dr Barnado set up children's homes and John Snow made the connection between a particular water pump in Broad Street, and the outbreak of cholera and was attributed with promoting early anaesthetics. These contributions have been influential on the health of children today.

It is evident that historical events have facilitated the shaping of society to enable access to basic hygiene and to develop strategies to educate the population. All of these visions or actions have enabled children to be safer, have better security and an enhanced quality of life, which continue as clear themes through to Maslow's hierarchy of needs and contemporary legislation and policies such as United Nations Convention on the Rights of the Child, the Children Acts and the National Service Framework for Children, Young People and Maternity Services (see Table 1.1).

20TH CENTURY: POLITICAL DRIVERS AND INFLUENCES OF WAR

Jolley (2011) identifies that the First World War (1914–1918) had a strong influence on society as the consequences of war led to child health issues becoming a focal point for the development of governmental policy. Jolley (2011, page 18) identifies that this led to the provision of a range of special schools and hospitals to provide 'good nutrition, good exercise and fresh air' but this paternalistic action had not considered the provision for feeling wanted and loved.

Ramsay (2008) highlights that during the Second World War concerns were raised relating to the effects the hostilities had on children in urban areas and, to that end, a programme for the evacuation of children was put in place to keep them safe from harm. In less urbanised areas, children stayed at home, yet women were required to return to the workforce to maintain the war effort, which had an impact on the supervision of their children. Ill health due to hostilities could not be ruled out with children and young people being admitted to hospital. There are personal stories, accounts or

Table 1.1 Timeline of historical political drivers

1834	Poor Law
1848	**Public Health Act**
	National schools The development of national schools was 'patchy' and was reliant on communities identifying the need for a school
1870	**Education Act** The development of boarding schools for children age 9–14 years by local boroughs
1906	**Children Act**
1909	**People's Budget**

CASE STUDY REVIEW 1.1

What if Rhys lived in the 18th or 19th century?

Had Rhys been living during the 18th or 19th century, there would have been very different health outcomes for him:

- Workhouses for those who were impoverished and homeless.
- The Industrial Revolution changed lives for the majority of people and for some it cost them their life.
- Society believed in the sanctity of marriage and although divorce was possible, it was rare.
- Working-class people had lower incomes and those who were more affluent were regarded as having more social standing.
- Churches offered alms.
- Social welfare systems were not in place.
- There was no children's hospital until the end of the 19th century.
- Consumption (contemporary name tuberculosis) was prevalent.
- Environmental factors impacted on health in some areas, such as smog in big cities.

---

anecdotes of experiences of being in hospital during the Second World War (see Voices 1.1). Joyce recalls her experiences of being in hospital during this period. Food as a resource was rationed due to the war effort and choices of food were limited. Assumptions could be made that the bike had been borrowed to facilitate Joyce's dad's visit. It is clear from this recollection that even during times of hostilities actions of compassion were evident (see Voices 1.1).

VOICES 1.1 Recollections of Joyce (aged 79 years)

'I was in hospital when I was 13 [years], in an isolation hospital, in a little room. They gave me Marmite on toast, which I still hate to this day. I had tonsillitis, quinsy and rheumatic fever. I remember my dad coming to see me on a bicycle and saw him coming round the roundabout on a bike that was too big for him. He had been given compassionate leave from the army, because I was weak and sickly and not expected to make it.'

21ST CENTURY: CONTEMPORARY ISSUES

Poverty and Healthcare Inequalities

There are similarities between contemporary issues facing parents, children and young people in the 21st century and those that were prevalent during the 19th century. Child poverty is relative to its society and although it is acknowledged that there are higher standards of living, poverty has been redefined in the context of contemporary society. As far back as the 1950s it was understood that there is a higher rate of admission of children to hospital from disadvantaged, lower socioeconomic group families. There have been reports to consider the impact of health inequalities over time with the publication of the Black Report (1980) and the Acheson Report (1998). Brewer et al. (2011) identified that relative child poverty will rise from 20 per cent currently to 24 per cent by 2020/21. Brewer et al. (2011) highlighted

CASE STUDY REVIEW 1.2

What if Rhys lived in wartime or the post-war period?

If Rhys lived in a rural area, then it is likely he would have stayed at home to be with his family and remain safely away from hostilities.

If Rhys lived in an urban area that was potentially under attack, then it is likely that he would have been sent to a safer area as an evacuee. It is likely the Rhys would have been taken to someone he had not built a relationship with and he would potentially be feeling scared.

If Rhys had needed hospitalisation during this era, it is likely that the hospital ward would have been a wartime temporary structure, based on a Florence Nightingale design, with an air-raid shelter incorporated into the design. Although these were built as temporary structures, some have remained into the 21st century. The private funding initiative through the modernisation of the NHS has begun a programme to replace them in some areas with facilities to meet the demands of 21st century healthcare.

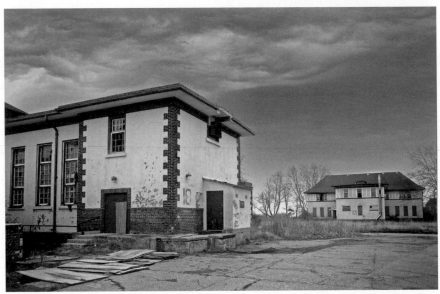

that this is significantly higher than the 10 per cent target within the Child Poverty Act 2010. The theme of healthcare inequalities has been linked with poverty throughout time. To this end, when considering high-quality care for all, the Department of Health (DoH) (2008) acknowledges that greater autonomy is needed to deliver health promotion strategies and reduce healthcare inequalities. However, Brewer et al. (2011) indicates that the proportion of children in absolute poverty is forecast to rise to 23 per cent by 2020/21, compared with the 5 per cent target. This poses a contemporary issue for the children's nurse to consider.

Child Welfare

Brannen and O'Brien (1996) inform us that in the 19th century the state was concerned with getting children off the streets and reducing the numbers of children at work, young offenders and children seen in regards to the Poor Law 1834 (National Archives). This was not purely altruistic, rather it was a mechanism to keep the 'unfortunates' in their place. It was also seen as a measure to reduce crime by offering apprenticeships and trades and a way of earning an income. With the firm establishment of industrialisation by the middle of the 20th century, children were no longer seen as economic necessities and the sizes of families reduced. Brannen and O'Brien (1996) acknowledge that this began the development of child welfare policy and legislation over a century.

Stress and Unemployment

Inequalities in resources and rising unemployment have led to impoverishment and poor living conditions and, when coupled with increased stress caused by financial burden and poor coping strategies, this could be interpreted as predictive factors for

ACTIVITY 1.1   Defining poverty

Research the terms 'relative poverty' and 'absolute poverty'.

Access the following web links to read more about children in poverty in the 21st century and make notes using the headings culture and ethnicity, social circumstance and financial issues and write a summary of your findings:

http://www.jrf.org.uk/publications/child-and-working-age-poverty-2010-2020

http://www.legislation.gov.uk/ukpga/2010/9/notes/division/3

http://www.barnardos.org.uk/poverty_full_report_07.pdf.

child abuse. Wilson and James (2009) point out that child abuse can arise from four main areas:

- relations between caregivers (intermarriage, marital disputes, step-parents/co-habitee or separated single parent)
- relations to children (spacing between births, size of family, caregivers' attachments to and expectations of their dependants)
- situational stressors (poor living environments and income)
- issues with the parent–child relationship (such as being unwanted)
- a child with a disability or behavioural issue.

For children to live healthy and well-adjusted lives, they need to live in a healthy and emotionally supportive environment even though society is in a constant state of change.

Child Focus and Perspectives

There are also differences from the 19th century compared to the present day in relation to listening to and hearing the voices of children. Within 19th-century society the adage 'children should be seen and not heard' existed and children were powerless to make changes or even express their views. Over time, child rearing practices have changed due to an increase in working mothers. James and Prout (1996, page 49) provide insight into the way in which children were beginning to be seen from the 1970s by regarding, 'children as complex actors in, and interpreters of, a complex world'. There has been a cultural shift in recent years to empower children and young people to express their views.

Technological Revolution and New Challenges

In considering the 21st century, a different kind of revolution is taking place. An information technological revolution has changed the lifestyles and expectations of society in which information is available through the internet, which is itself available through a range of devices. It would seem that contemporary lifestyles are dependent on the information technology revolution with access to information, music, games and social media. In the right context, these technologies can be beneficial for parents and children, as information regarding options for the treatment and management of conditions can be retrieved.

Technologies may also have a negative effect on a child or young person as this may impact on care, development or bring about lifestyle changes and increase stress levels in children, young people and their parents. The internet has the capacity for children and young people to access material that is inappropriate. They may thereby be exposed to 'cyber-bullying' and grooming, which could have an impact on the mental health of the vulnerable child or young person. Children and young people need protecting from the negative aspects caused by the availability of such technology. It is acknowledged that while the internet has a valuable place on a children's ward to facilitate the continuation of education for young people, the children's nurse and other members of the interprofessional team play a pivotal role in monitoring the online activities.

ACTIVITY 1.2 21st century childhoods

List the ways in which information technology may impact on 21st century childhoods.

Consider the list you formulated. Were there any considerations that children and young people's nurses should be aware of?

SOCIAL PERSPECTIVES: FAMILIES AND FAMILY DYNAMICS

Having considered the historic timeline of children's nursing, it would seem that there are similarities and differences between the 19th, 20th and 21st centuries in relation to the issues facing children and young people in contemporary society. For approximately 40,000 children, the Second World War meant that they were evacuated to parts of the country that were considered safer in order to protect them from the air raids. Jolley and Shields (2009) acknowledge that this led to suffering and concerns related to the separation of children from their parents and sometimes siblings. Evacuees experienced varying degrees of care from the volunteers who were responsible for them. Even when the volunteers were caring for the evacuees, it was not the same relationship as being with their parents. Contemporary society still includes victims of violence and aggression from war-torn countries or where there are issues of genocide, hostile political environments or famine. These children and their families may need to flee to find refuge and as a result become asylum seekers and need care by children's nurses in hospital.

ACTIVITY 1.3 Hospitalisation in times of war

Reflect on and write what it would have been like had Rhys been an evacuee during the war and also required hospitalisation.

During the war, women played a key role in the 'war effort' by taking on work roles usually associated with men and to provide support for the war, grow food, become drivers or operate heavy machinery. With the men returning from war, many women relinquished their role as breadwinner and supporter of the war effort returning to their role of housewife and mother. After the Second World War mothers traditionally stayed at home and played a pivotal nurturing role within the family, some mothers worked part time and fewer mothers worked full time. Traditionally, the family has been viewed as a basic unit of society as a 'nuclear' or 'traditional' family of two parents with children. The term 'family' at this point may seem a straightforward concept but although families have values and traditions, they are influenced by society and cultural 'norms' that do not exist in isolation. These families could be considered to be patriarchal with the father as figurehead and breadwinner.

FAMILY THEORIES AND DYNAMICS, EXPECTATIONS AND IMPACTS

What is a Family?

Within the United Kingdom during the past 70 years there have been many changes to society, which have been influenced by many factors. There have been changes to the ways in which families evolve and family dynamics can add complexities for healthcare practitioners to consider. Factors include migration of populations either by choice, or nationally or internationally or enforced migration; family regroupings; political drivers to find employment or social mobility drivers. The movement of people has impacted on family dynamics and how the family is depicted.

The notion of a nuclear family still exists in the 21st century. Browne (2011) highlights that during the 21st century the 'cereal packet family' is the image that the media tend to give as a representation of the family, and shows a first-time marriage where the father is depicted as the financial resource or breadwinner and is often depicted as being more important by being in the foreground of the picture or standing taller than the woman. The woman is depicted as a homemaker or 'stay-at-home mum' with two children, often a male and a female child. Browne (2011) further identifies that the 'happy family stereotype' portrayed by the 'cereal packet family' represents only 5 per cent of households.

VOICES 1.2 Grace's family (aged 7 years and a bit)

Grace and her parents have given permission for her name to be used.

Grace is part of a nuclear family and has drawn her family showing mummy and daddy with herself at the centre. Grace has clearly put distinguishing features into her figures, such as hair length and hair texture. There is clear recording of anatomy, such as facial features and fingers. Interestingly, Grace sees herself as of similar size to her parents. Many interpretations could be made: could it be that Grace sees herself as of equal importance to her parents in her unique family? Grace has clearly expressed her feelings and emotions within her picture denoting a heart alongside every family member's name, indicating her emotions and the love that exists between each family member (see Figure 1.2).

During the past 50 years, social attitudes to marriage, co-habitation and divorce have changed (ONS 2012). There has been a steady increase in the numbers of children born outside marriage. During 1971 8.4 per cent of births were outside marriage rising to 30.2 per cent of births being outside marriage during 1991 (ONS 2012). This has resulted in the provision of social support through the benefits system and protection through the provision of law (ONS 2012). Where couples choose to marry, there has been a change in society to ensure that women have more rights than their ancestors. Divorce, remarriage and single-parent status have added new complexities to the family unit. These are further complicated by economic circumstances including 'downturns' and recessions, increasing the necessity for parents to work.

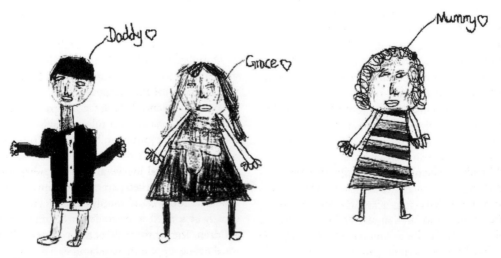

Figure 1.2 Grace's family

PRACTICAL GUIDELINES 1.1

There is an increasing number of grandparents involved in the daily care of grandchildren. The children's nurse needs to have an awareness of all types of family dynamic in order that they are prepared for the admissions process. Noah began a reception class aged 4 years and was asked to draw a picture entitled 'Who I live with' and his mother helped him by labelling the people in his drawing and encouraging him during the drawing process. Noah and his family have given permission for his drawing to be included and you can see it in Figure1.3. It is clear that Noah has a number of people who could act as 'enablers'.

It is also useful for teachers to have an understanding of the family dynamics in order that they may understand the support networks that children and young people may have to aid their journey through the educational system and enable them to participate in either a formal or informal home–school working agreement.

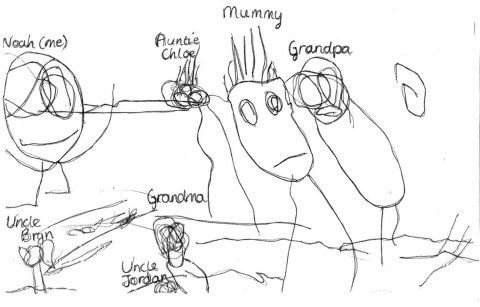

Figure 1.3 Noah's extended family

During the past decade there has been an acceptance of civil partnerships in the UK. This has meant that the changes needed to be subjected to revisions in the law to include legal provision for civil partnerships. To this end, the Civil Partnership Act 2004 was formulated, making it possible for single-sex couples to marry from December 2005. These changes in legislation have made civil partnerships legally binding and accepted in society with amendments to the Civil Partnership Act and the formulation of further provisions. From December 2005 to December 2009 there were 40,237 such partnerships (ONS 2011). This has led to a new genre of parents accessing children and young people's services with their family.

The nature of English society has changed since the 19th century, mainly due to migration of people to and from other parts of the world. Influence of culture and diversity will give rise to differences in the assumptions held about families by different groups of people and assumptions made about *what a family is*. Britain is a multicultural society and families live in different structures. Browne (2011) identifies that South Asian families live together in patriarchal groupings. These families are considered to be *vertically* extended family where three generations live together in a single household. Browne (2011) also identifies that West Indian households live together in matriarchal groupings and that there is a high number of lone parents heading West Indian households. There are differences in the ways these groups of people view the concept of the family and they hold different types of family value. Conflict occurs when individuals do not understand the culture of a particular family grouping. Therefore, it is important for children's nurses to be culturally aware of family grouping profiles. Faith values and rules may also be a part of family life and will need consideration during children's hospital journeys, such as kosher fridges to facilitate the separation of particular food groups or provision of kosher and halal foods into hospital menus. Hospitals have traditionally incorporated a chapel but these have now become faith rooms to respect the provision for needs of all faiths.

It would appear from the evidence presented that family types are becoming increasingly diverse, and that there is no one typical family type in Britain. Moules and Ramsay (2008) note that there are challenges in identifying 'the family' due to its complex and changing nature. Higham (2011) identified that families are more fluid and diverse and operate as a 'family' according to their own criteria. This will impact on the way in which children and families are perceived.

Due to circumstances, events or relationship breakdown, it is not always appropriate for families to stay in hospital as a 'family unit'. According to the Department for Education (2011) there was a total of 65,520 looked-after children at 31 March 2011 which represented a 2 per cent rise from 2010 and an increase of 9 per cent since 2007. The Department for Education (2011) identifies that 350 of the looked-after children had mothers aged 12–16 years old who were looked-after children themselves. This figure had decreased from 390 in 2010. The Department for Education (2011) further clarifies that, of these mothers 49 per cent were under 15 when their first child was born, and a further 35 per cent were aged 16 years. This reality will pose further complexities for the children's nurse when caring for children and young people, particularly related to issues of consent. Due to often being long distances away from home, the looked-after child is particularly vulnerable.

CASE STUDY REVIEW 1.3

Rhys Jones's family, theory and practice issues

Rhys and his family are a unique family unit, with their own health and family values. When children and young people are admitted to hospital for treatment or admission, it is easy to assume that family members are still legally related, and healthcare practitioners are required to clarify family dynamics as this may present legal complications if formal consent is required for procedures or treatments due to the issue of parental responsibility. Using a family systems approach it is evident that Rhys is supported by a family network and 'belongs' within the wider community. These concepts fit with the idea of Bronfenbrenner's ecological theory through viewing the contributions of the community as supporting Rhys and family (see Table 1.2).

Table 1.2 Concept of family

	What is a family?	How does this relate to Rhys and his family?	Implications for practice
Concept 1	A family system is a part of a larger supra-system and is also composed of many subsystems Part of the local community Parental system Sibling system Family systems have emotional boundaries that help to establish what is inside the system and what is outside it	Considering Bronfenbrenner's ecological theory, as most families, the Jones family live in a community with a supportive infrastructure such as support groups, educational and health provision and transportation links Rhys lives with his mother and her husband and appears to have a stable relationship Rhys has a 'second family' when he visits his father, Anthony, and Anthony's wife, Ellen who also appear to have a stable relationship This appears to be a supportive mechanism but due to potential tensions between two family units this could be a disruptive influence Family dynamics can be complex and confusing Rhys has a full sibling, and also a step-brother with whom he has developed a relationship Rhys is waiting for the arrival of a half-sibling Rhys could benefit from a widening in his range of experiences of family ethos, values and guidance. There is also room for confusion and conflict by two sets of 'family rules'	Accurate nursing and medical histories, care and management and communication skills are required to provide seamless care within the hospital setting and liaison with community support on discharge Accurate documentation of • typical daily routines • key relationships • key professionals • individualised care • intentional rounding (see nursing assessment)

	What is a family?	How does this relate to Rhys and his family?	Implications for practice
Concept 2	The family as a whole is greater than the sum of its parts. Family's wholeness is more that just the addition of another member Understand an individual better by understanding the way his/her family works	Rhys has parents, step-parents, grandparents and step-grandparents to gauge what his needs are	Accurate documentation Parental responsibility for potential consent issues
Concept 3	A change in one family member affects all family members Illness of a child impacts on all roles and relationships within a family; mother, father, their relationship, siblings' roles and their relationship to the parents and to the sick sibling	Rhys has needed to cope with the impact of divorce, remarriage and the arrival of new family members. The birth of the new half-sibling from Amanda and Huw will further add to the complexities of his family structures	Rhys may be thinking about/missing Bethan and his extended family Attempts to maintain the sibling's relationship are important
Concept 4	A family is able to create a balance between change and stability Always change within families as individual members develop and change Families adjust continually to incorporate these changes and maintain some stability Family can be dominated by change at times and dominated by stability at other times	Rhys has both parents as active participants in his life	Rhys has experienced previous hospital episodes and the family will have rehearsed strategies for coping with hospitalisation and maintenance of family units Alternatively, Rhys may have had a poor experience which has resulted in fear and anxiety
Concept 5	Family members' behaviour is best understood from a view of circular rather than linear causality	There may be many reasons why Rhys is wetting the bed Rhys may genuinely be having a bad dream/nightmare Rhys may have concerns about being in hospital Rhys may have concerns about not seeing his friends Rhys may have concerns about the arrival of the new half-sibling Rhys may be realising that his parents are not going to 'get back together'	Conversations with Rhys and actively listening to his views may be crucial to the process of detecting the cause. These must consider age appropriate language (see LEARNER)

Source: adapted from Glasper and Richardson (2006)

Changes to life experiences can cause stress to a greater or lesser extent at any point. The amount of stress a person can manage will be relative to life experiences, resilience and coping strategies and will vary according to the individual family member. Duvall (1977) formulated a family lifecycle theory, which was expanded by Carter and McGoldrick (1989), and which recognises that as families develop and grow they enter different stages of life. Each stage of life presents different stressors, the more stressors presenting to an individual or family the greater the potential for stress (see Table 1.3). Individuals' capacity in coping strategies varies.

Table 1.3 Family lifecycle theory: Rhys Jones and his family

Duvall's and Carter and McGoldrick's ideas on family lifecycle theory		Rhys Jones's family
Stage I: Marriage and an independent home: joining of families	Establishment/ re-establishment of couple identity. Realign relationships with extended family, make decisions about parenthood	Anthony and Amanda marry and establish a new identity as a couple Relationships with extended family further developed and maintained Have two children, Rhys and Bethan Anthony and Amanda decide to divorce Amanda and Huw marry and decide to have a further child of their own. Amanda is 7 months pregnant Anthony and Ellen marry Anthony takes on the role of Ben's step-father
Stage II: Families with infants	Integrate infants into a family unit Adjust to new parenting/ grandparenting	Amanda and Huw are preparing to enter this stage with the imminent birth of their child
Stage III: Families with preschoolers	Socialise children. Parents and children adjust to separation	Bethan is preparing to begin her school life
Stage IV: Families with school age children	Children develop peer relations Parents adjust to peer and school influence	Rhys has friends at school
Stage V: Families with teenagers	Adolescents develop increasing autonomy. Parents focus on midlife marital and career issues, shift towards concern for the older generation	
Stage VI: Families as launching centres	Parents renegotiate marital relationship; young adults establish independence	
Stage VII: Middle aged families	Reinvest in couple identity with concurrent development of independent interests Realign relationships to include in-laws and grandchildren Deal with disabilities and death of older generation	Marge will be at this stage
Stage VIII: Ageing families	Shift from work role to leisure and semi-/full retirement Maintain couple and individual functioning while adapting to ageing process Prepare for own death and dealing with loss of spouse, siblings, peers	

CASE STUDY REVIEW 1.4

Reflecting on the Jones family dynamics

Reflecting on the Jones family dynamics, it is apparent that three of the family-cycle stages are applicable. Rhys appears to have a stable relationship with both his natural parents and Anthony is also forging a step-father–child relationship with Ben. Amanda and Huw have formed a new family unit and are awaiting the birth of their first child and have the added stressors of Rhys experiencing acute exacerbation of asthma. Anthony and Ellen have formed a new family unit and maintain close relationships with Rhys and Bethan. Amanda and Anthony appear to have set their personal emotions aside to avoid conflict and maintain an amicable relationship to benefit Rhys and Bethan.

Sibling relationships are the longest relationships a human individual can experience. Rhys benefits from a sibling relationship with Bethan and a step-sibling relationship with Ben. The forthcoming birth of a half-sibling provides Rhys with a new relationship and added responsibility of being a 'big brother', which may be causing him some anxiety.

GENOGRAMS

Medical genograms provide a useful context for evaluating health risks in a diagrammatic format using symbols to denote meaning. Knowledge of diseases and conditions that occur within a family can give the healthcare team invaluable information that may aid a swift accurate diagnosis and treatment of health problems. Reading large sections of text in order to ascertain information about a family in relation to denoting gender, pregnancy and death is a time-consuming process. Genograms provide a diagrammatic and symbolic way of recording information. Shapes are used to denote meaning and lines are added to the connection between two people to denote whether relationship is present or finished. Age or years can also be added (see Figure 1.4).

PUBLIC AND POLITICAL PERSPECTIVES OF NURSING CHILDREN AND YOUNG PEOPLE

Research into the care of children began to inform the way in which society treated children at times of separation and hospitalisation. Bowlby (1951) found that children bonded with their parents and formed an attachment to them at an early age. From the 1950s to the early 1990s a number of reports had been undertaken into the care of children in hospital. Robertson (1952) demonstrated on film (*A Two Year Old goes to Hospital*) the responses of one particular hospitalised child. When children were separated from their parents during hospitalisation, they displayed signs of protest, despair, withdrawal and detachment (see Chapter 2). Lindsay (2011) suggests that changes had already begun to take place prior to the early 1950s. It is likely that mothers were inconsistently permitted on the ward and policy was dependent on the viewpoints of the hospital. In 1957 Robertson and MacCarthy gave evidence to the Committee on the Welfare of Children in Hospital (the Platt Committee) (Lindsay 2003). Subsequently, the Platt Report was published. Lindsay (2003) considers that the changes to the way in which children are cared for has been a gradual process rather than one of sudden change. Reports traditionally include a set of recommendations yet these are not always acted on or given due priority. Recommendations within many reports had not been fully considered or implemented to form firm foundations of children's nursing (see Table 1.X).

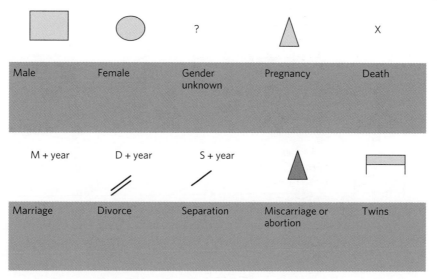

Figure 1.4 Genogram symbols

Source: Politics UK, 4th ed., p. 530 (Jones, B. 2001), Pearson Education Limited. © 2001 Pearson Education Limited.

VOICES 1.3 Grace's family (2)

Grace and her parents have given permission for her drawing to be included.

At 7 years old, Grace has drawn her family, yet in doing so, it is clear that she sees her family in a much wider context. Grace has drawn a 'family tree' yet looking further it can be seen that Grace has included family members who have died and still recognises them as her family. It is interesting to note that Grace has drawn living relatives larger than those who have died. Family is important to Grace. In natural and simple terms, Grace has drawn a genogram of her family history (see Figure 1.5).

ACTIVITY 1.4 Using a genogram to demonstrate a family tree

1. Beginning with the Queen, formulate a genogram that demonstrates three generations of the royal family.
2. Formulate a genogram of Rhys and his family.

Between 1991 and 1993 Beverly Allitt killed four patients on the children's ward at Grantham and Kesteven Hospital and other children received catastrophic injuries. Media reporting of Allitt's crimes drew attention to previous government reports and questioned why these had not been fully implemented. Allitt was diagnosed with Munchausen syndrome by proxy, which is now known as fabricated or induced illness (FII) but this is no excuse for the heinous crimes she committed (Department of Health 2008a). An inquiry followed this event and the subsequent Clothier Report (1994) aimed recommendations at tightening procedures for safeguarding children in hospital and preventing similar events (see Table 1.X and Chapter 14).

A number of events concerning children identified that there was confusion with the existence of many laws that determined how children were treated in law. These laws were challenging to navigate, causing confusion. The Children Act 1989 brought together public and private laws in order to strike a balance between the rights of children and the rights of parents to maintain their parental responsibility. Following the tragic deaths of Victoria Climbié and Lauren Wright in 2000 there was a public outcry and it was felt necessary to revise the laws to

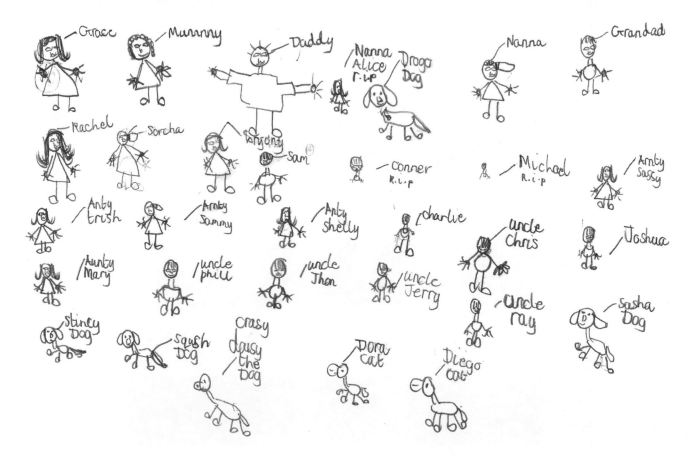

Figure 1.5 Grace's family tree

include an interprofessional focus and identify a change in the way child protection was managed, leading to the Children Act 2004. For a number of years in the UK there was a tendency for a reactive approach to policymaking.

POLICYMAKING

According to Jones (2001) policies convey a set of ideas and proposals to be acted on culminating in a government decision. Policies convey political decisions to support political agendas that can be used to guide healthcare provision and healthcare delivery. Policies may arise from top-down approach from government, where there is a reliance on political, economic and/or moral power to ensure change occurs. In terms of change management, this would be a power–coercive approach. Policies may also arise from a middle-of-the-road approach where knowledge is the source of power and key players are guided by reason, and justify that it is in the interest of children and young people to formulate policy or legislation in a particular area. In terms of change management, this would be a rational–empirical

approach. Policies may arise from a bottom-up approach where normative–re-educative processes involve children, young people and their families who can lobby for changes in legislation and policies. It is essential that policies from modernisation agendas or reform do not have a 'patchwork' effect on children's nursing but are orchestrated in such a way as to provide a seamless service of care (see Tables 1.4 and 1.5 and Figure 1.6).

POLITICAL ADVOCATES

There were other significant changes with the political modernisation agenda. For the first time in 2005, a Children's Commissioner was appointed, Aynsley Green, a doctor, who listened to the views of frontline workers, managers and children from around the country to formulate the National Service Framework for Children, Young People and Maternity Services NSFCYPMS. During 2010 the second Children's Commissioner, Maggie Atkinson, was appointed from an educational and social work background. One of her concerns is that the age of criminal responsibility is too low. Later during 2010 a review of the Office of the Children's

Table 1.4 Layers of policymaking

General public

Some of the ways the voices of the general public can be heard through:

- speaking to Members of Parliament in their constituencies
- writing in books, newspapers, online blogs and social networking to gain the support of others
- reality documentaries to raise their plight
- petitions and surveys
- contacting the government directly by post or online **https://email.number10.gov.uk/**

The involvement of children, young people and their families is relatively recent. The views of children, young people and their families was sought and considered in the development of the National Service Framework for Children, Young People and Maternity Services(NSFCYPMS)

Cause groups, media and academics

- charities such as Asthma UK, Bliss, Action for Sick Children, Together for Short Lives (and many others) influence policymaking
- on one level, the media can expose areas in which there are gaps in policies or bring issues forward
- on another level, the media can expose issues and lobby to gain support by petitions. Sarah's Law would have been an example of this (BBC News 2011)
- the research film *A two-year old goes to hospital* could be in keeping with this section

Extra-parliamentary parties, party groupings

Parties in the opposition can be consulted with or exert their views to influence policy

Parliament, party sources, select committees, the opposition

Although the political structures and process may have been different in the 1950s, it may be assumed that the Committee on the Welfare of Children (Platt Committee) would fall into this section

Ministers, civil servants, inquiries, key economic groups, think tanks

This is the most likely point at which the minister for children and children's commissioners could influence policymaking for *Every Child Matters*, NSFCYPMS, Laming Inquiry, Leveson Inquiry, Modernising NHS Careers

Prime Minister, Cabinet, cabinet office, policy unit, policy advisors

Policies are planned, debated, formulated and processed in line with the strategic vision of the government. The children's commissioner has influence at this level and acts as an advocate for children and young people

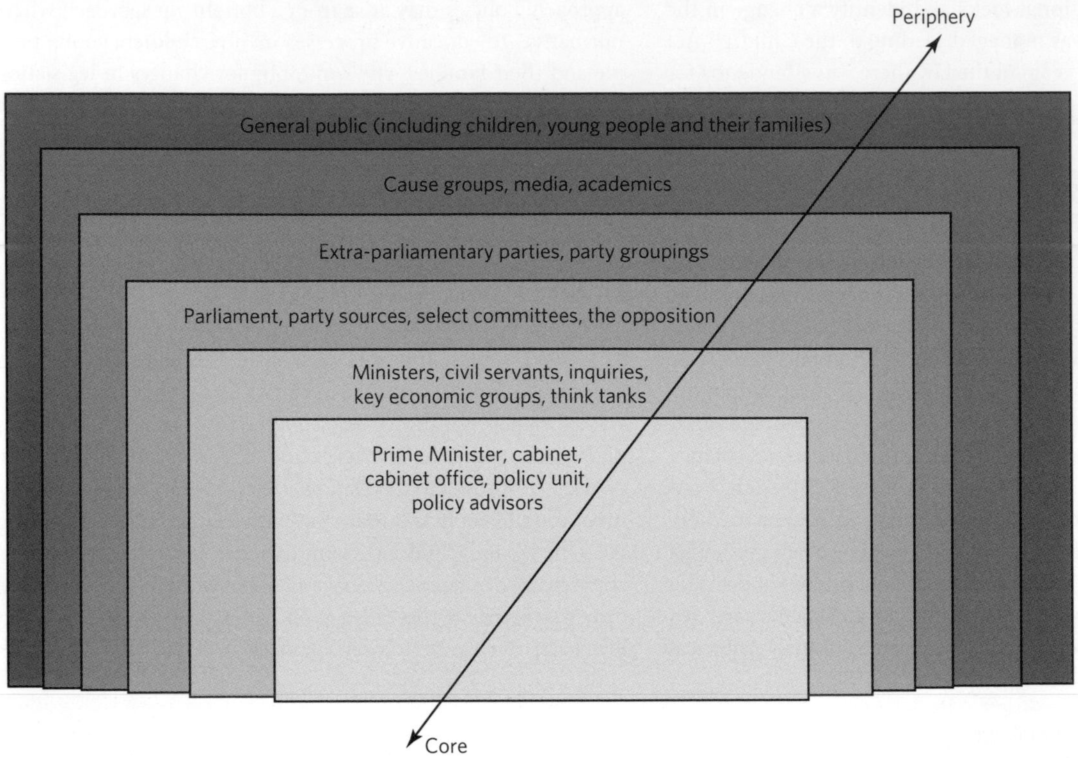

Figure 1.6 Political layers
Source: Jones (2001)

Table 1.5 Timeline of contemporary political drivers

1959	**Welfare of Children in Hospital (Platt Report)**
	First of many reports aimed at alleviating the stress of hospital admission for sick children by recommending that children should be cared for in an appropriate environment by specialist practitioners
1976	**Fit for the Future: Child Health Services (Court Report)**
	Improvements in child health services could only come through an integrated service
1989	**Children Act**
	The main principle of the Act detailed in this document is that, whenever possible, children should be brought up and cared for within their own families, but that children should be safe and protected by effective intervention if they are deemed to be in danger
1991	**Just for the Day (Thornes)**
	The underlying philosophy of this report was in its belief that in admitting children as day patients, the integrity of the family was maintained
1991	**Welfare of Children and Young People in Hospital (Department of Health, HMSO, 1991)**
	This document is still the industry standard for the care of children in hospital and recommends minimum numbers of registered children's nurses
1993	**Bridging the Gaps**
	This report highlighted ambulatory care for children as a growing discipline
	The main thrust of the findings was related to improving the inadequacies of the interfaces between hospital and home
1993	**Children First. A study of hospital services**
	This report by the Audit Commission investigated NHS trust compliance with previous reports and studies.
	It revealed that, all too often, reports related to children were slow to be implemented

1994	**Care of Sick Children. A review of the guidelines in the wake of the Allitt Inquiry**
	The Allitt Inquiry (Clothier Report)
	The Allitt Inquiry recommended that the Department of Health should take steps to ensure that the 1991 welfare document was more closely observed by NHS trusts. The heinous crimes of Beverley Allitt will never be forgotten and will continue to act as a reminder of how important it is to adhere to government and professional guidelines relating to the care of sick children
1995	**Listening to Children: Children, Ethics and Social Research**
	This publication was in many ways a forerunner to the recommendations made following the events at Alder Hey and Bristol. The report identifies 10 key topics relating to research ethics and children
1996	**Child Health in the Community**
	This companion to the 1991 welfare document concentrates on the management of sick children in their own homes
1996	**Patients Charter – Services for Children and Young People**
	Part of the government's commitment to accountability in public service
1997	**House of Commons Health Committee Reports on children and young people**
	Official responses to the House of Commons Health Committee Reports are in many respects an endorsement of other published reports related to the welfare of sick children and young people
1998	**Youth Matters. Evidence-based best practice for the care of young people in hospital**
	This document was designed to raise awareness of the plight of young people in hospital. The number of adolescent beds in UK children's hospitals/units is still relatively lower compared to the number of children's beds
2001	**Royal Liverpool Children's Inquiry**
	Failure to gain consent and the storage issues related to body parts caused public outcry. Obtaining body parts for research purposes without consent proved to be wider than a single children's hospital
2001 and 2002	**Bristol Inquiry and Kennedy Report**
	The Bristol Royal Infirmary (BRI) and the Bristol Royal Hospital for Sick Children (BRHSC) were and are teaching hospitals associated with Bristol University's Medical School. They looked after patients with heart disease: adults, children and infants. In this report, we are concerned particularly with congenital heart disease: babies born with heart problems and their subsequent treatment
2003	***Every Child Matters***
	Cross-government's agenda for every child, whatever their background or their circumstances, to have the support they need to be healthy, stay safe, enjoy and achieve, make a positive contribution and achieve economic well-being
2004	**Children Act**
	A children's commissioner to champion the views and interests of children and young people and changes:
	• a duty on local authorities to make arrangements to promote cooperation between agencies and other appropriate bodies (such as voluntary and community organisations) in order to improve children's well-being and a duty on key partners to take part in the cooperation arrangements
	• a duty on key agencies to safeguard and promote the welfare of children
	• a duty on local authorities to set up local safeguarding children boards and on key partners to take part
	• provision for indexes or databases containing basic information about children and young people to enable better sharing of information
2004	**National Service Framework for Children, Young People and Maternity Services**
	A 10-year blueprint for nursing children and young people
2004	**Choosing Health: Making Healthy Choices Easier**
	This White Paper sets out the key principles for supporting the public to make healthier and more informed choices in regards to their health. The government will provide information and practical support to get people motivated and improve emotional wellbeing and access to services so that healthy choices are easier to make

(Continued)

2006	**Acutely or critically sick or injured child in the district general hospital**
	An intercollegiate working party outlines HDU provision in district general hospitals
2010	**Child Poverty Act**
2010	**Review of the Office of the Children's Commissioner (England)**

Commissioner (England) made recommendations to change the role through legislation by strengthening its remit, powers and independence (DoE 2010). This document identifies that within the statutory framework of the Children's Commissioner, the *Every Child Matters* outcomes must be replaced by United Nations Convention on the Rights of the Child 1989.

At this point, a children's minister was appointed to advocate for children and young people with the government decision makers. This was the first time a minister could speak directly to government about issues that concerned children and young people. Due to changing political parties being in government a number of people have undertaken this role, including Margaret Hodge (2003); Beverly Hughes (2005); Dawn Primarolo (2009); and Sarah Teather with Tim Loughton as Junior Minister (May 2010).

LEADERSHIP, MANAGEMENT AND TEAM WORK

Contemporary Family-Centred Care and Partnership

There is a wealth of literature related to the development of family-centred care, therefore, the purpose of this section is not to rehearse family-centred care but to set it into the context of debates currently presenting in the literature. The notion of contemporary family-centred care has evolved over the past six decades and is a significant element of healthcare (Coleman 2010). Coleman also suggested that family-centred care is socially constructed in the time and place that it is being practised. Casey (1988) considered that working in partnership with the parents was crucial. Many authors published work to demonstrate the values and applications of including parents in the care of their children (see Figure 1.7).

The term 'family-centred care' is synonymous with children and young people's nursing. Coleman (2010) informs us that the notion of children being active participants in their own care journeys is pivotal to family-centred care. Bradshaw and Coleman (2007) identify that parents have a role of being active participants and decision makers in their child's care rather than being passive. They consider that coupled with the notion of family-centred care is the notion of the therapeutic relationship between the children's nurse and the child and family. By combining these two concepts, the notion behind family-centred healthcare has been reframed.

Children and young people with long-term conditions (e.g. asthma) manage their condition at home for long periods of time, only attending hospital when their condition is

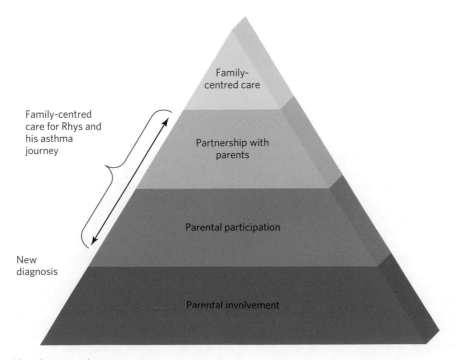

Figure 1.7 Hierarchy of family-centred care
Source: Hutchfield (1999)

not effectively responding to the treatment at home. If Hutchfield's (1999) hierarchy and Smith, Coleman and Bradshaw's (2010) continuum of family-centred care are applied to Rhys and his family situation, then the parents are working in partnership with healthcare professionals for the majority of the time. When the child comes into hospital and the management of care changes, it is likely that the parents will be at the participation level due to the new regimens and working in conjunction with the healthcare professionals. At the point of diagnosis, it is likely that the parents are at the involvement level with the care led by the nurse. Family-centred care can only be achieved when the parents and child are leading care (see Figure 1.8).

Reflecting on the scenario, it is unclear why Amanda thought she would be unable to stay with Rhys, yet this may have been his first admission into hospital. The children's nurse cannot assume that a long-term condition equates to previous hospital experiences (see Figure 1.8 and Table 1.6).

There is a growing contemporary debate over the need for further research into family-centred care. There may be many reasons for this debate such as lack of definition, relevance to staff and families and how family-centred care is embedded in clinical practice. Family-centred care must be negotiated and parents must want to participate in care, however, this is not always the case and parents are left feeling imposed on or may even think the children's nurse is being 'lazy'. Children's nurses need to ensure that family-centred care is not addressed in a tokenistic way and that the child and family are central to care. The National Service Framework for children, young people and maternity services (DoH 2004) and High-quality care for all (DoH 2008) clearly identify a political agenda to take family-centred care forward by demanding that services are designed around children, young people and their families and a personalised service is delivered. Smith et al. (2010) have made further adaptations to the continuum of family-centred care to cover the time from pre-diagnosis to bereavement.

More recent authors have identified that managers need to provide adequate resources, education and research to fully embed family-centred care. Shields (2010) points out that family-centred care is almost impossible to achieve. There are distinct benefits for the child to have a parent with them in hospital yet, ultimately, family-centred care has to be in the child's best interest (see Research notes 1.1 and 1.2).

NURSING PRACTICE, NURSING SKILLS AND DECISION MAKING

Higham (2011) identifies that the word 'family' is used in everyday language and meaning is apparent but identifies the need for children's nurses to 'problematise the concept'. By 'problematising' key points, the children's nurse raises questions for which answers can be found and/or strategies implemented. In order to 'problematise' the condition, it is essential to have some knowledge about it. Asthma UK (2011) considers that 40 per cent (i.e. some 33,285 hospital admissions) were children and young people under the age of 15 years. Asthma UK (2011) estimate that 1.1 million children and young people in the UK have asthma, with a higher incidence in the northwest of England. Asthma UK (2011) also point out that approximately 75 per cent of children, young people and adult asthma hospital admissions could have been avoided by routine care and effective care management. There are many ways and many tools relating to care planning. For ease and clarity, some have been teased out to identify concepts and processes that have been embedded in practice and work together.

	At the initial diagnosis	Participating in adaptations to care following hospitalisation	Managing asthma condition at home	
No involvement	Involvement	Participation	Partnership	Parent/child led
Nurse led	Nurse led	Nurse led	Equal status	Parent/child led

Figure 1.8 Continuum of family-centred care
Source: Coleman et al. (2007)

Table 1.6 Family-centred care timeline

1988	Casey	Believed that parents continue to provide care for their child in hospital, family care Nurses would provide nursing care and could enable them to adapt to the current health situation
1994	Darbyshire	Undertook research related to parent participation in family-centred care and considered views of parents and nurses
1999	Hutchfield	Considered that working in partnership did wholly reflect the relationship parents developed when their child was in hospital Offered a concept of family-centred care and identified that there was a hierarchy of family-centred care There was a holistic element and a functional element to family-centred care
2003, 2007, 2010	Smith, Coleman and Bradshaw	Believed that family-centred care should be seen as a continuum and parents can choose which stage of the continuum to be on, and that this can change during a hospital journey depending on the issue or area of need This model can also be used to consider the range of healthcare journey a child may follow both in and out of hospital
2004	Franck and Callery	Suggested that maybe it is time to rethink the way in which children and young people are cared for, suggesting that perhaps the care should be more appropriately titled child-centred
2005, 2006, 2010	Coyne	Has written extensively about family-centred care and undertaken research in the area
2010	Shields	Questions the relevancy of family-centred care from past and contemporary literature seeking the answer to five specific questions and concluded research into family-centred care is needed (see Research note 1.1)
2011	Coyne	Research demonstrated that nurses have clear understanding of the essential components of family-centred care and have positive attitudes towards the philosophy yet they experience difficulties practising family-centred care due to organisational and environmental conditions The research identifies that nurses need adequate resources, facilities and managerial support to be able to deliver optimal family-centred care and to meet families' needs appropriately (see Research note 1.2)

[This timeline is not exhaustive.]

RESEARCH NOTE 1.1

Questioning family-centred care
(Shields 2010)

There has been a growing trend to try to formulate a single statement to define family-centred care. Family-centred care appears to be a western phenomenon that is socially constructed to the time and place. Shields et al. (2006) wished to contribute to the family-centred care debate and sought answers to five questions using past and current literature and existing research following a discursive design in order to gain further insights into family-centred care:

- Is family-centred care relevant now?
- Is it relevant only in western countries?
- What does it mean to implement family-centred care?
- Is family-centred care implemented effectively?
- Does it make a difference?

Effective communication and negotiation skills are pivotal to providing family-centred care and it is not clear whether family-centred care makes a difference to the child's health outcomes. Service provision considers the size of the workforce in relation to the patient needs. This is underpinned by Article 3 of UNCRC (UN 1989). Managers need to acknowledge that the process of negotiating with families requires more time and that providing family-centred care impacts on service provision, with requirements of higher staff–patient ratios. Further education of staff regarding family-centred care and how it works would benefit practice. Parents and families would also benefit from education about family-centred care through media sources, pre-hospital programmes, consumer groups, on admission to hospital or at the first healthcare visit.

The study concludes that the notion of family-centred care is idealistic and almost impossible to implement. There is a lack of evidence to prove family-centred care works and further research is required.

RESEARCH NOTE 1.2

What does family-centred care mean to nurses and how do they think it could be enhanced in practice?
(Coyne 2011)

In this survey, nurses caring for children identified their practice and perception of family-centred care. International research has identified inconsistencies with the provision and application of family-centred care in practice. Existing research studies illustrate barriers to family-centred care including nurses' attitudes to families and a lack of support and resources for the philosophy. A descriptive survey design was employed to collect data in 2008–2009. The nurses completed a 47-item questionnaire that examined nurses' perceptions and practices of family-centred care. While nurses accept family-centred care as an ideal philosophy for the care of children and their families, the implementation of family-centred care in practice would seem to present challenges for nurses. The majority in this study indicated that they required further organisational and managerial support fully to implement family-centred care practices. Two interrelated themes were identified: the components of family-centred care and enhancing family-centred care. To provide good-quality family-centred care nurses need adequate resources, appropriate education and support from managers and other healthcare disciplines.

Nursing/Clinical Process

Orlando (1961) first identified the nursing process with five stages encountered when delivering care:

- assess
- diagnose (not used in England)
- plan
- implement
- evaluate

Within the UK, four stages of the nursing process are considered in the caring process and the word diagnose is omitted. During the 1970s the nursing process was introduced in the UK and has been embedded into practice over the past 40 years. Since Orlando's nursing process was generated, the nature of healthcare has changed and, to that end, Casey (1988) identified that other healthcare professionals use similar ideas and suggested that it is the 'clinical process' (see Figure 1.9). Using the same terminology may help to break down the barriers to interprofessional working. Casey (1988) points out that when learning about the complexities of nursing, it is useful to consider a diagram or model to understand how things fit together and the relationships between each component part.

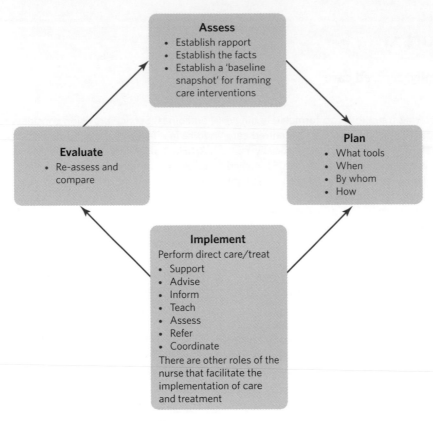

Figure 1.9 Nursing/clinical process
Source: after Casey (1988)

Models of Nursing

Models of nursing began in the United States and came to the UK during the 1980s. Models of nursing are frameworks for applying care and also offer a framework that can coexist with the nursing/clinical process. There have been many models of nursing and this demonstrates that there are many ways of viewing care.

Each model of nursing is presented in a unique way but there are shared components of models that influence practice. According to Pearson et al. (2005), each model has a belief or philosophy about nursing practice, patients' care and their health and environments. Each model of nursing will identify goals according to the situations in which care is given. Pearson et al. (2005) also identify that each nursing model has goals related to what nursing is aiming to achieve. Knowledge to care for patients will arise from a range of sources and all care is required to have an evidence base. Pearson et al. (2005) further identify that knowledge is essential to provide nursing care. This knowledge informs, directs and provides strategies for addressing care needs.

Casey's Model

The philosophy of Casey's model is that 'the care of children, sick or well is best carried out by their families with varying degrees of help from suitably qualified members of the health care team whenever necessary' (Casey 1988). Casey (1988) identifies the **child** as an individual who is growing, developing and functioning in five areas: physically, intellectually, emotionally, socially and spiritually. Children develop along a continuum from dependence on carers for fundamental needs

at conception to interdependence and self-caring at maturity. Casey (1988) believed that optimum **health** included physical and mental well-being. The child will develop healthily in a caring and nurturing environment and will have the best opportunity to meet her full potential. Each child and family will view health on a continuum from wellness to ill health. Ill health affects growth and development and may result from physical, social and/or psychological dysfunction. Casey (1988) identified that all stimuli from external sources are absorbed and processed by the child. Therefore, the child needs a conducive **environment** for development. Influences that can impact on development include: ethnic, socioeconomic, psychological, physiological, racial and cultural, all of which can also affect parenting. From the time of conception, the family mediates between the child and the environment.

Casey (1988) believed that one of the main goals of nursing were carrying out **family care** (the care usually carried out by the family to meet the child's needs on a daily basis). Family care would have been established from the child's birth and will adapt with growing independence and the increasing of children's rights and responsibilities according to their age and stage of development. Casey (1988) believed that **nursing care** (the extra care required to meet the child's needs in relation to a health problem) was to help meet the needs of sick children so that they can achieve their full potential. Casey (1988) believed that children's nurses should **support** sick children and families by helping them cope and continue to function as a family unit when the stresses caused by the disease or condition impact on family life. The children's nurses will **teach** knowledge and skills to help the child and family move from dependence to interdependence from the care team. In cases where care demands expertise from outside the nursing discipline, the children's nurse will **refer** the child/family to and liaise with other members of the healthcare team. One of the criticisms about Casey's model is that it can appear too vague and, to make it more robust, it is used in conjunction with another model.

Roper, Logan and Tierney's Systems Model

The Roper et al. model covers five lifespan changes: infancy, childhood, adolescence, adulthood and old age. The children's nurse cares for children from birth to transition into adult services and many children's wards use this model alongside Casey's model of nursing to provide a robust mechanism for care management. The model considers that care is organised around 12 activities of daily living and these are influenced by biological, psychological, sociocultural, environmental and politico-economic factors. Here there are similarities with Casey's model.

APPLYING THE NURSING/CLINICAL PROCESS, CASEY'S MODEL AND ROPER, LOGAN AND TIERNEY'S MODEL OF CARE

The next section will briefly consider the clinical process, Casey's model and the Roper et al. model in relation to the nursing care of Rhys and his family. Nursing assessments will vary according to the disease process and the context of the setting in which they occur (see Chapter 7).

Generalised Assessment

Contemporary children's nurses focus on a holistic approach to care rather than an assessment of a set of symptoms. A generalised assessment will vary according to the healthcare needs and social circumstances. The generalised assessment will draw from a broad range of knowledge from nursing and may have been 'borrowed' from other disciplines and contexts. During a generalised assessment, it is important to establish rapport with Rhys and his family. The nurse may find some common ground on which to base the conversation, which could be related to a toy or design on clothing. Crawford (2011) suggests that children's nurses are adept at undertaking observations while reading stories or playing with a teddy; this is because it facilitates the addressing of the fears and anxieties that Rhys may have and will provide an opportunity to have immediate concerns addressed.

As the conversation progresses, the children's nurse will establish historical and social facts about Rhys that will be relative to the acute exacerbation of his asthma diagnosis. Rhys and his family may require some explanation as to the nature of asthma (see Table 1.7 and Figure 1.10).

Focused Assessment and Planning

Once the assessment stage has established a 'baseline snapshot', the care planning process begins. Table 1.8 demonstrates a brief

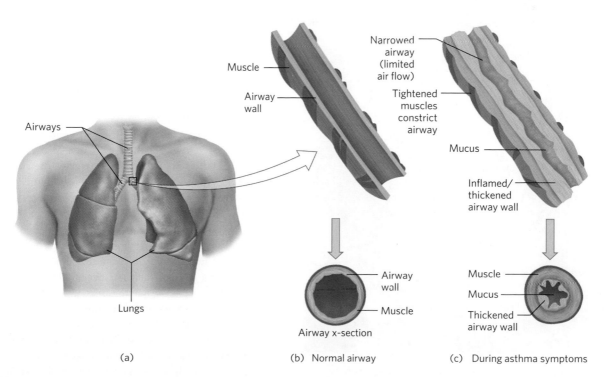

Figure 1.10 Comparison of normal airways with those of children with asthma

Table 1.7 Key points about Rhys and his asthma

Why asthma can cause breathing difficulties	Children have a relatively large tongue and smaller airways compared to those of adults. Children also have large tonsils, particularly in the case of Rhys as he is less than 5 years old. Proportionally children have smaller airways so therefore these are more susceptible to any swelling
	Children have a comparatively large head and occiput region which can contribute to increasing risk of airway obstruction. As Rhys is under 8 years of age his larynx is likely to be funnel shaped with a narrowing at the cricoid cartilage
What is asthma?	Asthma can be triggered by a number of factors that include infection, allergy or exercise. It is more widespread in urban than rural communities. In children under the age of 5 years, around nine out of 100 boys and six out of 100 girls are currently being prescribed inhalers
Signs and symptoms of asthma	May include: • wheezing • cough • breathing difficulty • chest tightness
Treatment	According to severity and the needs of individuals may include: • corticosteroids: inhaled, orally or intravenously • bronchodilator therapy: preventers and relievers • oxygen and pulse oximetry • chest X-ray

assessment using the 'activities of daily living' of Roper et al. which form part of the focused assessment process.

Asthma UK (n.d.) identifies that there are challenges about measuring how effectively the lungs are working when children are under 6 years old. Asthma UK (2011) suggests that a peak flow meter is a useful way of measuring lung capacity and function in children over 6 years (see Figure 1.11). As with any

measurement, it is essential that this information is compared to a nomogram, that appropriate courses of action are identified and that everything is recorded accurately within documentation (see Figure 1.12).

It is essential to ensure that attention is given to timings when planning care. Medications need to be given at a specific time. Measurements of vital signs are often planned pre- and post-delivery of medication administration in order to evaluate the effectiveness of the treatment.

Implementation and Evaluation

Once a management regimen has been confirmed, the treatment is undertaken through the most appropriate methods. Younger children often require the use of a spacer (Figure 1.13) and older children are often able to master the correct technique of taking an inhaler without the use of a spacer device (Figure 1.14). The administration of medicines is seen as a nursing duty within the hospital setting but, in other settings, the self-administration of medication or parental administration of medication will continue. Rhys may still require the information, help and support of both the nurse and parents in coping with his asthma (Casey 2006). If Rhys and his family were not able to effectively administer the inhaler medication then the nurse would offer advice and teach them the correct technique (Casey 2006). If the treatment was assessed to be less effective then Rhys could be referred to the medical team or the clinical nurse specialist for asthma. The coordination of care is crucial.

Whenever care is given, an evaluation should be undertaken. A reassessment of the vital signs should be made and

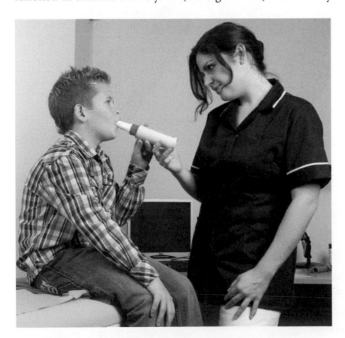

Figure 1.11 Assessing breathing function using a peak flow meter

Table 1.8 Roper, Logan and Tierney's activities of daily living

	Assess	Plan
Maintaining a safe environment	Ensure identification bands are in place Oxygen and suction in working order Bed space is tidy and fit for purpose	To check equipment and observe for signs of deterioration
Communicating	Communicate with Rhys using age-appropriate language according to his stage of development	To explain what is going to happen Answer questions
Breathing	Rate Depth Type For signs of deterioration Peak flow Need for a spacer device	Monitoring of vital signs Ensuring use of appropriate risk assessment tools Pulse oximetry Peak flow monitoring
Eating and drinking	Whether breathing affects ability to eat and drink Discuss with the doctors whether intravenous fluids are required	Encourage quieter activities to facilitate recovery
Eliminating	Whether Rhys is independent for toileting or whether he needs assistance	Orientate Rhys to the ward environment facilities
Personal cleansing and dressing	Whether Rhys requires help to wash and dress Whether Rhys will have his parent staying with him or whether the nurse needs to provide family care	To maintain normal routines as far as possible
Controlling body temperature		
Mobilisation	Whether breathing is affecting mobilisation	Encourage rest to aid recovery Encourage movement and play activities as able
Working and playing	Whether breathing affects ability to play	Provide toys around the bed space which promote quieter activities to promote rest
Expressing sexuality		
Sleeping	What Rhys's normal sleeping patterns and bedtime routines are	To maintain routines as far as practicable
Dying		

this should be compared with previous recordings to see if there are any trends emerging. It may be that Rhys is responding to treatment as expected or that the responses are at a slower pace than expected. It may be that the treatment needs to be reviewed or other treatments included. Making clinical judgements is about reaching a conclusion about what is (probably) going on. Once a clinical judgement has been made the clinical decision making process can be used to choose an appropriate course of action in relation to the current health needs (see Chapter 14).

DEVELOPING A PROFESSIONAL THERAPEUTIC RELATIONSHIP THROUGH DELIVERY OF NURSING SKILLS

Shared Knowledge

Nursing interlinks with a number of other disciplines in caring for children and to this end, the shared knowledge is

PAEDIATRIC NORMAL VALUES
PEAK EXPIRATORY FLOW RATE
For use with EU / EN13826 scale PEF meters only

Height (m)	Height (ft)	Predicted **EU** PEFR (L/min)	Height (m)	Height (ft)	Predicted **EU** PEFR (L/min)
0.85	2'9"	87	**1.30**	4'3"	212
0.90	2'11"	95	**1.35**	4'5"	233
0.95	3'1"	104	**1.40**	4'7"	254
1.00	3'3"	115	**1.45**	4'9"	276
1.05	3'5"	127	**1.50**	4'11"	299
1.10	3'7"	141	**1.55**	5'1"	323
1.15	3'9"	157	**1.60**	5'3"	346
1.20	3'11"	174	**1.65**	5'5"	370
1.25	4'1"	192	**1.70**	5'7"	393

Figure 1.12 A peak flow nomogram (google)

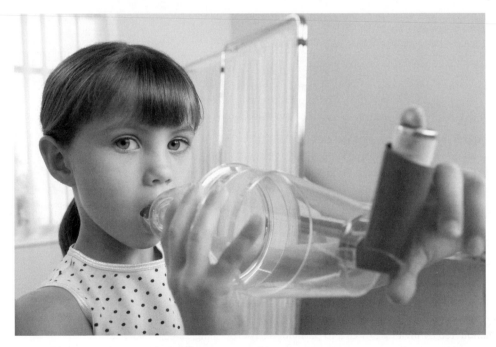

Figure 1.13 Using a spacer device

formulated into a policy (see this chapter). The National Service Framework for children, young people and maternity services (DoH 2004) enables nurses to act in accordance with expected practice unless the needs of the child or young person determine a deviation. In order to further assist practitioners, the Department of Health created exemplars to provide further illustrations to how the National Service Framework would fit with practice.

The National Service Framework for children, young people and maternity services gives an overview of managing asthma as a long term condition and how the interprofessional team have a part to play (see Chapter 14).

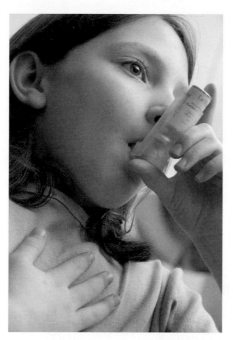

Figure 1.14 Using an inhaler without a spacer device

Nursing Knowledge

There have been many authors who have written extensively about nursing knowledge. Carper (1995, 1978) believed that there were many perspectives of nursing and has described it as being both an art and a science. Johns (1995, 2004) has included Carper's ways of knowing into reflection strategy within his reflective tool (see Tables 1.9 and 1.10). Parker (2002) believed that by linking aesthetics, knowing and nursing values, this would provide a structure and process for the formulation of aesthetics expressions in nursing. Nursing activities or nursing itself can be described by using Carper's ways of knowing. Carper's ways of knowing may lead to Rhys receiving prednisolone, a corticosteroid medication.

Framing the Roles of the Nurse

The work of a children and young people's nurse is varied. During the process of caring for children and young people, the nurse will undertake a range of activities that will relate to a

---

RESEARCH NOTE 1.3

Nurse-led asthma services for children and young people: a survey of GPs' views
(Frost and Daly 2010)

The aim of the research was to investigate GPs' views about children's asthma care in primary settings and their support for a nurse-led asthma service. The study took place between 2005–2007. GPs were invited to participate from four primary care trusts in a large cosmopolitan area within the East Midlands. Seventy per cent of the GPs were of black or Asian descent. In order to ascertain whether GPs would favour, refer to or value a nurse-led asthma service, a survey was conducted by inviting 541 GPs to participate. There were 236 responses to the survey which used a 17-item questionnaire.

The study found that nurse-led services were already being provided by 90% of the GPs. Eighty-nine per cent of GPs believed patients benefited or would benefit from attending a nurse-led asthma clinic. The authors considered that this may

be attributed to Choose and Book which facilitates referral to the hospital-based nurse-led asthma clinics. Eighty-four per cent of GPs would consider referral to a nurse-led asthma clinic; 79% of GPs would consider referral to a satellite nurse-led asthma clinic. The study identifies that, irrespective of whether it was a single-handed practice or part of a group practice, the nurse-led asthma clinics were highly valued and have been considered best practice in Making a Difference (DoH 1999) and Modernising Careers (DoH 2006).

The study concludes that clinical effectiveness for asthma patients could be improved by better communication and referral networks. The study provided a springboard for further discussion to set up a nurse-led asthma clinic with contributions from specialist asthma nurses working in hospital and primary care trusts.

Table 1.9 Carper's ways of knowing (i)

Empirical	The science of nursing, evidence-based
Ethics	The moral component, judgements about what is right and good
Personal knowing	Use of self, self-awareness and empathy
Aesthetics	Art of nursing, the intuitive expert (Benner 1984)
Sociopolitical context of knowing	The sociopolitical context of the persons (nurse and patient)
	The sociopolitical context of nursing as a practice profession, including both societies
	Understanding of nurses and nursing
	Understanding of society and its politics

Table 1.10 Carper's ways of knowing (ii)

Empirical	Knowledge of dosages, side effects, absorption rates
Ethics	What do you do if a child refuses to take the medicine?
Personal knowing	Relates to one's self and personal feelings about taking medicines and the administration of medicines which may have unpleasant side effects or 'after taste'
Aesthetics	Approach and manner towards child and family, masking unpleasant tastes
Sociopolitical context of knowing	Challenge why a particular treatment is not being given due to financial constraints when there is clear evidence that it is effective

---

ACTIVITY 1.5 Prednisolone, ways of knowing

Relate Carper's ways of knowing to the administration of prednisolone in liquid preparation to Rhys.

---

particular way care is 'framed' or identified as 'roles of the nurse'. While undertaking the care process the nurse will take on various roles which are required by children, young people and their parents/carers. During the process of assessment, the children's nurse will demonstrate being 'a skilled planner' and may need to 'refer' to other healthcare professionals. One aspect of nursing children is to build a therapeutic relationship with children and young people, yet in order to do this the children's nurse must establish rapport with the child and gain her trust in a short space of time. It is useful to observe the child's body language and watch for signs of distress and consider age appropriate approaches and language. Finding 'common ground' to initiate conversation is a useful strategy particularly if the child has a toy with her or is wearing a picture of a character from a film, TV programme or cartoon on her clothing. Children and young people would find it useful to know the geography of the ward in order to become oriented to the ward environment and routines.

Involving parents in conversation is essential to the building of a therapeutic relationship in order to gain their unique knowledge about their child. This enables the children's nurse to plan the care of the child more effectively. The parent(s) will also benefit from being oriented to the ward environment in order to feel a sense of acceptance. The children's nurse should seek clues and cues from parents in relation to their child's particular words for things such as 'dummy', 'pacifier' or 'plug', which will facilitate the child's being understood and minimise the potential frustration when the child is not understood. It is equally important to observe how the parents interact and speak with the child as this will demonstrate the state of their relationship.

Children's nurses must be approachable and sensitive to the needs of the child or young person. Showing respect to the child and family helps to form a firm basis for a two-way therapeutic relationship when caring for the child or young person. From a child or young person's perspective it is equally important to keep updated with current characters or topics of interest to children and young people. Caring for children and young people requires the children's nurse to take on different roles. The Department of Health (2010) indicates that the nurse should deliver care that shows compassion and empathy in a respectful and non-judgemental way. Over time, many authors have contributed to frame these different roles (see Practical guidelines 1.2 and Research note 1.3).

Reflecting on the scenario, it is clear that Paige, the student nurse, had received conflicting instructions from her mentor and another qualified member of staff. Paige is feeling uncomfortable with the situation and from her own assessments did not agree with the second request yet may have not felt confident enough to challenge the other nurse's judgement (see Chapter 14).

PRACTICAL GUIDELINES 1.2

Framing the roles of the nurse

Roles of the nurse	Author	Year
Advisor	Smith, Coleman and Bradshaw	2006
	Moules and Ramsay	2008
Advocate	Lee	2004
Care deliverer	Smith, Coleman and Bradshaw	2006
Communicator	Peplau	1952
	Smith, Coleman and Bradshaw	2006
Decision maker	Smith, Coleman and Bradshaw	2006
Educator	Casey	1988
	Smith, Coleman and Bradshaw	2006
	Moules and Ramsay	2008
Empowerer	Lee	2004
Encourager	Smith, Coleman and Bradshaw	2006
Evaluator of care	Smith, Coleman and Bradshaw	2006
Facilitator	Lee	2004
Information handling	Smith, Coleman and Bradshaw	2006
Leader	Smith, Coleman and Bradshaw	2006
Listener	Collier	2013
Negotiator	Corlett and Twycross	2005
	Smith, Coleman and Bradshaw	2006
Process linker	Smith, Coleman and Bradshaw	2006
Referrer	Casey	1988
Resourcer	Casey	1988
Skilled planner	Smith, Coleman and Bradshaw	2006
Supporter	Casey	1988
Surrogate	Peplau	1952
Teacher	Casey	1988
Technical expert	Peplau	1952

[The list is not exhaustive.]

Privacy and Dignity

Children's nurses are bound by the professional code to respect their patients and maintain their confidentiality (NMC 2008). The Department of Health (2001) identified a tool for benchmarking privacy and dignity within the essence of care agenda. The Department of Health (2008) organised a research survey through a market research company on adult service users related to privacy and dignity issues. The services users were surveyed on topics including cleanliness, quality of food, design of wards and adaptations of Nightingale wards and hospital garments. Information for children and young people must be interpreted from extrapolated data in the absence of similar research being undertaken.

The Department of Health, Nursing and Midwifery Council and Royal College of Nursing (2010) formulated a joint document 'The principles of nursing practice'. One of these principles relates to nurses treating patients with 'dignity and humanity'. The Department of Health (2010) issued further guidance relating to the essence of care. Factor 6 of this relates to privacy, dignity and modesty and essence of care, one of the criteria identifies that children and young people should 'be protected from unwanted public view for example, by using curtains, screens, walls, clothes and covers'. There have been several strategies for addressing issues of dignity, which included laminated 'no entry' signs and red pegs with varying degrees of success. It is useful to have systems embedded into practice. It is possible to incorporate information into a panel of a curtain: 'Please respect my privacy' and 'Clean hands saves lives' have been incorporated into the design of the curtain fabric (see Figure 1.15).

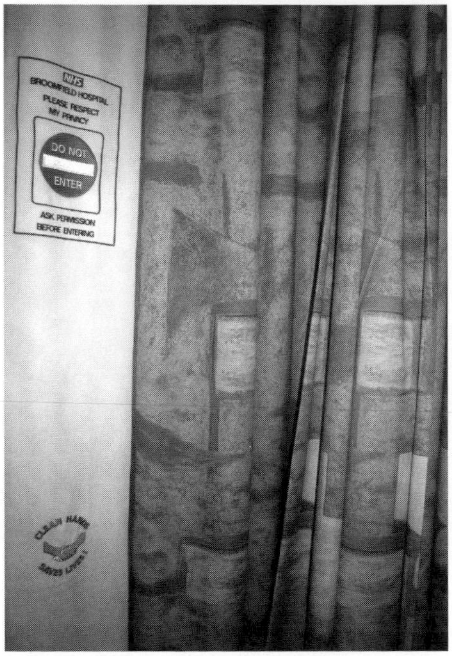

Reflecting on the scenario, it is clear that Rhys has wet the bed and the reason for this is not clear, although there are potential reasons why this may be. First, the scenario does not make it explicit whether Rhys was already incontinent at night due to nocturnal enuresis. If this was the case, then strategies could be explored with his mother. It may simply have been that no one was aware of his need for continence aid and Rhys's mother omitted to say. Alternatively, it may be that Rhys had experienced a nightmare, which is common with this age group with thoughts of monsters, dinosaurs and dragons (see Chapter 2). It could be due to the stress of being in hospital, missing other members of his family. The important thing would be to respect his vulnerability and prevent potential embarrassment by offering reassurance.

Figure 1.16 contains the NHS Asthma Care Journey data for continuing and linking care.

Communication and Interpersonal Skills

The Nursing and Midwifery Council exists to protect the public from harm by ensuring that there are good standards and guidelines in place to provide nurses and midwives with guidance and proficiencies to meet. The NMC Code: Standards of conduct, performance and ethics for nurses and midwives (2008) directs

Figure 1.15 Privacy messages on curtains

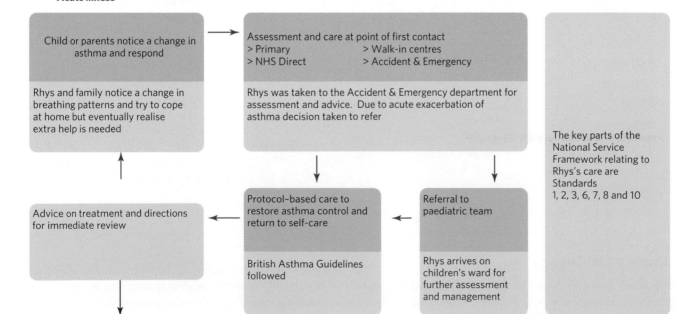

Acute illness

Child or parents notice a change in asthma and respond

Rhys and family notice a change in breathing patterns and try to cope at home but eventually realise extra help is needed

Assessment and care at point of first contact
> Primary   > Walk-in centres
> NHS Direct   > Accident & Emergency

Rhys was taken to the Accident & Emergency department for assessment and advice. Due to acute exacerbation of asthma decision taken to refer

The key parts of the National Service Framework relating to Rhys's care are Standards 1, 2, 3, 6, 7, 8 and 10

Advice on treatment and directions for immediate review

Protocol-based care to restore asthma control and return to self-care

British Asthma Guidelines followed

Referral to paediatric team

Rhys arrives on children's ward for further assessment and management

Figure 1.16 Asthma Care Journey
Source: Department of Health (2004)

Linking care

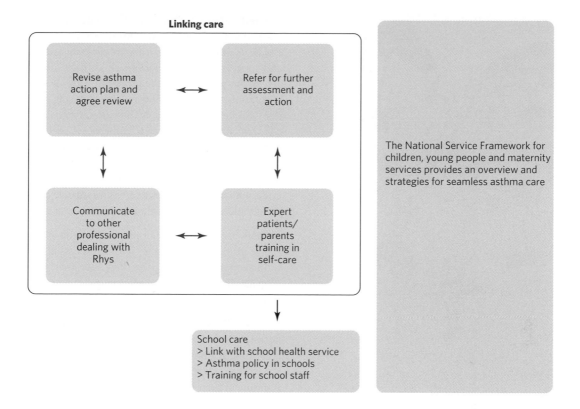

children's nurses to key areas of knowledge, skills and behaviours for professional practice. The NMC has considered the provision of guidance on professional conduct for nursing and midwifery students (NMC 2011).

ACTIVITY 1.6 NMC Code

Access the NMC Code: Standards of conduct, performance and ethics for nurses and midwives (2008) to revise its contents and make short notes as required (**http://www.nmc-uk.org/Publications-/Standards1/**).

Access the Guidance on Professional Conduct for nursing and midwifery students. Revise its contents and make short notes as required (**http://www.nmc-uk.org/Documents /Guidance/Guidance-on-professional-conduct-for-nursing-and-midwifery-students.pdf**).

Berlin and Fowkes (1983) proffered a communication framework that took into account the interaction between nurses and their patients. Berlin and Fowkes (1983) indicate that each letter is a representation of a word. The original LEARN communication framework provides a mnemonic that could serve as an 'aide memoire' for the children and young people's nurse. The nature of nursing has changed over the past 30 years and there is now a stronger emphasis on collaborative working with other healthcare workers and external liaison to facilitate seamless care. The NMC (2008, 2010) has developed guidelines that require nurses to share information confidentially and

appropriately to maintain accurate records. To this end, the letters ER have been added to create the LEARNER mnemonic to adapt the communication framework in order to consider communication and interpersonal skills during child and family healthcare (see Figures 1.17 and 1.18).

Listen

The NMC (2008) is clear that children and young people should be listened to and their preferences taken into account during healthcare interventions. The NMC (2008) clarifies that information should be presented in a way the child or young person will understand. This is underpinned by the United Nations Convention on the Rights of the Child (UNCRC) (1989). United Nations Conventions on the Rights of the Child (1989) direct society to ensure that children have the right to be consulted, have their views heard and to be responded to in an appropriate way.

In order to listen to children and young people, the children's nurse needs to develop a rapport and trust. With this in mind,

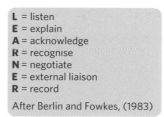

L = listen
E = explain
A = acknowledge
R = recognise
N = negotiate
E = external liaison
R = record

After Berlin and Fowkes, (1983)

Figure 1.17 LEARNER communication

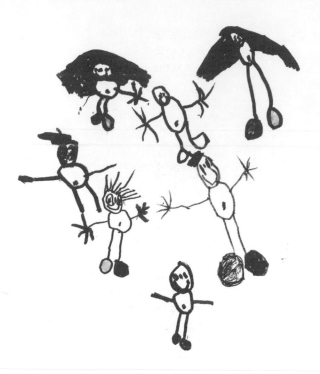

Figure 1.18 Charlie's family

children's nurses are required to develop a range of interpersonal skills from which particular approaches can be selected for use according to the situation being addressed. The children's nurse will also need knowledge of developmental milestones and be able to recognise where there are deviations from expected criteria. As the young person develops independence, he is afforded additional rights and responsibilities by his parents and steps are taken toward autonomy. As a result, the nature of communication with him changes to show maturity and change. In considering Rhys and his exacerbation of asthma, it will be essential to actively listen to his understanding of what is happening to him and listen to his fears and anxieties (see Tables 1.5 and 1.6).

Children's nurses are required to act as an advocate for all children or young people and speak on their behalf. At times, the child or young person will be required to give informal consent for some aspects of healthcare. This is a frequently occurring element of the children's nurses' role where they are required to have an understanding of the need for cooperation. Informal consent could be merely holding an arm out to facilitate venepuncture, participation in X-ray or a CT scan. This is underpinned by evidence within Article 12 which clearly states that children have the right to be heard during procedures:

> The child shall in particular be provided with the opportunity to be heard in any surgical or administrative proceedings affecting the child directly; or through a representative body. UNCRC (1989)

Explain

Children's nurses develop rapport with the child and family when establishing a therapeutic relationship. The chronological age and developmental stage the child or young person has reached will influence how information is shared with them. A children's nurse may want to administer an antibiotic to a child and conveys this message to the child. The nurse will know that an oral preparation is to be given but without stating the mode of administration, the child may be thinking that the medication will be administered by injection, when in actual fact the children's nurse is planning to dispense an oral preparation. It is important that the child or young person receive a clear explanation to reduce fear and anxiety. Explaining procedures and activities may include using play, pictures or drawings. This is underpinned by the evidence within Article 12 which clearly states children have the right to express views:

> State parties shall assure to the child who is capable of forming his or own views the right to express those views freely in all matters affecting the child, the views of the child being given due weight in accordance with the age and maturity of the child. UNCRC (1989)

Play is the work of children and time will be spent during a hospital journey undertaking activities such as games, painting, colouring or drawing. This is known as normative play. Play is an excellent tool for giving explanations or increasing understanding of their medical condition. This is known as therapeutic play (see Chapter 2). This is underpinned by the evidence in Article 12 and has the potential need to involve the interprofessional team at point of care delivery:

> For this purpose, the child shall in particular be provided the opportunity to be heard in any judicial and administrative proceeding affecting the child, either directly, or through a representative or an appropriate body, in a manner consistent with the procedural rules of national law.

Acknowledge

When communicating with children it is important to consider the influence that the culture may have on the interaction between the children's nurse and the child. The children's nurses should consider how communication with a child who is deaf may be different and may use Makaton or British Sign Language. Children's nurses can learn some of the Makaton system in order to communicate with their patients. There are some children's television programmes that sign using Makaton.

Children who are blind or have sight deficits can be taught communication using Braille. The signage in a large number of children's wards fails to make provision for children to navigate around the ward environment using Braille. Communication with the child who has a learning disability will be challenging particularly if they are preverbal or have no verbal communication skills. These children may still be able to understand or use pictures to communicate. Nursing could learn from methods of communication in school for those with educational needs and implement visual timetables for the day. For some children speech is made possible through electronic or hand held devices. Children are sensitive to nonverbal clues, which mean the children's nurse must ensure that mixed messages are not communicated.

Recognise

Article 3 directs organisations to act in the child's best interest and this also fits with the Children Act (1989, 2004). Risk assessments are undertaken to ensure that the child is cared for in a safe environment. Children's nurses develop interpersonal skills and interpretive skills. Children sometimes have hidden knowledge, thoughts or feelings that the parents are unaware of (see Voices 1.4).

RESEARCH NOTE 1.4 Therapeutic relationships in day surgery: a grounded theory study (Mottram 2009)

Therapeutic relationships are considered to be a core component of nursing practice; however, relationships are developed over time and this could be hindered with short hospital episodes. A major theme from the research was the development of a therapeutic relationship. The research was conducted using Glaserian grounded theory. Semi-structured interviews with 145 patients were conducted during a 2-year period. Although the research was conducted on adult patients, there are interpretations to be extrapolated from the data for the children's nurse. Currently, similar studies on children do not exist, yet family-centred care acknowledges the parent as part of the caring process.

The study identifies the category of therapeutic relationship has four subcategories: presence, extra special, befriending and comfort giving. Therapeutic relationships can be developed in day surgery and in a relatively short period of time. Patients have little time to familiarise themselves with their surroundings and the interaction of the nurse–patient relationship was supportive.

VOICES 1.4 'I am not going in there'

Parents may believe they have knowledge of their child's understanding of life and healthcare events. Unless a child talks about their experiences, adults can make assumptions about their child's level of understanding.

Walking towards the local health centre, a conversation took place between a boy aged 4 years, and his mother:

Boy: 'I am not going in there [health centre].'

Mother: 'Why not?' [surprised]

Boy: 'They hurt you.'

Mother: 'When did they hurt you?' [rather puzzled]

Boy: 'The nurse pinched my arm.'

[short pause] [Recalling the last immunisation experience]

Mother: 'The nurse gave you some medicine that will work in your body and was helping you to stay well for a long time.'

Negotiate

Family-centred healthcare with the child or young person encourages the choice of self-care, family care or nursing care providing it is appropriate for the child. Negotiation and empowerment work together. Negotiation should be desired by the child or family and not enforced. Negotiation should not demonstrate tokenism or assumptions.

External Liaison and Records

Effective communication and interpersonal skills will enable the children's nurse to collaborate with those in other healthcare settings to facilitate continuous care. Parent-held child records provide ongoing written communication when working in interprofessional partnerships with school nurses and other healthcare professionals in the community setting, social work, education or early years curriculum. The nature of communication with health professionals has a different focus and time efficiency can be crucial in summoning help for children and young people. Inexperienced staff find it challenging to know which information to present first. This can mean that the conversation meanders before the crucial points are stated. One disadvantage of this is that the priority information is missed. To this end, the NHS has devised a communication strategy that provides a framework facilitating succinct information giving.

The NHS has devised SBAR (situation, background, assessment, recommendation) as a succinct and methodical approach to communication and a means of summoning help appropriately, with due consideration to priorities and in a timely manner (see Figure 1.19). Care can be compromised if an incorrect or incomplete message is shared, therefore, it is in the child and young person's best interest to ensure this does not occur.

Communication is a key theme throughout children's nursing from the point of beginning a care journey to the point of discharge planning, facilitating seamless care with the interprofessional team

CASE STUDY REVIEW 1.5 (FINAL)

There are a number of systems in place within healthcare to ensure that Rhys remains safe in hospital and that all his care is underpinned by evidence-based practice, law, policies and guidelines. There is clear guidance how to manage asthma through the National Service Framework exemplar. This facilitates parity with the management of the long-term condition to provide seamless care and parity in case management.

Although Amanda and Anthony have ended their relationship as husband and wife they have remained amicable for the sake of their children. Both Amanda and Anthony have accepted one another's new relationships.

Exacerbation of acute asthma can be a frightening experience. A change in medicine regime and improvement of inhaler techniques enable Rhys to return home after a brief hospital stay.

Situation
I am (name), (X) nurse on ward (X)
I am calling about (patient X)
I am calling because I am concerned that…
(e.g. BP is low/high, pulse is XX temperature is XX, Early Warning Score is XX)

Background
Patient (X) was admitted on (XX date) with
(e.g. MI/chest infection)
They have had (X operation/procedure/investigation)
Patient (X)'s condition has changed in the last (XX mins)
Their last set of obs were (XX)
Patient (X)'s normal condition is…
(e.g. alert/drowsy/confused, pain free)

Assessment
I think the problem is (XXX)
And I have…
(e.g. given O$_2$/analgesia, stopped the infusion)
OR
I am not sure what the problem is but patient (X) is deteriorating
OR
I don't know what's wrong but I am really worried

Recommendation
I need you to…
Come to see the patient in the next (XX mins)
AND
Is there anything I need to do in the mean time?
(e.g. stop the fluid/repeat the obs)

Ask receiver to repeat key information to ensure understanding

The SBAR tool originated from the US Navy and was adapted for use in healthcare by Dr M. Leonard and colleagues from Kaiser Permanente, Colorado, USA

Figure 1.19 SBAR communication tool

for ongoing care. It is equally important to ensure that the care is appropriately documented in the patient record (NMC 2009).

CHILDREN AND YOUNG PEOPLE'S VOICES

During the past 30 years, there has been a substantial recognition of children's rights and how they should be listened to (Children Act, Her Majesty's Government 1989). The United Nations Convention on the Rights of the Child (UNCRC) (1989) was introduced to the United Kingdom during 1991 and it identified 40 substantial rights of children, which are incorporated into a range of laws (Alderson 2008). Webb et al. (2009, page 434) state that 'the UNCRC is a powerful tool and driver to improve the health and welfare of children and young people and the health services we provide for them.' As far back as the Community Care Act 1990 there has been a drive to involve service users in consultations. The involvement of service users has been included in several reports including the NHS plan.

The Department for Children, Schools and Families (2003) have identified five useful, key outcome goals for children: being healthy, staying safe, enjoying and achieving, making a positive contribution and achieving economic well-being. The United Nations Convention on the Rights of the Child (UNCRC) (1989) formulated 54 rights afforded to children and young people. These rights of the child serve to underpin government policy within the *Every child matters* agenda. UNICEF UK and the Department for Education (2006) overtly mapped the rights afforded children against the five *Every child matters* outcomes. The *Every child matters* agenda has been archived and new political direction is awaited. Greig et al. (2007) assert that the rights afforded to children are the minimum expectation in society and that the majority of parents and the wider big society would expect more for children than their predecessors.

SUMMARY OF KEY LEARNING

The Department of Health (2004) asserts that services should be designed around the child/young person and their families. As consumers of healthcare, children and young people were invited to participate in the formulation of the National Service Framework for children, young people and maternity services by sharing their views. Coad et al. (2008) have also influenced the development of children and young people's advisory groups/health councils. Coad and Shaw (2008) highlight that children and young people want to have a greater say in the design of appropriate hospital and community healthcare services. Heath et al. (2009) suggest that young peoples' lives are circumscribed by age-specific policies and laws but they are also shaped by hospital experiences over time.

The National Health Service Regulations (2010) require service users or their representatives to be involved in matters that affect public health. To that end, Myers and Collier (2010) undertook a consultation project involving children and young people in choosing décor for a regional children's burns ward. The views of children and young people were gained in relation to colour and thematic design and this was carried through to the new décor.

FURTHER RESOURCES

Asthma

http://www.asthma.org.uk/

http://www.asthma.org.uk/health_professionals/schools_early_years/index.html

Action for Sick Children: **http://actionforsickchildren.org/index.asp?ID=261**

Communication

SBAR: **http://www.institute.nhs.uk/safer_care/safer_care/SBAR_escalation_films.html**

Civil Partnership Act (2004)

http://www.legislation.gov.uk/ukpga/2004/33/contents

Poverty

http://www.jrf.org.uk/work/workarea/child-poverty

Education

http://www.education.gov.uk/

Children's rights

UNICEF: **http://www.unicef.org/crc/**

Children's rights: **http://www.unicef.org/rightsite/files/rights_leaflet.pdf**

Children's Commissioner for England: **http://www.childrenscommissioner.gov.uk/**

Children's Commissioner for Wales: **http://www.childcom.org.uk**

Children's Commissioner for Scotland: **http://www.sccyp.org.uk/**

Children's Commissioner for Northern Ireland: **http://www.niccy.org/**

Single parents

http://www.gingerbread.org.uk/content.aspx?CategoryID=365

ANSWERS TO ACTIVITIES

ACTIVITY 1.1 Defining poverty

Research the terms 'Relative poverty' and 'absolute poverty'

Absolute poverty: It refers to a set standard which is consistent over time and between countries. The absolute poverty measure trends noted previously are supported by human development indicators, which have also been improving.

Relative poverty: Relative poverty views poverty as socially defined and dependent on HYPERLINK "http://en.wikipedia.org/wiki/Social_context" \o "Social context" social context, hence relative poverty is a measure of income inequality. Usually, relative poverty is measured as the percentage of population with income less than some fixed proportion of median income. Relative poverty measures are used as official poverty rates in several developed countries. As such these poverty statistics measure inequality rather than material deprivation or hardship. The measurements are usually based on a person's yearly income and frequently take no account of total wealth. The main poverty line used in the HYPERLINK "http://en.wikipedia.org/wiki/OECD" \o "OECD" OECD and the HYPERLINK "http://en.wikipedia.org/wiki/European_Union" \o "European Union". European Union is based on 'economic distance', a level of income set at 60% of the median household income.

ACTIVITY 1.2

Q: List the ways in which information technology may impact on 21st century childhood.

Consider the list you formulated. Were there any considerations children and young people's nurses should be aware of?

A: The NMC (2012) has clear guidelines for the appropriate behaviours of social networking and has related them to the Code. It would be prudent for children's nurses to be mindful of dangers of the Internet in order to be more vigilant and be able to protect children and young people from harm in hospitals.

ACTIVITY 1.3 Hospitalisation in times of war

Q: Write some thoughts of what it would have been like had Rhys been an evacuee during the war and also required hospitalisation.

A: From being evacuated, Rhys may:

- be feeling homesick and missing his family
- be separated from his sibling, Bethan
- be separated from his step-sibling, Ben.

From being hospitalised, Rhys may:

- be feeling really scared
- have heightened feelings of missing his family
- be missing the comfort of his support.

These ideas are not exhaustive.

ACTIVITY 1.4 Using a genogram to demonstrate a family tree

1. Beginning with the Queen, formulate a genogram that demonstrates three generations of the royal family.

2. Formulate a genogram of Rhys and his family.

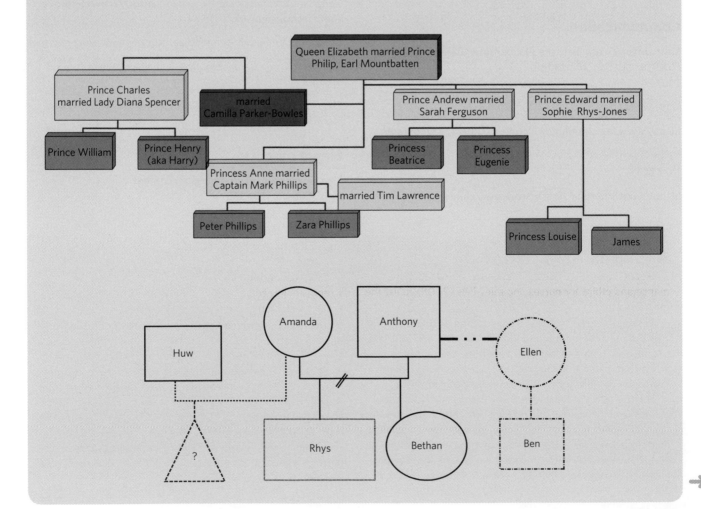

ACTIVITY 1.5 Carper's ways of knowing and administration of prednisolone

Empirical	Type: oral systemic steroid Knowledge of dosages: TBC	Side-effects: Absorption rates:
Ethics	What do you do if a child refuses to take the medicine? Estimate how much has been wasted, inform the healthcare professional or mentor, record the outcome of the medicines administration.	
Personal knowing	Relates to one's self and personal feelings about taking medicines and the administration of medicines which may have unpleasant side-effects or 'after-taste': • Do not disclose personal feelings about prednisolone. • Be honest with the child if she has no previous experience of taking prednisolone and tell her that there will be an 'after-taste'. • Prepare a coping strategy such as a sticker or a similar reward. • Offer a choice to have the prednisolone in a medicine pot or an oral syringe.	
Aesthetics	Approach and manner towards child and family: • Establish rapport. • Communicate clearly. • Explain what the medicine is and its purpose. • Recognise that the family may have experiences of administering the prednisolone at home. Masking unpleasant tastes: • Children should be aware of the need to take prednisolone; covert masking of unpleasant tastes may cause the child to mistrust. • Do not try to disguise prednisolone in a drink as the child may not consume all the drink or medication. • Record all refusal of prednisolone.	
Sociopolitical context of knowing	Challenge why a particular treatment is not being given due to financial constraints when there is clear evidence that it is effective.	

ACTIVITY 1.6 NMC CODE

Access the NMC Code: Standards of conduct, performance and ethics for nurses and midwives (2008) to list the main points:

• respect and advocate for patients
• maintain confidentiality
• listen to people in your care
• be mindful of mental capacity and act in the best interest of the patients
• maintain professional boundaries
• share information appropriately
• be a team player
• use the best evidence possible
• be up to date with skills
• act with integrity
• deal with problems of patients
• maintain accurate records.

Access the Guidance on Professional Conduct for nursing and midwifery students. Revise its contents and make short notes as required.

Has strong similarities with the NMC Code: Standards of conduct, performance and ethics for nurses and midwives (2008) as above, as expected but also identifies the need for good health, good character and maintaining confidentiality within assignments.

SELECTED REFERENCES

Acheson, D. (1998) The Acheson Report.

Afridi, A. (2011) Social networks: their role in addressing poverty, Joseph Rowntree Foundation: **http://www.jrf.org.uk/sites/files/jrf/young-people-education-attitudes-full.pdf**

BBC News (2011) 'Sarah's law' scheme covers all England and Wales: **http://www.bbc.co.uk/news/uk-12952334**

Beaumont, J. (2010) Social trends 41, households and families, Office for National Statistics: **http://www.ons.gov.uk/ons/rel/social-trends-rd/social-trends/social-trends-41/index.html**

Benner, P. and Tanner, C. (1987) Clinical judgement: how expert nurses use intuition. *American Journal of Nursing*, 87(1), 23–31.

Berlin, E.A. and Fowkes, W.C. (1983) A teaching framework for cross-cultural health care. *Western Journal of Medicine*, 139(6), 934–938.

Black, D. (1982) *Inequalities in health: Black Report*. Penguin Books: London.

Brewer, M.J., Browne, J. and Joyce, R. (2011) Child and working-age poverty, Joseph Rowntree Foundation: **http://www.jrf.org.uk/sites/files/jrf/children-adult-poverty-welfare-summary.pdf**

Bricher, G. (1999) Paediatric nurses, children and the development of Trust, *Journal of Clinical Nursing*, 8, 451–458.

Brooks, G. (2000) Children's competence to consent: a framework for practice. *Paediatric Nursing*, 12(5).

Browne, K. (2011) *An introduction to Sociology*, 4th ed. Polity Press: Cambridge.

Casey, A. (1988) A partnership with child and family. *Senior Nurse*, 8(4).

Children Act (1989) **http://www.legislation.gov.uk/ukpga/1989/41/contents**

Children Act (2004) **http://www.legislation.gov.uk/ukpga/2004/31/contents**

Clement Clarke International (n.d.) Peak flow nomogram: **http://www.peakflow.com/top_nav/home/index-2.html**

Clemow, R. (2006) Care plans as the main focus of nursing handover: information exchange Model.

Coad, J. and Coad, N. (2008) Children and young people's preference of thematic design and colour for their hospital environment. *Journal of Child Health Care*, 12, 33–48.

Coad, J. and Shaw, K.L. (2008) Is children's choice in health care rhetoric or reality? A scoping review. *Journal of Advanced Nursing*, Review Paper, 64(4), 318–327.

Coad, H., Flay, J., Aspinall, M., Bilverstone, B., Coxhead, E. and Hones, B. (2008) Evaluating the impact of involving young people in developing children's services in an acute hospital trust. *Journal of Clinical Nursing*, 17, 3115–3122.

Coleman, V., Smith, L. and Bradshaw, M. (2007) *Children's and Young People's Nursing in Practice: A Problem-Based Learning Approach*. Palgrave Macmillan: Basingstoke.

Corlett, J. and Twycross, A. (2006) Negotiation of parental roles within family-centred care: a review of the research.

Coyne, I. (2006) Consultation with children in hospital: children, parents and nurses' perspectives. *Journal of Clinical Nursing*, 15(1), 61–71.

Coyne, I. (2008) Children's participation in consultations and decision-making at health service level: a review of the literature.

Crawford, D.A. (2002) Keep the focus on the family. *Journal of Child Health Care*, 133–146.

Darbyshire, P. (1994) Living with a sick child in hospital: the experiences of parents and nurses. London.

Department for Children, Schools and Families (DFES) (2003) *Every child matters*. Stationery Office: London.

Department for Education and Skills and Department of Health (DFES/DoH) (2004) National Service Framework for children, young people and maternity services: asthma.

Department for Work and Pensions (2010) State of the nation report: poverty, worklessness and welfare dependency in the UK. Cabinet Office: London.

Department for Work and Pensions (2011) Households below average income 2009/2010. Figures are after housing costs. Cabinet Office: London.

Department of Education (2010) Review of the office of the Children's Commissioner (England), Stationery Office, Norwich: **https://www.education.Gov.Uk/Publications/Eorderingdownload/Cm-7981.Pdf**

Department of Health (2001a) Good practice in consent implementation guide: consent to examination and treatment.

Department of Health (2001b) Seeking consent: working with children.

Department of Health (2001c) The expert patient a new approach to chronic disease management for the 21st century. Department of Health: London.

Department of Health (2003) *National Service Framework for children, young people and maternity services*. Department of Health: London.

Department of Health (2004) Patient and public involvement in health, the evidence for policy implementation, a summary for the results of the health in partnership research programme. Department of Health: London.

Department of Health (2008a) Safeguarding children in whom illness is fabricated or induced: a review of implementation 2002 Guidance within the NHS. Department of Health: London.

Department of Health (2008b) High-quality care for all: NHS next stage review final report. Department of Health: London.

Department of Health, Nursing and Midwifery Council and Royal College of Nursing (DoH, NMC and RCN) (2010) *The principles of nursing practice*. Department of Health: London.

Egan, G. (1994) *The skilled helper: a problem-management approach to helping*, 5th edn. Pacific Grove, CA: Brooks/Cole Publishing Company.

Eiser, C. (2000) The psychological impact of chronic illness on children's development, in A. Closs (ed.) *The education of children with medical conditions*, pp 27–38.

Fletcher, T., Glasper, A., Prudhoe, G., Battrick, C., Coles, L., Weaver, K. and Ireland, L. (2011) Building the future: children's views on nurses and hospital care. *British Journal of Nursing*, 20(1), 39–45.

Forbat, L., Hubbard, G. and Kearney, N. (2009) Patient participation: patient and public involvement: models and muddles. *Journal of Clinical Nursing*, 18, 2547–2554.

Franck L.S. and Callery, P. (2006) Re-thinking family-centred care across the continuum of children's health care. *Child Care, Health and Development*, 30(3), 265–277.

Frost, S. and Daly, W. (2010) Nurse-led asthma services for children and young people: a survey of GP's views. *Paediatric Nursing*, 22(8), 32–36.

Glasper, E.A. and Richardson, J. (2006) *A textbook of children's and young people's nursing*. Churchill Livingstone Elsevier: Philadelphia.

Hharp Hospital Admissions Records Project **http://www. hharp.org/library/gosh/nurses/catherine-jane-wood.html**

Higham, S. (2011) Family-centred care and the evolving role of fathers, in R. Davies and A. Davies (eds), *Children and young people's nursing: principles for practice*, Hodder Arnold: London.

Hutchfield, K. (1999) Family-centred care: a concept analysis. *Journal of Advanced Nursing*, 29(5), 1178–1187.

Johns, C. (2005) Expanding the gates of perception, in C. Johns and D. Freshwater (eds), *Transforming nursing through reflective practice*. Oxford.

Jolley, J. (2007) Now and then: Florence Nightingale and children's nursing. *Paediatric Nursing*, 19(8).

Jolley, J. (2011) The development of children's nursing, in R. Davies and A. Davies (eds), *Children and young people's nursing: principles for practice*. Hodder Arnold: London.

Jones, B. (2001) The policy-making process, in B. Jones, D. Kavangh, M. Moran and P. Norton (eds) *Politics UK*, 4th edn. Pearson Education Limited: Harlow.

Kintrea, K., St Clair, R. and Huston, M. (2011) The influences of parents, places and poverty on educational attitudes and aspirations, Joseph Rowntree Foundation: **http://www.jrf. org.uk/sites/files/jrf/young-people-education-attitudes-full.pdf**

Laming Report (2003) The Victoria Climbié Inquiry Report **http://www.dh.gov.uk/en/publicationsandstatistics /publications/publicationspolicyandguidance/dh_ 4008654**

Lee, P. (2004) Family involvement: are we asking too much?, *Paediatric Nursing*, 16(10), 37–41.

Loudon, I.S.L. (1979) John Bunell Davis and the universal dispensary for children. *British Medical Journal*, 1, 1191–1194.

Lumsden, E. (2010) The new early years professional in England. *International Journal for Cross-Disciplinary Subjects in Education*, 1(3).

Makins, V. (1999) In the heart of the city; early years; profile. Thomas Coram Foundation, TES, 23 July.

Mottram, A. (2009) Therapeutic relationships in day surgery: a grounded theory study. *Journal of Clinical Nursing*, 18, 2830–2837.

Moules T. and Ramsay J. (2008) *The textbook of children's and young people's nursing*, 2nd edition. Wiley-Blackwell: Oxford.

Myers, J. and Collier, S. (2010) Bridging the gap between children and adults in the interior decor of a children's burn ward. Unpublished poster presented to the Australian and New Zealand Annual Scientific Meeting, October 2010.

National Health Service (Strategic Health Authorities: Further Duty To Involve Users) Regulations (2010) No. 423, The National Archives: **http://www.legislation.gov.uk/ uksi/2010/423/contents/made**

National Institute for Clinical Excellence (2010) Ta10 asthma (children under 5)–inhaler devices: understanding NICE. Guidance: **http://guidance.nice.org.uk/index .jsp?action=article&o=32077**

Nursing and Midwifery Council (2009) *Record keeping guidance for nurses and midwives*. NMC: London.

Office for National Statistics (2012) *Lone parents with dependent children*.

Parker, M.E. (2002) Aesthetics ways in day-to-day nursing, in D. Freshwater (ed.) *Therapeutic nursing, improving patient care through self-awareness and reflection*. Sage Publications Ltd: London.

Picard, C. (2002) A praxis model of research for therapeutic Nursing, in D. Freshwater (ed.) *Therapeutic nursing, improving patient care through self-awareness and reflection*. Sage Publications Ltd: London.

Priddis, L. and Shields, L. (2011) Interactions between parents and staff of hospitalised children. *Paediatric Nursing*, 23(2).

Rolfe, G. (2009) Writing up and writing as: rediscovering nursing scholarship. *Nurse Education Today*,

Scottish Intercollegiate Guideline Network and British Thoracic Society (2011) British guideline on the management of asthma: a national clinical guideline: **http://www.sign. ac.uk/pdf/sign101.pdf**

Sharma, N. (2007) It doesn't happen here – the reality of child poverty in the UK, Banardo's, Ilford: **http://www.barnardos. org.uk/poverty_full_report_07.pdf**

Shields, L. Pratt, J. and Hunter, J. (2006) Family-centred care: a review of qualitative ???and studies

Smith, L., Coleman, V. and Bradshaw, M. (2010) *Child and family-centred healthcare: concept, theory and practice*. Palgrave: Basingstoke.

Twycross, A. and Powls, L. (2005) How do children's nurses make clinical decisions? Two preliminary studies. *Journal of Clinical Nursing*, 15, 1324–1335.

UNICEF UK and Department for Education (DfE) (2006) Every child matters – the five outcomes and the UN Convention on the Rights of the Child (UNCRC): **https://www.edu-cation.gov.uk/publications/standard/publicationdetail /page1/32016**

United Nations (UN) (1989) United Nations Convention on the Rights of the Child (1989) Geneva: UN.

Webb, E., Horrocks, L., Crowley, A. and Lessof, N. (2009) Using the UN Convention on the Rights of the Child to Improve the Health of Children. *Paediatric and Child Health*, 19(9), 430–443.

CHAPTER 2
Using Developmental Theories to Enhance Holistic Care

Steve Bilham

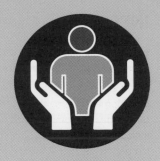
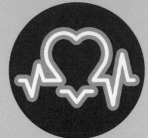
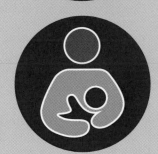

LEARNING OUTCOMES

On completion of this chapter, the reader will be able to:

- Describe the factors that may result in variations to the growth and development of children and young people.
- Reflect on the role of the family in the development of children and young people.
- Explore the theories of play in relation to the growth and development of children and young people and discuss their value in practice.
- Understand physical growth and maturation of children and young people in the assessment and planning of care.
- Use theories of child development and play to reflect on the care that respects the child and young person's ability and developing autonomy.

TALKING POINT

'Pupils with special educational needs have learning difficulties or disabilities that make it harder for them to learn than most pupils of the same age. One in every five pupils has a special educational need; about 1.7 million. This is a large and very important group of young learners.'

DoE (2010)

INTRODUCTION

This chapter will explore the social construction of childhood, alongside basic genetics and variations in growth and development; examination will also include assessment of physical and developmental growth to include discussion of developmental milestones. Important developmental theories will be discussed including Piaget, Freud, Vygotsky, Erikson, Bronfenbrenner, Skinner and Watson, from birth to adolescence. Attachment theories will also acknowledge Bowlby, while language development will include Chomsky, Brunner and developmental theorists. Alongside this moral development, we reflect on Piaget, Kolhberg, Berryman and Gilligan. A child's temperament and the value of an understanding of normative play will also be highlighted.

When thinking about growth and development the terms may seem interchangeable; however, they are two separate concepts. Growth can occur with or without development and an understanding of this will help when considering how development is assessed.

Distinction should also be made between the different types of development: organs develop in complexity and ability (this may be better described as maturation); however, growth in size may not always mean that there is corresponding development – this would be the case in unrestricted growth as in cancer. When considering the topic of child development taking in all of these areas, together they form an exciting journey into the development of ourselves.

This chapter will define the terms most commonly used in child development and bring them together in a way that will help the student of children and young people's nursing to apply them to the care they give. It should be stressed that not all the answers are here, but there is encouragement to 'go and find out more'. For example, an introduction to Sigmund Freud is made, but what is more exciting is that there is so much more to know. Think of this as an introduction to an adventure.

The following scenario (Case Study 2.1) will be referred to throughout the chapter in order to help the student apply the topics discussed.

CASE STUDY 2.1

Chris and Hannah are in their late 30s and have been trying for many years to have children. After undergoing many tests, Hannah finally conceived after undergoing in vitro fertilisation (IVF).

Thomas and Isaac were born at 34 weeks' gestation. They were cared for in the special care baby unit (SCBU) for two weeks before being discharged into the care of the community team.

When the babies were 6 months of age, Chris and Hannah noticed that Thomas and Isaac were not developing the same skills at the same time.

GROWTH

Growth describes the physical trajectory of a child from conception to maturity. Of course, when reaching maturity a person continues to grow and for many this is a constant source of personal conflict (links with health promotion and obesity/eating disorders). In biological terms, growth refers to the increase in the number of cells and the resulting increase in the size of the whole or parts of the whole. This is perhaps best illustrated at the time of conception when individual life commences with the joining of a male sex cell and one female sex cell – and from this physiological event to implantation in the uterus. The fertilised zygote represents a new single-celled individual and the process of mitosis (division) and growth begins. Distinction should be made between the development of organs and development of skills and this will be examined in more depth later.

The prenatal period (pregnancy), which usually lasts approximately 40 weeks (around 9 months), is usually divided into three trimesters of around 3 months. Several terms are used but generally the term zygote describes the fertilised egg, which constantly divides and at around day 3 when the term morula is used (see Figure 2.1). Continual development transforms this into a hollow blastocyst, which implants into the wall of the uterus. From about the third week after fertilisation until the end of week eight the term embryo is used to be replaced by foetus from week nine to birth. There is some contention about the use of terms and some organisations choose to use the term baby to describe the unborn child (links with cultural aspects).

Measurement of Growth

Growth is critical at all stages of life, from the point of conception through to old age, and it is important that growth, lack of growth or too much growth is measured. Accurate measurement of weight is critical in paediatric care for the administration of medicines and fluids; measurement of height can be critical in assessing the growth of children and head circumference measurement can be important in identifying consequences of birth trauma.

The Child Growth Foundation (**www.childgrowthfoundation.org/default.htm**) recommends a programme of weight, height and occipital frontal circumference (OFC) measurement. Figures 2.2, 2.3, 2.4, 2.5 and 2.6 and Table 2.1 will give you an idea of some of the measuring devices used but this does not provide an alternative to 'hands-on' experience.

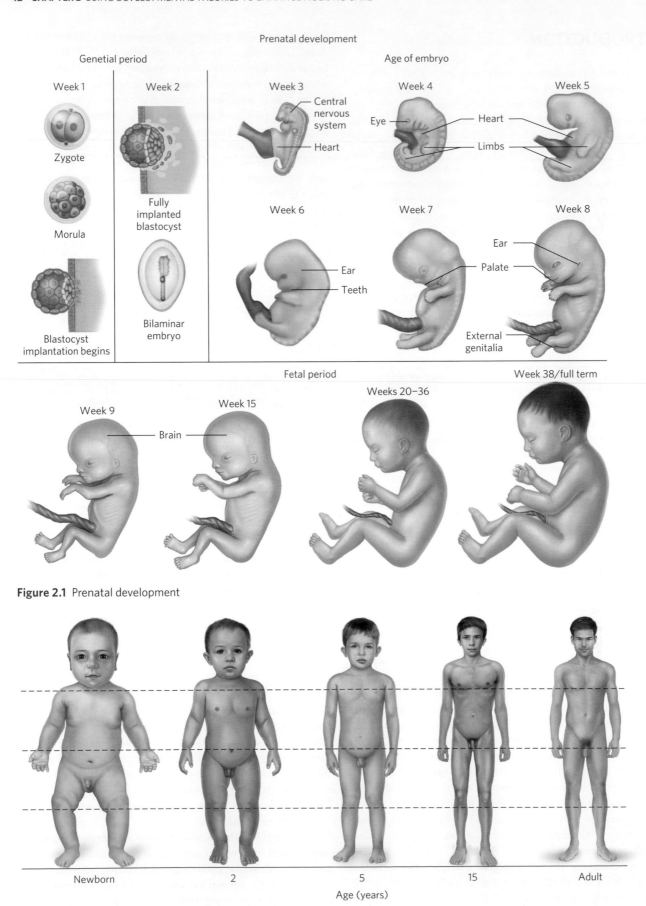

Figure 2.1 Prenatal development

Figure 2.2 Physical growth over time

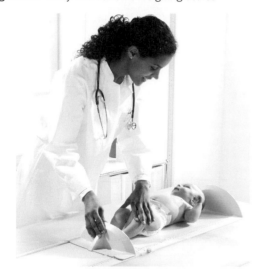

Figure 2.3 Baby in electronic weighing scales

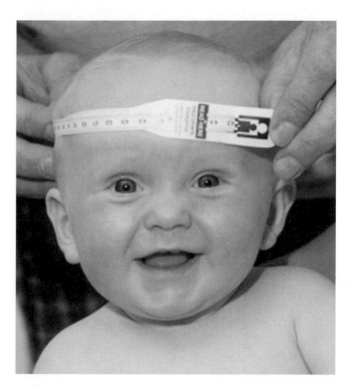

Figure 2.6 Use of the Lasso-o head circumference measuring tape

Figure 2.4 Estimating or measuring length/height

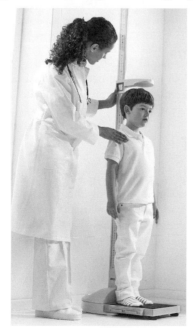

Figure 2.5 Child height measurement

Although there is some discussion about the validity of estimating body mass index (BMI) in children, it is still among one of the recommendations that is made. It is important that the BMI is not considered in isolation from other factors. The National Obesity Observatory (NOO) provide a guide for assessing BMI in children (available at **www.noo.org.uk/.../vid_11601**).

Following estimation of growth, measurements are entered in the personal child health record (PCHR) of the child. Within the PCHR, there are growth charts for boys and girls that are reproduced from World Health Organization (WHO) data sets (see Figure 2.7). The current growth chart was updated in 2009 to account for new data which were specifically related to breastfed babies.

ACTIVITY 2.1

Why is it important to have two different charts, one for boys and one for girls?

Pregnancy

Growth is measured throughout pregnancy by estimation of foetal size; midwives and obstetricians are trained to estimate through clinical examination. More accurate estimation of size is made by ultrasound, which can also be used to make prenatal diagnosis of congenital conditions that may affect the foetus. Hannah would have been monitored throughout her pregnancy and any concerns would have been investigated further.

Table 2.1 When should growth be monitored?

Years	Contact	Age	Weight	OFC	Length/Height	BMI
0–1	1	Birth	X		X [or 10 days]	
		24/30 hours		X		
	2 and 3	5 days and 10 days	XX			
	4	14 days		X		
	6	6–8 weeks	X	X	X	
	7	12 weeks	X			
	8	16 weeks	X			
	9	6–8 months	X		X	
	10	12–15 months	X		X	X
1–5		2 years	X		X	X
		3 years	X		X	X
		4 years	X		X	X
		Primary school				
5+		Reception	X		X	X
		Year 6	X		X	X
		Other years				
		Secondary school				
		Optional				
			X		X	X

Source: adapted from **http://www.childgrowthfoundation.org**

Infancy to Two Years

The neonate is measured at birth, usually weight and head circumferences are recorded. The health child programme suggests that infants are weighed without clothes or nappies until 2 years of age; scales should be accurate and the weight plotted on latest growth charts (see Figure 2.7). It is important that careful explanation of the relevance of growth charts is given to Hannah and Chris as parents to Thomas and Isaac as the charts can be a cause of anxiety. Height is measured as necessary and has become a less reliable measure of infant and child health. Growth is more rapid in the first year of life.

Two to Five Years

Growth of Thomas and Isaac may be monitored if there is concerns about the children's weight and parental concerns should be taken seriously. Children are usually measured at school entry.

Five Years Onwards

Throughout school, growth is not routinely monitored unless concerns are raised by parents or school and health staff.

DEVELOPMENT

Development is measured in practice using a number of tools, the most commonly used measure being that developed by Mary Sheridan (2008). Development is looked at most carefully in the first five years and health visitors have been central to the delivery of the healthy child programme (Chapter X).

Four major areas of development are assessed:

- gross motor
- fine motor
- speech and language
- social skills

EXISTING AND NEW GROWTH CHARTS COMPARED

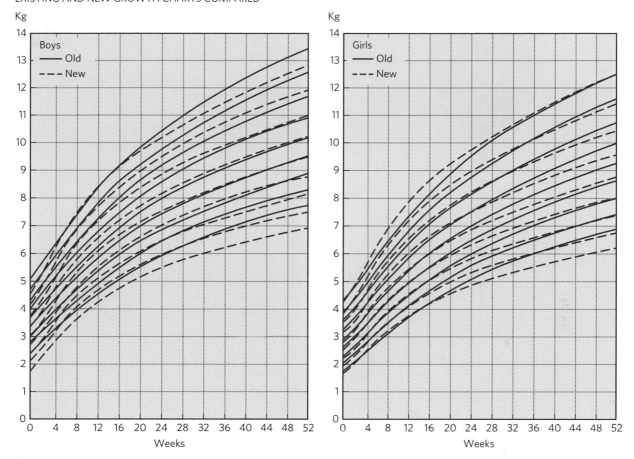

Figure 2.7 Child growth charts

Generally, professionals in primary healthcare will assess whether a child has reached her *developmental milestones* at a particular age.

Developmental Milestones

There are a number of tools available for assessing development and there are also a wide variety of resources available to parents and professionals. The NHS has recently produced a web-based resource for new parents (**www.nhs.uk/parents**), which provides information about what to expect from birth onwards. The website contains videos and text-based resources and also an interactive approach using text messaging linked to the baby's age. A timeline is given, which is closely linked to the healthy child programme (HCP) and gives parents the major developmental milestones.

HISTORICAL PERSPECTIVES

What is the point of looking back at historical perspectives of childhood? The whole area of childhood will be looked at in far more detail elsewhere but a brief introduction to the concept of childhood helps in understanding how the early theorists viewed childhood and children.

Aries (1962) argued that in the past children were seen as small adults and uses examples from the Middle Ages when children were sent, as young as 6 and 7 years old, to learn a trade and even in art were depicted as being of adult proportions and dressed in adult clothing. This has been argued against by writers such as Shahar (1990), Orme (2001) and Ozment (2001) who comment that parents viewed each of their children as unique. Until the invention of the microscope, the sperm was believed to contain a fully formed human being: this was known as the Homunculus (see Figure 2.8).

Two early writers on children, John Locke and Jean-Jacques Rousseau provided contrasting views of children. Locke proposed that children were born as a blank slate, that the mind should be viewed as a *tabula* rasa, which was written on with experience and thus the child developed. Rousseau countered this by suggesting that the child grew according to a plan whereby they developed different capacities at different ages. The two views led to different approaches to the education of children, with Locke declaring that required behaviour should be rewarded and he was opposed to any form of physical punishment. Rousseau proposed a child-centred education whereby the child's interests took precedence, removing harmful objects so the child could be allowed to explore and learn to think for themselves.

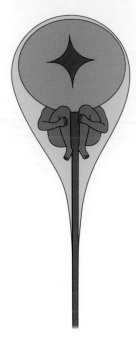

Figure 2.8 Homunculus

Charles Darwin observed his son, William for the first year of his life and published what was to become known as the *Baby biography*. Due to Darwin's prominence, he was taken seriously and contained within the 'biography' are Darwin's observations of his son's development in terms of social, emotional and linguistic levels. Although Darwin's theories are contentious, there is no doubt that this form of observation is fundamental to child development theory.

G. (Granville) Stanley Hall specifically identified adolescence as a time of 'storm and stress' and although this is the subject of some debate, it did bring the adolescent period to the forefront of people's minds. Gesell, one of Hall's students, developed maturation theory, by which he meant the biologically determined natural order of growth. Gesell echoed the theories of Rousseau in that he believed that without any outside interference the child would develop through an inbuilt process of maturation.

Development is described as being:

cephalocaudal: a child gains control of the head and neck before the trunk and limbs

proximodistal: arm movements are controlled before hands

general to specific: this simply means that there is a progression from crawling and walking before skipping.

This view of the lifespan shows that there has been an understanding of stages of development since Shakespeare and very probably before that. Although there is only the distinction between the infant and the child before reaching adolescence, this does provide us with a starting point. As shall be demonstrated, development is viewed from a descriptive, normative approach, with developmental theorists describing what they see and putting forward theories as to what is happening. The seven ages of man described by Shakespeare seem to reflect the theories of Freud, Erikson and Piaget, although

VOICES 2.1

As You Like It, Act II, scene vii

All the world's a stage, and all the men and women merely players: They have their exits and their entrances; And one man in his time plays many parts,

His acts being seven ages. At first the infant,

Mewling and puking in the nurse's arms. And then the whining school-boy, with his satchel

And shining morning face, creeping like snail

Unwillingly to school. And then the lover,

Sighing like furnace, with a woeful ballad

Made to his mistress' eyebrow. Then a soldier,

Full of strange oaths and bearded like the pard,

Jealous in honour, sudden and quick in quarrel,

Seeking the bubble reputation

Even in the cannon's mouth. And then the justice,

In fair round belly with good capon lined,

With eyes severe and beard of formal cut,

Full of wise saws and modern instances;

And so he plays his part. The sixth age shifts

Into the lean and slipper'd pantaloon,

With spectacles on nose and pouch on side,

His youthful hose, well saved, a world too wide

For his shrunk shank; and his big manly voice,

Turning again toward childish treble, pipes

And whistles in his sound. Last scene of all,

That ends this strange eventful history,

Is second childishness and mere oblivion,

Sans teeth, sans eyes, sans taste, sans everything.

they do provide far more explanation of their theories (and of course, Shakespeare was not putting forward a theory of development).

THEORIES OF DEVELOPMENT

Theories of development can be considered in a number of ways but broadly they fall into biological and cultural (or social) theories of development. Quite simply the nature vs. nurture debate (see Ridley 2004 for a full discussion on this subject). It is not in the scope of this chapter to provide an answer (not that there is one) but to sow the seeds of debate and to give the reader the opportunity to ask questions and also to begin to look at the manner in which the major theorists arrived at their conclusions.

In addition, a number of developmental theorists will be explored; it is important to note that these theorists will appear in relation to a number of other disciplines such as learning theory in the case of Vygotsky and psychoanalytic theory with Freud. Many of the theorists appear to 'borrow' or develop ideas from one another and it should be remembered that much of the theory is developed from observation and, although a number of experimental studies do exist, the variables are such that generalisations become difficult. One point that is important to bear in mind is that all the theorists have observed child development and all contribute to an understanding of what may have influenced the child. Perhaps the biggest mistake would be to subscribe to one theory alone as 'the' answer (see Tables 2.2 and 2.3).

Jean Piaget (1896–1980)

Jean Piaget was a Swiss developmental psychologist who is regarded as one of the most influential developmental theorists and many will be aware of his theories, whether or not a study of child development has been made (see Figure 2.9). Piaget's theory is described as a 'stage theory' as he describes stages that the child goes through – the role of 'maturation' figures strongly in this and the work of other cognitive theorists. Children are active learners who construct their own understanding of the world and, according to Piaget, pass through each of four stages in order, each of which correspond to changes in their understanding of the world around them. The four stages are **sensorimotor, pre-operational, concrete operational and formal operational**. The length of each stage may differ but Piaget stressed that each stage is passed through in this order.

Piaget used a term for the mental operations or structures that the child uses to apply to objects, beliefs, ideas and anything within the child's world – he referred to this as a **schema**.

Schemas are evolving structures that progress through the stages. Piaget developed this concept further by describing the **organisation** of schemas and their **adaptation** through **assimilation** and **accommodation**. It is not within the scope of this chapter to describe these in detail but an overview of the stages is given in Table 2.4: a number of texts are also referred to and should be consulted to gain more information about Piaget and the other theorists discussed here.

Critics of Jean Piaget state that there is weakness in his theory as much of his observation was carried out using his own children.

Sigmund Freud (1856–1939)

Sigmund Freud is equally venerated and berated but it cannot be denied that he is perhaps one of the most referred to of all psychotherapists, and his contribution to the study of child development and understanding of later difficulties cannot be underestimated. The term 'Freudian slip' is part of many people's vocabulary, although it is not always clear that it is fully understood.

Freud was born in Freiburg and was the first of eight children from his father's second marriage. He studied medicine in Vienna and his original interest was in histology and neurophysiology; he wanted to be a scientist rather than a doctor of medicine. He was given the opportunity to study under Charcot, a French neurologist, during which time he was exposed to fairly unorthodox ideas about hysteria (among other mental health disorders). This became the source of debate between Freud and Charcot, with Freud arguing that hysteria could be psychological in nature and Charcot putting forward a physiological cause. Freud continued to be heavily influenced by the ideas of Charcot. Freud proposed a psychosexual theory of development in response to the treatment

Table 2.2 Fields of child development

Theory	Broad definition	Major theorists
Psychoanalytic theory	Freud believed that behaviour (personality) was influenced by childhood experiences and unconscious desires	Freud Erikson
Cognitive theory	Looks at the way children think and solve problems – thus moving on to solve more complex and difficult problems	Piaget
Behavioural theory	Focuses on the external forces that influence the child's development	Skinner Pavlov Watson
Sociocultural theory	Looks at the settings in which development takes place; the environment is seen as the main driver in the child's development	Bowlby Bandura Vygotsky Bronfenbrenner

Table 2.3 Major developmental theorists

Developmental theorists	Brief overview of theory
Piaget	Piaget is noted for cognitive–developmental theory where the child is an active learner and constructs his/her own understanding of the world
Erikson	Was a follower of Freud and constructed his 'psychosocial theory', where the child needs to successfully negotiate stages where conflicts arise before moving on to the next stage
Vygotsky	Emphasised the influence of older more experienced members of a culture who were able to help children learn – developed the zone of proximal learning (ZPL)
Freud	Developed psychoanalytic theory but described development as being in stages where pleasure is concentrated on a particular part of the body
Bronfenbrenner	Developed ecological systems theory where the importance of different environments on the child's development is stressed
Kohlberg	Developed a theory of moral development by posing a series of moral dilemmas to children at different ages
Gesell	Gesell followed the works of Darwin and contended that the child's development was determined by biological or genetic factors in a predictable manner
Bandura	Bandura's social learning theory suggests that children and people learn from each other and development is by observation, imitation and modelling. It is suggested that his theory bridges the gap between cognitive and behaviourist approaches
Pavlov	Pavlov was researching into the physiology of the digestive system but developed the theory of classical conditioning, learning and development by means of a conditioned response
Skinner	Skinner built on the work of Pavlov and suggested that learning takes place by another form of response, which he termed operant conditioning

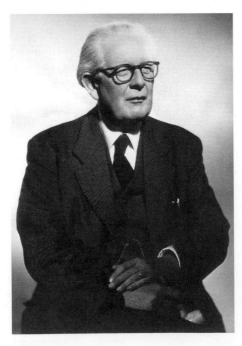

Figure 2.9 Piaget

of patients with phobias and linked these (put in a simplistic way) to the suppression of innate inborn sexual drives. Freud's contention is that all development is linked in some way to sexual development, hence, his theory of psychosexual development.

Development, according to Freud, is expressed in five stages: oral, anal, phallic, latency and genital; he also proposed that each stage had an erogenous zone related to it. Alongside this, Freud identified three facets of personality: the id, ego and superego (see Table 2.5).

In arguing that there were five stages in personality development, Freud caused controversy among his peers and early and perhaps later criticism is that he avoided experimental approaches to his work, somewhat surprising considering his early career. It is important to note that Freud did not set out to describe child and personality development but was interested in psychological explanations for phobias and the treatment of patients. Josef Breuer (1842–1925) described the case of Anna O, who presented with symptoms of a severe nervous cough, squint, visual disturbances and paralysis of the right

Table 2.4 Stages of cognitive development according to Piaget

Stage	Approximate age (years)	Characteristics
Sensorimotor	0–2	The infant knows about the world through actions and sensory information Infants learn to differentiate themselves from the environment Begin to learn causality in time and space and develop the ability to form internal mental representations
Preoperational	2–7	Through the symbolic use of language and intuitive problem solving the child begins to understand about classification of objects But thinking is characterised by geocentricism, children focus on just one aspect of a task and lack operations like compensation and reversibility By the end of this stage, children can take another's perspective and can understand the conservation of number
Concrete operational	7–12	Children understand conservation of mass, length, weight and volume, and can more easily take the perspective of others; can classify and order, as well as organise objects into series The child is still tied to the immediate experience, but within these limitations can perform logical mental operations
Formal operational	12+	Abstract reasoning begins Children can now manipulate ideas; can speculate about the possible; can reason deductively, and formulate and test hypotheses

Source: Smith et al. (2003)

Table 2.5 Facets of personality proposed by Freud

Facet	Characteristics
Id	This is identified as the inherited component which is biologically influenced and demands immediate satisfaction of need
Ego	The ego is influenced by the environment and is emerging. It regulates the id's desire for immediate gratification and acts as a social stabiliser
Superego	Often referred to as the 'policeman' and acts as the 'conscience' – may often be in conflict with the desires of the id

arm and neck. She also had a speech problem which meant she could understand when spoken to in German but often replied in English; she was also subject to hallucinations. Anna was a 21-year-old woman who had a very strict upbringing; the symptoms started when her father became seriously ill. Breuer used what he termed the cathartic method to treat Anna, whereby he traced symptoms back to where they first began. Although at the time Freud did not seem impressed with this method, it was to have a profound influence on his theory. He persuaded Breuer to collaborate on a book, *Studies in hysteria*, which was published in 1895.

Freudian psychoanalysis suggests that by understanding early childhood experiences and unconscious thoughts, the analyst can help the subject to deal with neuroses and other psychological difficulties. The stages according to Freud explain time's development when particular aspects of personality are prevalent; the stages are briefly described in Table 2.6.

What is the relevance of an understanding of Freud's psychosexual stages for nursing children and young people? Rather than trying to apply the theory directly, as was mentioned earlier, an understanding of the various theories allows the nurse both to question care of children and also leads to a deeper

Table 2.6 Freud's psychosexual stages

Stage	Age	Description
Oral	Birth to one year	The first year in life, according to Freud, is where pleasure is centred on the mouth and feeding
Anal	1–3	In the second stage of development, pleasure is centred around the anal region of the body
Phallic	3–6	Between the ages of 3 and 6, Freud asserts, pleasure is centred on the genital region
Latency	Six to puberty	In this stage of the theory of psychosexual development occurring during middle childhood, pleasure and energy are directed outside the body
Genital	Puberty onwards	In Freud's final stage of psychosexual development, pleasure is again focused on the genitals and genital stimulation such as in sexual intercourse

Source: Patterson (2008)

understanding of the mind of the child. There is no 'one-size-fits-all' approach to child development and, taken together, all theories add to a body of knowledge.

Erik Erikson (1902–1994)

Erik Erikson was born in Germany but spent most of his life and academic career in the United States of America (see Figure 2.10). He had a background in psychoanalysis and developed a theory of development; it differs from Piaget in that his theory covers the lifespan. He agreed with Freud about innate ability but he attributed

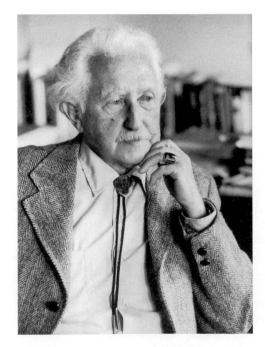

Figure 2.10 Erikson

a much greater role to cultural and environmental influences on personality development (see Figure 2.11). Erikson described eight stages of development and these are characterised by conflicts within each stage – each stage must be successfully negotiated before progressing to the following stage. Erikson's theory is referred to as a psychosocial theory.

Although the stages are referred to as conflicts or crises, Erikson considers each stage to be a task to be successfully negotiated. As in the first stage, Erikson places trust against mistrust, the infant depends on the caregiver for the basic needs of food, warmth and comfort. Although not always immediately responsive or timely, the needs of the infant are addressed, if not, the infant will become distrustful of the caregiver and others and will become withdrawn. If the infant is responded to and has an environment of trust, he will be more responsive and be willing to meet new situations. It was Erikson's contention that successful resolution of each conflict or crisis will lead to appropriate development, with the child and later adult being well balanced and well equipped to deal with whatever life has to offer (see Table 2.7).

Unlike Piaget, Erikson studied many different cultures and was able to compare his theory in different cultural contexts. Erikson offered perhaps his greatest insights into adolescence when he describes the important task of the search for identity (identity vs. role confusion).

Lev Vygotsky (1896–1934)

Lev Vygotsky was born and worked in Russia, significantly at the time of the Russian Revolution (1917) and is credited with developing a psychosocial theory of child development (see Figure 2.12). Understandably, Vygotsky stressed the importance of the culture and social group to which the child was exposed. In contrast to Piaget, who saw children as solitary or independent learners, Vygotsky saw development as a social process in which cultural groups identify tasks for learning.

Erikson's stages of personality development

Stage	1	2	3	4	5	6	7	8
Oral	Basic trust vs. mistrust							
Anal		Autonomy vs. shame, doubt						
Phallic			Initiative vs. guilt					
Latency				Industry vs. inferiority				
Genital					Identity vs. role confusion			
Young adulthood						Intimacy vs. isolation		
Adulthood							Generativity vs. stagnation	
Maturity								Ego integrity vs. despair

Freud's stages of personality development

Figure 2.11 Comparison of Freud's and Erikson's stages of development

Table 2.7 Erikson's eight developmental stages

Normative crisis	Age	Major characteristics
Trust vs. mistrust	0–1	Primary social interaction with mothering caretaker; oral concerns; trust in life-sustaining care, including feeding
Autonomy vs. doubt and shame	1–2	Primary social interaction with parents; toilet training; 'holding on' and 'letting go' and the beginnings of autonomous will
Initiative vs. guilt	3–5	Primary social interaction with nuclear family; beginnings of 'Oedipal' feelings; development of language and locomotion; development of conscience as governor of initiative
Industry vs. inferiority	6 to puberty	Primary social interaction outside home among peers and teachers; school age assessment of task ability
Identity vs. role confusion	Adolescence	Primary social interaction with peers, culminating in heterosexual friendship; psychological moratorium from adult commitments; identity crisis; consolidation of resolutions of previous four stages into current sense of self
Intimacy vs. isolation	Early adulthood	Primary social interaction in intimate relationship with member of opposite sex; adult role commitments accepted, including commitment to another person
Generativity vs. stagnation	Middle age	Primary social concern in establishing and guiding future generation; productivity and creativity
Integrity vs. despair	Old age	Primary social concern is a reflective one: coming to terms with one's place in the (now nearly complete) lifecycle and with one's relationship with others; 'I am what survives of me'

Source: Smith et al. (2003)

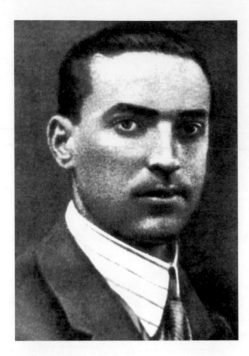

Figure 2.12 Vygotsky

Vygotsky emphasised the importance of learning from more experienced peers and adults. He described the zone of proximal development (ZPD) where tasks that cannot yet be performed independently are attained with the help of more experienced adults. Another concept that he proposed was that of 'scaffolding' where adults provide the right amount of help to enable children to succeed; the important aspect here is that the *right amount* of help is given. Too much and the child does not learn, too little has the same result.

One area of Vygotsky's research that is perhaps less well known is related to children's play. He stated that cognitive development is facilitated by children's play; not only do they play what they know but learn new things through play. He asserted that when children play, they are operating in the ZPD and again he differs to Piaget in that he suggests that they are operating within the next level of development rather than reflecting their present stage (Kalliala 2008).

Ivan Pavlov (1849–1936)

Pavlov was a Russian physiologist who was awarded the Nobel Prize for medicine for his doctoral thesis on the centrifugal nerves of the heart in 1904. His main area of research for most of his life was the digestive process and it was this work which led to his major contributions to the field of developmental psychology. It was while investigating the digestive process that Pavlov described classical conditioning. He knew that when food was placed in the mouth of a dog, it salivated, an involuntary response. He later noted that at the sight of food, the dog began to salivate. What had begun as a reflexive behaviour, salivating at the taste of food, had become responsive to new

conditions, the sight of food, and as Pavlov noted, to the sound of footsteps bringing food. This was the starting point for Pavlov's experiments. He began pairing something that naturally gave a particular response with something to which the animal showed a neutral response.

In one experiment, he placed the dog in a dark room and turned on a light; after less than a minute the dog was given food and the process was repeated many times. Eventually the dog would salivate as soon as the light was turned on. The food was referred to by Pavlov as the *unconditioned stimulus* (as it usually made the dog salivate) and the light as a *conditioned stimulus*, as the dog responded to it as it would to food. The dog salivating in response to food is termed the *unconditioned response* (as this would normally happen) and the dog salivating to light he called the *conditioned response*. This is the basis of classical conditioning.

John B. Watson (1878–1958)

The behaviourist theorists maintained that rather than focus on internal processes the external should be concentrated on. Among the foremost of the behaviourists was John Broadus Watson who considered children to be pliant and famously said:

> Give me a dozen healthy infants, well-formed, and my own specified world to bring them up in, and I'll guarantee to take any one at random and train him to become any type of specialist I might select, doctor, lawyer, artist, merchant chief, and yes, even beggar-man and thief, regardless of his talents, penchants, tendencies, abilities, vocations, and race of his ancestors.
> (Watson 1924, page 82)

Watson was keen to develop the work of Pavlov in order to demonstrate that infants learned through classical conditioning. His well-known, and now unethical, experiment with Little Albert and the rat goes some way to demonstrating this. Little Albert was presented with a white rat to which he showed no alarm; however, over time at the same time as being presented with the rat, a loud noise was created nearby. After repeating the experiment several times, Albert began to show alarm, until he showed alarm at the sight of the rat without the noise. It was subsequently noted that Little Albert showed alarm at other white furry objects such as a rabbit and a fur coat.

Burrhus Frederick Skinner (1904–1990)

Among behaviourists, Skinner is perhaps one of the most famous and he developed the theory of *operant conditioning*. He postulated that an animal or a person will repeat certain behaviours that are followed by favourable rewards; if the rewards are not favourable then those behaviours will be avoided. Skinner referred to the process of giving rewards as *reinforcement* and it was his contention that humans learned to carry out many everyday behaviours through continual reinforcement.

Urie Bronfenbrenner (1917–2005)

Bronfenbrenner developed what is known as the ecological systems theory of development. He saw the child's development as unfolding within a complex system of relationships with the child in the centre of multiple environments. Not only are those systems diverse, they are also related in a number of ways. The value of Bronfenbrenner's work is that he describes a model in which children are influenced at various levels. The model is often shown as a series of concentric circles with the child at the centre. Moving outwards, he describes first the microsystem which includes the family, school, peers and so on. The mesosystem comprises of connections between the various organisations within the microsystem, the interactions between people at home, school and neighbours that will all have an effect on the child. Bronfenbrenner describes an exosystem that includes those settings that, although not inhabited by the child, do have an effect, for example, mass media, family friends and neighbourhood services. These are areas that, although not directly associated with the child, do have an effect on the lives of children. Finally, Bronfenbrenner describes the macrosystem, which can be seen as the cultural aspects of the child, social class and ethnicity that will have an effect on the child (see Figure 2.13).

Bronfenbrenner also described how time has an effect on the development of the child; he termed this the chronosystem, recognising that there are changes as the child grows older and the historical aspects of time such as the influence of war or natural disasters.

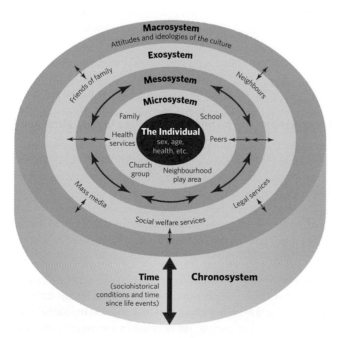

Figure 2.13 Bronfenbrenner's ecological model of development

LANGUAGE ACQUISITION

Many theorists have attempted to explain how children acquire language, especially the exponential growth of language in the early years. The theoretical approaches include behaviourist, nativist and social interactional; these will be introduced and further discussion encouraged by suggested reading.

B. F. Skinner (1904–1990)

Skinner falls into the behaviourist group of theorists and argued that children acquire language in much the same way that they learn other behaviours. He suggested that children learn labels for objects and, through repeated pairing of the object with the label, learn language.

Noam Chomsky (1928–present)

Unlike Skinner, Chomsky focused on the innate or inborn capacity rather than the process of learning language (the nativist theory of language acquisition). He argued that humans are born with an understanding of the fundamental structure of language. He termed this the language acquisition device (LAD), which is a set of mental capacities within the human brain. He proposed that infants are born with a set of universal rules – which he called universal grammar – allowing children from all language backgrounds to develop language skills. Put simply, the words may be different but the rules are constant. It is important to remember that he did not suggest that words were innate, only the rules – the grammar.

Social Interactionist Viewpoint

From this point of view, language is seen as essential for communication and social interaction and language is seen from the cultural as well as from the local conventions that may affect language acquisition. There are many who argue against this position although most researchers do agree that the acquisition of language is probably affected by both innate ability and environmental factors – nature vs. nurture.

Michael Halliday (1925–present)

Halliday suggested the child's language acquisition has seven stages with functions attached to each stage (see Table 2.8).

MORAL DEVELOPMENT

It has been suggested that the development of *moral reasoning* is closely associated with cognitive development. Piaget studied children's moral development by posing simple stories and asking them to tell him which child had been naughtier:

A little boy who is called John is in his room. He is called to dinner. He goes into the dining room. But behind the door

Table 2.8 Halliday's stages of language acquisition

Stage	Function
The first four stages help the child satisfy his/her physical, emotional and social needs	
Instrumental	The child uses language to express needs and get what she wants
	Her first words are mainly concrete nouns, e.g. want drink
Regulatory	Language is used to tell others what to do
	The child realises that language is a useful tool and by using language he can get what he wants, e.g. go away
Interactional	Language is used to communicate with other people and form a relationship
	The child begins to realise that language goes beyond what is needed, e.g. love you, daddy, thank you
Personal	When the child uses language that expresses feelings and opinions
	She realises that language is more than demanding and can be praised for using language, e.g. me good girl
The next two stages help the child come to terms with the environment	
Heuristic	This is when language is used to gain information about the environment and the world
	The child begins to question everything and is always seeking an answer, e.g. what that tractor doing?
Imaginative	Language is used to tell stories and to create an imaginary situation
	The child is able to recognise that an object can be called many things, e.g. creating an imaginary friend
The last stage is the representational stage when the child uses language to convey facts and information	
Informative	The child uses language to talk about brand new things
	They learn to represent themselves using language, e.g. telling a story about what has happened to them

Source: adapted from **http://www.thestudentroom.co.uk/wiki/Revision**

there was a chair, and on the chair there was a tray with fifteen cups on it. John couldn't have known that the chair was behind the door. He goes in, the door knocks against the tray; bang go the fifteen cups, and they all get broken!

Once there was a little boy whose name was Henry. One day when his mother was out he tried to get some jam out of the cupboard. He climbed up onto a chair and stretched out his arm. But the jam was too high up and he couldn't reach it and have any. But while he was trying to get it he knocked over a cup. The cup fell down and broke. (Piaget 1932/1925, page 122) (from Patterson 2008)

When asked about these two stories, younger children generally said that John was the naughtier child as he broke more cups. Older children chose Henry as he broke the cup through an act that was felt to be 'naughtier'. From this, Piaget concluded that there were two kinds of moral reasoning, *morality of constraint* and *autonomous morality* – the former shown by preschool children and the latter by school age children.

Perhaps the most widely recognised theory of moral development is that proposed by Lawrence Kohlberg (1927–1987) who developed the ideas of Piaget. It is suggested that Kohlberg developed his interest in moral development when working on freighters following the Second World War. He was involved in smuggling Jewish refugees through British blockades into what we now know as Israel – placing him in situations where he would be facing real life *moral dilemmas*.

Kohlberg approached his study of moral development in children by interviewing children about their reactions to moral dilemmas. Perhaps the most widely recognised of these is the story of 'Heinz and the drug':

In Europe, a woman was near death from a special kind of cancer. There was one drug that the doctors thought might save her. It was a form of radium that a druggist in the same town had recently discovered. The drug was expensive to make, but the druggist was charging ten times what the drug cost him to make. He paid $200 for the radium and charged $2000 for a small dose of the drug. The sick woman's husband, Heinz, went to everyone he knew to borrow the money, but he could only get together about $1000, which is half of what it cost. He told the druggist that his wife was dying and asked him to sell it cheaper or let him pay later. But the druggist said 'No, I discovered the drug and I'm going to make money from it.' So Heinz got desperate and broke into the man's store to steal the drug for his wife.

Should the husband have done that? (Kohlberg 1963, page 19)

Kohlberg studied a group of boys aged between 10 and 16 and asked the boys to give an answer to Kohlberg's question and, not only that, he asked the boys their reasons for their answers. He was not really interested if the boys thought Heinz should steal the drug or not – it was their *reason* for their answer. From

this, he was able to put forward a theory of moral development, which, in common with that of Piaget and of Erikson described development in stages (see Table 2.9).

PLAY THEORY

The theoretical perspectives of play and the importance of play in the way children develop and learn have been described since the late 19th and early 20th century. There are a number of important figures who have been involved and a brief overview will be provided; it is recommended that the student takes a deeper look into this subject as the role of play in the nursing care of children and young people cannot be understated.

Table 2.9 Kohlberg's stages of moral development

Level	Stage	What is right
Pre-conventional	**Stage 1:** heteronomous morality	To avoid breaking rules backed by punishment, obedience for his/her own sake, avoiding physical damage to persons and property
	Stage 2: individualism, instrumental purpose, and exchange	Following rules only when it is to someone's immediate interest; acting to meet one's own interests and needs, and letting others do the same Right is what's fair, an equal exchange, a deal, an agreement
Conventional	**Stage 3:** mutual interpersonal expectations, relationships and interpersonal conformity	Living up to what is expected by people close to you or what people generally expect of people in your role 'Being good' is important and means having good motives, showing concern about others and keeping mutual relationships, such as trust, loyalty, respect and gratitude
	Stage 4: social system and conscience	Fulfilling the actual duties to which you have agreed Laws are to be upheld except in extreme cases where they conflict with other fixed social duties Right is contributing to society, the group or institution
Post-conventional or principled	**Stage 5:** social contract or utility and individual rights	Being aware that people hold a variety of values and opinions, that most values and rules are relative to your group but should usually be upheld in the interest of impartiality and because that is the social contract Some non-relative values and rights like life and liberty, however, must be upheld in any society and regardless of the majority opinion
	Stage 6: (hypothetical) universal ethical principles	Following self-chosen ethical principles Particular laws or social agreements are usually valid because they rest on such principles. When laws violate these principles, one acts in accordance with the principle Principles are universal principles of justice: the equality of human rights and the respect for the dignity of human beings as individual persons

Source: Smith et al. (2003)

Table 2.10 Major theorists in relation to play

Theorist	Contribution
Friedrich Froebel (1782–1852)	Froebel is recognised for his insights into the importance of early education on the child's later educational achievement
	He is famous for developing the 'kindergarten' movement, which literally translated means 'child garden'
	He focused on the importance of play from within the child and the careful provision of support from outside
Herbert Spencer (1820–1903)	Spencer saw play as the use of 'surplus energy'
	In his view, when the immediate necessities of life have been met, the nervous system, rather than remaining inactive, stimulates play
	His approach has been termed a 'surplus energy' theory
Karl Groos (1861–1946)	Groos was a critic of Spencer in that, although he agreed that surplus energy might provide a favourable condition for play, he thought that play had a more definite function than the mere use of excess energy
	He observed that play provided exercise and the development of the skills needed for survival. This has become known as an 'exercise' or 'practice' theory of play
G. Stanley Hall (1844–1924)	Hall argued against Groos's theory and suggested that play was an outworking of our primitive or evolutionary past
	He stated that the function of play was cathartic in nature, allowing the playing out of instincts from earlier human history
	This became known as a 'recapitulation' theory and received very little support
Maria Montessori (1870–1952)	Montessori saw the value of self-activated activity in young children under the guidance of adults
	She saw the importance of acting out real life by providing appropriate materials
Jean Piaget (1896–1980)	Piaget saw play as a reinforcing and consolidation of existing skills. Within Piaget's theory this would be described as relating the processes of accommodation and assimilation
Sigmund Freud (1856–1939)	Although Freud did not write much on the subject of play, it has become very much part of the 'psychoanalytic' movement with 'play therapy'
	Play has been seen as a safe place in which to work through anxieties, fears and traumatic events
Susan Isaacs (1885–1948)	Isaacs held the view that play was essential to the emotional and cognitive growth of the child
	This was combined with a belief in the emotional benefits of play that is contained within the psychoanalytic tradition
	She felt that active play was a sign of positive mental health
Lev Vygotsky (1896–1934)	Vygotsky saw play as a chance for the child to liberate herself from her immediate situation and thereby lead to development. This was especially so in the preschool years
Jerome Bruner (1915–present)	Bruner has suggested that play serves as practice for the mastery of skills and serves as an opportunity for trying out new forms of behaviour in a safe context
Brian Sutton-Smith (1924–present)	Sutton-Smith has argued that play occupies an ambiguous position and that play is organised by adults as a way of controlling children, this is somewhat contrary to many theorists' approaches to play

Source: adapted from Smith et al. (2003)

Table 2.10 summarises a number of past and current play theorists. Of one thing, there is some certainty: play has been part of the child's repertoire for many years. Hugh Cunningham (2006) quotes from Bede's life of St Cuthbert who:

> Loved games and pranks, and as was natural at his age, loved to play with other children . . . He used to boast that he had beaten all those his own age and many who were older at wrestling, jumping, running and every other exercise. (Cunningham 2006, page 42)

PERCEPTUAL DEVELOPMENT

During a trip to the Grand Canyon, Eleanor Gibson wondered if a baby would be scared of the drop in the same way an adult would be. In order to test this theory, she constructed an experiment that would become known as the 'visual cliff' (see Figure 2.14).

The Healthy Child Programme (HCP)

The healthy child programme was introduced in 2009 by the Labour government and updated in 2010 by the coalition government of Conservative and Liberal Democrats. There are two key documents (Department of Health 2009a, 2009b), the first covering pregnancy and the first five years and the second covering the years from 5 to 19. Both documents draw on the work of Hall and Elliman (2006), which sets out recommendations for a universal programme of health and development surveillance. One note of caution at this point: each provider of health services interprets the guidance in a different way and although examples of the implementation can be given, local services will need to be accessed.

A clear message is included in the introduction to the programme that:

> The HCP offers every family a programme of screening tests, immunisations, developmental reviews, and information and guidance to support parenting and healthy choices – all services that children and families need to receive if they are to achieve their optimum health and well-being. (Department of Health 2009a, page 8)

The HCP recommends that developmental assessment and review is carried out at birth, 6 to 8 weeks, 1 year and 2 to 2½ years of age. As mentioned before, the detail and content of the review is given in more detail in the document. Health reviews in the first five years are focused primarily on development and the detection of delay. The focus of health review for school aged children is more focused on surveillance for problems

---

ACTIVITY 2.2

Access a copy of the healthy child programme and consider the scenario of Chris and Hannah. How would differences in the development of Thomas and Isaac be identified?

---

with growth such as obesity and, later on, eating disorders such as anorexia nervosa.

HOW DO THEORIES OF DEVELOPMENT ENHANCE CARE?

Consider some of the developmental theorists who approach the subject of child development from a number of different perspectives. The obvious question to ask at this point is 'so what?' How can the care given as a children and young people's nurse be enhanced by knowledge of child development? Quite simply, this understanding allows the appreciation of the complexity of child and human development. This short introduction has only been able to give an overview of child development.

Within the care context, it is of vital importance to be able to identify where a child is meeting her developmental milestones and, equally important, to be able to identify where she may not. The scenario at the beginning of the chapter has not been referred to until now, for a very good reason. The importance of the parents in identifying where a child may not be developing should not be underestimated. Parents know their children far better than any professional could ever hope to. The role of the healthcare professional is to investigate the concerns that parents may have about their children. This may take seconds when reassuring the parent that there is nothing to be concerned

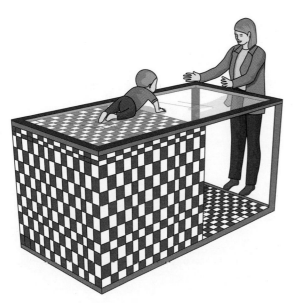

Figure 2.14 The visual cliff

CASE STUDY REVIEW 2.1

Support for Chris and Hannah; actions of the health professional

- It is important to take their concerns seriously and to take a full and clear history.
- The twins were born prematurely and this will have a bearing on the development of both children.

- The use of development assessment tools such as Sheridan (see Table 2.11 for milestones at 6 months) will enable the professional to make an initial assessment.
- Ask yourself whether twins develop at exactly the same rate or whether there are differences in development.

Table 2.11 Progress of infants and young children

Posture and large movements	Lying on back, raises head from pillow
	Lifts legs into vertical and grasps foot
	Sits with support in cot or pram and able to look around him
	Moves arms in brisk and purposeful fashion
	Holds arms up to be lifted
	When hands grasped braces shoulders and pulls himself up
	Kicks strongly, legs alternating
	Can roll over, front to back.
	Held sitting, head is firmly erect and back straight
	May sit alone momentarily
	Placed downwards on face lifts head and chest well up
	Can support himself on extended arms
	Held standing with feet touching hard surface, bears body weight
Vision and fine movements	Visually insatiable: moves head and eyes in every direction
	Eyes move in unison: squint now abnormal
	Follows adult's movements across room
	Immediately fixates interesting small objects within 6–12 inches, e.g. toy, bell, wooden cube, spoon, sweet
	Stretches out both hands to grasp objects
	Uses whole hand in palmar grasp
	When toys fall from hand over edge of cot forgets them
Hearing and speech	Turns immediately to mother's voice across room
	Vocalises tunefully and often, using single and double syllables, e.g. ka, muh, goo, der, adah, er-lah
	Laughs, chuckles and squeals aloud in play
	Screams with annoyance
	Shows evidence of response to emotional tones of mother's voice
	Responds to baby hearing test at one and a half feet from each ear
	Correct visual localisation, but maybe slightly brisker response on one side
	(Tests employed – voice, rattle, cup and spoons, paper, bell)
Social behaviour and play	Hands competent to reach for and grasp small toys
	Most often uses a two-handed, scooping-in approach
	Occasionally uses a single hand
	Takes everything to mouth
	Beginning to find feet interesting and even useful in grasping
	Puts hands to bottle and pats it when feeding
	Shakes rattle deliberately to make it sound, often regards rattle closely at same time
	Still friendly with strangers
	Occasionally shows some shyness if mother is out of sight

Source: adapted from DoH (2000)

SUMMARY OF KEY LEARNING

It is important that we understand how we gain an understanding of what is expected by growth and development. As has been discussed in this chapter, we have access to growth charts that have been established internationally (WHO 2009); the same is broadly true of development. Although there is no easy access to 'development charts', there is a broad recognition of what we call 'milestones'. For instance, the majority of children will walk between the ages of 9 and 18 months. There are examples of children who walk before that age but very few. It is also recognised that a few children are not walking unaided by 18 months – those who are not are generally investigated. A good place to start with an understanding of the major developmental milestones is the text by Mary Sheridan (2008).

The care that is given to children, young people and their families is enhanced by the nurse's having a working knowledge of the development of children and young people. An understanding of the developmental theorists will help the nurse to have a critical awareness of the way in which the child may view the wider world and enable the nurse to care for the child and young person in an appropriate way.

about, and this will reflect the experience and knowledge of the professional. There will also be times when the professional will have to investigate further and make full use of their knowledge and skills.

FURTHER RESOURCES

Healthy child programme

http://www.dh.gov.uk/en/Publicationsandstatistics
/Publications/PublicationsPolicyAndGuidance/
DH_107565

Information on the role of the health visitor: http://www.northeast
.nhs.uk/_assets/media/pdf/Health_visitor_role_-_key
_messages.pdf

The Child Growth Foundation (CGF)

UK's leading charity focusing on children's growth and endocrine issues. On this site, you can find helpful information whether you are a parent whose child has a suspected or diagnosed growth problem, an adult or family member of someone with a growth or endocrine disorder or a medical professional: http://www
.childgrowthfoundation.org/

Mission statement

Infertility Network UK is committed to providing a comprehensive support network to its members and to all those affected by infertility by actively promoting Infertility Network UK services.

As well as providing authoritative information and practical and emotional support, it is Infertility Network UK's mission to raise the profile and understanding of infertility issues in all quarters and to strive for timely and consistent provision of infertility care throughout the UK: http://www.infertilitynetworkuk
.com/?id=14755&gclid=CIrKmYC2-7ACFYzbfAodDT7tfg

Visible Embryo

Visual guide through fetal development from fertilisation through pregnancy to birth. As the most profound physiologic changes occur in the 'first trimester' of pregnancy, these Carnegie stages are given prominence on the birth spiral: http://www.visembryo
.com/baby/

Assessing children in need and their families: practice guidance

This publication is a companion volume to the guidance on the *Framework for the Assessment of Children in Need and their Families*. It is a significant contribution to a major programme of work led by the Department of Health to provide guidance, practice materials and training resources on assessing children in need and their families. This is to assist in the achievement of one of the government's key policy objectives in children's services, delivered through the Quality Protects programme, to ensure that referral and assessment processes discriminate effectively between different types and level of need, and produce a timely response. The focus is the Sheridan framework to assess child development: http://www.crin.org/docs/assessing%20
children%20in%20need%20and%20their%20families-%20
practice%20guid.pdf

Child development

As the flagship journal of the Society for Research in Child Development (SRCD), *Child Development* has published articles, essays, reviews and tutorials on various topics in the field of child development since 1930. Spanning many disciplines, the journal provides the latest research, not only for researchers and theoreticians, but also for child psychiatrists, clinical psychologists, psychiatric social workers, specialists in early childhood education, educational psychologists, special education teachers and other researchers. In addition to six issues per year of *Child Development*, subscribers to the journal also receive a full subscription to *Child Development Perspectives* and *Monographs of the Society for Research in Child Development*: http://www.blackwellpublishing.com/journal.
asp?ref=0009-3920

ANSWERS TO ACTIVITIES

ACTIVITY 2.1 Why is it important to have two different charts, one for boys and one for girls?

The specific charts used will depend on the child's age, which determines whether the child will stand for measurement of height or lie down for measurement of length. The measurements will be plotted on growth charts in the Boy's Growth Record or the Girl's Growth Record so that trends can be observed over time and any growth problems identified. It is important to use the Growth Record for the correct sex since boys and girls grow to different sizes.

ACTIVITY 2.2

Access a copy of the healthy child programme and consider the scenario of Chris and Hannah. How would differences in the development of Thomas and Isaac be identified?

In leading and delivering the healthy child programme (pregnancy through to 5 years) the health visitor will provide and/or oversee the health team that provides a service to all families that includes:

- prenatal visit/family health assessment/preparation for parenthood
- new birth visits – parenting, feeding, health checks – planning future healthcare
- first-year contacts: formal health programme immunisation, physical and developmental checks, information, support, feeding, parenting, safety, relationships
- one to three years: formal health programme, dental health, keeping safe, nutrition, speech, language and communication, play
- three to five years: a formal health programme for school entry.

Specific services for families when there is an issue affecting health and well-being. Health visitors use their expert professional judgement to agree appropriate levels of additional support, building on parents' strengths. Some of this support is provided by them, some they delegate or refer to the appropriate professional or practitioner.

Examples of common needs and services are:

- relationship counselling
- maternal mental health/prenatal depression

- parenting advice on family health and minor illness
- sleep problems
- feeding/weaning problems
- preschool behaviour
- speech/communication problems.

Ongoing additional services for vulnerable children and families. Health visitors are skilled at identifying families with high-risk and low-protective factors, enabling these families to express their needs and deciding how they might best be met. This may include:

- offering evidence-based programmes
- encouraging the use of the Common Assessment Framework
- referring families to specialists
- arranging access to support groups, for example, those provided in the local Sure Start children's centre
- organising practical support, for example, working with a nursery nurse on the importance of play
- delegating focused contacts to a team member and monitoring effectiveness.

Contribution to multidisciplinary services in safeguarding and protecting children. Health visitors are trained to recognise risk factors, triggers of concern and signs of abuse and neglect, as well as protective factors. Using this knowledge, they can concentrate their activities on the most vulnerable families. Through their preventative work, they are often the first to recognise that the risk of harm to children has escalated to the point that safeguarding becomes paramount.

SELECTED REFERENCES

Aries, P. (1962) *Centuries of childhood: a social history of family Life*. Vintage Books: New York.

Cunningham, H. (2006) *The invention of childhood*. BBC Books: London.

Department of Health (DoH) (2000) *Assessing children in need and their families*. Practice guidance.

Department of Health (DoH) (2009a) *Healthy child programme: pregnancy and the first five years of life*. Department of Health: London.

Department of Health (DoH) (2009b) *Healthy child programme: from 5–19 years old*. Department of Health: London.

Hall, D. and Elliman, D. (2006) *Health for all children*, rev. 4th edn. Oxford University Press: Oxford.

Kallialia, M. (2008) *Play culture in a changing world*. Open University Press: Maidenhead.

Patterson, C. (2008) *Child development*. McGraw-Hill: Boston, MA.

Ridley, M. (2004) *Nature via nurture gene, experience and what makes us human*. Harper Perennial: London.

Sheridan, M.D. (2008) *From birth to five years: children's developmental progress*, 3rd edn. Routledge: London.

Smith, P.K., Cowie, H. and Blades, M. (2003) *Understanding children's development*, 4th edn. Blackwell: Oxford.

Watson, J.B. (1924) *Behaviorism*. University of Chicago Press: Chicago, IL.

CHAPTER 3
Health Promotion Needs of Children and Young People

Hilary Collins

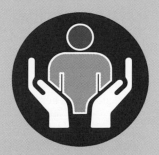
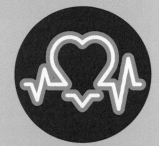
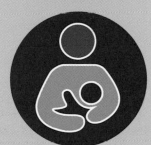

LEARNING OUTCOMES

On completion of this chapter, the reader will be able to:

- Identify issues in child health promotion and understand the role of the health professionals in addressing these.
- Describe the legislation and/or policies and research that influence the health trends and targets for children and young people.
- Understand the health professionals' role in enabling the care of children and young people with long-term health needs and their families.
- Reflect on the role of the health professionals as part of an interprofessional team when promoting the health and well-being of children and young people.
- Identify approaches to health promotion that are appropriate to children and young people and consider their relevance and effectiveness.

TALKING POINT

Do you want to know if you might live to age 100?

If you are aged between 17 and 50 years then the ratio of probability is 1:5.

This ratio rises to 1:8 for 51 to 65 year olds and 1:10 for 66 to 99 year olds.

Young people under 16 have a 1:4 possibility of living to over 100.

Department of Work and Pensions (2011)

INTRODUCTION

This chapter aims to raise awareness of the multiplicity of factors that may impact on the health and well-being of children in contemporary society and evaluate the role of the health professional as a health promoter. The emphasis on holistic care, healthcare legislation and policy and other developments have encouraged health professionals to examine practice, to use research and to approach change in a dynamic way. If children and young people's nurses are proactive as well as responsive to children, young people and their families/carers, successful health improvement outcomes can be achieved

---

CASE STUDY 3.1 Sinead and her daughter

Sinead is 14 years old. Her daughter, Chloe, was born at term, but was admitted to the neonatal unit. Sinead's parents did not want her to live with them, because she has been going to parties and has come home drunk on several occasions.

Sinead and Chloe are living with Sinead's grandmother. Sinead is struggling to assert her independence in caring for Chloe as her grandmother takes over the baby's care and is always giving advice. Sinead is seeking support and reassurance about her knowledge and abilities in caring for her baby

Sinead is reluctant to return to full-time education as she is worried about her grandmother caring for Chloe, but she does not have contact with Chloe's father and does not know where he is living.

Sinead started smoking when she was 12 years old. Her parents and grandparents smoke. She reduced the number of cigarettes she smoked during her pregnancy but she has started to increase the number again. She tries not to smoke when she is with Chloe. Sinead's grandmother does not smoke when she is with Chloe.

Sinead will be attending the outpatients' clinic for follow-up after discharge from the NNU.

Therefore, at the age of 14, Sinead and her baby might live to 100. Already she has made many more life-changing decisions that affect her health and well-being than many other girls of her age. She has been in an intimate relationship and conceived her baby. She has chosen to have the baby and to keep her rather than have her adopted. She did not use contraceptives. Her baby's father has decided not to continue to see her or the baby. Sinead wants to remain healthy and wants Chloe to be healthy. She is exploring what health means for both her and her baby.

CONCEPTS OF HEALTH AND ILLNESS

Concepts of health are defined through theoretical perspectives that have developed from the lived experiences of people including children, young people and their families. The theoretical perspectives give a framework for health professionals to work through and a structure for health promotion activities. This is confirmed by Piper (2009) when he discusses health as subjective and presents it as a continuum:

                              Total
    Illness I_____I Healthy

Individuals' location on the continuum depends on their perceptions, which are influenced by the absence of illness. Therefore health is relying on illness for its definition. This approach is usually described as the medical model. The medical model of health (Evans et al. 2011) views the patient in terms of her diagnosis or health problem. This provides a structure within which healthcare can be organised as healthcare providers segregate their services according to the medical specialities, for example paediatrics. The patient is seen by a medical practitioner who is an expert in relation to her health issues.

Tones and Tilford (2001) describe this approach as reductionist. Sinead and/or her baby as the client are seen as bodies with parts that when ill are not functioning, due to micro-organisms or disease. They would see the medical practitioners who have expertise in that field of practice and their role is to repair the body or mind. This approach can give the medical practitioners a sense of authority in healthcare and clients are expected to be passive and accept the medical practitioner's option. However, the medical diagnosis and speciality must not restrict the health professional's vision of the holistic needs of the patient. Children and young people's nurses need to work within these organisational structures but not allow their influence to restrict their view of the patient as a whole, because other aspects of the patients' life could be affected by the health issues.

The application of the medical model of health is clearly seen in the outpatient department (OPD). Sinead will be attending the paediatric clinic and this could generate confusion about whether she is the patient or the mother of the patient. Nurses working in the outpatient department have previously been seen as working without much autonomy under the authority of the medical practitioner (Brenchley and Robinson 2001). However, the nurse in the OPD may be the first children and young people's nurse that Sinead has met. This visit offers an opportunity for the nurse to discuss health promotion issues for Sinead, as well as Chloe. As the nurses in OPD have relinquished some routine aspects of care such as urinalysis and weighing patients to supportive appropriately trained HCAs this enables them to develop more specialist roles such as enuresis advice (for incontinence and bedwetting) or skin prick allergy testing. Sinead's ability to attend her outpatient's appointments will be influenced by her finances to pay the transport costs and her ability to access transport with a baby in a buggy.

The determinants of health consider the factors that will influence the individual's health and her view of her health. These include factors such as employment, age, gender, ethnicity, disability and social class (Green and Tones 2010). Income or poverty are often seen as the key factor as they influence many of the other determinants. The Health and Social Care Act (Department of Health 2012a) identified that poverty has an impact on life expectancy, which can vary by seven years, between wealthier and poorer families. In poorer families, people are more likely to experience negative health effects as a result of consumption of excess alcohol, taking drugs and smoking and suffer from mental health issues and disability.

The other issue to be considered in healthcare provision is inequality, which is seen as any variation and inequities in service delivery that can be avoided (Whitehead 2010 in Green and Tones 2010). One of the aims of the Health and Social Care Act (2012) is the reduction in inequalities, sometimes referred to as the 'postcode lottery'. That is defined as health provision you receive being affected by the part of the country in which you live, with variations of services and therefore health outcomes, for example *The Times* newspaper online in 2009 cited Nick Hornby, an author and a father of a child with autism: 'The average age of diagnosis varies from under three years to as old as seven years depending on the local authority', information released under a freedom of information request by the charity found. Public Health England is the body that will be responsible for reducing inequalities as the legislation requires it to work with the NHS commissioning boards and clinical

commissioning groups. They will be working with the secretary of state to address these inequalities and promote partnership working.

Increasing the responsibilities and involvement of local authorities is one aspect of the Health and Social Care Act (Department of Health 2012a). The local authorities will be responsible for some of the determinants of health that contribute to the inequalities, such as housing, and the improvement of the local areas. Also the local authority will be responsible for transport provision and this gives an example that would affect Sinead as she tries to access transport with her baby buggy.

The close collaboration between local authorities, the National Health Service and adult social care is shown in Figure 3.1. The impact of these changes on children's services is not specified yet. However, better integration of services is one of the aims as it has been identified that the handover of care between providers is not always managed well. These issues have been explored in the book. The inclusion of children and young people's educational services is not mentioned in the briefing papers.

For Sinead, her returning to school needs to be considered. The example of inequality in relation to nursery provision for Chloe would be that some nurseries for teenage mothers are closer to schools than others. The inequity would be if the nurseries nearer the school charged more because they were nearer the school. However, it must be remembered that Sinead is more than a new mother with a young baby. Her age and social circumstances must be considered. She is likely to wish to attend

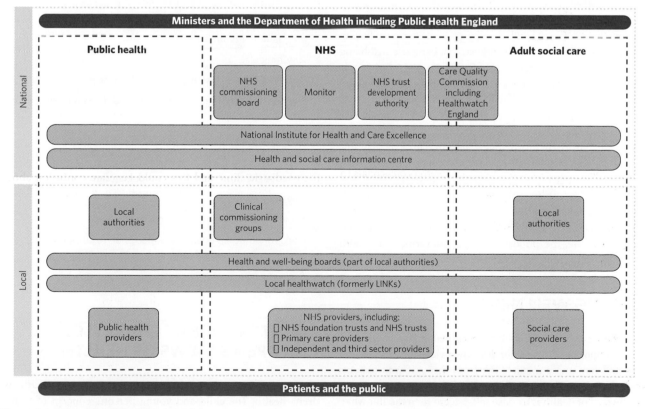

Figure 3.1 Overview of health and social care structures in the Health and Social Care Act 2012

appointments with a friend (Moyse 2009) rather than her grandmother or alone. She will need to build up trust in the children and young people's nurses before she will disclose her concerns.

Some patients require interventions in more than one field of medicine. This is an area in which the health professional can facilitate the referral and intervene to ensure that all the patient's healthcare needs are addressed. As a teenage mother, Sinead remains a patient although she has no medical diagnosis requiring treatment and cure (Evans et al. 2011) due to her age and the potential for health problems for her and the baby. However, she has other issues that are considered in other models of health.

The holistic model of health (Evans et al. 2011) encompasses the World Health Organization's (WHO 1948 in Evans et al. 2011) definition of health: 'Health is a state of complete physical, mental and social well being and not merely the absence of disease.' Consideration is given that there are more aspects to health but the definition does not recognise that the patient can be healthy even when they continue to have a disease or health problem, because there is a concentration on the absence of disease. However, this approach encourages the consideration of physical, mental and social aspects. It could be argued that the spiritual aspects of health have not been considered in this definition. The health professional needs to consider the impact of the health problem on all aspects of the patient's life. Some patients may not wish to disclose information about their social and mental well-being. The professional relationship that the health professional develops will be vital in encouraging the patient to disclose this information.

Sinead has concerns about asserting her independence due to her grandmother's involvement. This situation is creating a tension about whether she should return to education. This will affect her mentally and socially and, thereby, prevents her from having complete well-being. It could be argued that complete well-being is not possible due to the tensions of the relationships that people experience. Therefore, a model of health that can adapt to changes in life circumstances would provide a resource for living.

The wellness model of health (Evans et al. 2011) was developed alongside the WHO's (1986 in Evans et al. 2011) changing definition of health as it provides a 'resource for everyday life, not the objective of living. It is a positive concept emphasising social and personal resources, as well as physical capabilities.' This concept of health encompasses the choices that individuals are making in behaviour that will affect their health. The impact of luck or chance in health is dismissed by Ewles and Simnett (2003). Therefore, the philosophy of empowerment in health choices that underpins this model is vital.

DEFINING WELLNESS

When working with children and young people in a health context, it is important to consider your own views of wellness and health and how these might differ from those of your patients and clients.

If the goal of health is to raise self-esteem then the 'But why?' approach could be used with Sinead.

ACTIVITY 3.1 Consider your own views of wellness and health

Write down two or three health issues that you think would be important to young people.

Now compare your issues with the ones listed by the young people in Figure 3.2, which shows the issues that *they* think are important in health (from the National Children's Bureau 2011). How do the two compare?

ACTIVITY 3.2 Application of the But Why? approach used in Towards a Healthy Future

Add your own ideas about the factors that might contribute to Sinead's health.

Why did Sinead have a baby?

She did not use contraceptives for her first experience of sexual intercourse.

Anything else…

But why did she not use contraceptives?

She thought that she could not get pregnant as it was her first time.

Anything else…

But why did she think she couldn't get pregnant?

Her friend had told her that she has had sex and didn't get pregnant on her first time.

Anything else…

But why did Sinead listen to her friend's advice?

She has had very limited education about relationships and sex.

Anything else…

But why has she had very limited education?

Because she does not attend school regularly.

Anything else…

But why doesn't she attend school?

Her grandmother does not expect her to attend because she rarely attended school.

Anything else…

MAINTENANCE OF LIFESTYLE AND CHILDREN'S VIEWS OF HEALTH

The health decisions made by parents will impact on their children's health. The child and young person's concept of health will be linked to their age and stage of development. Sinead's

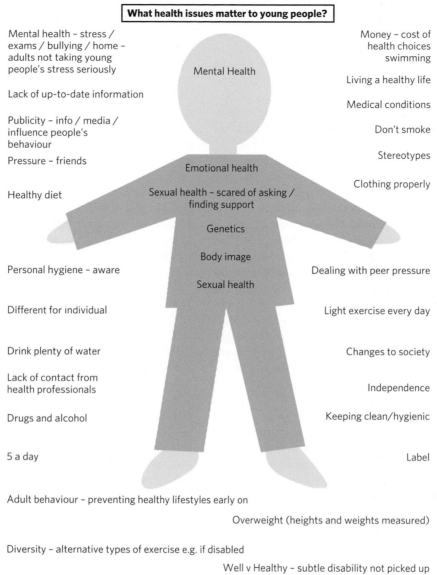

Figure 3.2 What health issues matter to young people
Source: National Children's Bureau (2011)

decision to proceed with her pregnancy is the first influence on Chloe's health. During pregnancy, mothers are given health promotion advice by their midwife. As Sinead's health behaviour included alcohol consumption, smoking and possibly an inadequate diet these could have a negative effect on the developing foetus. The teenager's view of what is risky behaviour will be influenced by their family's views. Hubley and Copeman (2008) acknowledge the influence of the family on health choices, especially in relation to nutrition. Families will influence their children's health and then their health decisions during their childhood. Furthermore, the media and health professionals will influence them all.

The influences on children's behaviour change as they start school. The views of teachers and peers start to impact as children and young people start to take more responsibility for their own actions. Within peer groups, comparisons are made by the children in relation to size, appearance and clothes and abilities such as learning to read (Hubley and Copeman 2008). The influence of peer pressure begins to emerge as children learn what behaviour is expected and acceptable. At the preoperational stage (from 2 to 7 years), Piaget suggests that children rely on external clues about their behaviour, as they cannot yet determine what health means and are relying on others to tell them (Moules and Ramsay 2008). They interpret this information into an absolute meaning that they think of themselves as either healthy or ill. Therefore children who are told that they do not look well will lie down whether or not they feel ill as they think that sick people lie down. This behaviour can be reinforced by parents who expect children who say they are not well to stay in bed in case they are making up an excuse not to attend school.

The national child measurement programme (NCMP) (National Health Service (NHS) 2005) monitors children's weight and height and notifies parents if their children are underweight, overweight or obese. However, the definition of these categories can be open to interpretation between health professionals. Cole et al. (2000) commented that there was no international definition. They recommended the use of centile charts and developed a table of body mass indexes relating to gender and age. Charts have been produced by the Child Growth Foundation (2012).

Children in reception class aged 4 to 5 years at Piaget's preoperational stage (2 to 7 years) (Moyse 2009) would be measured in the NCMP. They are usually unable to determine how healthy they are and often rely on others to tell them (Moules and Ramsay 2008). They see health as an absolute therefore they are either healthy or they are not and they are not able to relate behaviour to health. Therefore children in this age range who are told they are overweight or obese will not know what to do about this, as they are unable to relate behaviour to its consequences. The parents of children who are identified as overweight or obese by the NCMP receive a letter offering advice about strategies to reduce the child's weight. Strategies for families include the Change 4 Life Programme (NHS 2009). Campaigns such as the Healthy Schools Toolkit (Department of Education 2010) also impact on what children eat at school.

Children in year 6 aged 10 to 11 years are also measured by the NCMP. According to Piaget, children in the concrete operational stage (aged 7 to 11 years) view health and illness more as a total body experience (Moules and Ramsay 2008). They are developing their thoughts according to what they can do if they are healthy and may think that being fit and able to run is an example of health. As their thinking now allows two different states to exist at the same time they can be part healthy and part unhealthy. This enables them to consider the possibility that what they eat and how much exercise they do contribute to their weight loss or gain. Children in this age range can appreciate the purpose of health promotion.

Sinead at 14 years would be classified by Piaget as in the formal operational stage (aged 11 to 16 years). She would be considering her own health as well as Chloe's and this might be contributing to her struggle to assert her independence. Sinead would be able to recognise the changes in physical and mental health that may have occurred during her pregnancy and postnatally. Her health visitor will have undertaken a mental health assessment with her and would offer advice that Sinead would need to think was achievable in order for her to consider following it. Sinead would be referred to her general practitioner (GP). However, Sinead would be aware of her own role in health promotion for herself and Chloe. Upton and Thirlaway (2010) recognise that communicating the risk associated with behaviour may start with the individual considering how to change that behaviour.

The idea of the planned teenaged pregnancy needs to be discussed, as Sinead may have considered pregnancy as a route out of the circumstances in which she finds herself living. Cater and Coleman (2006) researched the motivations for teenagers becoming pregnant. Many of the teenagers interviewed thought that pregnancy would give them purpose and help to improve their lives. The media portray teenaged pregnancy as a problem, with headlines aimed at selling newspapers, for example: 'the teenage pregnancy problem or epidemic'. Teenaged parents should not be labelled or stereotyped in this way. Duncan et al. (2010) have researched the circumstances of teenaged parents and found that the pregnancy had less impact on many teenagers' circumstances at the age of 30 than expected. Conversely, there is evidence that teenaged parents do experience greater poverty, exclusion and more mental and physical health issues. Hall and Hall (2007) conclude that these issues arise due to the young people's circumstances when they became pregnant. Therefore, the pregnancy may have resulted from their circumstances as well as contributed to them. Society's views about teenaged pregnancy have changed over time. In the past Sinead would have been expected to give her baby up for adoption and probably not have seen her again.

The Family–Nurse Partnership Programme (Department of Health 2012b) was introduced in England in 2007 following research in the United States of America. The concept is a preventive programme aimed at first-time young mothers. Therefore, Sinead could be eligible to be included. The family nurse builds a supportive professional relationship with Sinead and empowers her to change her health behaviour. This would promote a healthier lifestyle for her and baby Chloe. The early evidence (Department of Health 2012b) suggests an improved outcome for the young first-time mothers and the programme is working alongside other initiatives, especially Sure Start children's centres.

Young People's Views about Teenage Pregnancy

Cater and Coleman (2006) recorded the views of one teenager:

> I had a really, really bad childhood – I was in care and my parents aren't very good parents so I just thought a baby would give me that stability and also give me something that would love me unconditionally – never thought it would leave me and – 'cos it'd be mine – nobody could take it away…I was the only kid at the age of 9, planning to have a baby…I was desperate for [baby son] and I've enjoyed him so much…[He] gave me my purpose and my place in life, and my goal. (mother, 13)

For some new mothers, the plans they have made do not work out as they thought. MIND (2012) reminds us that postnatal depression is very common (see Table 3.1).

The Department of Health (2011) guidance gives the 'You're welcome' quality criteria for making health services young people friendly. This toolkit gives the opportunity for health service providers to undertake a self-assessment using the 'You're welcome' criteria.

Table 3.1 Mental health assessment

At the booking visit, Sinead would have been asked:

- During the past month, have you often been bothered by feeling down, depressed or hopeless?
- During the past month, have you often been bothered by having little interest or pleasure in doing things?

  A third question would be asked if she had replied yes to either of the first two:

- Is this something you feel you need or want help with?

  She would have been asked about her past history of mental illness and previous treatment.

The guidelines mention adolescents especially and include the note that they are entitled to confidentiality and their rights must be respected. Consent must be obtained, while considering the adolescent's understanding and safeguarding issues.

Source: (NICE 2007)

RESEARCH NOTE 3.1   Healthy lives, healthy people: young people's views on being well and the future of public health (NCB 2011)

Young people are interested in participating in projects relating to health in their school and colleges and through other agencies. During one of these consultations the National Children's Bureau (NCB 2012) reported that young people view health professionals as 'information dictators'. Interestingly, their report identifies that the majority of young people viewed their parents as 'information providers'. However, these findings came from a study of children and young people with cancer, which will have influenced the respondent's perceptions. Health professionals should be considering how to make the health service more user friendly for children and young people. Ideas supported by the NCB's findings include further information for parents that they can explain in the language their child best understands. However, the children and young people want information to come directly from the healthcare providers too. The report identified that young people are most reluctant to access sexual health and mental health services. These could be services that they may not wish to discuss with their parents; therefore, this information must be accessible to them in language they can understand. Children and young people with long-term health issues want to have health services delivered in their own home. Those children and young people who visit health centres or hospital want them to be child-friendly environments, with services that are flexible and personalised.

ACTIVITY 3.3   Using the 'You're Welcome' criteria

Use the 'You're Welcome' (Department of Health 2011) criteria to review the service provision for children and young people in the area where you work:

- highlight what is good practice in the area
- highlight practices that need to be improved.

'You're Welcome' criteria

- Accessibility: ensuring services are accessible to young people and barriers to access are identified and removed.
- Publicity: need for effective publicity to raise awareness of the services available and the fact that these can be accessed confidentially.
- Confidentiality and consent: ensuring that young people are aware that they will be treated in confidence and of the limit of confidentiality linked to safeguarding.
- Environment: ensuring that the health environment and the atmosphere (e.g. staff's attitudes and actions) are young people friendly.

- Staff training, skills and values: staff need to receive appropriate training and supervision in understanding, engaging and communicating with young people.
- Joined-up working: where possible co-locate services for young people and when that is not feasible ensure that other relevant professionals are informed about the service young people have received.
- Involvement in the monitoring and evaluation of the patient experience: young people need to be routinely consulted about current service, service development and reviews of service provision.
- Transition: the need to consult young people on transition issues, both universal ones (e.g. sexual and reproductive health) as well as those specific to young people with specific long-term needs.
- Specialist child and adolescent mental health services (CAMHS): ensuring that these standards apply to CAMHS services as well.

HEALTH EDUCATION AND HEALTH PROMOTION

The debate about the relationship between health education and health promotion continues and Ewles and Simnett (2003, page 23) recognise that it could become time consuming to argue about the meanings of the words. However, they focus on the WHO (1984 in Ewles and Simnett 2003) definition of health promotion: 'Health promotion is the process of enabling people to increase control over, and improve their health.' Ewles and Simnett (2003, page 24) give their own definition of health education as: 'working with people to give them knowledge to improve their own health and working towards individual attitude and behaviour change'.

History of Health Promotion

There is a clear link between government policy and health promotion initiatives. Changes in government generate changes to these initiatives as reorganisation of government departments occurs and there are changes to the ministers who run them. However, the impact of health promotion on the health of children and young people may not be apparent until they are in their 50s (Craft 2005). Craft continues by commenting that as the term of office for a political party would be time limited, their interest in the long-term investment could likewise be limited. White and Wills (2011) discuss the impact of the New Labour government on health promotion. They remind us that health districts had health promotion teams or health education units in the 1980s and these developed with the establishing of health action zones. However, reorganisation and the establishing of the primary care groups in 1999 contributed to the end of many of these teams.

There were fewer specialised health promotion staff members in the primary care trusts, which had been developed by 2005. More recently, local authorities have become responsible for health improvement using funding that has been ring-fenced. Other factors that prompt the development of government policy are events that generate public concern, for example the death of Victoria Climbié and the subsequent Laming Report (Moyse 2009). This contributed to the development of the National Service Framework (NSF) for children and young people (Department of Health 2004). Tannahill (2008) reminds us that the language of health promotion has been changing as well. He confirms the move from the term health education and its context of prevention to the term health promotion and its context of health improvement. However, the international recognition of health promotion continues and even though the language may change, the focus and activity will remain.

Tannahill (2008, page 1389) gives a new definition of health promotion:

Sustainable fostering of positive health and prevention of ill-health through policies, strategies and activities in the overlapping action areas of:

- socio, economic, physical, environmental and other factors
- equity and diversity
- education and learning

- services, amenities and products
- community-led and community based activity.

Morgan (2006) urges a review of the drivers that influence health promotion activities in his discussion of the health assets model. Whiting and Miller (2008) contrast the health deficits model and the health assets model. The health deficits model is often applied after the poor health has developed. The individual or community is often blamed for this poor health in a negative way. Then the individual or community is faced with the need to justify the resources that might be required to assist in addressing the poor health. They confirm that interventions may be required after the poor health has developed but encourage the proactive approach of the health assets model. Morgan (2006) gives the overview of the health assets model by suggesting that the individual or community have positive health ideas and these should be the focus. He concludes that this approach raises the self-esteem of the individual or community and the need for professional support is reduced.

Approaches to Health Promotion

The NHS Future Forum has recommended that health professionals 'make every contact count' (2012). Therefore, the issues of diet, alcohol and smoking should be mentioned during each contact with clients. However, mentioning the issues may not be enough to encourage clients to change their behaviour, therefore, a collaborative approach is needed. When children and young people's nurses are working with other members of the interprofessional team, they need an approach or model that they can all utilise. A number of models have been developed but none is specific to children and young people, although they can all be adapted for use. Health promotion models are often considered to be either 'top down' or 'bottom up' in their application within the hierarchy of decision making and information forwarding. In the top-down models, the health professional holds the information and knowledge and shares this with the client at the time decided by the health professional. In the bottom-up approach, the client or a group of clients either have the knowledge or decide what information they require and when they require it. Naidoo and Wills (2010, page 63) expand this concept when discussing the 'implementation gap'. They describe this as the disparity between what is planned and what happens in practice. Examples of the health promotion models will be applied in the later sections on sexual health, smoking and drinking alcohol.

ACTIVITY 3.4

The National Service Framework for children, young people and maternity services (NSFCYPMS; Department of Health 2004) provides the framework for healthcare for children and young people. However, if children and young people are the service users then the information from the Framework needs to be available to them in a format they can understand.

Design an information leaflet for a child that explains the National Service Framework.

Healthy Child Programme

The healthy child programme (Department of Health 2007) uses *Health for all children* (Hall and Elliman 2003) as its point of reference but states that it is intended to continue the work started as a result of this work. However, it does supersede the previous NHS child health promotion programme. It is the guidelines for the implementation of Standard 1 of the NSFCYPMS (2004). At each age or life stage the guidelines provide a framework for health promotion activities.

PRACTICAL GUIDELINES 3.1

During early pregnancy, Sinead would have been assessed. The generic indicators would have identified that Sinead and her baby were at risk of multiple problems.

Sinead's risk factors are:

- Her young age and lack of educational attainment.
- She is not in education, training or employment.
- She is living in potentially unsatisfactory accommodation.
- She has an unstable relationship with her baby's father.
- She has low social capital.
- She may have suffered stress in pregnancy.

PRACTICAL GUIDELINES 3.2

During the birth to 1-year stage, Sinead and Chloe would be assessed by the 14th day after birth.

Sinead and Chloe's risk factors are:

- Any health problems.
- Any problems resulting from lack of social support.
- Being a first-time mother.

The following areas will be addressed:

- sensitive parenting promoted
- infant feeding
- parents who smoke
- sudden infant death.

Every Child Matters

The impact of changes in government policy on the ongoing healthcare of children and young people is illustrated in the suspension of the White Paper *Every child matters*. This was developed following the Laming Report into the death of Victoria Climbié (Moyse 2009) and has been the framework for the implementation of the Children Act. However, in 2010 there was a change in policy due to reorganisation following the change in government. This policy has been archived and the Department of Education (2012) states that it 'should not be considered to reflect current policy or guidance following the closure of the Department of Children, Schools and Families'. However, it still influences practice as it has a structure that is clear to remember and a focus that applies in most situations. The National Health Service (NHS) continues to refer to *Every child matters* in the National Service Frameworks (National Health Service 2012a). Part of the rationale for the development of the NSFCYMS was to apply *Every child matters*.

The recent White Paper of 'Healthy lives, healthy people' (DoH 2010) aims to build on the work undertaken through *Every child matters*. The White Paper is being implemented through the establishing of Public Health England. The White Paper acknowledges the role of local authorities in developing public health initiatives. This gives opportunities for health professionals to work closely with their local authority colleagues. However, some services will be mandatory, such as sexual health services, NHS health checks, national child measurement programme and public health advice. The operating model for Public Health England has been published and its rollout is being planned (DoH 2012c) (see Table 3.2).

Table 3.2 Public Health England mission statement and functions

Public Health England mission

'Public Health England's overall mission will be to protect and improve the health and well-being of the population, and to reduce inequalities in health and well being outcomes.' (DoH 2012)

Public Health England functions

1. Delivering services to national and local government, the NHS and the public.
2. Leading for public health
3. Supporting the development of the specialist and wider public health workforce.

Source: (DoH 2012c)

ACTIVITY 3.5

Figure 3.3 (from the Public Health England operating model) gives an overview of how the structure will fit together.

Select a child health service delivery and explore how the operating model will be applied.

Diet

You are what you eat **http://www.phrases.org.uk/mean ings/you%20are%20what%20you%20eat.html**

This slogan carries the reminder that diet does contribute to health and well-being. The diet available to Sinead will be determined by the family income and the family eating patterns. Therefore, income and family practices has an indirect effect on health as well. Contrasting the effect of financial poverty and affluence on the diet demonstrates that the income for both social groups could contribute to obesity (Fraser and Edwards 2010). The family in poverty may be buying cheaper high-fat, high-sugar and high-calorie foods to satisfy hunger but the affluent family can afford the luxury items that also contribute to obesity. Children's portion sizes have increased. 'The eating patterns established in childhood could continue into adult life and establish a cycle that contributes to obesity' (Stamatakis et al. 2005).

As Sinead lives at home, she will be relying on her grandmother who may still be buying and preparing her food. The family eating pattern will influence Chloe. The tradition of young people learning to cook at home has been reduced by parents working longer hours and cooking more convenient quick meals (Roberts 2011). Legal standards for school meals were introduced in 2006. This followed the School Meals Review Panel report (2005 from School Food Trust 2012a), which identified that school food was not meeting children's nutritional needs and that the children were not choosing healthy food to eat.

Guidelines for early years settings were launched in January 2012 with the Eat better, start better project (School Food Trust 2012b). The aim of these guidelines is to influence the menus offered to younger children.

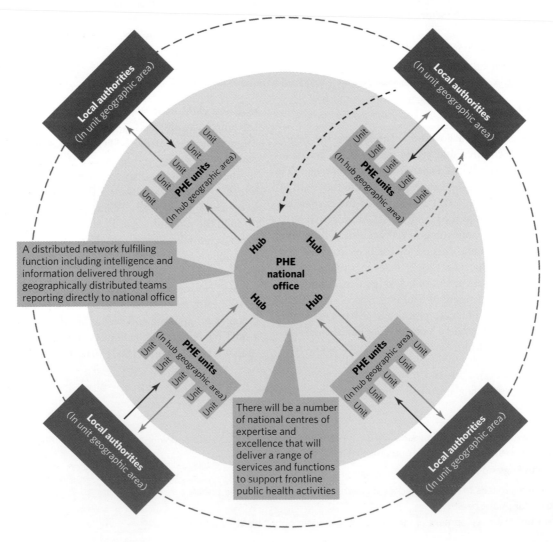

Figure 3.3 Public Health England operating model

PRACTICAL GUIDELINES 3.3

Roberts (2011) confirms that if children learn cooking skills at school it will prepare them for becoming independent and every child should have this opportunity. 'Let's Get Cooking' clubs offer this opportunity and children and young people are being empowered to learn cooking skills at school. Many of these children and young people transfer this knowledge to their home environment and influence the approaches to food preparation at home. Pictures and visual learning aids can assist in the education of children about healthy eating (see Figure 3.4).

Exercise

If exercise were a pill, it would be one of the most cost-effective drugs ever invented. (Cavill 2012)

The family's view of exercise will impact on Sinead and Chloe. If her family are not encouraging her to exercise then she increases the risk of premature death due to major chronic diseases like cancer, stroke, diabetes and heart disease (Naidoo and Wills 2010). NICE (2006) recommend that the primary care team briefly offer frequent advice about exercise. This provides opportunities for charities, government-sponsored initiatives and commercial organisations to offer exercise plans. (See resources for examples of diet plans and exercise suggestions.)

Sport England goals for 2012–17 are:

- Every one of the 4000 secondary schools in England will be offered a community sports club.
- County sports partnerships will be given new resources to create effective links locally between schools and sport in the community.
- All secondary schools that wish to do so will be helped to open up, or keep open, their sports facilities for local community use.
- At least 150 further education colleges will benefit from a full-time sports professional.
- Three-quarters of university students aged 18 to 24 will get the chance to take up a new sport or continue playing a sport they played at school or college.
- A thousand of our most disadvantaged local communities will get a DoorStep club.
- Two thousand young people on the margins of society will be encouraged to gain a new life skill.
- £100m will be invested in facilities for the most popular sports, for example new artificial pitches and upgrading local swimming pools.
- A minimum of 30 sports will have enhanced England talent pathways.

ACTIVITY 3.6

Compare the exercise that you do with the national averages.

View the Sport England Active People Survey results: **http://www.sportengland.org/research/active_people_survey/active_people_survey_6/key_results_for_aps6q2.aspx**.

- 15.3 million adults (aged 16 and over) participated in sport at least once a week for 30 minutes at moderate intensity during the period April 2011 to April 2012
- comparison of 2005/6 (Active People Survey) and the latest results to April 2012, shows that sports participation among adults with a limiting disability/illness has increased from 1.317 million to 1.662 million.

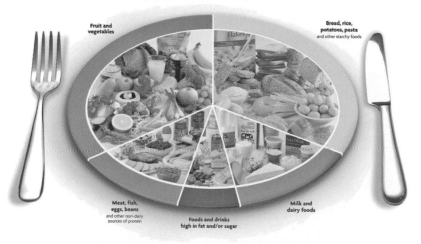

The eatwell plate

Use the eatwell plate to help you get the balance right. It shows how much of what you eat should come from each food group.

Figure 3.4 Picture of a range of food as a visual learning aid

Sexual Health

The promotion of sexual health for young people links with the issues discussed in sexual health. Sexual health promotion needs to be meaningful to the young person and the messages clear from all the health professionals involved. The use of a collaborative approach using a health promotion model enables the interprofessional team to work together.

Tannahill Model: Preventive Care

In preventive care, the health promotion advice to be given to individuals includes three levels of intervention (see Figure 3.5).

Primary prevention

Health promotion in this area aims to encourage positive health and reduce the behaviour that may have a negative effect on health.

Secondary prevention

This includes the screening processes aimed at detecting illness or poor health.

Tertiary prevention

This aims to treat any illness and prevent complications (see Table 3.3).

Tannahill Model: Protection

Protection in Tannahill's (2008) model of health promotion includes the support and control available in the community. The legislation relating to sexual activity is the Sexual Offences Act (2003). Other controls including fiscal controls might have applied to Sinead' access to contraception. However, she would be entitled to free supplies and advice. She may not know this and the health professionals have a duty to ensure that she has the information she needs. The other controls and

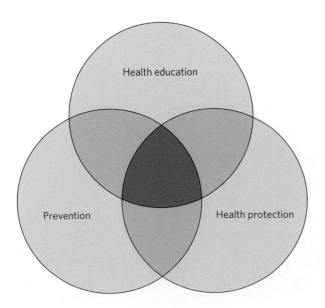

Figure 3.5 Tannahill's (2008) model of health promotion with three overlapping areas of activity

voluntary codes of practice are mentioned in the model. This could include access to condoms in schools and whether they are available in the school toilets.

Tannahill Model: Education

This includes all types of education, not just education for health but also life skills and building self-esteem. The use of the 'bottom-up' concept applies when individuals and communities become involved in addressing the health imbalances with their own solutions. This leads into the concept of HealthWatch. The Health and Social Care Bill (DoH 2012a) includes the principle of 'no decision about me without me'. Local HealthWatch will enable service users and professionals to work towards developing local provision. The local Health-Watch will take over responsibilities from local involvement networks (LINks).

Tannahill's model could be described as simplistic (Kozier et al. 2008), but its structure makes it popular with health professionals as it can be used across the interprofessional team. The model recognises that aspects of health promotion overlap. In application to Sinead, it would be noted that her social and economic circumstances are not included. Therefore it would not have been noted that she lives with her grandmother and has limited income to cover the travel costs to clinic.

Smoking

The effects of smoking on health are well documented (Royal College of Physicians 2010). Most young people start smoking between the ages of 14 and 15 (Swan et al. 1990) and most

Table 3.3 Topics for sexual health promotion for Sinead

Primary prevention	Contraceptive advice
Secondary prevention	Chlamydia testing when she is 16 years old
Tertiary prevention	Social support from other teenaged mothers

smokers start as children or young people. Therefore, Sinead is among the 27 per cent of secondary school pupils in England who have at the very least tried a cigarette. Girls are more likely to smoke than boys, with 9 per cent of girls and 6 per cent of boys smoking and 5 per cent of young people being regular smokers (Information Centre 2011). Assistance for smokers to give up is available free from the National Health Service (2012b). However, health professionals working with children and young people need to include health promotion activity that reduces the number of young people who start smoking.

Some success in preventing young people from starting to smoke has been reported by Fidler and Lambert (2001). They sent their target group of young people three monthly updates of age-appropriate leaflets about the advantages of not smoking. They used surface mail for their leaflets; however, with advances in media there could be scope for the use of email and text messages. The British Heart Foundation (2012) confirms that advertising cigarettes contributes to young people starting to smoke. Their current campaign to have cigarettes sold in plain packages is focused at removing the impressions that cigarettes in gold or silver colourful packages are interesting or trendy.

The health professionals' approach to young people who are smoking could utilise the health action model (Tones and Tilford 2001). The health action model includes two aspects. First, Sinead's intention to start a change in behaviour and, second, whether she continues with the changed behaviour. The factors that influence her intention to change behaviour include her knowledge and understanding of the required behaviour and her ability to make the decision or solve the problems required to change her behaviour. The role of the health professionals is to provide the information and explanation to assist her to make the decision to change behaviour. However, they need to be aware that Sinead may block this information due to beliefs and values she already holds. Tones and Tilford (2001) call this 'defensive avoidance'. This blocking behaviour could arise because change is challenging and there is a comfortable feeling about continuing with familiar patterns of behaviour. Sinead may think she will put on weight if she gives up smoking; as her enjoyment of the taste of the food returns she may eat more.

Sinead's decision to continue with her change in behaviour will be influenced by motivation and the reduction of any barriers which could inhibit her changed behaviour. Tones and Tilford (2001) suggest that this motivation can be subconscious but influenced by beliefs, motives and social pressure. Sinead may smoke after a meal and she is used to completing her meal with a cigarette. If she changes this behaviour then she may feel her meal is incomplete. However, it may be the tactile experience of holding a cigarette that Sinead will be missing as well as the nicotine intake. Health professionals should advise Sinead about the QUIT Kit resources available from the National Health Service (NHS 2012b).

The health action model aims to promote self-worth and self-esteem, through advocacy and empowerment. Tones and Tilford's (2001) model assists the health professional to consider the stages of health behaviour change (Kozier et al. 2008). If Sinead recognises the benefits of change this will increase her motivation to give up smoking. However, Sinead may need the encouragement of others to assist her to give up smoking. If her grandmother joined her this could be of benefit to both of them, as they could encourage one another. Tones and Tilford's (2001) model acknowledges the barriers to change that Sinead may be feeling. Her desire to protect Chloe from the effects of passive smoking could be the final incentive because she reduced her smoking while she was pregnant. The health professionals need to motivate Sinead, capturing her keenness to care for herself and for Chloe.

ACTIVITY 3.9

Design an information leaflet about smoking, targeting young people to encourage them not to start smoking.

Chloe could be exposed to tobacco through passive smoking, even if Sinead does not smoke near her. The Royal College of Physicians (2010) has made links between the development of some diseases and passive smoking. General practitioners estimate that passive smoking contributes to the development of a number of conditions including middle ear infections and asthma and is estimated to have resulted in over 300,000 consultations each year in the United Kingdom.

Alcohol and Illegal Drugs

Young people are attracted to behaviours that are restricted or illegal in their exploration of their increasing freedom and maturity. They may want to experiment with risky behaviour including drinking alcohol and taking drugs. They are influenced by those they view as role models which includes their celebrity heroes, as well as family members and friends. The young person's understanding of the risks involved is developing as the areas of their brain continue to develop during adolescence (Blackmore 2007). Therefore, the controls they will learn as adults are not yet in place. Healthcare professionals can support the young person during this period of development. They will have access to resources including the Alcohol Learning Centre (2012) and FRANK – the National Drugs Information Service (2012). The health professionals could use a health promotion model such as Beattie's (1991 in Moules and Ramsey 2008) (see Figure 3.6).

Beattie recognises there are two aspects to health promotion. These are called the *mode* and the *focus*. The *mode* is where the knowledge and control sits. This control can be with the expert or with the client. The *focus* is the target of the intervention. This can be the individual or the community, government or an institution as a structure. Beattie identifies four areas of health promotion activity. Piper (2009) clarifies the application of these areas into four models that stand separately as they are relevant to the health professional and client.

Health persuasion is directed to the client by the expert. Piper (2009) considers this to be led by the expert and is a top-down approach. The information that the experts are using is developed from their knowledge base and research relating to the effects of behaviour and the development of illnesses or side-effects. This information could be delivered by media adverts, but is likely to be most effective through the one to one discussion.

Personal counselling is led by the client and the professional responds. Piper (2009) remarks on this as a bottom-up approach as the client is enthused to participate in health-promoting activities. This could include training offered by organisations such as Catch-22 (2012). This approach would assist Sinead to ignore peer pressures about drinking alcohol or taking drugs.

PRACTICAL GUIDELINES 3.5

This could mean that Sinead attends a course run by the substance misuse team, i.e. client centred and individual.

Legislative action is led by experts and aimed at structures or corporate bodies. Piper (2009) describes this as a top-down intervention. This could be the recommendations of a Green Paper being presented for the development of legislation about underage drinking, i.e. expert led and structural.

Community development is client centred and aimed at structures or corporate bodies. Piper (2009) describes this as bottom up in its application.

PRACTICAL GUIDELINES 3.4

This could be the children and young people's nurse talking to Sinead about the effects of alcohol on breast milk when she is breastfeeding, i.e. expert led and individual.

The Alcohol Learning Centre (2012) gives an extensive range of projects targeting drinkers including young people. In Greater London, 40 young people have been trained as peer educators and are working in a peer outreach team. They are working alongside other agencies in London and offer advice and help at structural level as well as to individuals. Legislative action could be the recommendations of a Green Paper being presented for the development of legislation, i.e. expert led and structural. Community development could be the parents lobbying their MP for school crossings, i.e. client centred and structural.

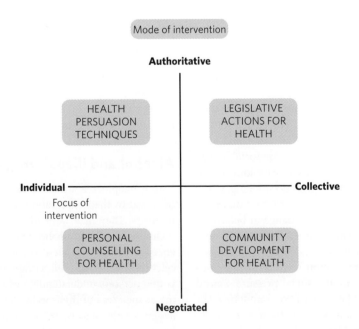

Figure 3.6   Beattie's model

PRACTICAL GUIDELINES 3.6

This could be the teenage parents' group that Sinead belongs to lobbying the local council to prohibit the drinking of alcohol in the local park near the children's play area, i.e. client centred and structural.

Beattie's model considers the issues that underpin health behaviour and considers such issues as income and social circumstances (Kozier et al. 2008). The broader issues are considered such as impact of local and national politics. This model could form part of any local and national initiatives and give the interprofessional team a broader picture of the issues. The model will prompt discussion about the changes and encourage clients to see how their behaviour impacts on their health.

ACTIVITY 3.10   Access the web pages of the alcohol learning centre or Catch-22 and review the projects in your area

Catch-22 is a local charity with a national reach **(http://www. catch-22.org.uk/?gclid=CMi00LmO5LACFcQKfAod2Hg 6zA)**. We work with young people and others who find themselves in seemingly impossible situations. Our services help them develop the confidence and skills to find solutions that are right for them – whether it's getting back into school or training, choosing to stay out of trouble, finding a safe place to live in or helping them to live independently after leaving care or custody. As young people become more positive, productive and independent, the whole community benefits. We believe every young person deserves the chance to get on in life.

CASE STUDY REVIEW 3.1

Attending outpatients

Sinead will be attending the outpatients' clinic for follow-up after Chloe's discharge from the NNU. This is the best time to have an informal conversation, as Sinead and Chloe are living with Sinead's grandmother. Sinead is seeking support and reassurance about her knowledge and abilities in caring for her baby and needs a named key worker who can support her in making her decisions.

Arranging an interprofessional meeting

It would also be valuable to have an interprofessional meeting in which the nurse, health visitor, teaching staff and school nurse could work with Sinead and her grandmother to develop an action plan for supporting caring for Chloe.

Returning to full-time education

Sinead needs to know about the options for returning to full-time education and whether there is a resource in the area that means she can bring the infant to the school or college nursery. Other options may include a home tutor or course that can be undertaken at home.

Sinead started smoking when she was 12 years old

Her desire to protect Chloe from the effects of passive smoking could be the final incentive because she reduced her smoking while she was pregnant. The team needs to motivate Sinead, capturing her keenness to care for herself and for Chloe.

SUMMARY OF KEY LEARNING

The factors that impact on the health of children and young people are diverse. Some of these have changed as views in society change, for example teenage mothers keeping their babies and not being expected to give them up for adoption. The role of children and young people's nurses in health promotion is changing, because practice is advancing and because of changes in legislation and policy. This change brings opportunities for developments using existing approaches such as models of health promotion and collaboration with different members of the interprofessional team. Recent legislation is going to change healthcare delivery and management in the future and the implications for the care of children and young people will need to be monitored by children and young people's nurses.

FURTHER RESOURCES

Pregnancy

Family Nurse Partnership Programmes. These programmes are the current licensed initiative under research by the Department of Health to empower first-time young mothers: **http://www. familynursepartnership@dh.gsi.gov.uk**

Diet and Exercise

Young people have the opportunity to discuss their views on healthcare. Watch and listen to the young people talking about their experiences about diets and weight: **http:// www.youthhealthtalk.org/young_people_health_and_ weight/**

View the Department of Health recommendations for exercise for children and young people: **http://www.nhs.uk/chq/Pag-es/819.aspx?CategoryID=52&SubCategoryID=142**

One of the NHS strategies for promoting the increase in exercise is Change 4 Life: **http://www.nhs.uk/Change4Life/Pages/ change-for-life.aspx**

One of the NHS strategies for promoting the intake of fruit and vegetables is Five a Day: **http://www.nhs.uk/ LiveWell/5ADAY/Pages/5ADAYhome.aspx**

Commercial organisations are also offering advice. This advice gives suggestions for the foods included in five-a-day and portion sizes. Asda: **http://health.asda.com/nutrition/food/**

5-a-day-the-easy-way.aspx; Tesco **http://www. tescorealfood.com/healthy-eating/5-a-day.html**; Sainsburys: **http://www2.sainsburys.co.uk/food/healthylifestyle/ healthy_balance/5-a-day/5adaypage1.htm**

An information source about exercise: HENRY (Health Exercise Nutrition for the Really Young): **http://www.henry.org.uk/**

One example of how other non-health organisations are promoting healthy activities: National Trust plan for 50 things for children to do before they are $11\frac{3}{4}$: **https://www.50things.org.uk**

One example of an approach to increasing exercise for the whole family: MEND (Mind Exercise Nutrition Do It!): **http:// www.mendcentral.org/**

Smoking

Resources on the Action on Smoking and Health (ASH) web pages: **http://www.ash.org.uk/information/resources/ school-resources**

One organisation assisting individuals to give up smoking is GASP, the one-stop shop for stop smoking, smoke-free and tobacco education resources: **http://www.gasp.org.uk/**

One organisation assisting individuals to give up smoking: the National Centre for Smoking Cessation and Training: **http://www.ncsct.co.uk/**

QUIT: This is the UK charity that helps smokers to stop and young people never to start: **http://www.quit.org.uk/**

ANSWERS TO ACTIVITIES

ACTIVITY 3.1

Two or three health issues important to young people could include

1. awareness of sexual health issues
2. awareness of effect of behaviour on health such as smoking
3. impact of media on health issues such as advertising.

All these issues are mentioned by the young people in the National Children's Bureau's research.

ACTIVITY 3.2

Why did Sinead have a baby?
She did not use contraceptives for her first experience of sexual intercourse.
She wanted to experience what it would be like to have a baby.
But why did she not use contraceptives?
She thought that she could not get pregnant as it was her first time.
She thought that contraceptives would interfere with her experience.
But why did she think she couldn't get pregnant?
Her friend had told her that she has had sex and didn't get pregnant on her first time.

She wasn't worried about getting pregnant.
But why did Sinead listen to her friend's advice?
She has had very limited education about relationships and sex.
She wanted to believe her friend.
But why has she had very limited education?
Because she does not attend school regularly.
Her parents and grandmother had not given Sinead any advice.
But why doesn't she attend school?
Her grandmother does not expect her to attend because she rarely attended school.
She could not see the value of schooling.

ACTIVITY 3.3

Use the 'You're Welcome' (DoH 2011) criteria to review the service provision for children and young people in the area where you work.

'YOU'RE WELCOME' CRITERIA

- Accessibility: ensuring services are accessible to young people and barriers to access are identified and removed.

  Lifts enable all children and young people access to the ward.

- Publicity: need for effective publicity to raise awareness of the services available and the fact that these can be accessed confidentially.

  Service provision is clearly signposted. Services are offered with confidentiality.

- Confidentiality and consent: ensuring that young people are aware that they will be treated in confidence, and of the limit of confidentiality linked to safeguarding.

  Confidentiality is discussed with patients.

- Environment: ensuring that the health environment and the atmosphere (e.g. staff's attitudes and actions) are young people friendly.

  The young people's views have been included in the design of the ward.

- Staff training, skills and values: staff need to receive appropriate training and supervision in understanding, engaging and communicating with young people.

Regular staff training occurs.

- Joined-up working: where possible co-locate services for young people, and when that is not feasible ensuring that other relevant professionals are informed about the service young people have received.

  Services are not co-located but there is clear communication in the interprofessional teams.

- Involvement in the monitoring and evaluation of the patient experience: young people need to be routinely consulted about current service, service development and reviews of service provision.

  Young people are consulted.

- Transition: the need to consult young people on transition issues, both universal ones (e.g. sexual and reproductive health) as well as those specific to young people with specific long-term needs.

  Young people are consulted.

- Specialist child and adolescent mental health services (CAMHS): ensuring that these standards apply to CAMHS services as well.

  These standards apply to CAMHS.

ACTIVITY 3.4   National Service Framework leaflet

The leaflet is available at **http://www.wales.nhs.uk/sites3/docmetadata.cfm?orgId=441&id=101606**.

ACTIVITY 3.5

This is a hub and spoke structure with the central hub as Public Health England (PHE) national office (probably) in London.

The spokes will be the PHE units locally (probably) in Essex based in local government.

The local authorities are in the unit geographical areas (possibly) in Chelmsford.

ACTIVITY 3.6

Daily walk of at least 15 minutes.
Weekly swim.
This is less than the Active People Survey.

ACTIVITY 3.7

Add some suggestions of your own to this list.

Primary prevention	Contraceptive advice. Advice about sexually transmitted infections.
Secondary prevention	Chlamydia testing when she is 16 years old. Cervical screening.
Tertiary prevention	Social support from other teenage mothers. Follow up with members of the interprofessional team.

ACTIVITY 3.8

Reviewing the policy about access to sex education in secondary school

A government review of how the subject is broached in schools recommends that sex education should be compulsory. Schools now offer emergency contraception and sexual health advice. These advice services are usually staffed by experienced school nurses, family planning or sexual health nurses.

Do you think sex education should be compulsory?

Do you think any individuals should be able to opt out?

Do you think sexual advice and contraception should be offered in school?

What is currently available to young people?

There is no right or wrong answer; however, sexual education gives the young person the information to make an informed decision. Some local secondary schools have condoms available from machines in the toilets. The school nurse can offer advice, support and contraception.

ACTIVITY 3.9

Anti-smoking leaflet

See Figure 3.7.

Available from **http://www.gasp.org.uk/p-ten-top-reasons-to-stay-smokefree.htm**.

10 TOP reasons to stay SMOKE FREE
Say no to tobacco

Many smokers die before their time. On average 5.5 minutes of life is lost for every cigarette smoked. Smokers die upto 23 years earlier than they should. Smoking is like commiting suicide slowly and peacefully.

Live 1 Longer

Cash 2 not ash

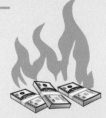

A 20 a day smoker spends around $1.5K a year. Surely there are better things to spend your cash on. Clothes, CDs, holidays, computers, anything in fact.

Figure 3.7 Anti-Smoking Leaflet

ACTIVITY 3.10

Addenbrookes Hospital Fetal Alcohol Syndrome (FAS) Research Study and Pocket Guide (0WBC)

Drinking alcohol during pregnancy can result in a number of disorders in the baby collectively referred to as fetal alcohol syndrome (FAS) or fetal alcohol spectrum disorder (FASD). Characterised by minor facial abnormalities, growth retardation, behavioural problems and neurological signs, it is totally preventable by maternal abstinence from alcohol.

Alcohol Learning Centre (2012) local initiatives available at **http://www.alcohollearningcentre.org.uk/Localinitiatives/projects/index.cfm?sectorIDs=45&keywords=&pct=&pageLength=10&page=1**.

SELECTED REFERENCES

Action on Smoking and Health (2012) School resources: **http://www.ash.org.uk/information/resources/school-resources**

Alcohol Learning Centre (2012) Topics and resources: **http://www.alcohollearningcentre.org.uk/**

Allergy UK (2012) Skin prick testing: **http://www.allergyuk.org/diagnosis-testing-of-alleargy/skin-testing**

Blackmore, S. (2007) The social brain of a teenager. *The Psychologist*, 20(10), 600–602.

Brenchley, T. and Robinson, S. (2001) Outpatient nurses: from handmaiden to autonomous practitioner. *British Journal of Nursing*, 10(16) 1067–1072.

British Heart Foundation (BHF) (2012) Policy statement on tobacco advertising: **http://www.bhf.org.uk/pdf/Tobacco%20marketing%20policy%20statement%20Sept%202011.pdf**

Brykcznska, G.M. and Simons, J. (2011) *Ethical and philosophical aspects of nursing children and young people*. Wiley-Blackwell: Chichester.

Catch-22 (2012) Projects and services: **http://www.catch-22.org.uk/services**

Cater, S. and Coleman, L. (2006) 'Planned' teenage pregnancy: views and experiences of young people from poor and disadvantaged backgrounds, Joseph Rowntree Foundation: **http://www.jrf.org.uk/publications/planned-pregnancy-views-and-expereinces-young-people-poor-and-disqdanvtaged-bac**

Cavill, N. (2012) Benefits of exercise: **http://www.nhs.uk/Livewell/fitness/Pages/whybeactive.aspx**

Child Growth Foundation (2012) Recommended growth monitoring: **www.childgrowthfoundation.org**

Cole, T.J., Belizzi. M.C., Flegal. K.M. and Dietz W.H. (2000) Establishing a standard definition for child overweight and obesity worldwide: international survey. *British Medical Journal*, 320(7244), 1240.

Cox, J.L., Holden, J.M. and Sagovsky, R. (1987) Detection of postnatal depression. Development of the 10-item Edinburgh postnatal depression scale. *British Journal of Psychiatry*, 150, 782–786.

Craft, A. (2005) The National Service Framework for Children. *Archives of Disease in Childhood*, 90(7), 665–666.

Department of Education (DoE) (2010) Healthy schools toolkit: **http://www.education.gov.uk/schools/pupilsupport/pastoralcare/a0075278/healthy-schools**

Department of Education (DoE) (2012) Every child matters: **https://www.education.gov.uk/publications/standard/publicationDetail/Page1/CM5860**

Department of Health (DoH) (2004) National Service Framework: **http://www.dh.gov.uk/en/PublicationsandstatIstics/Publications/PublicationsPolicyAndGuidance/DH_4089100**

Department of Health (DoH) (2007) Healthy child programme: **http://www.dh.gov.uk/en/Publicationsandstatistics/Publications/PublicationsPolicyAndGuidance/DH_107563**

Department of Health (DoH) (2010) Healthy lives healthy people: **http://www.dh.gov.uk/en/Publicationsandstatistics/Publications/PublicationsPolicyAndGuidance/DH_128120**

Department of Health (DoH) (2011) 'You're Welcome' quality criteria: making health services young people friendly: **http://www.dh.gov.uk/en/Publicationsandstatistics/Publications/PublicationsPolicyAndGuidance/DH_126813**

Department of Health (DoH) (2012a) The Health and Social Care Act: **www.dh.gov.uk/healthandsocialcarebill**

Department of Health (DoH) (2012b) The family nurse partnership programme: **http://www.dh.gov.uk/en/Publicationsandstatistics/Publications/PublicationsPolicyAndGuidance/DH_11853**

Department of Health (DoH) (2012c) Public Health England's operating model: **http://www.dh.gov.uk/en/Publicationsand statistics/Publications/PublicationsPolicyAndGuidance/DH_13188**

Department of Work and Pensions (DoWP) (2011) Number of future centenarians by age group: **http://www.dwp.gov.uk**

Duncan, S., Edwards, R. and Alexander, C. (2010) *Teenage parenthood: what's the problem?* Tufnell Press: London.

Evans, D., Coutsaftiki, D. and Fathers, C.P. (2011) *Health promotion and public health for nursing students*. Learning Matters: Exeter.

Ewles, L. and Simnett, I. (2003) *Promoting health. A practical guide*, 5th edn. Baillière Tindall: Edinburgh.

Fidler, W. and Lambert, T.W. (2001) A prescription for health: a primary care based intervention to maintain the non-smoking status of young people. *Tobacco Control*, 10, 23–26.

FRANK (2012) The National Drugs Information Service: **http://www.talktofrank.com/**

Fraser, L.K. and Edwards, K.L. (2010) The association between the geography of fast food outlets and childhood obesity rates in Leeds, UK. *Health and Place*, 16(6), 1124–1128.

Green, J. and Tones, K. (2010) *Health promotion*, 2nd edn. Sage: London.

Hall, D. and Elliman, D. (eds) (2003) *Health for all children*, 4th edn. Oxford University Press: Oxford.

Hall, D. and Hall, S. (2007) The 'family–nurse partnership': developing an instrument for identification, assessment and recruitment of clients: **www.dera.ioe.ac.uk/6740/1/DCSF-RW022.pdf**

HM Government (HMG) (2007) The smoke-free regulations: **http://www.legislation.gov.uk/2007?title=smoking**

Hubley, J. and Copeman, J. (2008) *Practical health promotion*. Polity: Cambridge.

Information Centre (2011) Statistics on smoking – England 2011: **http://www.ic.nhs.uk/pubs/smoking11**

Kozier, B. et al (2008) *Fundamentals of nursing. Concepts, process and practice*. Pearson: Harlow.

MIND (2012) Understanding post-natal depression: **www.mind.org.uk**

Morgan, A. (2006) Needs assessment, in W. Macdowell, et al. (eds) *Health promotion practice*. McGraw-Hill Education/Open University Press: Maidenhead.

Moules, T. and Ramsay, J. (2008) *The textbook of children's and young people's nursing*, 2nd edn. Blackwell Publishing: Oxford.

Moyse, K. (2009) *Promoting health in children and young people. The role of the nurse.* Wiley-Blackwell: Chichester.

Naidoo, J. and Wills, J. (2010) *Developing practice for public health and health promotion.* Bailliére Tindall: London.

National Children's Bureau (NCB) (2011) Healthy lives, healthy people: young people's views on being well and the future of public health: **http://www.ncb.org.uk/media/37997/ vss_publichealth_report.pdf**

National Children's Bureau (NCB) (2012) Listening to children's views on health provision. A rapid review of the evidence: **www.ncb.org.uk/policy-evidence/research-centre/ research-projects/a-z-research-projects/listening-to- children%E2%80%99s-views-on-health-provision- %E2%80%93-a-rapid-review-of-the-evidence**

National Health Service (NHS) (2005) National child measurement programme: **http://www.nhs.uk/Livewell/child- health1-5/Pages/ChildMeasurement.aspx**

National Health Service (NHS) (2009) Change 4 life: **http:// www.nhs.uk/Change4Life/Pages/change-for-life-fami- lies.aspx**

National Health Service (NHS) (2012a) National Service Frameworks: **http://www.nhs.uk/NHSEngland/NSF/Pages/Chil- dren.aspx**

National Health Service (NHS) (2012b) Why quit?: **http:// smokefree.nhs.uk/**

National Health Service Future Forum (2012) Summary report: **http://healthandcare.dh.gov.uk/forum-report/**

National Institute for Health and Clinical Excellence (NICE) (2006) Four commonly used methods to increase physical activity: **http://guidance.nice.org.uk/PH2**

National Institute for Health and Clinical Excellence (NICE) (2007) Antenatal and postnatal mental health. Clinical management and service guidance: **http://www.nice.org. uk/guidance/index.jsp?action=bypublichealth&PUBLIC HEALTH=Mental+health&page=2\#/search/?reload**

Piper, S. (2009) *Health promotion for nurses.* Routledge: London.

Roberts, B. (2011) School food trust contribution to the review of the national curriculum: **http://www.schoolfoodtrust. org.uk**

Royal College of Physicians (RCP) (2010) Passive smoking and children: **http://bookshop.rcplondon.ac.uk/contents/ pub305-e37e88a5-4643-4402-9298-6936de103266.pdf**

School Food Trust (2012a) Turning the tables: transforming school food: **www.schoolfoodtrust.org.uk/partners/ reports/turning-the-tables-transforming-school-food**

School Food Trust (2012b) Eat better, start better: **www.school- foodtrust.org.uk/parents-carers/for-parents-carers/ eat-better-start-better**

Sport England (2012) Active people survey: **http://www.sport- england.org/research/active_people_survey/active_peo- ple_survey_6.aspx**

Stamatakis, E., Primatesta, P., Chinn, S., Rona, R. and Falascheti, F. (2005) Overweight and obesity trends from 1974 to 2003 in English children: what is the role of socioeconomic factors? *Archives of Diseases of Childhood*, 90, 999–1004.

Swan, A.V., Creeser, R. and Murray, M. (1990) When and why children first start to smoke. *International Journal of Epidemiology*, 19, 323–330.

Tannahill, A. (2008) Health promotion: the Tannahill model revisited. *Public Health*, 122, 1387–1391.

Tones, K. and Tilford, S. (2001) *Health promotion effectiveness, efficiency and equity*, 3rd edn. Stanley Thornes: Cheltenham.

Upton, D. and Thirlaway, K. (2010) *Promoting healthy behaviour. A practical guide for nursing and healthcare professionals.* Pearson: Harlow.

Welsh Assembly Government (2008) Your guide to the national service framework for children, young people and maternity services: **http://www.wales.nhs.uk/sites3/page.cfm? orgId=441&pid=33013**

White, J. and Wills, J. (2011) What's the future for health promotion in England? The views of practitioners. *Perspectives in Public Health*, 131(1), 44–47.

Whiting, L. and Miller, S. (2008) Traditional, alternative and innovative approaches to health promotion for children and young people. *Paediatric Nursing*, 21(2), 45–50.

CHAPTER 4
Cultural Aspects for Children and Young People

Steve Bilham

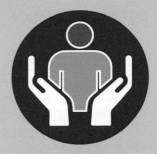

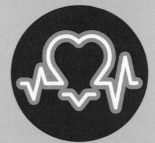

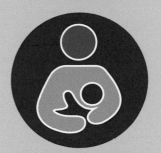

LEARNING OUTCOMES

On completion of this chapter, the reader will be able to:

- Reflect on society's views of the role and position of the child and young person and the implications for practice.
- Reflect on how personal beliefs and cultural practices impact on the delivery of holistic care to children and young people and their family.
- Explore how children's nurses can offer culturally appropriate nursing care.

INTRODUCTION

An understanding of culture helps to equip the health professional with beliefs and values that give individuals a sense of identity, self-worth and belonging, as well as providing the rules for behaviour. This enables the child or young person to physically survive and provide for the welfare and support of the members of a particular culture and therefore its healthcare system, including the values, beliefs and practices that group members possess about health promotion and illness prevention. Culture can also help establish the cause, detection and treatment of illness. As a result, concepts of health, illness and care are integral parts of general cultural values, beliefs and practices. By the professional recognising her own cultural biases, she can learn about or remove unintentional influences. This awareness process must involve examination of her own prejudices and biases towards diverse groups, as well as an in-depth exploration of her own cultural background.

Several years ago when teaching a group of child branch nursing students, the subject was cultural issues in children's nursing. Introducing the session included asking the group members to tell one another about their own culture. Silence. After what seemed like an age (about three minutes in real time) one of the group stated boldly that she could identify the culture of the group. This student came from the Caribbean and proceeded to tell her peers all that she could identify about their culture and it was not all cricket and cream teas.

Ridley (2004) gives an interesting slant on what culture is when he suggests that, when asked about culture, people think either of 'being cultured', that is, to be exposed to and enjoy opera or art, or of ethnic cultures where tribes engage in alien behaviours such as dancing around a fire. He explains that the meaning of the word came from the French enlightenment, where *la culture* meant *civilisation*. In Germany, *'die Kultur'* was the Germanness that separated it from other cultures. In England, following from the response to the theories of Darwin, culture was what was not human nature but the essence that separated man from the ape.

Why Look at Culture?

Anthropologists view culture as actually the complete heritage of humans; it is what makes humans who they are. They may even go so far as to say that in order to understand the self there must first be an understanding of the person's own culture. This is where the going gets tough . . . it may be evident that, at the end of this chapter, there remain more questions than answers; if that is the case, then the goal aimed for has been achieved.

What this Chapter is Not

This chapter is not going to provide a handbook of other cultures, religions and cultural practices, although there may be a few examples for comparison; however these are easily found on the web and in existing textbooks. The chapter is about provoking the reader to explore the implications of culture on nursing practice. By the end of this chapter, the reader will be seeking out information about children and families contacted during practice and will be able to give care that respects their culture and enables the family to feel comfortable.

Whiting (1999) suggests a number of points to consider when gaining knowledge of a patient's culture:

- Develop an understanding of the concept of culture (Leininger 1978).
- Develop an appreciation of your own culture (McGee 1992).
- Have a desire to facilitate effective communication (Murphy and Macleod-Clark 1993).
- Appreciate the differing perceptions of health, illness and treatment in different cultures (McGee 1992).
- Have a desire to work with patients in consideration of their cultural values (Lipson and Meleis 1985).

CASE STUDY 4.1

Melena was admitted to the children's observation ward with a fever and a history of being unwell for several days.

Her father was found scratching her back. He was asked to stop by the nursing staff and when questioned about the incident he explained that he was practising 'cao gio', also known as 'coin rubbing' a form of dermabrasive therapy, which is used to treat a number of illnesses such as pain and fevers and is common in a number of South Asian cultures.

LINKS BETWEEN CULTURE AND DIVERSITY

Is this more about an understanding of the law related to valuing diversity or not causing offence? The code (NMC 2008) clearly sets out how nurses are to 'treat people as individuals':

- You must treat people as individuals and respect their dignity.
- You must not discriminate in any way against those in your care.
- You must treat people kindly and considerately.
- You must act as an advocate for those in your care, helping them to access relevant health and social care, information and support. (NMC 2008, page 3)

All staff within the National Health Service are required, as part of mandatory training, to undertake equality and diversity training. This may take the form of e-learning or may be a classroom session. Within this there is a strong recognition of the law related to equality and diversity. It should be noted that 'equality and diversity' relates to all aspects of employment, sex, race, religion, disability and sexual orientation. In order to fully understand this it is important that all professionals working in health and care professions have an understanding of their own background and culture (see Table 4.1).

Culture is often viewed as something that is to be attained, if one is described as 'having culture'; this is seen as somewhat elitist. An often cited definition of culture is that of Helman:

> To some extent, culture can be seen as an inherited 'lens', through which the individual perceives and understands the world . . . and learns how to live within it. Growing up within any society is a form of enculturation, whereby the individual slowly acquires the cultural 'lens' of that society. (Helman 2000, page 2)

It has been noted that cultural studies is a relatively new discipline but the study of culture has been a main focus of anthropology for many years (Naidoo and Wills 2008). From Helman's definition, we have a view that culture is something that has influence on the individual, both from the way in which the world is perceived and also from the effect that the culture has on the individual.

Table 4.1 Definitions of culture

Theorist/source	Definition
Giger and Davidzhar (2004)	A patterned behavioural response that develops over time as a consequence of imprinting the mind through social and religious structures and intellectual and artistic manifestations
Leninger (2002)	The learned, shared and transmitted values, beliefs, norms and lifeways of a particular group
Purnell and Paulanka (2003)	The totality of socially transmitted behavioural patterns, arts, beliefs, values, customs, lifeways and all other products of human work and thought characteristics of a population that guide their worldview and decision making
Spector (2004)	The nonphysical traits, such as values, beliefs, practices, habits, attitudes and customs that are shared by a group of people and passed from one generation to the next
Ridley (2003)	'Culture means at least two different things. It means highbrow art, discernment and taste: opera in a word. It also means ritual, tradition and ethnicity: dancing round the campfire with a bone through your nose'
http://www.languageshop.org/ glossary/culture.htm	An evolving mix of values, lifestyles and customs derived from social heritage. The culture of ethnic minority groups will be affected by the social, economic and political situation in the part of the country, in which they live and is not just about ethnic origin and religious beliefs. Day-to-day social, economic and political life will have a greater impact on some ethnic groups than on others for whom religion may be an almost all-embracing influence

Source: adapted from Ball and Bindler (2006)

DEVELOPMENT OF CULTURE

Within these definitions, there is a suggestion that culture is passed from one generation to the next. There is a suggestion that culture can be passed on in the form of *memes*, a term for a unit of cultural information such as a practice or an idea. This is not such a strange idea. To begin to understand the importance of genetic information being passed through the generations, this science is still very much in its infancy.

How Then is Culture Passed On?

Richard Dawkins (1976/2006) describes evolution as a competition between 'replicators', which are usually genes, and 'vehicles', bodies to carry them in. He suggests that for 'replicators' to survive they must have three properties – fidelity, fecundity and longevity. Susan Blackmore (cited in Ridley 2004) argues that many ideas exhibit longevity, are fecund (productive) and exhibit fidelity, that they are able to compete for brain space, hence the idea of a 'meme' and the ability of humans to imitate each other and therefore the ability to move ideas forward such as language and innovations. There is no proof for this theory but it provides an interesting perspective on an 'evolution' or 'natural selection' approach to the question of culture. Put quite simply, where a gene is the basic unit of biological inheritance, the meme is the basic unit of cultural inheritance.

There are many examples of how individuals and peoples have developed within a culture and their view of the world has been profoundly affected by this. For example, Turnball (1961) describes his experience with a man named Kenge of the BaMbuti pygmies. Kenge had lived all his life in the forest and when he was taken by Turnball to the plain and shown a herd of buffalo in the distance he said that he had never seen insects of that kind. When Turnball explained that they were buffalo and took Kenge closer, the 'insects' grew in size. Kenge explained this as witchcraft. The reality was that Kenge had no experience of judging the size of objects over great distances. In the same way, if we have no experience of other cultures, how are we to respond or react when we are faced with peoples from different cultures and backgrounds. The impact of this description is that where there is no experience of something, individuals from other cultures may just not 'get it' and the responsibility of the nurse to both understand and help is paramount. There is another issue which may arise for nurses working with children and young people. Where the children have grown up in one culture and the parents are from another there may be difficulties of cultural dissonance within families (this is referred to as 'intergenerational cultural dissonance' or ICD).

CULTURAL DEVELOPMENT OF CHILDHOOD

In the United Kingdom, a child reaches majority at the age of 18. That means that legally, until the age of 18, you are a child. However, the boundaries are rather blurred. Coram Children's Legal Centre publish a pamphlet 'At what age can . . . ? A guide to age-based legislation.' This pamphlet provides information for professionals, children and their families on the legislation that can have an impact on their lives. The most recent update was in 2010.

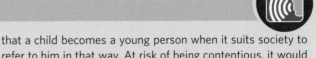

VOICES 4.1

Have you noticed the different ways of referring to children? You may have noticed that the title of this book is *Essential Nursing Care for Children and Young People*, but at what age does a child become a young person? It could be suggested that a child becomes a young person when it suits society to refer to him in that way. At risk of being contentious, it would feel wrong to give contraception to a child but would probably be acceptable to a young person.

Is there a different definition or concept of childhood that is culturally biased? The answer to this is probably yes and some examples of differing approaches to childhood will be explored below, with a consideration of some of the cultural definitions of childhood that may be familiar. Cultural constructions of childhood are drawn together briefly in several textbooks of children's nursing (Sidey and Widdas 2005). The suggestion is that childhood is both historically and culturally dynamic and at any time or place, childhood can be conceptualised in a different way. This is not as complicated as it first seems. Let's take the example of smacking as a punishment. In England, the law still allows for physical chastisement of children by their parents, however, in Scotland, *any* form of physical punishment is not allowed under law. Both time and distance are factors in this case. In the recent past physical punishment was being given out in schools by teachers in the form of either the cane or, in some cases, the edge of a rule. This is not meant to be in support of the action but merely to identify how times change. Not all countries have the same legislation and with an increasingly multicultural population, it can be found that there are differences in the approaches taken by different families and, also, with different generations within those families.

The International Labour Organisation (ILO) estimates that 215 million children work either part or full time (**http://www.ilo.org/global/topics/child-labour/lang-en/index.htm** accessed 29th April 2012). The majority of children involved in child labour are from low-income countries and, in these countries, there is a higher proportion of children not in primary education. One of the reasons given for this is that children are involved in working to bring income to the family (Giddens 2009).

The centrality and importance of children within modern western culture is seen in the way that children are often celebrated and shown by celebrities, for instance, the notorious episode in which singer Michael Jackson held his child over the balcony. It is possible that what Michael Jackson was trying to demonstrate will never be known, but to the casual observer he seemed to be 'showing off' his child. More recently, the children of sports or pop stars are often seen with their parents at high-profile events. It is important to ask the question as to the position of children in situations such as these and also to consider the rights of the child to privacy.

HISTORY OF CHILDHOOD AS A CULTURAL CONSTRUCT

Cunningham (2006) provides a thorough and entertaining description of the development of childhood over the last 1000 years. Alongside the history of childhood, the development of legislation related to children should also be considered. Philippe Aries (1962) provided an earlier history of the evolution of family life and how children are viewed. Although not without his critics, this book has remained a classic. In the chapter considering child development, there was the beginning of the view of different approaches to the study of child development and also, within that, we were able to see that childhood is invariably viewed with a contemporary lens (see later). What is learnt from looking at the child, and childhood in history, is that the improvement in both national and personal wealth is often reflected in the status of children. It was mentioned earlier in the chapter that time has an influence on culture and that what was acceptable several years ago may not be acceptable now. Corporal punishment used to be an acceptable way of dealing out discipline to children in schools; this is no longer acceptable within the United Kingdom. Another aspect of changing approaches to childcare can be seen in the stories that are told to children. Consider the tale of Struwvelpeter by Heinrich Hoffman.

The Story of Little Suck-a-Thumb

One day, Mamma said, 'Conrad dear,
I must go out and leave you here.
But mind now, Conrad, what I say,
Don't suck your thumb while I'm away.
The great tall tailor always comes
To little boys that suck their thumbs.
And ere they dream what he's about
He takes his great sharp scissors out
And cuts their thumbs clean off – and then
You know, they never grow again.'

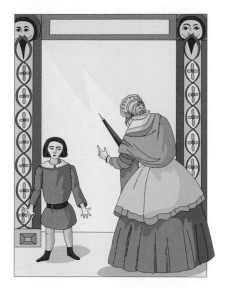

Mamma had scarcely turn'd her back,
The thumb was in, alack! alack!

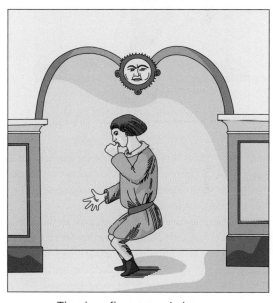

The door flew open, in he ran,
The great, long, red-legged scissorman.
Oh! Children, see! the tailors come
And caught our little Suck-a-Thumb.

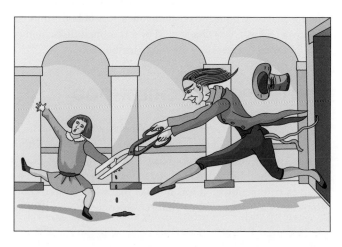

Snip! Snap! Snip! the scissors go;
And Conrad cries out – Oh! Oh! Oh!
Snip! Snap! Snip! They go so fast;
that both his thumbs are off at last.
Mamma comes home; there Conrad stands,
And looks quite sad, and shows his hands –
'Ah!' said Mamma, 'I knew he'd come
To naughty little Suck-a-Thumb.'

A cautionary tale of this nature would be frowned on in contemporary western culture; however, so-called fairy stories were often written to dissuade children from engaging in practices that were eschewed by parents.

Another aspect to consider is the relative status of boys and girls within a culture. The National Health Service (NHS) and legislation declares that equality of opportunity is central. It is not many years ago that this was not the case; some would argue that this is still not the case. Boys were sent away to boarding school or went to work with their fathers, while their sisters stayed at home and learnt how to manage a household. Of course, within the differing structures over the centuries, where the United Kingdom went from a feudal to an industrial society, how this worked in practice has changed. The point to bear in mind is that over time, the position and status of both children, and boys and girls has changed. (For a thorough discussion of class and society access any sociology textbook.)

CONTEMPORARY CHILDHOOD

While Cunningham considered childhood within a historical context, Layard and Dunn (2009) looked at childhood within a more contemporary frame. What is clear however, from this is that childhood is a dynamic state and many parents can be heard to comment that 'it was not like that when I was a child'. Brooks (2006) spoke to nine children in contemporary Britain

to give a view of how children are today in the British culture. This book is recommended to give an insight into child culture in Britain today.

United Nations Convention on the Rights of the Child (UNCRC)

The UNCRC was adopted by the United Nations General Assembly on 20 November 1989 and came into force on 2 September 1990. The key provisions covered in the convention can be broadly summarised within four categories:

- survival rights
- development rights
- protection rights
- participation rights.

In all, there are 54 articles that state parties are expected to incorporate within their own legal frameworks. The UNCRC was not ratified by the United Kingdom Government until 16 December 1991.

Importantly, Article 1 provides a definition of the child:

For the purposes of the present convention, a child means every human being below the age of eighteen years unless, under the law applicable to the child, majority is attained earlier.

The UNCRC gives a clear cross-cultural view on the definition of a child. This is irrespective of local descriptors such as 'young people', 'young adults' or 'adolescents'.

ACTIVITY 4.3

Consider your own definition of a child.

How would you define childhood?

How do We Look at Culture in the Caring Environment?

When considering a child or family's culture we often put people into categories by asking a number of questions; these usually include asking which religion people follow, what their ethnicity is and generally occupation (or at least we do with adults). The final question often gives an idea of the social class of the individual, although this is not always the case. It is useful to spend a little time considering these three questions and asking if they give a clear indication of culture, or at least some guidance.

Religion

Religion has been interwoven throughout the history of humankind and archaeologists have identified 'religious practice' as early as 10,000 years ago. What do we mean by religion ?

The Oxford Online Dictionary states that religion is:

The belief in and worship of a superhuman controlling power, especially a personal God or gods. **(http://oxforddictionaries. com/definition/religion?q=religion**)

Very often there seems to be a mix up between religion, ethnicity and culture, although some would argue that religion is invariably tied to both culture and ethnicity. We would refer to a whole group of people by their religion and, while religion seems to have an impact, it certainly does not provide us with the whole story. To attribute a set of cultural values to someone because he or she is 'a Muslim' would be plain inaccurate. There are many different groups in which Islam is the predominant faith, but the culture of the people may be very different. This is also the case with people who may refer to themselves as 'Christian'. Are they Roman Catholic, or Church of England,

Greek Orthodox, Baptist, Methodist . . . the list continues. These labels do not really tell the whole picture. It would be true to say that, while being aware of the religious practices of children and their families will invariably allow the children's nurse to give optimum care to the child, it will not tell her the culture of the child.

Effects on Culture of Major World Religions

This is perhaps one area in which it is pertinent to spend some time looking at the way in which culture and religions are often confused. Thinking back to the various definitions of culture it is possible to identify how important religion is to people's culture and how great an influence religion is. Another major difficulty in identifying religious influences on nursing practice is the differences in the practice of religion between groups.

ACTIVITY 4.4 Working with families who acknowledge their religion

If the family of a child identified their religion as Christian, what would be the attributes that could be given to the family?

Could it be that they were giving the expected answer that many people in the United Kingdom would do?

What if they were considered to be 'practising' Christians? How would their answer enable the nurse to plan the family's care or would there be no difference to the care given?

Table 4.2 Selected cultural and religious influences on nursing practice

Religion	Belief	Basis for belief	Implication for practice
Jehovah's Witness	Will not accept blood transfusions	Bible Acts 15:20 and 21:25, where followers are instructed to 'abstain from…blood'	Seek alternatives to blood based products
Islam	Do not eat pork	Specifically forbidden in the Qu'ran	Ensure that alternatives to pork are available and that medicinal products do not contain pork or derivatives (e.g. dressings)
Judaism	Do not eat pork	Specifically forbidden by the Kashrut, which is a biblical set of dietary restrictions	Ensure that alternatives to pork are available and that medicinal products do not contain pork or derivatives (e.g. dressings)
Rastafarianism	Do not cut hair – the wearing of 'dreadlocks'	Leviticus 21:5 – do not cut hair. Links to the lion's mane – Lion of Judah	May prove troublesome when infestations are suspected – great respect needed
Hinduism	Vegetarianism is common and many will not eat beef or pork	Vegetarianism is regarded as a high level of spirituality	Care should be taken to be clear what diet the person is following – make no assumptions
Buddhism	Some are strictly vegetarian, refusing any product containing or produced using animals	The first precept is 'I undertake the precept of refraining from taking life' but not all schools of Buddhism take this view	Care should be taken to ascertain what the dietary beliefs of the individual are

Taking this one step further, consider that the child became quite ill. What if both parents were insistent that no medical intervention would be welcome and they were going to rely on the benefits of prayer: would the answer that was given earlier take on a different significance? This question is in some ways impossible to answer, but in considering the possibilities the ability to begin to question the importance of religion and, in turn, culture on the care that is given needs to be recognised by the nurse. There are many influences on how healthcare is both delivered and received within the different cultures you will come into contact with during your career as a nurse. It is not possible to list each one within the scope of this chapter, however, a selection appears in Table 4.2.

As can be seen from Table 4.2 (and these are only a sample of the many and varied religious and cultural practices), the most important aspect is that care is taken to find out what are the beliefs or practices of the individual child, young person or family. An often cited example, or dilemma, is that of the Jehovah's Witness practice of not accepting any blood products. The dilemma that is faced by health professionals is when a parent refuses consent for a child to receive a blood transfusion. Within English law, should life-saving treatment be required, the wishes of the parents can be overruled, until such time as the child reaches competency (following the Gillick competence/Macpherson guidance) and can make the decision for himself. This in itself poses so many questions that will be dealt with in more depth in other chapters in this volume. Is it for the nurse to question the beliefs of the parents or is the role of the nurse to understand the reasons behind the belief? The development of a 'cultural reference manual' would help to answer many of these questions, and the benefit will be that it can be added to over time (see later in the chapter).

Other Cultural Practices

There are many arguments that have been rehearsed about whether humans are designed to eat meat or not. There are other aspects to choice of diet, choice of clothing, the way in which people choose to live, that may or may not be culturally defined:

- How far do definitions of culture allow nurses to go?
- What about vegetarianism?
- Is this cultural or could it be called a lifestyle choice?

Bronfenbrenner's ecological model gives some insight into the influences on children as they are growing up and perhaps this is a good way to look at why choices are made. As can be seen from the model (see Chapter 2) the child is seen to be directly influenced by her immediate family and moving away this other influences, however, the prime influence will always be the child's immediate family. Children tend not to grow up in isolation and are usually part of both an immediate and wider family.

Ethnic Diversity

Ethnicity is, again, not the whole picture. Often asking to record a child or family's ethnicity is required for statistical purposes.

VOICES 4.2

I remember that once I asked the father of a newborn baby how he would describe his ethnicity – he answered, somewhat surprisingly 'human'. Was this a misunderstanding of my question or was he trying to make a point? The family actually came from South Africa and I was required to collect this information for statistical purposes.

Ethnicity is generally accepted as being related to where an individual comes from, their country of birth. The NHS generally asks for a patient's country of origin and their colour. Giddens (2009) states that ethnicity 'refers to the cultural practices and outlooks of a given community which sets them apart from others'. This immediately leads to the question of how culture and ethnicity are seen as separate from this point of view. In fact, this reinforces the multifactorial nature of culture. A clearer picture can be gained by asking the purpose of collecting the information. The NHS collects ethnicity data in order to provide figures for national statistics; this should enable the nurse to provide culturally appropriate care.

It is important that ethnic data are collected and recorded, but to suggest that this then completely reflects the individual's cultural background would only form part of the picture. Many individuals are closely connected to their ethnicity as can be seen from the practices of people who have lived in other countries for all their life. St Patrick's Day parades in the United States, especially in New York, are examples of Irish heritage being celebrated by people who may never have even set foot on Irish soil.

One of the most striking aspects of contemporary society is that, although ethnicity may be fixed, it is very difficult to be a 'black African' when in fact you are 'white British': culture is more fluid. Globalisation, made possible by the communication revolution, enables all people to be exposed to all cultures, whichever ethnic group they come from. Take as an example the habit of young people to wear their trousers low, *gangsta* style. This has been taken from the prison culture of the United States where belts are removed from prison inmates, consequently, their trousers do not stay up. Many of the young men dressing in this way will never see the inside of an American prison, let alone have any ethnic similarities with the prison inmates. Although a simple example, it does help to give an insight into the potential effects of globalisation.

Social Class

Even within what may be thought of as a distinct culture there are many differences. We all move in different social circles, although it could be argued that with current technology and access to all aspects of people's lives through media publications, there are very few closed doors. We are fascinated by the way in which other people live their lives and through social media such as Facebook,© we are able to share, albeit vicariously, in those lives. Reality television allows access to all sorts of cultures and recent examples include *The only way is Essex*, *My big fat gypsy wedding* and *Made in Chelsea*. These productions afforded an insight into what for many of us may have been another world or, in the terms considered here, another culture.

Part of a lecturer's role when training as a health visitor (specialist public health nurse – health visiting) on a course shared with social workers was to ensure knowledge of different lifestyles was explored. *EastEnders* became required viewing for the social workers due to the issues that were being dealt with on a regular basis. Interestingly, over recent years there has been no need to view soaps, as the plethora of reality television shows has more than helped to expand the potential knowledge gap of the range of cultures in the United Kingdom.

One practical consideration is how social class is measured. It is surprising when colleagues are reluctant to ask parents' employment when admitting a child. When the practice was challenged, the rationale was that it was rude and intrusive. When the Black Report was published in 1980 (Townsend and Davidson 1982), class-based health inequalities were highlighted for the first time. The report showed that although Britain was a relatively wealthy country, there were still major disparities in health between the richest and the poorest. The report showed that people from higher socioeconomic groups are taller, stronger, experience better health and live longer. An updated report in the 1990s repeated the findings and also showed that the situation had not improved (Acheson 1998) and there has been no real change up to the present day.

It is important to consider the impact that social class has on health and even a brief review of the two reports just mentioned will confirm this. More recently, the Marmot Review was published (2010). Sir Michael Marmot was commissioned in 2008 by the Secretary of State for Health to investigate the most effective evidence-based strategies for reducing health inequalities in England. The second key message from the review follows:

> There is a social gradient in health – the lower a person's social position, the worse his or her health. Action should focus on reducing the gradient in health. (Marmot Review 2010, page 15)

At this point it is worth mentioning the political implications. The Black Report was commissioned by the Labour administration, but was published under a Conservative government. Giddens (2009) comments that the conservative government was dismissive of the findings. The Marmot Review was commissioned by a Labour government and published in February 2010; the coalition government came into power in May 2010. How historians view how this government tackles this issue will be of interest. It is important to develop a questioning approach to all aspects of life and for nurses to have a political awareness, as this will enhance the care given to patients.

Sex

What about the impact of sex in culture? Many cultures hold boys in higher regard than girls, for instance, the single-child policy that was established in China by Deng Xiaoping in 1979. The purpose of the policy was to limit population growth at a time when China's population was quickly outgrowing available resources. An analysis of data from 2005 by Zhu et al. (2009) showed that, in China, the number of males far exceeded that of females. Using an outcome measure known as the 'sex ratio', which means number of males per 100 females, it was found that there were between 108 and 124 males per 100 females (depending on age range).

The study found that this was mainly due to selective abortion of female foetuses. While this appears to be a fairly extreme example, there are other anecdotal consequences of this policy. With the 'one-child policy' comes a reported rise in the numbers of elderly people with no one to care for them. Chinese culture has long enjoyed a reputation for venerating old age, but this now seems to be changing. This example is given to show the impact that sex preference can have. Some cultures do indeed have preferences where care is involved and these should be respected where possible.

EFFECT OF CULTURE ON HEALTH

Browne (2005) provides a very clear diagram illustrating the cultural and material influences on health (Figure 4.1).

It can be seen from Figure 4.1 that there are many influences on the health of children, young people and families, and other chapters in this volume will provide further insight into this. There must be a point to understanding all the different cultures that surround individuals in society. It has been commented that the United Kingdom is one of the most culturally diverse countries in the world; if this is the case, what, then, are the implications for the care that is given within the different areas of practice? Whether in the hospital or community setting, it is important that the nurse understands the cultural background of the child, young person and family they come into contact with. By beginning to understand the many influences on or causes of ill health from the perspective of the child and family, there is more chance of culturally competent and effective care being given.

Dent and Stewart (2000) comment that there are not only differences between two different cultures; there are also differences *within* cultures. It is not enough to have a broad understanding of the different cultures; it is also important that there is a close understanding of the individual cultural needs of the child and family.

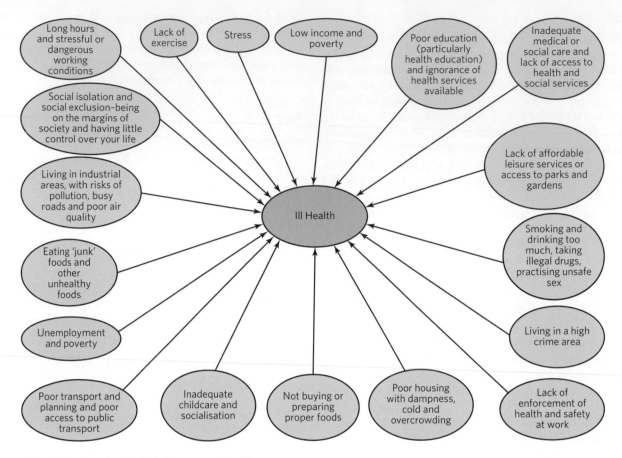

Figure 4.1 Cultural and material influences on health
Source: Browne (2005)

EXPLORATION OF TERMS

Cultural Competency

Cultural competence can be described as a professional or organisation's ability to work across a number of different cultural groups. Klossner and Hatfield (2006) suggest that in order to develop cultural competency the nurse should first learn to recognise his or her own cultural influences. By doing this the nurse will then be more able to recognise and accept the different (or indeed similar) aspects of another person's culture and be able to work effectively with Melena and her parents.

Cultural Identity

So how does the nurse ensure that a patient is able to maintain his cultural identity within the care environment? It is, of course, important to have an understanding of what a cultural identity is. In some ways, it could be simply described as something about the individual that demonstrates that he or she is part of a particular culture. It has been suggested that globalisation has made the issue of cultural identity less important; however, the Brandt Report (1980) declared that 'cultural identity gives people dignity' and, within the care environment, dignity is one of the measures of effective care. While the nurse may not understand 'cao gio', a form of dermabrasive therapy, there is a

need to maintain anti-discriminatory practice when exploring the practice and how it may affect Melena's recovery.

Cultural Integrity

So, having considered many of the definitions of and meanings of culture, aspects of the culture and how these affect our care of children and young people need to be fully understood. Cultural integrity is often seen as an important aspect of the care that is given by nurses, but are the implications of this clearly understood? The notion of cultural integrity means maintaining the culture of the person throughout the episode of care. It is not merely an acknowledgement of the person's culture but a conscious effort to enable the person to feel that her culture remains central to her care. For some, being able to celebrate or engage in activities that are part of their culture would be seen as 'cultural integrity'. For others, it may mean being able to dress in such a way as to maintain their cultural identity. While Melena is on the ward it is important to offer diet and treatment that is not in conflict with any cultural or religious beliefs.

Diversity

Diversity refers to the differing experiences of all people, individuals and groups and, within the context of healthcare, it has the added dimension of acknowledging these differences. Cultural differences in terms of expression of emotion are fairly well documented and the British have often been described as possessing a 'stiff upper lip' and suppressing their emotions. Differences have also been noted between male and female within British culture. Other cultures have been noted to be more expressive in their emotions.

There is, however, a theory of universality of expression and, in general, it is agreed that facial expression reflects the emotion of the individual. This appears to be the case across all cultures. The theory was first put forward by Charles Darwin (1872) and has been further explored and is supported by Joshua Susskind et al. (2008). Darwin suggested that facial expressions were useful physiological reactions. The six major emotions are anger, fear, disgust, happiness, surprise and sadness (see Figure 4.2). Susskind et al. confirmed that expressions of these emotions were similar across cultures. However, the nurse needs to listen to Melena's parents about whether she is in pain.

Benedict (2005), along with Mead (1975), observed that different patterns of culture would 'mould a child from the moment of his birth; the customs into which he is born shape his experience and behaviour'. This illustrates some of the contentions that

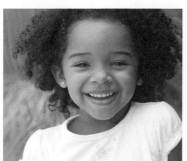
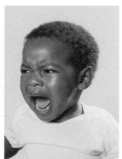
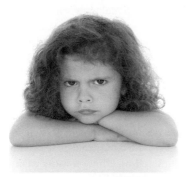
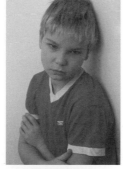
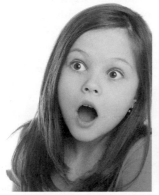
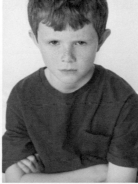

Figure 4.2 Children's expressions

ACTIVITY 4.5

Start to develop a 'cultural reference manual'. In it, you could:

- include descriptions of the cultures you come into contact with
- describe the different views on health, illness, diet and faith
- include links to websites with supporting information.

exist between the nature and nurture debate. Mead did accept that the temperament of the child may be related to genetics, however, the strongest link is with the cultural context in which the child is raised.

CULTURALLY COMPETENT CARE

Nurses are urged to consider cultural care preservation whereby care is organised in such a way as to allow patients to continue to carry out their distinct cultural practices. When nursing Melena, this may mean allowing the parents space to continue with their family routines. This is where there may be major problems: although patient-centred care is often proposed, there are still ward routines, mealtimes to be adhered to, consultant ward rounds and so on.

ACTIVITY 4.6

Consider the 'routine' of your most recent inpatient ward, for example, who decided where and when meals were served?

Cultural Views on Health

A definition of health is put forward in this book. The World Health Organization's is perhaps the most widely quoted definition and one that perhaps binds many healthcare systems. This definition moved away from our biomedical definition of health and acknowledged the social and cultural aspects of health. As can be seen from the short case study, treatments for disease in some cultures often represent a view of health and illness, rather than the altered physiology of the body due to the diseases.

Some authors argue that a cultural approach to the understanding of health and illness is essential if health promotion and disease prevention activities are to be effective.

Construal

A construal is defined as 'the way in which people perceive, comprehend and interpret the social world' (Aronson et al. 2010, page 36).

Naive realism

It is often commented that particular cultural groups are more 'outgoing' than others. For instance, people from North America will often strike up a conversation with a stranger on a train, but when they attempt this in England they may be greeted with silence. It was once commented about practice as a health visitor that offering to shake hands with all the clients, including children, was a 'man thing'.

ACTIVITY 4.7

Consider your own forms of greeting. Are these governed by your cultural background, your race or your sex?

Note that there is a difference between 'sex' and 'gender'. Sex is determined biologically and gender is often seen as a social construct. Put another way – sex is male or female, whereas gender is masculine or feminine.

Cultural Aspects of Growing Up

Childhood has been divided up by age and stage by many writers and researchers over the years. Let us consider puberty for a moment. It has been suggested that the 'attractiveness ideal' for a male is muscular and for a female it is ultra slim. During puberty, adipose tissue is laid down that moves away from the cultural ideal of 'attractiveness', thus leading to increased body dissatisfaction. There are many questions that can be asked at this point – what determines the 'attractiveness ideal', for instance – while it is not the place to expand on this. It is, however, important to begin to understand why some young people may feel pressured into taking health risks.

Erikson discussed role confusion and although he stated that identity was important throughout development, it was during adolescence that the most difficulties could be expected. As far back as the time of Plato and even that of Shakespeare, 'Sturm und Drang' has been linked to adolescence. We provide a more full discussion about the importance and challenges of the transfer of care between paediatric and adult services later. In this chapter, some time will be spent looking at the importance of culture in the adolescent period.

Coleman and Hagell (2007) discuss the issue of resilience and risk in adolescence and ask whether there are cultural or sex differences. Is there a *culture* among boys that leads them to take more risks or is it an expectation?

RESEARCH NOTE 4.1 Adolescent rites of passage

The Amish community who live mainly in Pennsylvania have a term for the period in which teens are 'set loose'. The term *rumspringa* literally means 'running around'. Contrary to popular belief, this period is not one of wild hedonistic partying as is sometimes portrayed in films and some articles. Many Amish youth live at home during this time, however, they are not yet full members of the Amish church and are not fully subject to the rules of the church. This is also a time of finding a partner and *rumspringa* finishes at marriage. Parents hope their children will live a 'moral' life and would wish their children to follow this path.

Some indigenous cultures mark the passage from child to adult by what we may consider barbaric means. East African herding tribes, for instance, will shave the young man's head and cut deep incisions in the skin reaching from ear to ear.

In South America, young men are laid over a red ant's hill and allowed to be bitten many times – a real man will not cry out.

This makes *rumspringa* seem quite tame by comparison and the attainment of a driver's licence as a rite of passage does not make the same impression.

NURSING ATTITUDES TO DIFFERENT CULTURES

Research into the different practices between cultures and the nursing attitude shows that we are still coming to terms with the relatively free movements of peoples around the world.

In 1993 Action for Sick Children conducted a study that explored the difficulties encountered by ethnic minority families when a child was admitted to hospital (see Table 4.3). The research was carried out by interviewing 77 families in Bristol, Birmingham and London.

RESEARCH NOTE 4.2 Providing transcultural care to children and parents: an exploratory study from Italy (Festini et al. 2009)

In a study looking at nurses' attitudes to transcultural care, Festini et al. (2009) found that effective communication was the most important aspect of providing culturally competent care. They identified language as a means of communication to be of the utmost importance to an effective nurse–patient relationship. This may seem to be stating the obvious but it will become increasingly evident as a nurse that communication will be a central role. Interestingly, Festini et al., while discussing immigration to Italy from countries including China, North Africa and eastern Europe, could also be referring to the United Kingdom.

Table 4.3 Summary of the findings from Action for Sick Children

The interviews showed that many families felt that their cultural needs were not always considered. The following were raised as areas of concern:
- information giving
- food
- facilities for parents
- facilities for religious observance
- staff attitudes
- availability of interpreters
- awareness of the need for multicultural play
- ignorance of naming systems
- care and services for children with blood disorders, such as sickle cell disease and thalassaemia

Source: Action for Sick Children (1993)

While it is acknowledged that this research was published some time ago, it serves as a useful guide as to what areas should be considered by the nurse when looking at culturally competent and considerate care. Writing in 1999, Whiting provides a very thoughtful consideration of caring for children of differing cultures.

Holistic Care

Holistic care is commonly accepted as treating or caring for the person as a 'whole' or 'complete' person and not as a distinct diagnosis or 'part'. There are many cultural implications of this point of view and it may be worth considering these briefly. It is important that all aspects of a child or young person's background are taken into consideration. Look back at the cultural and material influences on ill health. An individual's ethnicity may be one aspect, but this cannot be taken in isolation. This is really what is at the heart of holistic assessment and holistic care. Leininger also commented when defining culture that it was the shared 'beliefs, values and life-ways' of a particular group that made up a cultural identity. He further commented that these are also passed through the generations, giving a clear insight into the importance and centrality of the family.

When considering the cultural aspects of children such as Melena and their families, the nurse should seek to provide holistic care and, in order for this to be successful, it is important that a holistic assessment is carried out. As nurses caring for children and young people, there is a need to become familiar with asking a whole host of questions and of seeking a 'picture' of the patients. Very often, there are two questions that are asked and these tend to reflect the patients' culture: these are what their 'religion' and their 'ethnicity' are. It is important now to ask the question of whether this really reflects an individual's culture.

This exercise gives a clear insight into the complexity of culture and that it is not just a matter of ethnicity or religion, although these will undoubtedly have a bearing on culture. There will be demographic information that is required to be collected, but neither does this give the full picture.

Culturally Safe Practice

This is perhaps the most difficult aspect when considering culture, as it is possible to offer culturally unsafe care. By causing offence to Melena's family, the whole care experience could be compromised. It is important that nurses practise in such a way that does not compromise the culture of either the patient or the nurse. By understanding the culture of the patient, it is always possible to take reasonable measures to ensure that respect is afforded to cultural wishes. It is common practice to make a fuss of a child if they happen to celebrate a birthday when they are on the ward. Jehovah's Witnesses do not celebrate birthdays and would find this culturally unacceptable if their child were exposed to such a celebration. It is important to respect such families' wishes where possible. Referring back to the examples of religious and cultural influences on nursing practices, the nurse should be familiar with the practices of his or her patients. A very good resource is produced by Jogee (2004).

ACTIVITY 4.8 Sensitivity of assessment document to the patient's culture

Take an assessment document – a nursing admission form or whatever is used on the ward or area that is your current placement.

Identify all the questions and pieces of information that may give a clue to the patient's culture.

CASE STUDY REVIEW 4.1

Holistic nursing care for Melena needs to focus on the fever first and investigating the history of being unwell for several days.

However, as the family comes from a Southeast Asian culture, where elements of health belief may be different, it is important to ensure the nursing practice is supportive and culturally sensitive. Following a full assessment including questions about nationality, religion and parental occupation, the nurse can offer appropriate interventions including diet. The nurse needs to discuss the dermabrasive therapy and explore with Melena's father the safe way of undertaking the process.

SUMMARY OF KEY LEARNING

The United Kingdom is becoming increasingly multicultural and as a nurse working with children, young people and their families, it is vital that an understanding of the cultural factors is applied to practice. I hope that this chapter has given an insight into the development and complexities of culture and also an interest in seeking to find out more about the cultures and backgrounds of the people for whom we provide care.

FURTHER RESOURCES

Culturally competent care policy and guidance: **http://www.clusterweb.org.uk/UserFiles/CW/File/Childrens_Services/Specialist_Children/Culturally_Competent-19Dec07.pdf**

Caring for unaccompanied asylum-seeking children and young people, Eileen Fursland, BAAF, 2007.

Children's views on adoption, Morgan, CSCI, 2006.

Cultural diversity guide, Meridian Broadcasting, 2001.

Cultural competence in family support, a toolkit for working with black, minority ethnic and faith families, Husain, National Family & Parenting Institute, 2005.

Culturally competent care, a good practice guide for care management, Bijay Minhas and Navdeep Kaur, KCC, 2002.

Effective fostering panels, guidance on regulations, process and good practice in fostering panels in England, BAAF, 2007.

Learning difficulties and ethnicity, a framework for action, DoH, 2004.

Life story work, a practical guide to helping children understand their past, Ryan and Walker, BAAF, 2007.

Placements, decisions & reviews, Morgan, CSCI, 2006.

Promoting equality: challenging discrimination, Thompson, 2003.

Safeguarding children from abuse linked to a belief in spirit possession, every child matters, DCSF, 2007. **http//www.teachernet.gov.uk/publications**

Stopping places, a gypsy history of south London & Kent, Evans, 2004.

The colour of difference: the adoptee's experience of transracial adoption, Armstrong and Beveridge, ACWA conference paper, 2002.

Working with black children and adolescents in need, Ravinder Barn, BAAF, 1999.

ANSWERS TO ACTIVITIES

ACTIVITY 4.1 Provide a definition of culture

Spend a few moments thinking about your own culture.

What makes you different from your neighbour or peer?

Following on from this – what difference does this difference make?

- What language do you speak (usually English in the UK)?
- What religion (usually either C of E or none)?

- What sexual orientation are you (usually heterosexual)?
- What makes people different is family relationships, family belief, about health education and religion.
- Difference of life experiences related to culture need to be acknowledged by the nurse for herself so that caring for children from a different culture need an awareness of the different needs that might be required.

ACTIVITY 4.2

The definitions just given are taken from nurse theorists and describe a number of views of culture. How far do these definitions resonate with your own view of culture?

- Reflect on your answer compared to the description given.

ACTIVITY 4.3

Consider your own definition of a child.

- Is this an individual under 18 years of age?
- Or a child or young person who has no responsibility?

How would you define childhood?

- A society constructed time where children are protected before adulthood.

ACTIVITY 4.4 Working with families who acknowledge their religion

If the family of a child identified their religion as Christian, what would be the attributes that could be given to the family?

The term 'Christian' describes association with Christianity or is seen by the family as all that is noble, good and Christ-like. It is also used as a label to identify people who associate with the cultural aspects of Christianity, irrespective of personal religious beliefs or practices.

Could it be that they were giving the expected answer that many people in the United Kingdom would do?

What if they were considered to be 'practising' Christians? Practising Christians may also:

- have a Bible or read one
- pray on various occasions
- attend a Christian church (such as Catholic or Protestant)
- if they attend a Mormon temple (also called Latter-Day Saints) and believe in the book of Mormon, they are not practising Christians, they are practising Mormons or practising Latter-Day Saints, depending on their preference
- they are baptised (either immersion or sprinkling)
- they may have taken the Holy Sacrament, sometimes called the Lord's Supper. In Catholicism, it is called Mass.

How would their answer enable the nurse to plan the family's care or would there be no difference to the care given?

All nursing care should be culturally or religiously sensitive and therefore the only difference in care should be an acknowledgement of the specific needs of the child's culture or religion in regards to diet or treatment. This should wherever possible be negotiated with the child and her family.

ACTIVITY 4.5

Start to develop a 'cultural reference manual'. In it, you could:

- include descriptions of the cultures you come into contact with
- describe the different views on health, illness, diet and faith
- include links to websites with supporting information.

Use a notebook to reflect on the experience you have with families and use the information to develop your practice.

ACTIVITY 4.6

Consider the 'routine' of your most recent inpatient ward, for example, who decided where and when meals were served?

Usually it is the kitchen and catering staff who decide when food is served and where.

ACTIVITY 4.7

Consider your own forms of greeting. Are these governed by your cultural background, your race or your sex?

Is it 'hello' or 'hi'? Sometimes we greet people differently if they are men or women, sometimes a hug or a kiss or a shake of the hands.

What is your greeting on the ward; make sure that you say 'hello' to the child or young person as well as the parents.

SELECTED REFERENCES

Acheson, D. (1998) *Independent inquiry into inequalities in health*. Stationery Office: London.

Aries, P. (1962) *Centuries of childhood: a social history of family life*. Vintage Books: New York.

Aronson, E., Wilson, T.D. and Akert, R.M. (2010) *Social psychology*, 7th edn. Pearson: Boston, MA.

Ball, J.W. and Bindler, R.C. (2006) *Child health nursing partnership with children and families*. Pearson-Prentice-Hall: Boston, MA.

Benedict, R. (2005) *Patterns of culture*. Mariner Books: New York.

Coleman, J. and Hagell, A. (eds) (2007) *Adolescence, risk and resilience: against the odds*. John Wiley & Sons: Chichester.

Cunningham, H. (2006) *The invention of childhood*. BBC Books: London.

Darwin, C. (1872) *The expression of emotions in man and animals*. Murray: London.

Dawkins, R. (2006) *The selfish gene*, 30th anniversary edn. Oxford University Press: New York.

Dent, A. and Stewart, A. (2000) *Sudden death in childhood: support for the bereaved family*. Butterworth: Edinburgh.

Festini, F., Focardi, S., Bisogni, S., Mannini, C. and Neri, S. (2009) Providing transcultural to children and parents: an exploratory study from Italy. *Journal of Nursing Scholarship*, 41(2), 220–227.

Giddens, A. (2009) *Sociology*, 6th edn. Polity Press: Cambridge.

Helman, C. (2000) *Health, culture and illness*. Butterworth Heinemann: Oxford.

Independent Commission on International Development Issues, Brandt Commission (1980) *North–south: a program for survival*. MIT Press: Cambridge, MA.

Jogee, M. (2004) *Religions and cultures: a guide to beliefs, customs and diversity for health and social care services*, 6th edn. R & C Publications: Burntisland.

Klossner, N.J. and Hatfield, N. (2006) *Introductory maternity and pediatric nursing*. Lippincott: Philadelphia.

McGee, P. (1992) *Teaching transcultural care*. Chapman & Hall: London.

Murphy, K. and McLeod-Clark, J.M. (1993) Nurses' experiences of caring for ethnic minority clients. *Journal of Advanced Nursing*, 18(3), 442–450.

Naidoo, J. and Wills, J. (eds) (2008) *Health studies. An introduction*. Palgrave-Macmillan: Basingstoke.

Nursing and Midwifery Council (NMC) (2008) *The code*. NMC: London.

Ridley, M. (2004) *Nature via nurture*. Harper Perennial: London.

Sidey, A. and Widdas, D. (2005) *Textbook of community children's nursing*, 2nd edn. Elsevier: Edinburgh.

Susskind, J.M., Lee, D.H., Cusi, A., Feiman, R., Grabski, W. and Anderson, A.K. (2008) Expressing fear enhances sensory acquisition. *Nature Neuroscience*, 11, 843–850.

Townsend, P. and Davidson, N. (1982) *Inequalities in health: the Black Report*. Penguin: London.

Turnball, C.M. (1961) Some observations concerning the experiences and behaviour of the BaMbuti Pygmies. *American Journal of Psychology*, 74(2), 304–308.

Whiting, L. (1999) Caring for children of different cultures. *Journal of Child Health Care*, 3(4), 33–38.

Zhu, W.X., Lu, L. and Hesketh, T. (2009) China's excess males, sex selective abortion, and one child policy: analysis of data from 2005 national intercensus survey. *BMJ*.

CHAPTER 5
Safeguarding Children and Young People

Steven Walker

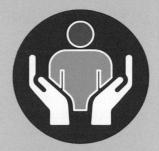
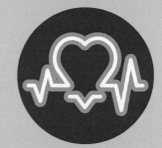
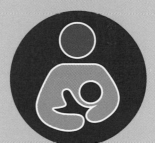

LEARNING OUTCOMES

On completion of this chapter, the reader will be able to:

- Describe risk and resilience factors in children and young people.
- Identify the signs, symptoms and effects of abuse.
- Understand how the interprofessional team can use protocols and policies related to children and young people at risk.
- Reflect on issues of confidentiality in regards to safeguarding children and young people.

TALKING POINT

'Recorded offences of gross indecency with a child more than doubled between 1985–2001 but convictions against perpetrators actually fell from 42 per cent to 19 per cent. Fewer than one in fifty sexual offences results in a conviction. In 2007–08 there were 20,000 recorded sex offences against children.' NSPCC (2009).

INTRODUCTION

In Britain, at least one child dies each week as a result of adult cruelty and it has been estimated that about 5000 minors are involved in prostitution in Britain at any one time. Nearly 23,000 children were being looked after by local authorities for the year ending 2007. About 60 per cent of these children had been abused or neglected with a further 10 per cent coming from 'dysfunctional families' (ONS 2008). In 2007 there were over 300,000 children in need in England. Of these, 69,100 were looked after in state care while the rest were in families or living independently. One quarter of all rape victims are children and 75 per cent of sexually abused children do not tell anyone at the time. Each year about 30,000 children are on child protection registers. Children with learning disabilities are at a greater risk of experiencing all forms of abuse and neglect.

The following scenario examines the skills that could be used when developing a safeguarding children plan and reviewing its progress. As a nurse, you have been requested to work jointly in a risky situation in which the mother is finding it difficult to trust anyone.

CASE STUDY 5.1 Ms B and her four children

Ms B is a depressed young Bangladeshi Muslim woman with three children under 5 years of age exhibiting disturbed behaviour and a 10-year-old at primary school with poor attendance. The family has experienced severe trauma in recent years. Her partner, who is 10 years her senior, has been involved with drug and alcohol abuse and is suspected of abusing her. She is terrified her children will be removed because she is unable to care for them properly or protect them from the violence of her partner. Ms B is hostile to social workers, health visitors and teachers who have expressed concerns about the welfare of all four children. She feels persecuted, does not want any involvement and resents any interference in her life. See Table 5.1 for a potential plan of safeguarding action for the family.

ACTIVITY 5.1

Together with a colleague, consider the case illustration and map out an action plan, including alternatives and the reasons for them.

THEORIES OF CHILD ABUSE

Nurses have instinctively been conditioned to link the words abuse with adults' behaviour towards children, yet recent research evidence has exposed another aspect of abuse that is beginning to impact on how we perceive our society and culture. Children under 18 years of age are now increasing in the numbers recorded as abusing other children physically, sexually and emotionally.

Solid data about the prevalence of child abuse are difficult to obtain but a reliable indication is that about 750,000 children will have been abused by the time they reach 18 years of age, with 400,000 having been sexually abused (Cawson et al. 2000). This NSPCC research suggests that about 30 per cent of girls have been sexually abused and about 15 per cent of boys. Reductions in the length of time children spend with their names on child protection databases seem to imply that child abuse is decreasing – which is not the case, rather they illustrate the shorter time spent on records consistent with the reported increase in deregistrations. In other words, the government target for shorter registration periods may be being achieved, but the consequence is that risk is being hidden.

The problem with child abuse is the often hidden nature and secrecy surrounding it combined with societal ambiguity about state intervention in family life. Crude structural and organisational changes to the way in which child protection services are delivered are the institutional knee-jerk response to

---

Table 5.1 Potential safeguarding plan summary for the B family

For mum	For dad	For the children
Ms B to attend domestic violence survivors' group	Partner to attend anger management course	Younger children to attend nursery daily
Ms B to play with the younger children once a day	Partner to attend drug counselling	Ms B to play with the younger children once a day
Ms B to take 10-year-old to school		Ms B to take 10-year-old to school
Family network to visit Ms B weekly		

RESEARCH NOTE 5.1

A growing body of research finds concordance between mothers' adult attachment and their attachment relationship with their child. It has been widely assumed that quality of the parent–child relationship is the linking mechanism – that adults who are securely attached themselves tend to provide a secure base for their children (Byng-Hall 1998). This is a strong protective factor in safeguarding assessment. It is also suggested that the relationship between the parents plays a central role in the generational transmission of working models of attachment. That relationship quality may play a causal role in affecting parenting style and children's adaptation. In other words, the family system plays a part as well as the dyadic parent–child relationship.

Extrapolating from recent research findings, some authors conclude that the transmission of attachment relationships from grandparents to parents to children is not simply a matter of parenting. When a person learns early on that he or she is worthy of love and that adults will be responsive and available in times of need, he or she is more likely to establish satisfying relationships with other people and to have the inclination and ability to work toward solving relationship problems and regulating emotions so that they do not escalate out of control (Mikulincer et al. 2002).

improving the safeguarding of children and young people in the wake of the damning Laming inquiry into the death of Baby P (DoH 2008), Victoria Climbié (DoH 2003) and the Bichard Report of the deaths of Holly Wells and Jessica Chapman (Home Office 2004). *Every child matters: change for children* (DoH 2004) established the new framework for building services around children in which previously separate services must work together in an integrated way.

Above all, these changes aimed to provide professionals with consistent ways of communicating about children's welfare. In many ways it is the most important because organisational change of itself cannot bring about shifts in entrenched attitudes, beliefs, customs and vocabulary. And despite repeated child abuse inquiries citing poor communication between agencies as one of the major reasons why children have not been properly protected, it remains difficult to get right (RCN 2007). Recent research also highlighted the paradox of the disproportionate investment in management performance recording templates, rigid timescales and IT systems resulting in a reduction in safety of systems and children rather than an increase in safety (Broadhurst and White 2009).

History of Abuse Cases

Despite the hyped publicity and modern media circus exploding around high-profile child deaths, historically, expectations of child protection staff have tended to be lower than they are nowadays. Up until 1914 around 250 children every year died in child protection cases that were known about – more perished without coming to the attention of professionals. By 1970 the number of deaths in child protection cases had shrunk but the impact of the cruel death of Maria Caldwell and the blaming of professional staff started a trend in public discourse that endures today (Munro and Calder 2005). Ironically, the better social workers have become at protecting children and preventing their deaths, the more bitter the public and political outcry

has become when this fails to happen (Ferguson 2004.) Poor interagency communication is usually cited in subsequent internal investigations and public inquiries.

Rather than trying to design ever more elaborate bureaucratic data systems, Reder and Duncan (2004) suggest that agencies need to put greater effort into understanding the psychology of communication in order to improve it. This means more than superficial and tokenistic exercises hosted by agency managers, but a fundamental reappraisal of the knowledge, values and personal beliefs held by every member of staff engaged in work with children and young people so that integrated working is actualised. The mental health and emotional wellbeing of children can be both a consequence of child abuse and a precursor. You must consider this aspect of your work in safeguarding children as much a priority as learning new procedures, computer data systems and legislative guidance.

Integrated working does not mean absence of disagreement – indeed, the evidence suggests closer proximity with other agency staff accentuates differences between professionals. But this need not be a problem, provided you work hard to appreciate each other's perspectives and not be so certain of your omnicompetence. Thinking about yourself as an equal part of an integrated system, rather than as an individual agency representative is a crucial reconceptualisation to make. Disagreement may actually be healthy and force staff to compromise or continue seeking a solution. At another level, such differences between professionals may reflect the dynamics in the family situation that produce splits. The mental health of a young person at risk of abuse can find expression in other family members through a process of identification and projection (Walker 2005).

Equally, you should be wary of rushing too quickly to agreement and consider whether the multiagency group are avoiding or denying some unanswered and complex issues because of the risk of exposing an argument. This could reflect the emotional dynamics within the family. Nurse self-awareness is one of the keys to managing the stress and strain inherent in working together to safeguard children (RCN 2007). This requires skilled and highly developed supervision skills from line managers and a willingness to expose your practice to scrutiny and to engage in reflective practice (Walker and Thurston 2006).

POLICY

Stages of the safeguarding process

It is possible to discern and identify the stages through which a safeguarding case may pass. Many cases do not pass beyond the investigation and initial assessment stage. Very few will reach the stage of legal proceedings. At each stage, the system asks whether the person has suffered, or is likely to suffer, significant harm. If the answer is yes, the case proceeds to the next stage. If no, the child or adult drops out of the system. At the same time, if the person is considered to be in extreme danger, at any stage of the process, a legal order may be requested (usually by social services from a magistrate's court) that can remove the person for a short period of time to a safer environment. The series of stages within any safeguarding system is as shown in Table 5.2.

Observation and Recognition

The Laming inquiry (DoH 2003) discovered several occasions when Victoria Climbié should have been included in the protection system but was effectively excluded by the practitioners who dealt with her. Dingwall et al. (1995) argue that there are certain belief systems that prevent practitioners from recognising the signs of abuse. The most influential of these is the rule of optimism, which leads to a belief on the part of an individual practitioner that child abuse would not happen in their class, patient list or caseload. A second factor that might hold a practitioner back from acting on a suspicion of significant harm is called cultural relativism. This is where the practitioner suspects that something is wrong, but this is excused as normal in that culture, family or community.

In Victoria Climbié's case, the poor relationship between Victoria and her great aunt was reframed as normal in West African families. At some time a threshold will be crossed when the practitioner will begin to suspect abuse and further evidence may then lead to subsequent referral. Often it is difficult for the practitioner to judge if that threshold has actually been passed, in which case it is advisable for the staff member to get help both from within her own agency and from the outside system. Paradoxically, practitioners who have had their awareness of

Table 5.2 Stages of the safeguarding process

- Observation and recognition
- Referral
- Investigation and initial assessment
- Conference
- Assessment and review conference

child abuse or elder abuse increased by study or by training can express fears that they will employ a rule of pessimism and see abuse in every person that they work with (Murphy 2003).

Referral

The referral stage is often the first stage of interagency cooperation and communication and can set the scene for the interactions that subsequently occur. Referrals can be made to social services, the NSPCC or to the police. When the referral is made a conflict of expectations sometimes arises. The referrer often comes from a non-social work agency or is sometimes a member of the family or the public talking with a nurse. Making such a referral is an unusual, often stressful event, during which they require reassurance and time to discuss their concerns. But the worker needs to elicit the maximum amount of hard information about the case in order to judge whether it is an appropriate referral or not.

Investigation and Initial Assessment

The first task of the investigation is to access as much information about that particular person and their family. Shared databases and records should always be checked. Access to education, health, and probation and police information will also be requested. Any specialist mental health involvement needs to be highlighted and investigated to ascertain the background and explanations for disturbed behaviour. In Britain, police checks reveal if any member of the household has been convicted of serious crimes against children (Schedule 1 offences). If it becomes known that the family had regular contact with any other agency relevant information from their databases would also be sought.

Most agencies have safeguards against disclosure of confidential information to third parties. However, the needs of the child, via the child protection procedures, supersede these safeguards, and relevant information is usually forthcoming. In practice, the test of relevancy and the breaking of confidentiality for some practitioner groups is still an area of some difficulty (Kearney et al. 2000). The risk of sabotaging sensitive therapeutic work addressing the child's emotional well-being, post-abuse, is balanced with the need to obtain reliable evidence to put into court. The gathering of all this information could take a substantial amount of time. There could be a considerable time delay between referral and actual investigative interview. This delay can increase anxiety in the child and the referrer (Murphy 2005).

Following the gathering of information the investigating social worker interviews sometimes jointly with the police or a nurse: the referrer; the child; the child's parents or carers; the alleged abuser; the child's brothers and sisters; any other person with relevant information to disclose. Although the interviews with relevant adults may be quite direct and detailed, the interviewers are conscious of the need to form a close working relationship or partnership with the adults who care for the child concerned. When interviewing children, great emphasis is now placed on not leading, suggesting or influencing the child's story in any way (Home Office 2001).

In British child protection systems, the medical examination commonly occurs in cases of physical and sexual abuse, and sometimes in the cases of neglect, organised and professional abuse. The child always has the right to refuse to be medically examined and the parent, in some circumstances, also has the right to refuse on their behalf. In practice, this refusal seldom occurs.

There are three reasons for the investigative medical examination:

- to inform other agencies about the likelihood of abuse having occurred
- to gather forensic evidence for use in legal proceedings
- to assess the immediate medical needs of the child or adult.

There can be significant differences between the medical examinations involved in physical and in sexual abuse. In physical abuse, the medical will frequently be undertaken by a hospital paediatrician. Signs of physical trauma can last for some considerable time but as far as forensic evidence is concerned, the medical examination needs to occur as soon after the abusive event as possible. In child sexual abuse, the examination will usually be done by a police surgeon. Forensic evidence in child sexual abuse needs to be gathered as soon as possible, often within 72 hours of the last occasion of abuse.

These investigative medical examinations have been criticised in the past for having been too intrusive (thereby re-abusing the child) and for being too inconclusive, thereby not giving the system any clear messages on which to work. However experienced practitioners can make the medical examination a non-intrusive, positive experience for the child concerned (Murphy 2005). They can, however, tend to focus on physical forensic matters and neglect the associated mental health and emotional issues.

The definition of significant harm is not precise but this can mean the term can be adapted to different circumstances. It is the harm that has to be significant, not the act that caused it. Thus, a sustained series of privations, not individually harmful as in the case of neglect over time, could amount to significant harm as far as the child's development was concerned. Not all harm will be significant, neither will significant harm in one context necessarily be significant in another. Ultimately, it is a matter for the court to determine whether the harm is significant for the particular child in question (Butler and Roberts 1997). The problem is that mental health and emotional wellbeing are difficult concepts for the criminal justice system to comprehend and measure. This is where your extra expertise and knowledge can significantly benefit the client by helping the court understand what psychological impact has occurred.

ACTIVITY 5.2

- Discuss a recent safeguarding assessment with a colleague/mentor and reflect back on how you did it. In retrospect, how do you feel your assessment went?
- Identify three areas for improvement and the means for doing so.

THE CHILDREN ACT 1989

The Children Act Report (DfES 2003) discovered that '30% of updated child protection plans were unsatisfactory . . . However all agencies accepted that they have a fundamental responsibility to ensure that children are safeguarded, and in most cases this was backed up with a firm commitment by senior managers to ensure that their agencies did so.' The DoH (2003) developed a straightforward document, 'What to do if you are worried a child is being abused', which progresses the childcare practitioner through a number of flowcharts highlighting the appropriate approach to take if you suspect abuse is occurring and how to work alongside other professionals.

Nurses have an opportunity to engage with CAMHS specialist staff who often assist with facilitative interviews as part of Section 47 assessments. This is an important role to which they can add their expertise into the process particularly with young children, traumatised children and disabled children. The Children Act aimed to consolidate a number of childcare reforms and provide a response to the evidence of failure in children's services that had been mounting in the 1980s (DHSS 1985). The Act provides the legislative foundation on which subsequent policy guidance has been built to inform planning and intervention in safeguarding children and young people. There is a specific legal requirement under the Act that different authorities and agencies work together to provide family support services with better liaison and a corporate approach.

The guidance is a key element of the Department of Health's work to support local authorities in implementing Quality Protects – the government's programme for transforming the management and delivery of children's social services. This has been incorporated into other government guidance on protecting children from harm – working together to safeguard children (DoH 1999). This has subsequently been augmented with the *Every child matters* (DfES 2003) programme of reforms aimed at developing more effective child protection work and the new Children Act 2004. The duties under the terms of the Children Act 1989 are straightforward and underpinned by principles as shown in Table 5.3.

Section 17 lays a duty on local authorities to safeguard, promote the welfare and provide services for children in need. The definition of 'in need' has three elements:

- The child is unlikely to achieve or maintain, or to have the opportunity of achieving or maintaining, a reasonable standard of health or development without the provision for the child of services by a local authority, or
- The child's health or development is likely to be significantly impaired, or further impaired, without provision for the child of such services, or
- The child is disabled.

The Act further defines disability to include children suffering from mental disorder of any kind. In relation to the first two parts of the definition, health or development is defined to cover physical, intellectual, emotional, social or behavioural development and physical or mental health. These concepts are open

Table 5.3 Summary of Children Act 1989

- The welfare of the child is paramount
- Children should be brought up and cared for within their own families wherever possible
- Children should be safe and protected by effective interventions if at risk
- Courts should avoid delay and only make an order if this is better than not making an order
- Children should be kept informed about what happens to them and involved in decisions made about them
- Parents continue to have parental responsibility for their children even when their children are no longer living with them

to interpretation of what is meant by a 'reasonable standard of health and development', as well as the predictive implications for children having the 'opportunity' of achieving or maintaining it. However, it is reasonable to include the following groups of children within this part of the definition of 'in need' and to argue the case for preventive support where there is a risk of children developing problems (Ryan 1999) (see Table 5.4).

Some children from these groups may be truanting from school, getting involved in criminal activities or have behaviour problems at school and/or home. Agency responses tend to address the presenting problem and implement an intervention to address this rather than the underlying causes. Assessment of the needs of individual children and families therefore is often cursory, deficit oriented and static. It should be more positive, enabling, build on strengths and be undertaken alongside family support measures. Mental health and emotional well-being needs should be fully explored.

Table 5.4 Children at risk of developing problems

Children living in poverty

Homeless children

Children suffering the effects of racism

Young carers

Children separated from parent/s

Young offenders

Refugee and asylum seekers

Source: adapted from Ryan (1999)

Care orders can be made in respect of children under Section 17 (see Table 5.5). This results in the child being placed in the care of the local authority which then assumes parental responsibility for that child. Parents still retain parental responsibility for the child but this is shared with the local authority.

Section 26 provides for a complaints procedure through which children and young people can appeal against decisions reached by social workers. There are informal and formal stages to the procedure with an expectation that an independent person is included at the formal stages. When these procedures have been exhausted a judicial review may be applied for within 3 months of the decision being appealed against (see Table 5.6).

Section 27 requires local education authorities and other organisations to assist in functions derived from Section 17.

Section 31 enables staff to apply for a care order or supervision order if the child is suffering, or is likely to suffer, significant harm or the likelihood of harm, which is attributable to the care being given the child not being what would be expected from a reasonable parent. The court decision is based on the balance of probability, which means a parent can lose the care of their child even though in a previous criminal court, they were found not guilty because the standard of proof is beyond reasonable doubt.

Section 43 enables staff to apply for a child assessment order from a court following parental lack of cooperation in a child protection assessment. The worker in situations like this, and in full care proceedings, has a crucial role in balancing the need to protect the child with the future consequences on them and their family of oppressive investigations and intervention.

Section 44 enables staff to apply for an emergency protection order where they need to investigate suspected child abuse

Table 5.5 Grounds for a care order

The child concerned is suffering significant harm, or is likely to suffer significant harm and the harm or likelihood of harm is attributable to:

- the care given to the child, or likely to be given if the order were not made, not being what it would be reasonable to expect a parent to give him/her or
- the child is beyond parental control

Table 5.6 Three grounds for succeeding with judicial review

- Ultra – the social services department did not have the power to make the decision
- Unfair – the decision was reached in a procedurally unfair manner, or by abuse of power
- Unreasonable – all relevant matters were not considered, the law was not properly applied or there was insufficient consultation

and access to the child is being refused. The order allows immediate removal of the child to a place of safety for 8 days.

Section 46 permits the police to remove and detain a child for 72 hours without reference to a court where they have reasonable cause to believe a child would otherwise be likely to suffer significant harm.

Section 47 gives the local authority a duty to investigate where they suspect a child is suffering or is likely to suffer significant harm. Guidance suggests the purpose of such an investigation is to establish facts, decide if there are grounds for concern, identify risk and decide protective action.

There is a very extensive body of government policy and practice guidance in relation to assessment in child protection. Research on assessment in child and family work affirms that mental health and emotional well-being apply specifically to childcare and child protection. However, it is clear that the overemphasis on risk control that followed the Children Act 1989 and various child protection failures preceding it have obscured the mental health aspects in these complex situations. One report concluded that child protection appeared to have a deskilling effect on staff who were only expecting to respond to families in crisis and where children were at risk of significant harm (SSI 1997; Thompson 2005).

Nurses typically find the policy emphasis is on reacting to child protection and looked-after children cases to the exclusion of support to other families of children in need. Therefore, too narrow a focus on danger can lead to neglect of the wider picture whereas a strategy of risk management that takes the wider context into account is more likely to effectively meet need. Or the policy emphasis swings towards more early intervention designed to prevent abusive situations developing.

THE CHILDREN ACT 2004

The Children Act 2004 offers recent guidance on how to develop your individual practice to safeguard children and provides a legislative spine for the wider strategy for improving children's lives and therefore their emotional well-being. This covers the universal services that every child accesses, and more targeted services for those with additional needs. The Act defines children and young people to mean those aged 0 to 19 but also includes those:

- over 19 who are receiving services as care leavers under sections 23c to 24d of the Children Act 1989
- over 19 but under 25 with learning difficulties within the meaning of section 13 of the Learning and Skills Act 2000 and who are receiving services under that Act.

The overall aim is to encourage integrated planning, commissioning and delivery of services as well as improved multidisciplinary working, removing duplication, increasing accountability and improving the coordination of individual and joint inspections in local authorities. The legislation is enabling rather than prescriptive and provides local authorities with a considerable amount of flexibility in the way they

implement its provisions. The Act set the seal on a series of developments for safeguarding children and young people's welfare that have radically changed the shape of provision and created a new organisational context for their protection.

Section 10 came into force in April 2005 and placed a duty on local authorities and relevant partners to cooperate in order to improve the well-being of children in their area. Well-being covers: physical and mental health; emotional well-being; protection from harm and neglect; education, training and recreation; the contribution made to society; and general well-being. These terms are not well defined and neither is the linkage between the separate elements. This could lead to very different perceptions from the variety of agency staff involved with the same child. The notion of cooperation includes working together to understand the needs of local children; agreeing the contribution each agency should make to meet those needs; effective sharing of information about individual children at a strategic level to support multiagency working; and the commissioning and delivery of services.

Schools and GPs have only recently been included in the specific list of 'relevant partners' in the Act mandated to cooperate. This had caused serious concern among nurses and child care organisations that feared the government's drive to increase the autonomy of schools would undermine the coherence and collaboration explicit in safeguarding policy. The National Youth Agency was disappointed that youth work is relatively ignored in this legislation despite evidence of the effectiveness of youth workers in safeguarding young people and managing mental health and emotional well-being. The government believes that other guidance implicitly expects all agencies to cooperate in safeguarding children and young people:

Sections 11 and 28 introduced a general duty of care on services to safeguard and promote the welfare of children. This applies to the children's services authority; schools; district council; strategic health authority; primary care trust; NHS or foundation trust; police authority; probation board; youth offending team; prison governor; and Connexions. The duty to cooperate is meant to lead to integrated services through: children's trusts; national outcomes for children and young people; the common assessment tool; information-sharing databases; and safeguarding children's boards.

Safeguard means prevention of and protection from maltreatment. Promoting welfare means ensuring children and young people have opportunities to achieve physical and mental health; physical, emotional, intellectual, social and behavioural development. However, current guidance on Section 11 fails to establish a clear line of accountability between children's trusts and safeguarding children boards or to make explicit how the two bodies relate to one another on child protection matters.

Section 12 provides for the creation of a database to facilitate a new identification, referral and tracking system. This was one of the key practical measures to emerge following the 2003 Laming Report and is an information system designed to enable all staff concerned about any child or young person to access a database to ascertain who else might be involved and contact them if necessary. However, the aim of encouraging

Table 5.7 Guidance that concerns need to be flagged

- A practitioner feels that others need to know the important information that cannot appear on the database
- That this information may affect the types of service made available to the child or young person
- The practitioner has completed an initial assessment under the common assessment framework and wants to discuss their findings

better interagency communication may well be at the cost of reducing the much valued confidentiality desired by young people in contact with sexual health, HIV and mental health services. There is no guarantee this information system will actually deliver better interagency communication and there is a real prospect of placing some young people at greater risk of harm if young people are deterred from seeking help because of fears that their confidential details will be exposed.

The system should only contain the child's name, address, gender, date of birth, a unique identifying number, plus the name and contact details of any person with parental responsibility or day-to-day care of the child, education provider and primary care provider. A flag will indicate that a professional working with a child has a cause for concern. The nature of the concern would not be described on the system. This has attracted criticism because there are no published threshold criteria for what constitutes reasons for concern. The fear is that this is likely to lead to a variety of definitions from staff in different agencies and result in defensive practice, whereby minor concerns are flagged to ensure legal cover, causing unnecessary work (see Table 5.7).

Security of this database has been questioned because of fears that a lack of staff training combined with the sheer numbers of staff able to use the system will invariably lead to a breach of security. Also users need to ensure compliance with the Data Protection Act 1998 and the Human Rights Act 1998 where client's rights will sometimes conflict with child protection procedures. Children and young people when consulted about this accept that information should be shared between agencies if it will help them gain access to the services they need. But they want to be consulted, know with whom it is being shared and to be reassured that the information is accurate, will be used properly and kept safe.

The government has proposed that a lead professional should be designated to act on information placed on the database, operate as a gatekeeper, decide whether information was merited and coordinate service responses. The recommendation is that this person should be someone from the agency with most day-to-day contact with the child. For most children, this person will be their school teacher but teachers are resisting taking on this scale of responsibility (see Table 5.8).

Sections 13 to 16 imply that now safeguarding children boards have been put on a statutory footing, their expanded role will cover monitoring of practice, training and service development. The majority of this membership will be drawn from police, education, social services and health. Health can be particularly well represented from paediatrics, hospital trusts, the new commissioning groups and child and adolescent mental

Table 5.8 Responsibilities of local safeguarding children boards

Developing local procedures

Auditing and evaluating how well local services work together

Putting in place objectives and performance indicators for child protection

Developing effective working relationships

Ensuring agreement on thresholds for intervention

Encouraging evidence-based practice

Undertaking part eight reviews when a child has died or been seriously harmed

Overseeing interagency training

Raising awareness within the community

health. The probation service, the Crown Prosecution service, Children and Family Court Advisory and Support Service, the magistrate's court, the NSPCC and other voluntary organisations are all likely to be represented (Murphy 2003).

Sections 17 and 26 introduce a new children and young people's plan (CYPP), which, from April 2006, is the strategic, overarching plan replacing the behaviour support plan, children's services plan, early years development and childcare plan, education development plan, Area Child Protection Committee business plan, teenage pregnancy strategy and youth services plan. The CYPP should set out the improvements that local authorities intend to make to meet the five outcomes for children and young people identified in *Every child matters* (2003) (see Table 5.9).

THE NATIONAL SERVICE FRAMEWORK FOR CHILDREN, YOUNG PEOPLE AND MIDWIFERY SERVICES 2004

The National Service Framework for children, young people and midwifery services (NSFCYPMS) is a 10-year programme intended to stimulate long-term and sustained improvement in children's health. It aims to ensure fair, high-quality and integrated health and social care from pregnancy right through to adulthood. Overall, the NSFCYPMS sets national standards for the first time for children's health and social care, which promote high-quality, women- and child-centred services and personalised care that meets the needs of parents, children and their families (see Table 5.10).

Table 5.9 Every child matters

Enjoying and achieving – this means getting the most out of life and developing broad skills for adulthood; attending school and achieving national educational standards; achieving personal and social development and enjoying recreation

Staying safe – being protected from harm and neglect and growing up able to look after themselves. Being safe from maltreatment, neglect, violence, sexual exploitation, bullying and discrimination. Protected from crime and antisocial behaviour. Learning and developing independent living skills

Being healthy – enjoying good physical health and mental health and living a healthy lifestyle. Being emotionally and sexually healthy and choosing not to take illegal drugs

Making a positive contribution – to the community and to society and not engaging in antisocial or offending behaviour. Making decisions and supporting community development and enjoying positive relationships. Choosing not to bully or discriminate, develop self confidence and manage challenges

Economic well-being – overcoming socioeconomic disadvantages to achieve their full potential. Engage in further education or training and prepare for employment, family life and independent living. Access to decent homes, transport and sustainable incomes

Table 5.10 National Service Framework

The framework requires services to:

- give children, young people and their parents increased information, power and choice over the support and treatment they receive and involve them in planning their care and services
- introduce a new child health promotion programme designed to promote the health and well-being of children from pre-birth to adulthood
- promote physical health, mental health and emotional well-being by encouraging children and their families to develop healthy lifestyles
- focus on early intervention, based on timely and comprehensive assessment of a child and their family's needs
- improve access to services for all children according to their needs, particularly by co-locating services and developing managed local children's clinical networks for children who are ill or injured
- tackle health inequalities, addressing the particular needs of communities, and children and their families who are likely to achieve poor outcomes
- promote and safeguard the welfare of children and ensure all staff are suitably trained and aware of action to take if they have concerns about a child's welfare
- ensure that pregnant women receive high-quality care throughout their pregnancy, have a normal childbirth wherever possible, are involved in decisions about what is best for them and their babies, and have choices about how and where they give birth

Standard 5 of the NSFCYPMS states that: 'All agencies work to prevent children suffering harm and to promote their welfare, provide them with the services they require to address their identified needs, and safeguard children who are being, or who are likely to be, harmed.' The responsibility for contributing to this new multiagency integrated framework rests with:

- health commissioners (previously PCTs), who are responsible for improving the health of their whole population
- NHS trusts, which are required to designate a named doctor and nurse to take a professional lead on safeguarding children
- ambulance trusts, NHS Direct and NHS walk-in centres, all of which must have similar arrangements in place
- local authorities, which must ensure there is a designated professional for safeguarding children in social services, housing and the education department.

Safeguarding and promoting the welfare of children should be prioritised by all agencies, working in partnership to plan and provide coordinated and comprehensive services. Agency roles and responsibilities should be clarified to ensure that harmed children are identified and assessed as soon as possible by appropriately trained staff with suitable premises and equipment. Under the NSFCYPMS, an up-to-date profile of the local population must be compiled to facilitate needs assessment and to provide integrated services to meet that need.

ACTIVITY 5.3

- Obtain a copy of your trust's safeguarding children procedures and practice guidelines or make sure you know where it is held.
- Make a note of the contents.
- Examine it carefully and make sure you know how and to whom you should refer in cases involving child protection.

INTERAGENCY WORKING

The much vaunted aim of joint working and closer collaboration has echoed throughout much of the past 30 years of public reports where people have been killed when problems in communication between agencies have occurred. In fact, it appeared much earlier in a 1945 inquiry report into the death of Denis O'Neill, often cited as the first child killed while subject to child protection agency involvement.

Guidance suggests that staff should receive more comprehensive safeguarding training that equips them to recognise and respond to a person's welfare concerns. Thus the policy aspiration to foster closer collaborative working between agencies involved in safeguarding people faces serious obstacles.

The principal reason given for failures in interagency cooperation is that one key individual within that system failed to fulfil their part of the process which resulted in a breakdown in the protective intervention. It is not the individual within the system but the *structure of the system itself* that is of key importance. That one individual within a system can be blamed for a child's injury denies the whole concept of collective interagency decision making and responsibility. Agencies can fall into the convenient practice of finding a scapegoat reflecting a societal individualistic culture and the adversarial legal system: 'In Britain, when things go wrong, the system encourages a blaming of individual agencies and practitioners' (Murphy 2000).

ACTIVITY 5.4

- Make an effort to link up with a practitioner from another agency and meet to discuss the above.
- Draw up an action plan to present to one another's teams to tackle the barriers to better collaboration.

HOW TO UNDERSTAND RISKS IN SAFEGUARDING CHILDREN

Assessment of risk and its management has always been a dominant theme in nursing. As with other aspects of the profession – such as the move to competence- and evidence-based practice – this has been a reaction to a wider demand for the greater public accountability of professionals in all spheres, and, particularly in nursing, several highly publicised failures to protect patients and the public from dangerous people. Lurid tabloid media stories have over the years initiated public moral panics and fuelled political posturing about mental health, youth justice and child protection policy.

Despite the fact that these failures – mainly in childcare and mental health work – represent a minority of cases, their impact on practice has been considerable. The death of one child can trigger a wholesale evaluation of the UK child protection system, regardless of the specific features of particular cases or the evidence of excellent practice elsewhere. This has led to policy and practice in relation to risk and its management becoming focused on dangerousness (particularly so in work with offenders and mental health) and significant harm (in relation to children and elders). Definitions of both concepts are ambiguous and widely agreed to be determined by social, cultural and historical factors (RCN 2007).

Nonetheless it is important that – in any other than purely philosophical debates – nurses are aware of and work with current definitions – regardless of how open to question they may be. Despite this relativism, there is always a tendency to subscribe to the conventional wisdom within oneself or part of a peer belief system that nurses must be aware of and consider carefully with considerable thought, consultation with managers and involvement of patients.

One interesting aspect of the moral panic about risk is that the risk to nurses from dangerous people and the adverse attention of politicians and the media has not been of such concern. In terms of its frequency, the risk of abuse and physical threat or attack for social workers is far more prevalent than similar risks to their service users. Nurses – particularly those in residential settings – are among those who share the highest risk of assault at work. The recognition of this risk should be a primary consideration for all nurses, their managers and the organisations within which they work.

As in other areas of practice – such as community care – the consequence of such pressures has been an obsession with the production of checklists such as eligibility criteria, assessment schedules and risk assessment scales. The tendency has been for practice to become narrowly focused on aspects of the individual (such as dependency or dangerousness) rather than on the whole person-in-context. This is counter to – and in extreme cases can threaten – the established values and practice of nursing, which emphasise individualisation, respect for the person and a holistic approach that takes full account of social and cultural context.

There is some evidence that effectiveness in assessment and intervention can be enhanced by the use of well-validated assessment scales – for example in relation to risk and its management with offenders or suicidal individuals. Additionally, in terms of accountability, nurses must be able to demonstrate that they are aware of and make appropriate use of all available aids to best practice. However, the consensus from research presently is that such tools are useful adjuncts to competent professional judgement, not substitutes for it.

In relation to the assessment and management of risk there is a need therefore to resist the reductionist tendency to focus exclusively on assessment of risk conceived as 'danger' and intervention as 'risk control'. Ironically, the danger of such practice is that in pursuing the ultimately unattainable goal of entirely risk-free practice workers may:

- overlook the risks attached to intervention
- neglect the rights of individuals in order to control the risks they pose to themselves or others
- lose sight of the individual-in-context, their strengths and the creative potential for development and growth this brings
- overlook the risk to themselves.

PRACTICAL GUIDELINES 5.1

Nursing intervention in safeguarding should be:

- optimally non-intrusive
- compatible with the promotion of individual potential and personal responsibility
- a balance of both rights and risks, care and control
- aware of risks to nurses.

ACTIVITY 5.5

Try putting an item on the agenda for your next team/ group meeting to discuss ways in which nurses pose a risk to patients/service users and how those risks could be minimised.

TWO APPROACHES TO RISK IN NURSING

As nursing develops its understanding and practice in relation to risk, two contrasting approaches have emerged, which have been described as:

1. The 'safety first' approach, which can be paraphrased as CYB – cover your back
   - Competent nursing should not be entirely defensive and preoccupied with covering your back.
2. The 'risk-taking' approach, which subscribes to the view that risks are an inherent part of social life and that if individuals are to be fully engaged in social life some risk is inevitable. Both terms are problematic:
   - Risk taking has connotations of an advocacy of taking risks that is counterintuitive to many and easily misconstrued as irresponsible in view of the vulnerability of many patients.

For these reasons, risk control and risk management are terms used here and some of the implications identified.

Safety Approach Nursing Intervention in Safeguarding and Risk Control

- Definition: risk is negative – danger, threat.
- Priority principles: professional responsibility and accountability.
- Practice: identification (assessment scales) and elimination (procedural, legalistic).
- Benefits: apparently unambiguous (clear categories of risk); routinised, standardised, quality assured (checklists);

defensible (evidence based); publicly understood (politicians, public and media).
- Drawbacks: risk is seen as static, unchangeable; context neglected; strengths unacknowledged; labelling, stigmatising, stereotyping; opportunities for development missed; practice is rule driven; assessment tools are imperfect; impossible to eliminate risk entirely; risks to nurses ignored.

Risk-taking Approach Nursing Intervention in Safeguarding and Risk Management

- Definition: positive – risk is part of life, balancing risks and benefits is part of individual's development, being self-determining and personally responsible.
- Priority principles: self-determination, anti-oppression.
- Practice: solution focused, partnership practice, empowerment.
- Benefits: in keeping with values and practice of modern social work; emphasises process of maximising benefits as well as minimising risks, rather than procedure of identifying and eliminating risk; builds on strengths; developmental rather than judgemental.
- Drawbacks: relies heavily on highly developed professional competence and judgement; requires commitment of client to partnership; requires intellectual/cognitive competence of client; involves ambiguity and uncertainty; is poorly understood by public; requires supportive management practice and organisational policy; risks to nurses ignored.

As understanding and practice in relation to risk develops, it becomes clear that there needs to be an integration of the best of both approaches.

Eliminating or Totally Controlling Risk is Impossible

It is undesirable to think of risk and the nursing task in relation to it in this way because evidence and intuition suggests it is impossible and thus resources are wasted. Risk is part of social life and the real world of everyday experience and should not be perceived as only of interest to specific client groups. Practice that is effective in terms of promoting individual responsibility and social competence cannot be reductionist – it must recognise the person-in-context and build on strengths (Walker 2012). NHS trusts and other providers have responsibilities in law in relation to certain client groups and you need to be very aware of legislative imperatives determining the scope of your powers. Individual nurses must neither neglect these responsibilities nor accept 'unlimited liability' – whether or not there are legal requirements.

It is very important to remember that the social and individual costs of control can outweigh the social and individual benefits thus highlighting your assessment and analytical skills. Nursing routinely brings its practitioners into contact with dangerous people and entails professional judgements that are potentially castigated by management, your work organisation, professional association and the media.

Minimising Risk is Possible

Competent nurses must be aware of the meaning of risk and its role in the personal development and social life of patients. Understanding the function and then appropriately employing well-validated risk assessment scales where they are available is useful in some cases. Ensuring practice is evidence based and in accordance with statute, government guidance and agency policy will provide you with a safe framework within which to practice.

Having the ability to handle stress and crisis situations or managing 'decision calls' is something that cannot be taught, but is learned through practice, reflection and skilled supervision. It is important when anxieties are escalating not to be rushed, but to ensure immediate safety of all parties involved, be appropriately assertive, be sure a decision has to be made and by whom, share responsibility, involve where possible and support the subject of the decision, report back to the referring agency, ensure continuity, debrief and reflect with a supportive manager/supervisor.

The Skills for Care and the Children's Workforce Development Council produced guidance on effective supervision in 2007. Further guidance due in 2012 was to specify minimum levels of supervision especially for newly qualified staff when national standards for employers will be published. Supervision is not a luxury; it is a critical priority and could mean the difference between life and death in some cases.

By clearly identifying specific risks and the contexts in which they might occur you can begin to sort out priority areas for more of your attention and intervention. This will be helped enormously by fully engaging clients and significant others as far as possible in risk assessment, management and recording. Differences will happen and these need to be openly acknowledged and recorded too. Multidisciplinary sharing of risk management with other involved professionals is advised and expected but you must be prepared for difficulties and the potential for conflict and disagreement. Everyone will claim to be making a professional judgement but these often sit on top of considerable personal anxieties and strongly held beliefs.

The recording of risk assessment and management plans and relating them to specific legal requirements as appropriate should be a matter of routine and many assessment schedules/forms will contain guidance on the statutory grounds for your intervention. It is important to ensure the availability of supervision and recording key decisions from it; otherwise, you will be vulnerable to charges of a cavalier approach to your work and open to disciplinary procedures. However, you also have a professional duty to object to and refuse to comply with activity that is not in your view in the best interests of the client. Professional codes of practice, RCN and trades union advice and support are all available to help you cope with and manage these situations.

PRACTICAL GUIDELINES 5.2

Skills and knowledge for safeguarding

This is an attempt to enhance integrated practice in safeguarding children. The main elements of the common core which you need to know about and become proficient in are:

- Effective communication and engagement – includes establishing rapport and respectful, trusting relationships; understanding non-verbal communication and cultural variations in communication; active listening in a calm, open and non-threatening manner; summarising situations to check understanding and consent; outline possible courses of action and consequences; ensuring people feel valued; understand limits of confidentiality and relevant legislation; reporting and recording information.
- Human growth and development – includes observing behaviour in context; understanding developmental

processes and mental health issues; evaluating circumstances in a holistic way and distinguishing fact from opinion; knowing when to refer on for further support; demonstrating empathy and understanding; supporting the person to reach their own decisions; taking account of different lifestyles; distinguishing between organic disability and poor parenting producing delayed development; understanding attachment patterns and the inter-relationship between developmental characteristics; being clear about your role and how to reflect on practice to improve it.

- Safeguarding and promoting the welfare of the child – includes ability to recognise overt and subtle signs that children have been harmed by considering all explanations for sudden changes in mood or behaviour; involving parents/carers in promoting welfare and recognising risk factors; developing self-awareness about the impact of child abuse; building confidence in challenging oneself and others; understanding legislation, guidance and other agency roles; sharing information in the context of confidentiality; appreciating boundaries of your knowledge and responsibility; responding appropriately to conflict, anger and violence; understanding that assumptions, values and prejudice prevent equal opportunity.

- Supporting transitions – includes recognising changes in attitudes and behaviour; empathising and reassuring to help the young person reach a positive outcome; considering issues of identity and the effects of peer pressure; understanding key areas affecting emotional well-being such as divorce, bereavement, puberty and family break-ups, primary to secondary school, unemployment, leaving home, disability and increasing levels of vulnerability; knowledge of local resources and how to access information.

- Multiagency working – includes effective communication by listening and ensuring you are being listened to; working in a team and forging sustaining relationships; sharing experience through formal and informal exchanges; developing skills to ensure continuity for the person; knowing when and to whom to report incidents or unexpected behaviour changes; understanding how to ensure another agency responds while maintaining a focus on the person's best interests.

- Sharing information – includes making good use of available information such as a common assessment; assessing the relevance and status of different information and where gaps exist; using clear, unambiguous language; respecting the skills and expertise of others while creating a trusting environment and seeking consent; engaging with people and their families to communicate and gain information; sharing confidential information without consent where a child is at risk; avoiding repetitive questions and assessment interviews; appreciating the effect of cultural and religious beliefs without stereotyping; understanding the principles governing young people's consent; distinguishing between permissive information sharing and statutory information sharing and their implications.

The activity that follows applies to all professionals involved in child protection and provides space for reflecting on the human cost of such stressful work. Knowing other professionals feel the same should help break down some of the barriers erected by bureaucratic systems.

ACTIVITY 5.6

Prior to your next planned supervision session let your line managers know that you want some extra time at the end of the agenda. Avoid explaining specifics.

In that extra time, express how your work in general or a specific high-risk case is affecting you emotionally. Stop your manager attempting to provide a quick fix or reverting to bureaucratic mode involving procedures for stress management.

Explain that you need them to listen, absorb what you are saying without comment, reflect in silence and resist feeling that you are criticising them.

THE EXPERIENCE OF INTERPROFESSIONAL WORKING

If new children's services ensure the availability of time that permits a reflective, considered atmosphere, this can optimise professional judgement. This contrasts with previous work experiences that can be characterised by reactive, unplanned and overburdened workloads permitting little time for considered judgements (Casey 1993). This welcome capacity to reflect, however, presents possible dilemmas in cases where, for example, some staff feel they may not, in the short term, be addressing the underlying causes of some children's problems, particularly where longer term input would be valuable.

Staff are under pressure to reduce waiting lists and respond quickly to emerging problems with early intervention of a short-term nature. The concern is that this may result in either early rereferral or may indeed result in an eventual need for help from specialist services if short-term input is inadequate or the situation deteriorates. Or having too much time to think about every detail of a child's circumstances can emphasise the complexity and multiple explanations available, leading to drift and ineffective decision making.

One evident strength of new team cultures is the potential for co-counselling and training support systems for these kinds of concern. Teams can learn to utilise the best aspects of skills mix using each other as resources of expertise and specialist knowledge to the advantage of vulnerable children and tackling the challenges in incorporating new ideas and different ways of approaching child and family difficulties. A consultation and training role now in place in many children and families teams offering support and advice to other professionals can also contribute to more interprofessional understanding, particularly in the health and education sectors where old contacts and relationships could be employed to positive effect. This next activity focuses on the challenges in interprofessional child protection work, and provides the chance to reflect and discover positive ways forward.

It is possible that, as new teams continue to train together, and develop generic working, there may be some resistance to relinquishing former roles, and even strengthening of the boundaries between professions. The challenge for service managers will be to preserve the distinctive individual professional expertise base but not at the expense of service

ACTIVITY 5.7

If you are working in a multidisciplinary team or know someone who is, think about the advantages and disadvantages you personally feel there are.

Now discuss in supervision your thoughts and list the practical differences you can introduce to reduce the disadvantages.

coherence. When attempting to engage children and families already suffering under the pressure of racism and discrimination it is important that children, families and carers have the maximum choice when engaging with services aiming to meet their needs (Bhui and Olajide 1999). In addition, new teams would benefit from formal service user involvement, especially children and young people separately from parents or carers, at the clinical audit, monitoring, review, and strategic planning levels of the service (Alderson 2000). Conventional uniprofessional services have tended to miss this opportunity for empowering patients.

We have seen that a child protection system will be influenced and formulated by the conflicting definitions of and perspectives on child abuse. This system will also be influenced by the shape of the existing professional network and by the roles that agencies take or are given within the process. The crucial dilemma, around which the system is built, is the child's right not to be abused and the parent's right not to be interfered with by agents of the state. Twenty years ago we heard a familiar lament – concerns about the childcare agents of the state doing too much, too coercively, and about them doing too little, too ineffectually, resulted in a wish for legislation and policy to attempt to proceed in two directions at once – both towards better protection of the child and better protection of the parent (Fox Harding 1991).

This is the key debate for all child protection systems in the post-Munro period: how well will they be able to hold these mutually antagonistic demands at the forefront of their work? How well will they be able to intervene to prevent serious abuse and to act in a non-interventionist way towards those families

ACTIVITY 5.8

Working with children and families across different professional groups has advantages and disadvantages. What information is required to enable a better understanding of how the overall picture of support services fits together?

where there is no threat of serious abuse? Or can a balance be struck between these two poles of behaviour or is constant conflict between the two inevitable? In the child protection system, interagency work is compulsory.

Unfortunately, doing interagency work well, and striving for good interagency practice, is not easy. Do we need a revolution in safeguarding practice or rely on an evolutionary process? Poor practice is shown by grudging communication with, and lack of inclusion of, other agencies (RCN 2007). It is also shown by the resistance behind the conviction that 'my agency or practitioner group knows best, and we have nothing to gain from the input of other agencies or practitioners'.

The journey towards good practice begins with the acknowledgement that all agencies and practitioner groups have something to offer to child protection work and is followed by striving to let others participate in the fullest possible way in the process, combating the urge to think and work in unilateral ways (Murphy 2003).

The responsibility for achieving good practice is a shared one. It does not rest with one agency or one particular practitioner group. Neither does it rest solely with individual practitioners or their managers – although the latter have an important role to play, they share that crucial responsibility with local childcare systems and with local and national political systems.

The level of achievement of good practice will vary over time, place and even between cases. It is important that we constantly strive to improve practice at all levels, remembering that positive interagency interaction is recreated with each new interaction and each new case that comes into the system: interagency collaboration requires constant attention, remotivation and energy (Murphy 2000). Positive interagency and multidisciplinary practice is not easy to achieve. In some ways the unilateral, single-agency path is easier to organise and to control. However, good child protection work itself is not easy to accomplish, but becomes more attainable in the context of positive systems-based interagency practice.

Each child is unique and therefore blanket policies and procedures will not support every child, rather a focused approach is required that acknowledges the rights of the child to have holistic and optimum growth and for the reader to be able to assess if abuse has occurred. Children, therefore, need to feel it is safe to communicate with professionals, which may lead to issues of confidentiality for the carers working with the child. In order to achieve a balance between family support and safeguarding individual children, the reader needs to consider the factors involved in the investigation and any intervention in child abuse.

CASE STUDY REVIEW 5.1

Engage Ms B by addressing her own needs for safety and protection

While the main focus of intervention must be on the care and safety of the children, practitioners also need to engage Ms B by addressing her own needs for safety and protection.

Domestic abuse interventions

She is aware that her partner will harm her if she asks him to leave so she is stuck in an impossible dilemma.

If he stays, the practitioner will allege she is failing to protect the children, if she tries to make her partner leave she will endanger herself as well as the children.

If staff acknowledge this dilemma in an uncritical way without blaming Ms B or by pretending that there is a simple solution, then they are more likely to begin the process of gaining her confidence and working collaboratively rather than coercively.

Encourage Ms B to attend a survivors' group.

Cultural understanding

The context of her culture and religion are important factors in seeking to understand the complexities of her situation.

The nurse needs to be open and direct about this without giving the false impression of knowing how she feels or by signalling discomfort or embarrassment at such sensitive matters.

Consideration should be given to employing an interpreter or translator even though she may be able to make herself understood, as this will signal a respectful approach and provide a cultural connection that will be emotionally supportive.

Being a parent

Engaging Ms B in a conversation about her experiences as a wife and mother in Bangladesh and comparing her life with how it is now will open up a rich seam of information that can simultaneously serve a therapeutic purpose.

Getting Ms B to list her worries and concerns about the children will enable her to demonstrate that she is a capable mother and help you appreciate the emotional aspects of her experiences.

Attempts to engage her partner need to be made but not at the risk of inflaming the situation or putting her and the children at greater risk.

You can then help her consider ways of tackling these worries in small, practical ways before addressing the major issue of her complex relationship with her partner.

Holistic overview of the review

The review needs to examine every element of the plan, check whether it is happening, which agency is responsible for what element, what impact the intervention is having on each child's development and whether additional needs have emerged or alternative interventions need to be considered.

The review should check whether the plan is addressing and meeting each individual child's developmental needs, mental health and emotional well-being, as well as their collective needs as a sibling group.

It also needs to examine the parenting capacity of Ms B on her own and conjointly with her partner.

The wider family context should be explored to see what pattern of relationships exists with a view to encouraging increased supportive contact.

If no immediate family exists then a wider definition of 'family' could identify religious, spiritual or social support networks.

In a safer environment the children's behaviour may regress and deteriorate so it is important to distinguish these temporary healing experiences from sustained developmental problems due to continued abuse.

Ms B may not be able to manage every aspect of the plan because it feels overwhelming. For example, the survivors' group may be poorly organised by unskilled people who cannot meet her particular needs. She may be the only Muslim and the target of racist abuse within the group. Thought needs to be given to finding the right group for her particular needs rather than just the first available resource. However, she may be succeeding in getting the older child to school and she must be genuinely congratulated for this. By establishing a solid platform for her to feel supported, empowered and capable of defining her children's needs she will be more likely to feel strong enough to deal with her violent partner.

Evaluating the family's progress

If the situation became more risky then the practitioner would need to confront Ms B with the likely consequences of inaction on her part. However, this needs to be done alongside offering maximum support by all agencies involved in a coordinated package. Effective review and closure will more likely happen if a collaborative relationship with Ms B has developed that will enable her to seek further help in future if required.

SUMMARY OF KEY LEARNING

Changes to the organisation and delivery of safeguarding services have followed legislative change and policy guidance that has evolved over many years in relation to vulnerable children and young people.

Children's trusts/services are becoming the core locus for the delivery of joined-up services for children and young people whereby staff from every agency will be expected to work collaboratively in multidisciplinary teams or virtual networks.

Nurses need to raise their awareness of new responsibilities implicit in legislation and new policy guidance. They also need to improve knowledge and skills in the emotional well-being of young people.

Nurses working with vulnerable children need to learn about, understand and engage critically but positively with other agency staff responsible for child protection. Different values, knowledge bases and skills in perceptions of the needs of children, who are or may be at risk of significant harm, need to be acknowledged.

FURTHER RESOURCES

Organisations that support vulnerable children and young people – NSPCC: **http://www.nspcc.org.uk/**

Action for Children: **http://www.actionforchildren.org.uk/?gclid=CMrbvqvs-7ACFVMTfAodAXXqNw**

Save the Children: **http://www.savethechildren.org.uk/**

National Children's Bureau: **http://www.ncb.org.uk/**

ANSWERS TO ACTIVITIES

ACTIVITY 5.1

Together with a colleague consider the case illustration and map out an action plan, including alternatives and the reasons for them.

   Example: While the main focus of intervention must be on the care and safety of the children, practitioners also need to engage Ms B by addressing her own needs for safety and protection. She is aware that her partner will harm her if she asks him to leave so she is stuck in an impossible dilemma. If he stays, the practitioner will allege she is failing to protect the children; if she tries to make her partner leave, she will endanger herself as well as the children. If staff acknowledge this dilemma in an uncritical way without blaming Ms B or by pretending that there is a simple solution, then they are more likely to begin the process of gaining her confidence and working collaboratively rather than coercively.

ACTIVITY 5.2

Discuss a recent safeguarding assessment with a colleague/mentor and reflect back on how you did it. In retrospect, how do you feel your assessment went?

   Identify three areas for improvement and the means for doing so.

ACTIVITY 5.3

Obtain a copy of your trust's safeguarding children procedures and practice guidelines or make sure you know where it is held.
   Make a note of the contents.

   Examine it carefully and make sure you know how and to whom you should refer in cases involving child protection.

ACTIVITY 5.4

Make an effort to link up with a practitioner from another agency and meet to discuss the above.

   Draw up an action plan to present to each other's teams to tackle the barriers to better collaboration.

   Example: There is a myth, subscribed to by most agencies and professional groups involved in child protection work, which suggests that while at work one can leave the self or the personal part of the practitioner at home. However, those personal histories and feelings travel to work with us every day. Unless we work with our conflicts, confusions, disgusts and deep satisfactions they will skew our work. Nothing makes us as aware of our sexuality and anger as sexual abuse (Walker

→

2012). Murphy (2000) reminds us that this split between the professional and the personal is largely false and the myth of the personal–professional split is likely to reduce rather than increase our individual and collective effectiveness. Child protection procedures implicitly presume that staff leave their individual selves at home and become truly selfless parts of the child protection machine. It is assumed that there is no need to care for staff who are engaged in child protection work, as that comforting process should take place solely in the private life of the individual concerned or somehow dissipate within the office or be absorbed in supervision (Murphy 2000). Our current understanding of personal history and personal reaction is more complicated than this. The severity of an individual's reaction is not just based on whether, or how badly, an individual has been abused. It is important to move away from the linear, compartmentalising way of understanding, towards one where we recognise that a multiplicity of personal factors affect our personal response to a given child protection case – as systems theory informs us.

ACTIVITY 5.5

Try putting an item on the agenda for your next team/group meeting to discuss ways in which nurses pose a risk to patients/service users and how those risks could be minimised.

Example: Be open and trust one another in a discussion about which patients make you feel angry or despairing and how you manage and process those feelings. You will find most other nurses have similar feelings. Sharing and reflecting on these feelings will make them much easier to handle and serve as important material for supervision from line managers.

ACTIVITY 5.6

Example: Supervision or being mentored or in whatever way your employer offers you time and space for reflection on your performance. Unfortunately, due to pressure of work and time, senior staff and managers tend to concentrate on basic housekeeping or critical incident reviews. The emphasis is usually on what went wrong rather than what went right. Mistakes happen but should not be used negatively to undermine you or for you to become defensive and verbally attack your employer. Reflection can be done in a non-judgemental way, be empowering and contribute to professional development.

ACTIVITY 5.7

If better communication is to happen, it is essential that the practitioner or agency concerned behaves in an assertive way by explaining the reasons behind a judgment or opinion to the rest of the interagency group. You must never attempt to take over another agency's role or sphere of activity. It is helpful to use the technique of predicting positive or negative outcomes for the proposed courses of action. Where possible, aim for compromise if not consensus. Where there is a sense that one side has forced a decision through, the probability of positive interagency cooperation being achieved around that decision is extremely low.

By being proactive about potential problems and difficulties, much goodwill can be generated and misconceptions dealt with before they occur during stressful situations. Acknowledging the powerful feelings aroused during this stressful work in a safe environment away from the frontline with a neutral facilitator can be very helpful in reducing all sorts of barriers to better communication. These training experiences are not add-on extras or self-indulgent experiential exercises. They are the real process by which learning takes place, practice improves and children are better safeguarded.

ACTIVITY 5.8

Establishing new teams in an existing professional network of statutory and voluntary providers within established agencies and a dynamic context of shrinking resources, austerity measures and multiple initiatives is not easy. There are opportunities for collaboration between these providers and new teams but there are also challenges in fitting in without duplicating or undermining existing good work. Changes in the wider system in areas such as school health provision, and fluctuations in the voluntary sector, emphasise the importance of collaborative meetings to enhance opportunities for maintaining and improving working together principles and integrated provision rather than causing confusion. Multidisciplinary teams require skilled management and supervision and constant monitoring using a systems perspective to note alliances, interactions and communication patterns.

There is some potential for confusion about specific services, however, because of the variety of voluntary and statutory agencies working in the broad area of family support, especially in disadvantaged locations (Hetherington and Baistow 2001). Church, voluntary, and charitable groups have existed in these locations for many years and created their own distinctive role within the diverse range of formal and informal provision of welfare services. There is in these circumstances the prospect of duplication of effort or worse, mixed messages to families from different agencies. The interprofessional nature of new teams carries the potential for enabling a better understanding of how the overall picture of support services fits together.

SELECTED REFERENCES

Bhui and Olajide (1999) *Mental health service provision for a multicultural society*. Saunders: London.

Broadhurst and White (2009) Error, blame and responsibility in child welfare: problematics of governance in an invisible trade. *British Journal of Social Work*, 39(1), 15–30.

Casey, A. (1993) Development of the use of the partnership model of nursing care, in G. Glasper and A. Tucker (eds) *Advances in child health nursing*. Scutari Press: London.

Cawson, P., et al. (2000) *Child maltreatment in the United Kingdom: a study of the prevalence of child abuse and neglect*. NSPCC: London.

Department for Education and Skills (DfES) (2003) *Every child matters: change for children*. Nottingham: DfES.

Department for Education and Skills (DfES) and Department of Health (DoH) (2004) *National Service Framework for children, young people and maternity services*. London. Department of Health.

Department of Health (DoH) (1999) *Lac circular, (99) 33. Quality protects programme: transforming children's services 2000–01*. HMSO: London.

Department of Health (DoH) (2003) *Laming inquiry into the death of Victoria Climbié*. HMSO: London.

Department of Health (DoH) (2004) *Every child matters: change for children*. HMSO: London.

Department of Health (DoH) (2008) *Laming inquiry into the death of Baby P*. HMSO: London.

Ferguson, H. (2004) *Protecting children in time: child abuse, child protection and the consequences of modernity*. Palgrave-Macmillan: Basingstoke.

Fox Harding, L. (1991) *Perspectives in child care policy*. Longman: London.

Hetherington, J. and Baistow, R. (2001) Supporting families with a mentally ill parent: European perspectives on interagency cooperation. *Child Abuse Review*, 10, 351–365.

Home Office (2004) *The Bichard Report of the deaths of Holly Wells and Jessica Chapman*. HMSO: London.

Munro, E. and Calder, M. (2005) Where has child protection gone? *Political Quarterly*, 76(3).

Murphy, M. (2000) The interagency trainer, in M. Charles and E. Hendry (eds) *Training together to safeguard children*. NSPCC: London.

Murphy, M. (2003) Keeping going, in Harrison, et al. (eds) *Partnership made painless*. Russell House: Lyme Regis.

NSPCC (2009) NSPCC research shows fifty recorded child sex offences a day, Press Release 1/09. NSPCC: London.

Office for National Statistics (ONS) (2008) *Looked after children*. HMSO: London.

Reder, P. and Duncan, S. (2004) Making the most of the Victoria Climbié Inquiry Report. *Child Abuse Review*, 13, 95–114.

Royal College of Nursing (RCN) (2007) *Safeguarding children and young people – every nurse's responsibility*. RCN: London.

Ryan, M. (1999) *The Children Act 1989: putting it into practice*. Ashgate: Aldershot.

Social Services Inspectorate (SSI) (2000) *Excellence not excuses. Inspection of services for ethnic minority children and families*. HMSO: London.

Thompson, N. (2005) *Understanding social work*. Palgrave: Basingstoke.

Walker, S. (2005) *Culturally competent therapy: working with children and young people*. Palgrave: Basingstoke.

Walker, S. (2012) *Effective social work with children and families – putting systems theory into practice*. Sage: London.

Walker, S. and Thurston, C. (2006) *Safeguarding children and young people – a guide to integrated practice*. Russell House: Lyme Regis.

CHAPTER 6
Caring for Children in a Variety of Settings

Sharon Clarke

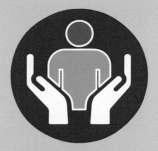

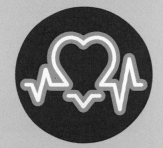

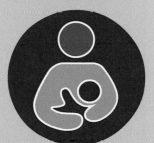

LEARNING OUTCOMES

On completion of this chapter, the reader will be able to:

- Identify issues in child health and explain the role of the children's nurse in a variety of settings.
- Explain the children's nurse's role in enabling the care of children, young people with long-term health needs and their families.
- Discuss the role of the children's nurse as part of an interprofessional team when promoting health and well-being of children and young people in the community setting.
- Identify approaches to healthcare that are appropriate to children and young people and consider their relevance and effectiveness.

TALKING POINT

When is a child not a child?

'A little bit good and a little bit bad.' A child caring for a child with a life threatening or terminal illness can isolate families from friends, extended family and their local community.

INTRODUCTION

Advances in medical technology have enabled increasing numbers of children with congenital impairments to survive (Glendinning et al. 1999; Kirk, 1998). This is due to improvements in survival rates for very premature infants, improvements in the care of children born with congenital abnormalities and advances in paediatric intensive care (Wang and Barnard 2004). Glendinning et al. (2001) estimated that there were 6000 children living at home in the UK who are technology dependent, that is, dependent on the use of ventilators, artificial feeding devices, haemodialysis and oxygen therapy.

One of the consequences of such advances is that there now exists a growing group of children with continuing medical and nursing needs, some of whom remain dependent on the very technology that enabled them to survive. This extension to the disabled and chronically ill child population has been accompanied by a move to care for such children at home rather than in hospital (Glendinning et al. 1999). This has occurred as a response to policies emphasising the community as the area for care for these children, but dilemmas of resource allocation and rationing of services still need to be addressed. The reality of these policies is that complex nursing care, involving highly technical procedures, is now being carried out in the home environment, frequently by parents.

CASE STUDY 6.1 Lily's journey through care

Lily is 13 years old. She was born at term in good physical condition (normal Apgar scores) in the local maternity unit and was discharged. Through course of the next 6 weeks Lily's mother Penny noticed that Lily looked grey at times and was not gaining weight. Visits from the health visitor confirmed concerns and an urgent review was undertaken by the GP. Lily was transported to hospital from the GP surgery by ambulance.

While being examined in the local children's A&E department, Lily required resuscitation and was transferred to a paediatric intensive care unit (PICU) for assisted ventilation and observation. Lily spent the next 2 weeks in PICU undergoing investigations, diagnosis and stabilisation. Lily was diagnosed with congenital central hypoventilation syndrome (CCHS). In order to establish stabilisation, a tracheotomy was fashioned.

Lily requires Bilevel Positive Airway Pressure (BiPAP) ventilation when she sleeps. A further 6 months was spent in the high dependency unit (HDU) for medical and nursing management in preparation for discharge home. In total, Lily was in hospital for 7 months. The hospital was 30 miles away from the family home. During this time, Lily's parents and siblings visited as often as possible, with Penny living in parents' accommodation for most of this period.

When Lily was born, Penny was 40 years old and working as a clerical officer. Her husband, Roger (Lily's dad), was 48 years old and is self-employed. They have two other children – Jason, aged 10 years and Emily, aged 8. They own their house in a rural area. Roger's parents live 20 miles away but are both in full-time employment. Penny's mother lives locally and is dependent on her daughter.

As in Lily's case, children who require long-term ventilation (LTV) support may or may not be disabled, but have the same range of needs for services and support as other disabled and non-disabled children. However, they also have additional care needs specifically related to the use of technology. They are alive through the use of complex technical equipment and the skilled intervention of highly trained carers.

VOICES 6.1 Congenital central hypoventilation syndrome (CCHS)

'I forget to breathe when I go to sleep' (a child with CCHS, aged 5).

Lily has congenital central hypoventilation syndrome (CCHS), a rare condition characterised by the failure of automatic breathing control in the absence of obvious anatomic lesions (Weese-Mayer et al. 2009).

Although there are no conclusive estimates at worldwide level, a recent French epidemiological study reported that the incidence may be estimated as one per 200,000 live births (Trang et al. 2005). One of the primary manifestations of the syndrome consists of alveolar hypoventilation and diminished tidal volume, which are more pronounced during sleep than during wakefulness.

Lily has problems in speech and concentration. Parents cited problems in producing sounds and speech in the age range 0 to 6 years old. This evidence could be explained by the fact that, during the first 6 years of life, 10 of 11 children (91 per cent) breathed through a tracheotomy, which interferes with the production of verbal messages. The results also show a reduced quality of sleep, with a considerable percentage affected by this in all the age ranges taken into consideration. Overall, the findings show that some clinical characteristics associated with CCHS may effectively influence these patients' quality of life. The results suggest that concentration and attention abilities are compromised throughout the entire developmental age, which would also be connected to some difficulties of learning reported in the school achievement. Overall, the findings are consistent with surveys in which developmental and motor and speech delays and learning disabilities were reported in more than 25 per cent of the CCHS population.

IMPLICATIONS FOR POLICY AND PRACTICE

The provision of healthcare services for children and young people who are technology dependent has been brought about by several political, economic and social drivers which have influenced the development and shaping of practice. The National Service Framework for children in hospital concerning disabled children and long-term conditions states that:

> Families need a seamless child and family-centred service that addresses all types of need, provides continuity across all transitions in the child's family life, and is not limited by separate agency roles and responsibilities. A diagnostic and assessment process carried out promptly and leading to an agreed multi-agency plan can best meet the family's needs. In particular, many children require the timely provision of therapy services and community equipment services to help encourage inclusion in local community and the best possible developmental progress. (Department of Health 2003a, page 28)

Over the last decade there have been numerous department policy developments to bring about multiagency working and integration within disabled children's services generally, as can be seen in Table 6.1. These policy developments have included children with disabilities and children with life-limiting conditions. The situation is further complicated with the introduction of the concept of technology dependence; these children may or may not be considered to be disabled, may or may not have any life-threatening condition and so may or may not be covered by either of these services, as can be seen in Figure 6.1. All are aimed at providing seamless services that start from user need and that involve children and young people with complex medical and nursing needs.

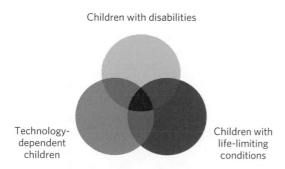

Children with disabilities

Technology-dependent children

Children with life-limiting conditions

Figure 6.1 Provision of seamless services

While the particular needs of children on long-term ventilation must be a distinct focus of the ongoing work of the development of the National Service Framework the impact of childhood disability within the family are manyfold, which cannot simply be defined or described in the context of a particular 'medical' diagnosis or prognosis.

Children's Rights: Education, Leisure and Cultural Activities

Health, social and education departments should aspire to implementing the rights outlined in the United Nations Convention on the Rights of the Child (1989), specifically those relating to children who are on long-term ventilation who have a right to:

- participate in family and community activities
- access to services that are culturally competent and sensitive
- basic health and welfare
- housing and social security
- civil rights and freedoms
- family life. (Noyes 2006)

> **ACTIVITY 6.1** Barriers to children's rights
>
> Consider the rights of children who are long-term ventilated and list the barriers that they may encounter.

PREVALENCE OF LONG-TERM VENTILATED CHILDREN IN THE UK

Lily has congenital central hyperventilation syndrome and requires long-term BiPAP ventilation. She also has a tracheostomy, which needs intermittent suctioning. UK children's long-term ventilation working party defined long-term ventilation as:

> Any child who when medically stable, continued to need a mechanical aid for breathing which may be acknowledged after a failure to wean, 3 months after the institution of ventilation. (Jardine and Wallis 1998)

Lily is part of a rapidly growing population of children and young people with a wide spectrum of impairments who require long-term ventilation. These children are often labelled 'technology dependent' and are not considered within the category of palliative care. According to Boosfield and O'Toole (2000) children may require ventilation for any of the following reasons:

- They were born prematurely and have developed severe, chronic lung disease.
- Their primary problem relates to instability of the upper airway.
- They have survived acute illness or trauma.

- They have neuromuscular disorders.
- They have complex long-term needs and have usually survived deterioration within a chronic disease or an acute and life-threatening illness, such as trauma or major surgery.

Over the last 10 years the incidence of children with chronic respiratory insufficiency has grown. Jardine et al. (1999) carried out a survey in 1998 that identified that there were 141 children receiving long-term ventilation. This survey was repeated in

Table 6.1 Policy specifically relating to the technology-dependent child

Disability Discrimination Act 1995	• It is unlawful to discriminate in relation to the provision of services against disabled people, including disabled children • Service providers have a duty under this Act to take reasonable steps to remove or alter physical barriers and to take reasonable steps to change practices, policies or procedures that make it impossible or unreasonably difficult for disabled people to use a service • Service providers should also take reasonable steps to provide auxiliary aids or services that enable disabled people to use a service or facilitate the use of such a service
Children Act 1989	• The Children Act 1989 provides a comprehensive framework for the care and protection of all children and young people in need, including those living away from home • Local authorities have a specific duty under section 22 of the Act to safeguard and promote the welfare of each child they look after • Under section 27 of the Act, local authorities are entitled to expect other authorities and certain NHS bodies to assist them in discharging their functions to children in need, looked after children and their parents and carers
Children Act 2004	Under section 10 of the Children Act 2004, PCTs are under a duty to cooperate with local authorities and other key partners in making arrangements to improve the well-being of children in their population and must have regard to guidance
Every child matters: Change for Children (DES 2003). Five outcomes: • be healthy • stay safe • enjoy and achieve through learning • make a positive contribution to society • achieve economic well-being	• Birth to age 19 • Aimed at the well-being of all children and young people in the UK • Protect children from harm and help them achieve in life • All children's services should: 　⊕ collaborate 　⊕ share information • Service user involvement in their care and service developments
National Service Framework for Children, Young People and Maternity Services (DoH 2004) Standards 1–5, apply to all children	Sets out standards for children's health and social care including: • promoting high quality • child-centred services • personalised care • meeting the needs of parents, children and their families
Standards 6–11 apply to specific groups of children	*Standard 8* Sets out the responsibilities of multiagency commissioners and service providers towards disabled children under the Disability Discrimination Acts (1995, 2005) and the Special Educational Needs and Disability Act (2001) Standard 8 of the Children's NSF highlights the importance of the role of a named key worker. Research has shown the benefits of having a key worker, commissioned jointly to work with families, who can: • provide information and advice • identify and address needs • improve access to services • improve coordination of services • provide emotional support • act as an advocate

National Framework for Children and Young People's Continuing Care (DoH 2010)	Home is the most appropriate place for the care of children with long-term health needs It focuses on the planning and provision of equitable, transparent and timely services for children who require complex care at home Consists of: ● a decision support tool (DST) to aid identification of continuing care needs in children and young people ● a continuing care pathway to help plan, design and deliver services. This care pathway is based on the Association for Children's Palliative Care Integrated Multiagency Care Pathway for Children with Life Threatening and Life-limiting Conditions
Aiming High for Disabled Children (DCSF 2008)	Provides evidence that families with disabled children often face particularly high stress and breakdown owing to the increased pressures of having a disabled child
Framework for the Assessment of Children in Need and their Families (DoH 2000a)	Provision of a comprehensive multidisciplinary needs assessment and joint planning of care with integrated provision to help maximise children and young people's development and achievement in life
Joint Planning and Commissioning Framework for Children, Young People and Maternity Service (DoH 2006)	Introduces a framework to help local commissioners (both PCTs and local authorities) to design a unified system in each local area for a joined-up picture of children and young people's needs and for collaboration to achieve best use of joint resources for better outcomes
Local Government and Public Involvement in Health Act (2007)	The voices of children, young people and their families are expected to inform local design and delivery arrangements of services which allows for the establishment of scrutinising and monitoring of health services and represent users' views

2008 and identified 933 children, a more than 600 per cent increase in 10 years (Wallis et al. 2011). Children are now surviving into adulthood, which is a likely contributor to the increase. A comparison of the census has been provided in Figure 6.2. The reasons behind this increase are likely to be the wider availability of improved paediatric home technology, i.e. ventilators and a changing ethos towards the benefits of home ventilation. This

increase in patient numbers has provided the impetus to develop individualised programs of care for these children outside an intensive care setting. This is not only important with regards to freeing up intensive care beds for other use, but also the needs of these patients which are better addressed in alternative care settings that can focus on growth and development, enhancing quality of life and the function of the child–family unit.

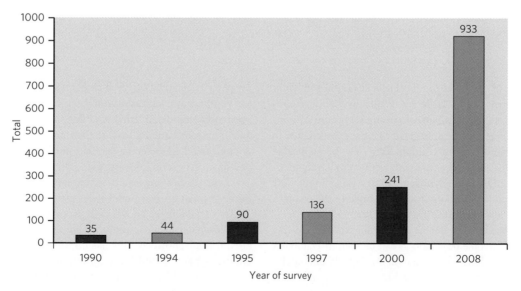

Figure 6.2 Comparisons of ventilated children in the UK by year
Source: Wallis et al. (2012)

Table 6.2 Comparison of LTV prevalence in 10-year period

	Jardine et al. 1999	Wallis et al. 2011
Number of children ventilated	141	933
Continuous positive pressure ventilation Ventilation by tracheostomy over 24-hour period	33 (24%)	88 (9.5%) ↓
Ventilation while asleep only	103	658
Ventilation by non-invasive mask	62 (46%)	704 (75%) ↑
Ventilation by tracheostomy	32 (24%)	206 (22%) ↓
Negative pressure ventilation	9 (7%)	–

Table 6.3 Diagnostic categories

Central nervous system	Congenital central hypoventilation syndrome
	Spinal injury
	Birth injury/cerebral palsy
	Acquired central hypoventilation syndrome
Musculoskeletal	Duchenne muscular dystrophy
	Congenital myopathy
	Myopathy
	Dystrophy
	Kyphoscoliosis
	Spinal muscular atrophy types I, II and III
	Mucopolysaccharidosis
Respiratory	Chronic lung disease
	Chronic lung disease (prematurity)
	Airway malacia
	Prader–Willi/obesity syndromes
	Upper airway obstruction
	Cystic fibrosis/primary ciliary dyskinesia

Source: Wallis et al. (2011)

A comparison of the data from Jardine et al. (1999) and Wallis et al. (2011) is provided in Table 6.2. While, overall, the numbers have increased, the numbers of children who are 24-hour ventilated have decreased for this group. This suggests that with increasing experience, many children can now be supported non-invasively; this makes the care management much simpler.

Lily has congenital central hypoventilation syndrome but there is a wide spectrum of disorders from the simple to the complex that require long-term ventilation, as can be seen in Table 6.3.

The study by Wallis et al. (2011) also highlighted the growing numbers of young people (*n* = 129) as can be seen in Figure 6.3. This represents a combination of survival through childhood plus an increasing contribution from the children with neuromuscular conditions such as Duchenne muscular dystrophy requiring the initiation of non-invasive ventilation (NIV) in their teenaged years. Consequently, programmes addressing the needs of these young people, particularly when their care is transferred to adult services, are required. An increasing number of children with disorders, previously considered lethal in childhood, will be transferring to adult physicians unfamiliar with their problems. Transitional programmes and adult service capacity for long-term care must be developed very soon to ensure a smooth transfer to adult services.

These studies suggest that there is a rising trend toward home ventilation from 68.5 to 92 per cent, as can be seen in Table 6.4 (Wallis et al. 2011). It is encouraging that children with complex chronic conditions are increasingly being looked after at home, however, this has important implications for the children's parents and local community services that support them. It is also likely to impact on local district general hospital resources and expertise that provide technical support and care during emergencies and intercurrent illnesses. Children with tracheostomies usually lived in the hospital.

Table 6.4 Location of care

	Jardine et al. 1999	**Wallis et al. 2011**
Home	93	844
Hospital	43	Acute hospital units = 34 PICU/HDU = 15

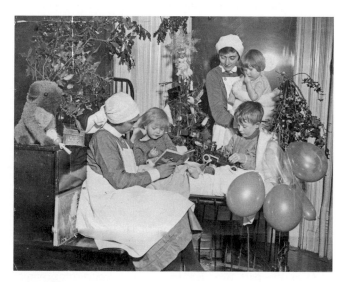

Prolonged hospitalisation: Christmas in the bronchoscopic clinic ward

Figure 6.3 Numbers of ventilated children by age
Source: Wallis et al. (2011).

Ever since the Platt Report in 1959, the negative impact of prolonged hospitalisation and separation from parents has been researched and documented (Ministry of Health 1959). Lily was in hospital for 6 months, a relatively shorter period of time, in contrast to the reported average lengths of time. Many children spent between 7 and 18 months (an average of 13 months) longer than medically necessary (Noyes 2000b). Long-term ventilated children who are unable to live with their families spend longer or indefinite periods in hospital. According to Ludvigsen and Morrison (2003) prolonged hospitalisation, especially in distant regional or tertiary hospitals, as in Lily's case, increases the risk of vulnerable families losing contact with their child and hence their chance of returning home. Parents and carers described their children as having become 'institutionalised' as a result of their prolonged hospitalisation.

Lily and her family endured periods of isolation while in hospital, which had impacted on her social and emotional development. Many research studies have shown that the emotional, social and psychological needs of this group of children are not being met and may, in fact, be made worse by their experience, as discussed in other chapters. The young people in Noyes' study also describe their boredom, apathy and hatred of hospitals. Whereas, in the study by Darvill et al. (2009), the children's stories and drawings of being sick were set in hospital. They did respond positively by drawing about happy things: feeling better, getting good news about going home and receiving presents. However, not everything that happened in hospital was seen positively and their stories revealed their suffering.

VOICES 6.2

'A sense of being in limbo and socially excluded' (a young person, cited in Noyes 2000).

RESEARCH NOTE 6.1 Enabling young 'ventilator-dependent' people to express their views and experiences of their care in hospital (Noyes 2000a)

A phenomenological study was carried out in England describing the views and experiences of young 'ventilator-dependent' people aged 6 to 18 years, regarding their health and social care, education, and aspirations for the future. Findings reveal that a significant number of articles in the United Nations (UN) Convention on the Rights of the Child were not respected or upheld. Young 'ventilator-dependent' people were discriminated against when trying to access health services because of their need for assisted ventilation. They were particularly excluded from making important decisions about their lives. Some young people were not able to maintain adequate contact with their families, first language, culture, nationality and religion. Almost all spent prolonged periods of time (in some cases years) in hospital when they no longer wanted or needed to be there. All those interviewed wanted to be discharged far sooner. Innovative methods of data collection were used with younger children and those who had a range of communication impairments.

SAFEGUARDING CONCERNS FOR CHILDREN IN HOSPITAL

In addition to the general safeguarding concerns, this group of children are vulnerable to neglect of their emotional, developmental, and educational and attachment needs that may be caused not by the action of an individual but by default. For example, while living on an intensive care unit children and young people may be routinely exposed to horrific incidents and frightening adult behaviour inflicted on critically sick and dying children (safeguarding; Chapter 5).

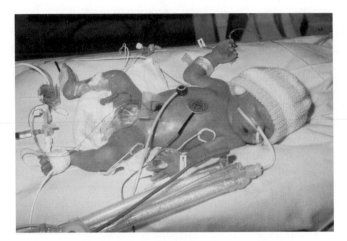

Paediatric intensive care unit

Paediatric Intensive Care and High-Dependency Care

Medically stable, ventilator-dependent children are often nursed in paediatric intensive care units (Murphy 2008). A PICU has a crucial part to play in helping the family gain trust in the expertise of the local specialists and to encourage flexibility with the routine so that it is truly focused around the child and family at home. Table 6.5 provides a framework for the degree of support and care required and demonstrates how the features of a HDU include; acting as a 'step-up' or 'step-down' unit between the level of care on the general ward and PICU, providing a continuum of care (Crawford and Powell 2004).

Many children such as Lily are socially and clinically ready to be at home but are often being cared for in an inappropriate environment. The health professional in the intensive care unit is primarily focused on medical and technical interventions in order to stabilise a child during an acute illness. In addition, staff are confronted with the pressure of acute admissions. Therefore, Lily often had to cope with inconsistencies in care, with either over or understimulation or lack of access to normal developmental experiences (Boosfield and O'Toole 2000).

This means there is often little time for developmental or social interventions and therefore not compatible with the long-term, dynamic and complex needs of a developing child. It is well recognised that the hospital represents both an unsuitable environment for a growing child and an inappropriate use of resources.

Ultimately, whatever the environment, parents and/or carers and the child or young person should be involved in the learning about procedures, processes and services that affect them. Health professionals need to be creative in providing opportunities for parents to be confident with their own skills outside the hospital environment and the support it provides.

Parental Distress in PICU

Lily's parents felt disempowered within the PICU environment and their role as the primary caregiver was initially taken on by the nursing staff (Colville and Gracey 2006). Lily's parents were faced with the shocking reality of their child in PICU and needed permission to touch and participate in her care. Lily's initial instability was further compounded by equipment, monitors, tubes and noise. Haines and Wolstenholme (2000) identified that parents feel a great deal of stress, grief and helplessness when their child is admitted to the PICU. While it is reasonable to accept that nurses undertake many technical aspects of Lily's care, consideration should be given to the preservation of the parent role wherever possible with sensitivity (Colville 2008).

Over the past two decades, research concerning parent stress in the high-technology PICU and NICU settings has demonstrated that medical technology and equipment have contributed to the experience of parental stress (Board and Ryan-Wenger 2003). Board (2004) found that all interviewed mothers with hospitalised children reported stress from hearing monitor alarms and viewing the heart rate on the monitor. Board and Ryan-Wenger (2003) found that 87 per cent of fathers reported stress related to sounds of their child's monitors in the PICU setting. However, Harbaugh et al. (2004) in a qualitative study of 19 parents with children hospitalised in the PICU, analysed parents' perceptions of nursing care and found that parents acknowledged the importance of medical technology and expected nurses to be competent at using this technology (Colville and Cream 2009).

Managed Local Children's Clinical Networks

All children and young people must have access to primary, secondary and tertiary medical services if and when they need them, whether they live close to, or remote from a centre of care. Managed clinical networks, both local children's networks and specialist clinical networks, are a means of ensuring this; they bring together the range of services. Managed clinical networks have been around for over 10 years and although each one is different, they all comply with the same core principles. The purpose of a managed clinical network is to link people across boundaries to improve services for the people using them. Very

Table 6.5 Stepping up and down of intensive care

Environment	Level of care / intervention	Advantages and disadvantages
Intensive care (Level 3 or above) (DoH 1997)	Children with two or more organ systems needing technological support, including advanced respiratory support, will need intensive nursing supervision at all times and will be undergoing complex monitoring and/or therapeutic procedures	PICU service providers are all required to provide a high-quality, integrated and comprehensive service organised with respect to the needs of the individual child and family and to the needs of the general population
Intensive care (Level 2) (DoH 1997)	These children will always need continuous nursing supervision. They may need ventilatory support, or support for two or more organ systems Sometimes the child will have one organ system needing support and one other suffering from chronic failure Usually children receiving Level 2 care are intubated to assist breathing	The service should be coordinated and seamless from the initial intensive care episode through a period of transitional care to eventual family home or a suitable community based alternative Many PICU centres have developed outreach services and training programmes for non-hospital-based staff
High dependency care (often described as Level 1) (DoH 1997)	Closer observation and monitoring than is usually available on an ordinary children's ward. For example, the child may need continuous monitoring of vital signs or single organ support (but not respiratory support)	Studies conducted found to be more private and restful, and also more accessible to visiting family and friends. It is also generally less noisy and not as technological as a PICU (Ruby et al. 1995)
Children's wards	Recently acute ward areas are frequently required to care for critically ill children or to support the respiratory needs of otherwise stable children (Haines et al. 2006).	District general hospitals have one major advantage, that of proximity to the child's home (Boosfield and O'Toole 2000) Most hospitals, however, are confronted only occasionally with a long-term ventilated child Nursing a medically stable but ventilator-dependent child on a paediatric ward challenges the traditional nursing routine and requires high flexibility, enormous commitment, and detailed planning and risk management Nevertheless, provision for a low-dependency care environment could be made close to the child's family home if he or she needs prolonged hospitalisation prior to discharge (Boosfield and O'Toole 2000)
High dependency care in the community	The original model for the care of long-term ventilation of children was hospital focused; it is increasingly being recognised that transitional care could also be provided in a community setting Several authors suggest that education and support may help prepare parents and other caregivers to adjust to the introduction of technology into their child's care while hospitalised (Ratliffe 2002)	There is considerable interest in promoting the provision of HDC in the community; however, there is the problem of providing adequate services in the community to allow for appropriate and timely discharge (RCN 2009) Community HDC care can be facilitated with appropriate support and careful planning, using the appropriate resources such as the national need assessment tool (NHS 2004)

few people are employed in managed clinical networks; rather, they achieve results by enabling participants to come together to work through what needs to change.

The local children's clinical network needs to take account of:

- **The characteristics of the child population**, measures of health need and the needs of vulnerable groups. This includes likely changes in numbers of children in the area, socioeconomic factors, transient and hard-to-reach populations, and the need for interpreting services.
- **Geography**, transport links and patient flows.
- **Staffing pressures** and **workforce issues**, in the current service and proposed models.
- **The need to increase the capacity of primary care** and skills to deliver a range of services to children, including chronic disease management, e.g. asthma, in line with the national target on chronic disease management.
- **Maternity, neonatal and accident and emergency services**: changes in acute service provision for children

have immediate impact on these services. Accident and emergency services are a vital component of ambulatory services.

Essential features of a managed clinical network are:

- clinical and managerial leadership and accountability
- trust between participants
- common protocols for care
- management of resources
- audit and governance.

ACTIVITY 6.2 Children's managed clinical networks

What are the components of a local children's clinical network?

RESEARCH NOTE 6.2 Impact on parents of a child's admission to intensive care (Colville and Cream 2009)

In this mixed methodology study, parents were asked which aspects of their experience of having a child in intensive care had caused them the most distress and how they continued to be affected by these experiences. Significant themes included the vividness of parents' memories of admission; the intensity of distress associated with times of transition; and the lasting

impact of their experience, in terms both of the ongoing need to protect their child and in relation to their priorities in life. Fathers reported different coping strategies, spent less time on the unit and were less likely than mothers to report fearing that their child would die.

VOICES 6.3

'It's a whole new world and new language for parents to learn if they have never had any experience before' (parent).

ACTIVITY 6.3 BiPAP ventilation

Lily has a tracheostomy and requires intermittent suctioning as and when needed. Lily is ventilated via a BiPAP when she is asleep, which was more frequent when she was an infant.

Why does Lily need ventilation?
What is BiPAP ventilation?

PARENTS, CHILDREN AND TECHNOLOGY IN THE COMMUNITY

Wang and Barnard's (2004) literature review on technology-dependent children encompassed research from 1976 to 2004 and addresses issues of the chronically ill paediatric patient and technological dependence. This review addressed various social aspects of care of the technology-dependent child in the

community that are important to note but may or may not be applicable to the inpatient setting. These issues include chronic illness as experienced by children, the impact of home care on children, the unique experiences of technology-dependent children and their families, and parents' experience of caring for the technologically dependent child in the home setting. The study concluded that both the presence of medical technology and healthcare professionals in the home may change the family's concept of 'home', as well as changing the parent's range of caregiving responsibilities, and change the relationships between the ill child, his or her family members, healthcare professionals and society (Wang and Barnard 2004, 2008).

A large body of research examines parents' perceptions of medical technology used in community settings. In one such study, researchers evaluated parents' responses to the use of medical technology in the home in the United Kingdom (Kirk et al. 2005). Parents of 24 children dependent on medical technology were interviewed. The parents reported the types of medical technology used in their homes included tracheostomy, oxygen, mechanical ventilation, IV medication, total parenteral nutrition (TPN), and dialysis, among others. Most parents reported a minimum of two types of technology being used in the home. Kirk and Glendinning (2004) found that the home itself could become a place in which there was tension between the need for a normal life and the equipment required to care for the child.

Noise was also found to be a problem, with alarms from the machinery causing disruption and noise from equipment, such as oxygen concentrators, being continuous in some homes. Some parents made efforts to try to normalise the home environment by camouflaging or hiding equipment so that it did not dominate and by covering hospital-style beds with brightly coloured bedding to try to distract from their medical purpose (Carnevale et al. 2006). Parents stated that the inclusion of medical technologies in the home changed the nature of their parenting. Many felt they took on the role of nurse in addition to the parental role, sometimes feeling that they were forced to switch between the two roles as circumstances required. This role change may also exist for the parent of the hospitalised child, who may feel that he takes on part of the role of the nurse,

particularly for the parents of chronically ill children who may become more familiar with medical technologies.

While there is a growing body of research that has examined children's experiences of disability and chronic illness, very few studies have focused on those whose lives are sustained by medical technologies. Kirk's (2010) qualitative study has explored how young people experience, understand and negotiate living a technology-assisted life. It has highlighted how children see medical technology as both a positive and negative presence in their lives. Interestingly, in the study by Darvill et al. (2009), the children clearly understood their technology in their own terms, as they are able to explain its purpose and how it functioned. The ventilators were described positively as easy, being good, helping with breathing and preventing death.

PRACTICAL GUIDELINES 6.1

Over a period of time Lily's parents became familiar and comfortable with the presence of medical technology during their hospital admission and gained comfort in knowing that their child was being closely monitored. Eventually, Lily's parents started to interpret some of the data output, i.e. low saturation readings. They became comfortable disconnecting Lily from the monitors to provide care, such as bathing or feeding. Although this could potentially have

negative consequences for the child, it may also be viewed as a sign that the parent is confident in his or her ability to 'monitor' the child without technology. Lily's parents had gained an understanding of the data the technology produces and incorporated these data into decision making about her care. Indeed, over the ensuing years, Lily's siblings took on responsibilities in suctioning and tracheostomy changes.

RESEARCH NOTE 6.3 Caring for ventilated children at home: the child's perspective (Darvill et al. 2009)

This study described the experiences of two Australian ventilator-dependent children who are cared for at home. A primary objective was to capture the voices of the children themselves. Data were generated with the children themselves, who drew pictures and told stories of children just like them.

The study confirmed that children can meaningfully contribute to research. Listening to the child's voice and their participation in their care is now acceptable practice.

VOICES 6.4

'For other parents in a similar situation, I want them to know that even though times can be tough, life can get better if you get the right support' (parent).

Benefits of the Child being at Home

The general health, wellbeing and development of children on [long-term ventilation] had significantly improved since being at home. (Margolan et al. 2004)

Many studies have discussed that the physical health of children improved significantly after they came home. The goals of home ventilation are:

● to enhance growth and development

● to sustain and extend quantity of life without compromising quality
● to improve or sustain physical and psychological function
● to provide cost-effective care
● to minimise disruption to family life.

Once home, Lily's parents described her as 'blossoming'; she gained confidence as well as making remarkable improvement in her developmental milestones. Her personality changed, she was able to smile and was clearly happy at being in her home environment with her family. The transfer home of technology-dependent children signals a shift in the balance of power from professionals to the parents. The parents are expanding their parenting role to include a complex nursing role. This challenges nurses to learn to manage this transition and indeed the development of the parent as the expert in order to foster a supportive partnership.

Studies have shown that children cared for at home had fewer hospital-acquired infections, such as MRSA, chest

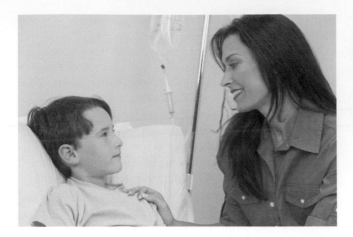

Benefits of the child being at home

ACTIVITY 6.4 Key goals in discharge planning

Reflect on Lily and her family's prolonged hospitalisation.

Consider what the key goals will be in discharge planning.

infections, diarrhoea, colds and coughs. The overall amount of time they spent on the ventilator was also reduced, with most of them requiring only night-time ventilation. Parents and carers highlighted the social and emotional benefits of home care. Attending school provided the children with opportunities to interact and play with other children, which again helped their sense of independence and belonging in the community.

PLANNING FOR DISCHARGE OF A CHILD FROM HOSPITAL

What the child really needs is to be out of hospital, to be in a home environment where they can be picked up and cuddled and played with, and have normal bedtimes and bathtimes and playtimes with the family and have their brothers and sisters around them. (Dr Gillian Halley, intensive care consultant)

Interprofessional discharge planning national standards recommend that efforts are made to discharge children home from hospital as quickly and safely as possible (Carlin 2010) and it is generally accepted that children fare much better at home. Table 6.6 details a number of research articles that highlight the discharge and the themes to be considered when discharging ventilated children. Navigating a discharge from hospital to home can be a protracted process, fraught with difficulties for a child with complex care needs. In preparation for discharge, the family needs to be empowered in their new role as primary carers. Family-related issues such as the ability of the family to cope safely with the child's care and other demands on the family, e.g., other children or work commitments need to be taken into consideration.

The Council for Disabled Children and the Department of Health produced guidelines on the discharge from hospital of children and young people with high support needs (Carlin 2010). These guidelines should be read in conjunction with the guidance issued by the Department of Health (2010) *National framework for children's continuing care*. Despite these policy initiatives, one of the most challenging aspects of improving the quality of services and the experience of children has been the lack of widespread implementation of best practice guidance in the assessment of need, the organisation of discharge of children from hospital and the effective continued management of a package of services to enable children and their families to live as near ordinary lives as possible at home.

PRACTICAL GUIDELINES 6.2

Preparing a technology-dependent child for discharge

Lily's parents could not imagine living at home without the level of nursing support and technical back-up provided by the intensive care unit. Initially, they requested that a team of highly trained children's nurses be employed to care for Lily at home, which was not appropriate or deliverable. Parents often have a better idea of their needs once they gain confidence and competence and have experienced some time at home with their child. Nonetheless, getting the right balance concerning the amount and type of care is very challenging. The principle here should be to find a balance that is deliverable in *practice*. It is often helpful for parents to know that there are flexibilities built into the care package that can be used when they require periods of additional support.

While the family could envisage the benefits of having Lily at home, Roger was also coming to terms with the prospect of having a constant presence of carers in their home.

The discharge plan is made following a framework for discharge planning that has been adapted locally. This includes planned and good advice on timescales, actions and responsibilities.

The community children's nurse (CCN) key worker provided a discharge-planning checklist that is individualised for Lily and her family; a copy is given to professionals involved in the process so all are confident that all aspects of Lily's discharge are clear about who is responsible for them. An agreement of care between the family and the community nursing service is drawn up and agreed with Penny and Roger. This

is a useful tool to help family needs and establish a working partnership between the family and community nursing team, to ensure clarification of roles, responsibilities and expectations.

Three unqualified carers were employed and underwent robust competency training, working within documented guidelines. They began working with Lily and her family within the PICU and then in the home. Once the family and the trained carers completed the training programme they were able to take Lily out of PICU for short trips and eventually home for the day.

During the first trips home the CCN keyworker accompanied Lily and her family. The day trips went well and, without any adverse incidents, the family's and carers' confidence in their abilities grew. Meanwhile, equipment and the associated supplies were now in place at home.

The first night at home was arranged with the CCN key worker and carer. It was a major hurdle for Penny and Roger but they were reassured that they had 24-hour access to speak to either medical or nursing staff in PICU, as well as having back-up from the CCN team.

Final discharge arrangements were agreed with parents and various members of the interprofessional team were involved. Emergency and utility companies were informed by the key worker.

The hospital play specialist had worked with Jason and Emily in preparing them to have their sister back at home.

Discharge from hospital can cause anxiety for parents, children and health professionals alike and therefore in order to manage the transition successfully sufficient information and planning is required. While there has been a significant number of studies that discuss the process and barriers to discharge (Table 6.6 provides an overview of research specific to the ventilated child), there has been very few that conveyed a sense of the parents' experiences and needs throughout the whole process.

ACTIVITY 6.5 Interprofessional responsibilities

Consider who would be involved with Lily's interprofessional discharge meeting and what are their key responsibilities?

Consider the difficulties in discharging a child with a tracheostomy and requiring long term ventilation.

The essential role of the interprofessional team in enabling the discharge cannot be underestimated and planning should begin at the earliest opportunity (see Table 6.7). Planning is

complex and requires pragmatic coordination from a nominated lead professional who has the time, ability and expertise to orchestrate this process and keep the child, family and interprofessional team regularly updated. As Figure 6.4 demonstrates, many concurrent activities need to be undertaken by the family and the interprofessional team before the child can be safely and quickly discharged. It is helpful to have a discharge coordinator in this role, where available. Timely interprofessional team meetings, involving hospital-based and community professionals may help to clarify roles, responsibilities and holistic action plans.

It is imperative that the child and family are central to the planning process and are involved throughout to respect their wishes and needs (Lewis and Noyes 2007). Transfer of information between relevant agencies is crucial, particularly where needs are complex and detailed planning is required, for example, for equipment or to ensure that training programmes can be continued at home. Indeed, most of the literature considering home ventilation refers to the technical education of parents as part of the process of discharge from hospital, although parents report variable training for themselves and other family members prior to taking their child home (Margolan et al. 2004).

Table 6.6 Articles relating to discharge of the long-term ventilated child

Study/Article	Themes of the article

Jardine and Wallis (1998)	• Discharge team
	• Discharge process
	• Needs assessment:
	  • funding
	  • equipment and supplies
	  • servicing and maintenance contract
	  • rehabilitation
	• Housing review
	• Home carers
	• Training programmes and risk management
	  • emergency procedures
	• Return to the education system in children of school age respite care

Lewis and Noyes (2007)	• Discharge process • Parental involvement • Equipment

Edwards, O'Toole and Wallis (2004)	• Common delays to the discharge process
	  • staff recruitment
	  • funding
	  • family issues
	  • housing
	• Benefits

Noyes and Lewis (2005)	• This guidance draws heavily on existing examples of best practice relating to the discharge and ongoing management of children who require long-term ventilation • The care pathway described in the guidance has been adopted as an exemplar within the National Service Framework for Children

Poorly coordinated planning prolongs the discharge process (Noyes 2002; Ludvigsen and Morrison 2003; Edwards et al. 2004). The main barriers to a rapid discharge are the difficulties in recruitment of home care staff, incomplete funding, unsuitable housing and local bureaucracy. Margolan et al. (2004) found that this delay causes considerable frustration and distress to parents who feel unwanted while on the PICU, aware that their child is potentially blocking a bed that could be used for an acutely ill child. Noyes also describes barriers, such as 'attitudes of professionals, lack of joint commissioning and accounting responsibilities, general poor management both within the health service and in collaborating with other services, complex social issues, housing problems and a general lack of auditing and outcome measures' (Noyes 2002, pages 2–11).

Ludvigsen and Morrison (2003) suggest that a framework known to both the community and hospital settings would offer better coordination and overcome major barriers to timely discharge such as funding and housing issues, and recruitment of supporting staff (Jardine et al. 1999; Noyes 2002). Lack of collaboration between services and issues of parental, medical and nursing responsibility also hinder the discharge process.

ASSESSMENT

A systematic assessment process is essential to ensure that the child's and family members' health is fully appreciated and the full range of needs addressed in partnership (DoH 2000, 2004, 2008). Getting the assessment process right for families is one of the most important factors in delivering an effective service that will meet individual and family needs; it is particularly relevant in the context of interprofessional and interagency working. A number of these more specialist assessment tools have been developed specifically for long-term ventilated children or children with complex care needs. Examples of best practice in assessment have been discussed in Chapter 14.

Burden of Care and a Normal Life

Some families cope well with the most distressing problem, whereas others are devastated by disabilities that in purely medical terms are less severe. The differences are to be found in the personalities and life experiences of the child and their parents, the functioning and strength of the family unit and the effectiveness of their network of support

Table 6.7 Roles of the interprofessional team

Speech and language therapist

Children requiring ongoing ventilation may have tracheostomies and frequently have specific speech and language difficulties. In addition, there are often issues concerning the safety of oral feeding and management of drooling in children with neuromuscular conditions. Speech therapists have a vital role to play in the assessment of and development of child-specific therapy programmes to develop their orofacial and communication skills. Ideally, this should be a speech therapist with skills and experience in these areas

Physiotherapist

The physiotherapist plays a role in the initial assessment of the child's suitability for a long-term ventilation programme. In the hospital, they have a role in the development of specific therapy in addition to the supervision of regular chest physiotherapy for the ventilated child. The hospital physiotherapist must liaise closely with both the community and school physiotherapists to ensure consistency of the treatment the child receives. They should evaluate the patient and equipment in the home setting on a monthly basis and whenever there is a change in patient status or possible concern of equipment malfunction

Psychologist

Psychology input may be required to help with the change in life circumstances, which could include the fostering process, helping the family and child to come to terms with the enormity of the life events that they are experiencing and this may take the form of full counselling. Children can present behavioural problems related to any trauma they may have experienced. A psychologist may be able to advise on strategies for caring for the child and family and how to ensure consistency of approach between all those involved with the discharge process. Psychology input allows a rational basis to the way the teams approach and manage the children and their disabilities. The psychologist would have a role in the assessment of the effect the child's disability has on the child and their family and advise on coping strategies. The clinical psychologist will have an ongoing role post-discharge to support the child, family and team and should work across the boundaries of hospital and home. They have a role to play both in the hospital and home setting. The need to assess and support the family is ongoing. In order to perform these assessments, they must understand the demands that caring for this type of child can place on the family. In addition, they provide the expertise to help families optimally access and utilise community resources and benefits in particular

Social worker

Although the child may well be known to social services in his own area, it is desirable to have a direct link to the hospital to facilitate statutory meetings and to advocate for the child and his family. Often the major block to home discharge is the suitability of the family property, and adaptation through grants may be required

among relatives, friends and professional services (Hall and Hill 1996, page 1).

VOICES 6.5

'When I'm looking after the boys on my own, life somehow has to fit around all of Charlie's procedures' says Tracey. 'It makes it very hard to do anything normal, from going to the supermarket to getting a decent night's sleep' (parent).

ACTIVITY 6.6

Consider and list some of the difficulties Lily and her family face in day-to-day life.

For Lily and her family, home life is far from easy. Families experience a considerable burden physically, psychologically, emotionally and financially when caring for a ventilated child at home (Margolan et al. 2004; Kirk et al. 2005; Rehm and Bradley 2005). Parents identified a range of emotionally exhausting issues. Some of the recurring themes in the literature about the emotional pressures experienced by parents are: sleeplessness; the strain of 24-hour vigilance; the experience of the healthcare system as a challenge not a support; the loss of privacy when nursing staff are providing care for a family member at home and associated problems of reliability of staff, theft and intrusion and constant domestic disruption.

Consequently, parents go to great lengths to try to increase the stability of family life. This involves constant monitoring of the condition of the ventilated child to detect and treat any deterioration in condition. By constant observation and adhering strictly to routines parents are aiming to avoid hospital admission and further disruption to family life (O'Brien 2001; Kirk et al. 2005). In addition, Heaton et al. (2005) found that parents stuck to a rigid routine as a way of controlling and normalising their lives. Routine was used by some parents to emphasise the similarities between their families and 'normal' families (Rehm and Bradley 2005). This rigid control allowed the child and siblings to participate in activities outside the home, such

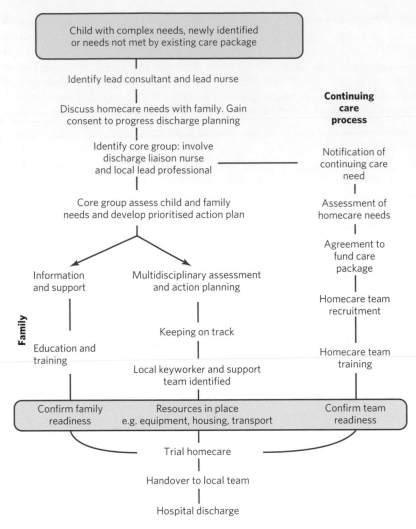

Figure 6.4 Algorithm for discharge of a child with complex needs

as schooling or social activities. There is also the added tension of balancing Lily's condition and risk with autonomy. If her parents are overprotective she may lose her independence and the opportunity to meet developmental tasks.

Kirk and Glendinning (2004) interviewed a total of 24 sets of parents with a child who is technology dependent. The researchers found that the lives of parents revolved around the technology so there was little opportunity to escape the reality of the situation they were in. Parents commented how important it is for them to have time with their child as a parent carrying out normal parenting activities. They view this time as distinct from the time spent undertaking nursing procedures such as suctioning. Carrying out painful and distressing procedures on their child and spending time in the nursing role has negative effects on how parents view themselves in the parenting role. Parents want to define themselves as parents, not nurses, which can be difficult due to the intensity of the nursing role (Kirk et al. 2005).

Most families who have children with serious illnesses eventually view their children and their lives as normal and manage

the illness-related demands successfully (Deatrick et al. 2006). Rehm and Bradley (2005) reported that for families like Lily's, denial was not possible because the continuous and intensive care giving required was a constant reminder to parents. One mother said: 'Every part of our conversation about future things, like where we want to be and where we want to live' was influenced by the need to provide optimal care for her daughter, 'because we can't live in places we might want to live if she were still alive with her situation. We'll never move away from the people here or her caregivers.' (Rehm and Bradley 2005, page 813). This can have a potential impact on the health of parents. Murphy et al. (2006) conducted a qualitative study on the caregiving experience, which is captured by five themes: the stress of care giving; the negative impact on caregiver health; sharing the burden; worry about the future; and caregiver coping strategies. Forty-one per cent of the caregivers reported that their health had worsened over the past year and attributed these changes to a lack of time, a lack of control and decreased psychosocial energy.

Many families are financially disadvantaged through caring for a technology-dependent child. Income can be substantially reduced when one parent is obliged to stop working to care for their child; in some cases, both parents give up work in order to share the care. Inevitably, single parents will also experience financial difficulties. Extra costs are incurred, for instance in travelling to clinics, providing additional heating in the home or purchasing special equipment, food or clothes. Such financial and employment problems and lack of social support put undue stress on families. While there are some entitlements, accessing them may be difficult. Parents are often unfamiliar with the benefits system and may not even be aware that financial assistance could be available to them. The financial situation of the family could be approached at assessment and the options explained. There are various avenues of help including care allowances, income support, travel grants, help with items such as nappies and charitable grants for items of equipment, holidays and other expenses. However, eligibility is generally means tested and rules governing this change frequently. As part of the agreed plan, the family's key worker could provide valuable help in obtaining financial assistance although it is vital that information is up to date (DoH 2004, 2009).

Equipment

Improving community equipment services provision to disabled children and their families requires action at a number of levels including: funding; broadening the scope of community equipment service (CES), improving access to CES, greater coordination between CES and housing adaptation services and strategic collection of information by services on the use and need of equipment. (Beresford et al. 2003, page 1)

Lily has significant equipment requirements to be cared for at home, to assist in meeting her daily living needs and promoting her independence (DoH 2004, 2007). Equipment is needed to support her daily life at home, in educational settings and to support her leisure activities. Equipment also enables children to become more independent, mobile, communicative and active and to live as fulfilling lives as is possible. Children's equipment is different from adults; not only is it likely to be smaller, it also needs to be adaptable to the changing development needs of the child as they grow. Unlike adults, children are likely to need considerably more ongoing support from professionals to ensure equipment and services fit emerging needs and wider family circumstances.

An early assessment and procurement of equipment can ensure that discharge is not unnecessarily delayed. Indeed, much of the research on discharging technology-dependent children highlights that one of the main obstacles to discharge has been identified as difficulty in getting agreement to fund a package of care to enable the child to live at home. The main reasons for these difficulties appear to stem from the lack of data concerning the costs associated with providing a package of services and the inability of various budget holders to agree on who should fund all or parts of the package. Discussions

on funding packages of care should commence early in the discharge process; it is important to involve those responsible for funding within the locality that the child will be discharged to. Poor local arrangements can result in delayed discharge from hospital, introduce unnecessary risks to the child at home and cause frustration for parents.

There is an expectation that community equipment services are integrated across health, social services and education ensuring multiagency arrangements are in place for the provision and maintenance of equipment and supplies (DoH 2004, 2007). Equipment chosen for home care should be portable and easy to use with the aim being not to transfer an intensive care unit to the child's home. The child must be well established and stable on the equipment that is going to be used at home while still in hospital. An itemised equipment list should be prepared according to the child's individual needs and all members of the management team should check this. The equipment list should include:

- purchased items
- leased equipment and servicing costs
- a monthly estimate of disposable supplies and consumables
- delivery or collection cost for the consumables
- revenue consequences including consumables and servicing costs.

The widespread adoption of mask interface and suitable bilevel devices for paediatric use has almost certainly contributed to this important change. The introduction of NIV for this group of children has significantly enhanced their respiratory management and, in some subgroups, has shown evidence of clinical and psychosocial benefits as well as a substantial increase in survival. It is anticipated that the use of NIV for paediatric neuromuscular disorders is likely to increase still further in forthcoming years. As the numbers grow, consideration will have to be given to the delivery of home healthcare and local hospital input, as tertiary centres will not be able to deliver the bulk of this service.

Risk Management

VOICES 6.6

'One of my biggest fears is the consequences of falling asleep and not knowing if there's a problem with the ventilator' (a parent).

Lily, like many children who are dependent on assisted ventilation, lives with a level of risk that other children do not. Risk management is the systematic process of identifying, evaluating and addressing potential and actual risk, and building up an organisational culture of being proactive towards safety (O'Rourke 2005). It is a valuable tool in supporting the assessment of eligibility for children's continuing care and for appraising options for care delivery. Risk management can be used to assess clinical or environmental

ACTIVITY 6.7   Types of equipment used in homecare services

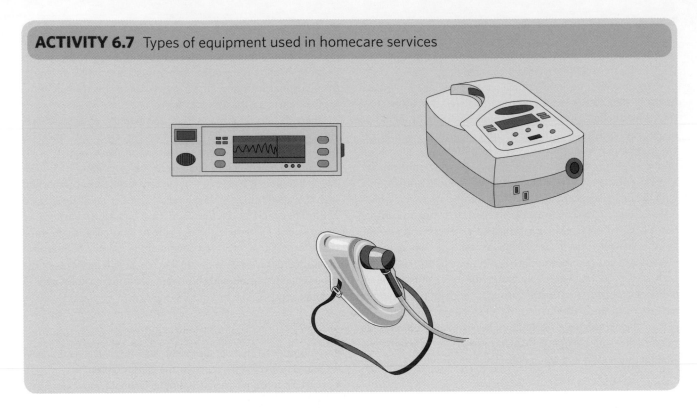

risk (see Chapter 15). Children with continuing care needs will receive care, support and education in a variety of settings. Risk management has the potential to enable inclusion or to be used as a justification for exclusion. The 'Dignity of Risk' (Lenehan et al. 2004) and 'Including me' (Carlin 2005) are key texts in using risk management to enable, rather than exclude, in social care and educational environments. In continuing care, risk assessment can be used to make informed decisions about staff levels and numbers, equipment and back up services. Organisations have a duty under the Disability Discrimination Act (2005) to overcome physical barriers and to take reasonable steps to change practices, policies or procedures, which make it impossible or unreasonably difficult for them to use a service. They must also be provided with auxiliary aids or services, which make it easier for them to use a service.

The lead nurse must address the requirement for a formal risk assessment of any equipment during the discharge process, as can be seen in Table 6.8. A written plan of training and

accountability is required and needs to be agreed on by the hospital, community team, family and carers. Careful documentation is important because of the medico legal implications. This would be in line with best practice and could support the family with respect to safety issues.

Minimising Clinical Risk

Many clinical interventions carry the risk of unexpected or unwanted outcomes and the cost of dealing with these is a significant burden on healthcare resources. Paediatric cases have their own specific problems, related to issues like physiological immaturity and patient size and complex family dynamics with third parties like guardians or parents. Techniques such as risk analysis and significant event audits can be used to develop strategies. Risk management brings benefits in reducing adverse clinical outcomes and litigation (O'Rourke 2005).

Care Closer To Home

VOICES 6.7

'When you are sitting here at home on your own at night and you are covered in vomit and you've got secretions stuck in your hair, you just think "Is this my life?" You know, and the pressure is on you.' (parent).

'Meaning and sense-making as key determinants of parent's experience when caring for children with disabilities and complex health needs' (Whiting 2009).

The National Service Framework for children, young people and maternity services (NSFCYPMS) (Standard 6) states that care for ill children should be timely and provided as 'close to home as

possible' (DoH 2004). This policy direction was confirmed with the later publication of the child health strategy, 'Healthy lives, brighter futures', which also advocated such care (DoH 2009b).

Table 6.8 Risk assessments may influence eligibility or care package design

Clinical risk	Parent and extended family training package will continue during the child's hospital admission in preparation for discharge home Competencies includes: • infection control • tracheostomy care • cardiopulmonary resuscitation • routine use of supplies and storage of supplies • using equipment and equipment failure – such as the ventilator

	For healthcare assistants:
	• a patient-specific training package should be devised
	• competencies includes:
	  ◦ tracheostomy care
	  ◦ cardiopulmonary resuscitation
	  ◦ routine use of supplies and storage of supplies
	  ◦ using equipment and equipment failure – such as the ventilator
	• carers should be deemed competent by the hospital unit and community staff, and the level of competence should be recorded in the patient's notes
	• the responsibility of carer training should never be placed on the parents although the parents will be involved in the training process

Staffing levels	• There should be annual assessment of Lily's and her family's holistic care needs, which are integral with the amount of staff required • There should be an annual review of cardiopulmonary resuscitation for the carers • Core team meetings need to be held regularly to address problem areas and discuss changing needs • This may include decisions regarding future resuscitation policies and the training of replacement carers
Moving and handling	For parents and carers this should include annual training and competencies in moving and handling patients and equipment
Environment of care	• Initially, there should be a negotiated secondment to Lily's local hospital to complete the training programme with a short familiarisation course at home • As Lily enters the education system there should be a negotiated secondment to her nursery/school to complete the training programme • Assessing storage of medical supplies • Electrical supply and location of sockets for electro-medical equipment • Lone working • Medical gas safety

Source: adapted from O'Rourke (2005) and Lewis and Noyes (2007)

Lily's care requirements will vary from those of other children and the level of support required in the home is best determined by a local interprofessional assessment with supporting advice from a PICU/transitional care unit. The makeup of the care team will depend on the level of need, recognising that the child's needs may vary over time. The focus is on helping children to lead a normal life to the greatest extent possible. The home team should consist of experienced community children's nurses (CCN) to coordinate clinical care, as well as supporting others, including professionals from outside the health services

such as teachers, parents and carers, in providing care for the child. CCNs would be responsible for the recruitment, training, supervision and quality assurance of the care provided by a team of healthcare assistants.

The provision of care for ill children outside hospital is perhaps most commonly recognised in the UK in the form of children's community nursing teams, whose presence in the NHS reaches back to the 19th century with the establishment of a home nursing service by Great Ormond Street Hospital for Sick Children. More than half a century later, after the advent of

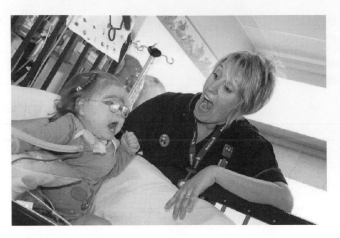

Community children's nurse

the NHS, home care for ill children was advocated in the Platt Report on the welfare of children in hospital (MoH 1959).

The need to reduce hospitalisation and shorten length of stay has prompted the development of specialist home-based nursing services for children with acute and chronic illnesses, to provide clinical review, support and education during the time of illness. It has been suggested that these services have the potential to reduce hospital admissions (Meates 1997), reduce length of stay (Whiting 1997) and facilitate early discharge by providing a continuum of care from the hospital into the home. Appierto et al. (2002) also suggest that children's physical outcomes are generally better when they are cared for at home and that this is a more cost-effective option for the NHS. They also provide opportunities to enhance primary care in the community through liaison with general practitioners (GPs) and

VOICES 6.8

'Without Lucy, we would have been in the situation of having to go home without any help which is not a good place to be in when you've got another two babies to deal with. It's reassuring to know you have someone like Lucy on your side.' (parent—Well Child Charity)

through links with other community-based health services (Fradd 1994). In addition, facilitating home care may assist in empowering children and their families; while in hospital, the power ratio is tipped in favour of healthcare staff and parents are visitors in an unfamiliar environment. This situation is reversed in the family home, as it is the healthcare staff who are the visitors (Taylor 2000).

Today, surveys of CCN provision indicate growth in the number of CCN teams with Whiting (2007) reporting 192 teams in England in 2007. Despite the increase in the number of teams providing care, there are still children who do not have access to a community children's nurse. In addition, the complexity of community children's nursing practice has been acknowledged (Sloper and Beresford 2006; RCN 2009). The CCN service should be an integral part of other primary

healthcare and community provision. Whiting (2007) has distinguished seven types of care provided via the CCN: neonatal care, acute care, supporting planned surgery, long-term care, follow-up and emergency care, care for disabled children and palliative care, as can be seen in Table 6.9. While CCN teams may differ in their remit of care, most share features in terms of their coverage, base settings, referral sources and care activities. Figure 6.5 illustrates the core attributes, as detailed in the research by Carter and Coad (2009).

Community children's nurses often adopt key worker roles for caring for children and young people with particular conditions. All long-term ventilated children should have access to an identified and effective key worker system, as outlined in the joint Department of Health/Department for Education and Skills guidelines, 'Together from the start' (DOH and DfES,

Table 6.9 Community children's nursing: differing roles

'Traditional' community children's nursing
Neonatal community nursing
Ambulatory/urgent care
Disability nursing
Special school nursing (and supporting children with complex needs in 'mainstream' school)
Palliative care
Diabetes care
Paediatric oncology outreach nursing (POON)
Continuing care
Advanced practice

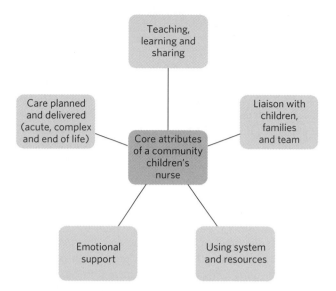

Figure 6.5 CCN core attributes
Source: Carter and Coad (2009)

- a way of working across agencies
- a way of working with families' strengths and ways of coping
- a way of working for the *family* as opposed to working for an agency (see Figure 6.5).

The community children's nurse's role as advocate may include representing to others the need for a carer who can meet the child's needs and accompany him or her to school, and for staffing and other resources, including transport, to be made available for extracurricular activities. Children who have complex health needs may also miss school more often than their peers because of the number of health-related appointments that they have to attend, as well as because of ill health. Nurses may be instrumental in emphasising to parents their right to request planning of appointments to minimise such interruptions (Hewitt-Taylor 2007). Nurses may have a role in supporting parents while they seek the right provision for their child and in explaining the steps (such as obtaining a statement of special educational need) that may be necessary to enable them to obtain appropriate support in school settings.

Lastly, an emphasis needs to be placed on supporting CCN development and ensuring that they receive sufficient ongoing training and updating in their field of expertise. (The keyworker role is discussed in more detail in Chapter 14.)

2003). A key worker or lead professional is responsible for coordinating the child's comprehensive care package, coordinating and liaising with all the professionals and services involved with the child and being a main point of contact for the family. The key worker will be responsible for undertaking a risk assessment of the home and of the education setting as appropriate, as illustrated in Table 6.8. Studies of key workers consistently report positive effects on relationships with services, fewer unmet needs and greater family well-being. However, fewer than one-third of families with severely disabled children have a key worker.

Key workers should be able to offer the child and family:

- proactive, regular contact
- a supportive, open relationship
- a family-centred approach

ACTIVITY 6.8 SWOT analysis of a CCN service

Lily's keyworker is a senior nurse within the children's community nursing team. In your experience, consider some of the issues for the children's community nursing service and undertake a SWOT analysis of the service you have experienced.

RESEARCH NOTE 6.4

Managing the caseload: a qualitative action research study exploring how community children's nurses deliver services to children living with life-limiting, life-threatening and chronic conditions (Pontin and Lewis 2008).

This qualitative action research study used in-depth interviews to determine how community children's nurses (CCNs) manage their caseloads.

The study generated a number of insights about the sorts of phenomena that contribute to CCNs' perceptions of workload. Themes included strategy, being proactive, purposeful visit and knowing families.

THE ROLE OF THE CARER

When Lily was initially discharged home, she had a team of carers to help with the amount of care that was required in the home. Her parents, relatives and friends could not help with

childcare unless they had been trained, so her parents relied on formal services to provide a break from caring. However, both parents and professionals described how accessing such support was one of the biggest problems families faced (Jardine et al. 1999; Noyes 2002; Margolan et al. 2004). Usual short-term care or home-based support services were inappropriate because of Lily's specialised nursing needs. Consequently, homecare workers were specially recruited and trained to support Lily at home and eventually at school, by providing a regular break during the day and/or overnight. This support could be required round the clock, if children had particularly intensive care needs. Other sources of help at home came from district nursing auxiliaries, Marie Curie nurses, voluntary agency workers, agency nurses, foster carers and family aides. However, the levels and sources of help with homecare seemed to be determined more by the area in which the family lived than their needs or those of the child.

The issue of whether the care should be provided by trained carers or qualified nurses complicates the provision of formal home-based respite care. The debate revolves around three main themes: competency of staff, training of personnel and accountability. Staff competency is frequently highlighted as an area of concern for families with the technology-dependent child (Kirk 1999; Noyes et al. 1999). Interestingly, the Kirk and Glendinning (2004) study found that parents did not object to homecare staff without professional qualifications, as long as they were familiar with the child and her treatment. Indeed, many parents thought they would be unable to sustain caring for their child at home without the support of home carers.

Carers will inevitably play a part in the child's emotional and physical development and that role has to be defined. The relationship between the carer and the family must be written down clearly and formalised prior to discharge. Assumptions should be avoided and the boundaries between the role of the family and carers must be clearly stated at the outset in order to avoid misunderstandings. Dybwik et al. (2011) carried out research that describes the challenges associated with working with long-term ventilated patients in their homes. Working inside a private residence was described as the biggest challenge and was the main trigger for the other challenges they described. Carers felt that they were merely guests in the patients' homes and this was something they had to be constantly aware of while at work. They held a low profile in order not to disturb peace in the home and thereby to avoid conflicts. The staff consciously kept a neutral demeanour, did not stand out, stayed quiet, closed their ears and held their tongues. They were, after all, in the patient's home and had to behave in keeping.

Education

Statutory Right to Education

All children have statutory rights to education under the UN Convention which should be directed towards 'the development of the child's personality, talents, mental and physical abilities to their fullest potential' (United Nations 1989). All education settings must comply with the Disability Discrimination Act 2005.

Education is a significant part of a child and young person's life. Education provides intellectual stimulation and development, social interaction and the attainment of qualifications that are key components in personal development. The value of education is reflected in the views of the young people in the study by Noyes et al. (1999). They reported significant examples of good practice and also disappointment at the discontinuity between hospitals, the low priority on education in some long-term medical settings, barriers to entering the school of their choice when living at home, insufficient classroom support, and sometimes damaging shortfalls in the communication facilities and staff skills that were essential in their education. Ludvigsen and Morrison (2003) state in their study that attending school provided the children with opportunities to interact and play with other children, which again helped their sense of independence and belonging in the community.

The intention is for all UK children to attend mainstream schools, unless their parents or guardians choose otherwise, or unless other children's education is compromised and there are no 'reasonable steps' that the school and local education authority can take to overcome this. Schools are obliged to treat all pupils equally and to make 'reasonable adjustments' to ensure that disabled pupils are not disadvantaged in relation to the full range of school activities.

In May 2010, the government set out its vision for disabled children and young people and those with special educational needs and their families in the Green Paper 'Support and aspiration: A new approach to special educational needs and disability' (DfE 2010) as can be seen in Table 6.10. The proposals have the potential to make a very positive impact on children who require continuing care from their families. In particular, the single assessment and education, health and social care plan could help to improve the integration and coordination of care for children and families. In addition, the introduction of a pooled and personal budget could, for those who want it, improve choice for families and consistency in approach for those providing services.

Table 6.10 Support and aspiration: a new approach to special educational needs and disability

- Children's special educational needs are picked up early and support is routinely put in place quickly

- Staff have the knowledge, understanding and skills to provide the right support for children and young people who have special educational needs (SENs) or are disabled wherever they are

- Parents know what they can reasonably expect their local school, local college, local authority and local services to provide, without them having to fight for it and are more closely involved in decisions about services

- Children who would currently have a statement of SEN and young people over 16 who would have a learning difficulty assessment have an integrated assessment and a single education, health and care plan which is completed in a shorter time

- Parents have greater control over the services they and their family use with:

  - every family with an education, health and care plan having the right to a personal budget for their support
  - parents whose children have an education, health and care plan having the right to seek a place at any state-funded school, whether that is a special or mainstream school, a maintained school, academy or free school

Source: DfE (2010)

However, there are some clear challenges. First, the single assessment and coordinated plan only refers to children and young people with a statement of special educational need (SEN). This will potentially exclude those children who are disabled, technology dependent or have a life-limiting condition, because they do not have a statement of SEN, including those very young children not in education or using early years' services. Second, the statutory regimes and funding systems in health and education are very different. While the Department for Education can bring legislation around a local authority duty to jointly plan and commission with local health services, the levers to make this happen in health are less clear. Local authorities are responsible for arranging to provide suitable education at school or elsewhere for children of school age who, because of illness, may not otherwise receive appropriate education. It will also be important for government to consider how to ensure pooling and personalising budgets does not add an administrational burden on families or undermine funding for vital services.

Health professionals liaising closely with the local authority, hospital, schools and home teaching services can make it possible for the child to receive some continuing education. Interprofessional care plans for children on long-term ventilation must acknowledge their educational needs and be clear about how these are to be met. This can enable the child's precise needs to be determined. It allows the opportunity for individuals as well as organisations to work collaboratively and to focus, as the social model of disability suggests, on removing barriers to participation, thus addressing concerns some education providers may have over their legal and professional responsibilities regarding aspects of a child's care, such as the administration of medication or tube feeding, as well as the practicalities of how this adds to their workloads.

Well-informed teachers, learning support assistants and other school staff are well placed to support the child or young person and enable them to have as 'normal' a life as possible by involvement in educational activities. Attention to pain management and symptom control services are primary considerations in order to help maximise the child's quality of life and the confidence of the family, schools and other providers. Services to provide appropriate advice and support to schools and other community services with regard to the administration of medication, management of personal care, counselling and risk management are further elements for consideration. However, for mainstream education to be truly inclusive, children with complex health needs must be able to engage meaningfully with their peers during a significant part of the school day and to participate in extracurricular and school time activities. If children have to leave lessons frequently, for example because of medication administration, tube feeding or airway suction, it can detract from their academic achievement and if they miss playtime activities it can make it difficult for them to socialise with their peers. If the parents of children with complex health needs have to come into school to meet their needs, it can set the child out as different from other children.

SHORT-BREAK CARE

VOICES 6.9

'Hannah's needs are so complex that it's rare for me to get a chance to spend any quality time with her brother in the school holidays, and when Hannah comes home it's wonderful to hear about the different activities she got involved with that day' (parent).

PRACTICAL GUIDELINES 6.3

By the time Lily was 3 years old, Roger and Penny felt that she was ready and would benefit from attending nursery. This would help her meet more children of her own age.

Lily attends a private nursery once agreement is reached between the local education authority and the health service commissioners about the provision of support being available to meet Lily's needs. Initially, Lily attends for two mornings a week; this is increased to three full days over time. Her package of care is adjusted to provide a carer to cover the nursery hours and transport to and from nursery.

Lily's key worker liaises with the nursery to provide information and training to staff regarding Lily's needs and helps the nursery manager undertake an assessment of risk using the principles of risk assessment. A health plan is developed.

The CCN team regularly visited the school to provide:

- competency training for school support workers in tracheostomy care and suctioning
- emergency care training in the event that Lily had an accident at school, i.e. emergency tracheostomy tube replacement and basic life support
- advice and support in minimising risk to Lily while maintaining her independence
- in conjunction with the speech and language therapist, providing practical advice on supporting speech and language development
- provision of written guidelines and ongoing assessments.

RESEARCH NOTE 6.5 Children with a tracheostomy: experience of their carers in school (Smith et al. 2003)

Tracheostomies in children are increasingly performed for chronic medical conditions. There are no published studies reporting the experience of children with a tracheostomy in school. Such information would be valuable in planning the care and education of these children.

The aims of this study were to identify those children with a tracheostomy in Nottinghamshire schools and determine the support they were receiving. A questionnaire survey was sent to families and school carers of 11 children with a tracheostomy.

The study concluded that children with tracheostomies can successfully and safely achieve full-time education in both mainstream and special schools. A dedicated multidisciplinary team, including input from the parents, is essential to achieve this goal. Regular revision of skills and information sessions for the teaching staff would be beneficial.

Lily and her family felt that it was at times stressful and intrusive having carers in their home; equally, they recognised their dependence on these workers. It was important for them to find a balance between privacy and the need for support (Ludvigsen and Morrison 2003). The children's NSFCYPMS states that: 'Good short term break services are associated with reductions in maternal stress and a reduction in marital problems and breakdown' and identifies short-term breaks as providing positive experiences for children and families (DoH 2004; Eaton 2008). 'Better care, better lives' identifies that services will be commissioned and provided to enable specialist short breaks with appropriate healthcare, nursing and medical input (DoH 2008).

Legal Duty

Services provided under Section 17 of the Children Act 1989 should 'safeguard and promote the welfare of children in need'. Services should be designed to minimise the effect on disabled children of their disabilities and give disabled children and their families the opportunity to lead lives that are as normal as possible. Such services include social or recreational activities, services to a child at home, help with holidays and where necessary the provision of accommodation.

The Children and Young Persons Act 2008 altered Schedule 2 of the Children Act 1989 so it requires that every local authority (in England and Wales) shall provide services designed to assist individuals who provide care for such children (disabled) to continue to do so, or to do so more effectively, by giving them breaks from caring.

Short-break care services are essential in care packages for these children and are an integral part of maintaining family well-being (Olsen and Maslin-Prothero 2001; Eaton 2008). Caring for the ventilated child at home can place wide-ranging, unrelenting, and sometimes overwhelming emotional, social and financial stressors on the family, and the burden of caring for a child with ineffective support can affect the well-being of all members of the family (Prilleltensky and Nelson 2000; Eaton 2008). Consequently, families require services to meet both their child's and their own support needs. According to a survey of parents of disabled children, a break from caring to be with their partner and/or other children is the single most important factor in helping their relationship (McConkey and Truesdale 2000). Davies et al. (2004) confirmed that parents reported benefits for themselves in terms of a break from routine, sleep, comfort, freedom, time for themselves, a sense of privacy and 'normalcy'. It also gave them time to spend with their other children. Freedom and comfort came from knowing their child was happy and well cared for, allowing them to relax. Some parents found that knowing that other families lived similar lives helped them feel that their life was 'not as weird' as they had believed. Laverty and Reet (2001) recommend that family members be empowered through short-break care and siblings shielded from being overshadowed by the child with complex health needs. The provision of short-break care is one such service that allows therapeutic opportunities, quality time, independence and the living of life for all family members (Laverty and Reet 2001; Eaton 2008). However, the provision and use of short-break care for children with complex health needs remains limited, mainly because many of these children are cared for at home and remain hidden in community profiling.

As stated in many studies, the value of a break from caring has been identified by parents as their greatest area of unmet need. Findings in the study by Noyes et al. (1999) suggest that being able to take a break was absolutely essential for parents and provision for short-break care needed to be included in the child's care package. Families have very different needs in terms of the nature, place and timing of breaks from caring. Many parents report a significant mismatch in terms of what they were offered and what they felt they needed, which highlights that breaks from caring must be carefully matched to individual parents and children. In addition, many parents reported that they simply were not offered enough breaks (Thompson et al. 2009). Packages of short-break care must be responsive to parental expressions of need.

Short-break care is often viewed as a crisis intervention, rather than part of a network of services to support the child and family. Consequently, some families express reservations that centre primarily on the stigma and guilt associated with respite provision and the quality of care. For some families, the concept of short-break care signifies an inability to cope with the caring situation, which consequently develops into guilt. It is essential for short-break care to be viewed in a more positive light; as a supportive and preventative service for families, rather than as a way of managing a crisis. In the study by McConkey (2008), some parents chose not to use short breaks as they saw the child as part of the family and wanted to take holidays and breaks together. Some were reluctant to use residential facilities due to the child having picked up infections on previous stays or unsuitable accommodation such as hospital-type wards and concern over high staff turnover.

ACTIVITY 6.9 Short-break care

List the different types of short break available.

RESEARCH NOTE 6.6 'I don't know how we coped before': a study of respite care for children in the home and hospice (Eaton 2008)

The aims of this qualitative study was to describe the experiences of families, whose children have life-limiting and life-threatening conditions and who have complex healthcare needs, of receiving respite care at home or in a hospice.

The areas of concern identified as significant to all the families were referral to respite service, service organisation, communication, relinquishing control to respite carers and satisfaction with service.

To conclude, within the provision of respite care, there needs to be more overt referral systems and criteria, negotiation of appropriate roles, continuity of care, regular assessment of need and acknowledgement of the difficulty that parents have in relinquishing control to respite carers.

EXPERT CHILDREN, YOUNG PEOPLE AND PARENTS

The Department of Health and the Department for Education and Skills have recognised that parent and children's views need to inform policymaking and practice. One of the key markers of good practice within Standard 8 of the NSF is that disabled children, young people and their families are routinely involved and supported in making informed decisions about their treatment, care and support, and in shaping services. Standard 2 of the NSF, 'Supporting parenting,' reinforces the importance of listening to parents' views.

Kirk and Glendinning (2004) found that families caring for a technology-dependent child often had considerably more specialist knowledge than the community-based professionals they encountered and this altered parent–professional relationships. Some parents felt primary and community health professionals, in particular, could be threatened by their specialist expertise. However, parents valued professionals who admitted the limitations of their knowledge; this honesty provided the basis for a trusting relationship. In contrast, parents' own expertise was not always acknowledged by professionals and parents described instances when their views had been ignored or dismissed. Continuity in parent–professional relationships was important in developing trust and mutual understanding of respective expertise. There was remarkable consistency between parents' and professionals' views of the types of support valued by families (Kirk and Glendinning 2002).

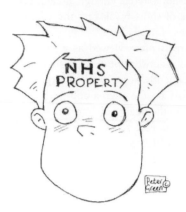

Young people (and their parents) said that nurses assumed an ownership of them

The young people said they felt they had no voice

Figure 6.6 A young person's views and experiences of medical care
Source: Noyes (2000a)

Information is one of the most valued services and parents and disabled children and young people consistently request more information about services and about the child's condition and treatment (see Figure 6.6). Parents from minority ethnic groups are least well informed. Efforts need to be made to provide information in appropriate formats and language. Duties under the Disability Discrimination Act need to be taken into consideration when considering the provision of information in appropriate formats and language (including sign language) (DoH 2004).

Children want staff to listen to them, ask them for their ideas, take notice of what they say and give them choices. Children can contribute unique and essential knowledge during decision making. Parents of disabled children also want to be involved in decisions about the services and treatments their children receive. Involvement of children and their parents in planning services results in the provision of more appropriate services. However, disabled children are less actively involved in decision making than children who are not disabled. Therefore, professionals should ensure that disabled children, especially children with high communication needs, are not excluded from the decision-making process. In particular, professionals should consider the needs of children who rely on communication equipment or who use nonverbal communication such as sign language (DoH 2004).

CASE STUDY REVIEW 6.1

Lily was finally successfully discharged from hospital after a period of 7 months. Once at home, the CCN key worker:

- managed the daily organisation of care
- liaised with the interprofessional team
- provided ongoing emotional, psychological and developmental support for Lily and her family
- developed ground rules for the carers
- developed policies and procedures to ensure the safety of everyone in the home
- coordinated hospital, clinic and therapy appointments
- organised and maintained equipment and supplies
- facilitated an annual reassessment of the care package and ongoing training, recruitment and retention of carers
- organised short breaks and holidays
- continually re-assessed interprofessional care plans should Lily need local hospitalisation.

At the age of 3 years, Lily attended nursery. This followed a process of agreeing and implementing an amended package of care. Lily had a carer in attendance at nursery. Lily enjoyed and thrived within this environment.

At the age of 5, Lily started full time in her local village primary school. Careful interprofessional planning and risk assessment was undertaken by the key worker and the school. Lily only required her ventilator at school for emergencies, as she no longer requires ventilation during the day. Lily progressed very well in school and joint reviews were changed as she became more independent. Her carers in school now had a dual role of supervising her health requirements but in the main were educational support assistants. Lily adjusted very well to life in school and she integrated well with her peers who were very supportive of Lily. Lily had ongoing speech and language assessments and occasional admission to a tertiary centre for sleep studies.

At the age of nine, following a consultation with her respiratory consultant, Lily had a successful trial period of using non-invasive mask ventilation. Lily had her tracheostomy closed. This was seen as a huge step for Lily and the family in achieving more independence and normality.

As Lily has grown, her package of care has been adapted according to her needs. Although Lily still attends consultation with her parents, she is increasingly more involved in making decisions about her care. As Lily is becoming more independent and taking on responsibilities for her healthcare, this poses difficulties for Roger and Penny. Roger is particularly worried that, as Lily grows older, she will take more risks. From his contacts with the support group, he is aware that these risks can be fatal.

SUMMARY OF KEY LEARNING

Collaboration and partnership are now at the heart of health and social care policies in the UK. Meeting the needs of these children locally has been challenging multiagency working over the past decade, and will continue to challenge as more vulnerable children survive prematurity, serious illness or congenital anomalies. Caring for technology-dependent children both in hospital and in the community requires a multiagency approach to planning and funding services, with good interprofessional collaboration at operational levels. Despite these policies, findings from various studies suggest that there is still disparity in the development of appropriate community-based services and medical and technological advances that now allow children with complex, intensive needs to be discharged from hospital. Although there has been a growth in the provision of children's community nursing teams, they are not universally available, and often appropriate and flexible community services are not readily available, and the funding and supply of equipment, consumables and medications is fragmented and poorly organised.

The literature throughout this chapter has often highlighted the many policies involved in supporting the care of the child and their family as well as similarities between the experience of caring for a technology-dependent child and that of a chronically ill or disabled child, but undoubtedly the former group requires medical and nursing care that is more specialised, complex and intensive. The studies have highlighted how transferring responsibility for the provision of clinical care was rarely negotiated with parents before discharge and although they had a strong desire to care for their child at home, their choices were constrained to some extent by the lack of alternatives to parental care giving. Similarly, there have been constraints in the provision of short-break care and the provision of training for carers.

When working with this group of children, young people and families, professionals need to recognise parents' particular knowledge and expertise in providing specialised nursing care and value their active participation in their child's care. Moreover, it is important that professionals are aware that learning and providing care of this nature for their child has a substantial emotional dimension for parents and does not only involve the competent performance of a set of nursing skills. Parents should be given the opportunity to discuss their feelings about providing care of this nature for their own child. There is a need to remember that they are parents first and foremost, *not* nurses or care workers, and that they may need support in developing and sustaining a parenting role with their child.

FURTHER RESOURCES

Long-term ventilation, information sharing and support for families and health professionals caring for children and adolescents: **www.longtermventilation.nhs.uk**

Royal College of Nursing (2009) A position statement – A child's right to care at home. RCN: London – **http://www.rcn .org.uk/__data/assets/pdf_file/0004/242248/Position_ statement_A_childs_right_to_care_at_home_-_finalem bargoed_3.pdf**

Support and aspiration: a new approach to special educational needs and disability – progress and next steps sets out a summary of the key responses to the consultation questions in the Green Paper, current progress and our further plans for the vision: **http://www.education.gov.uk/childrenandyoungpeo ple/sen/a0075339/sengreenpaper**

Parents of disabled children and young people care passionately about the services they receive. All services are now expected to consult with parents and involve them in planning and development.

This guide has been produced by Contact a Family and the Council for Disabled Children to address these issues and to help and support the many parents and professionals who want to work together to improve services.

Parent participation: improving services for disabled children: **http://www.cafamily.org.uk/pdfs/ParentParticipationGuide .pdf**

ANSWERS TO ACTIVITIES

ACTIVITY 6.1 Barriers to children's rights

Consider the rights of children who are long-term ventilated and list the barriers that they may encounter.

They face a number of barriers to exercising their basic human rights, including:

- prolonged and unnecessary hospitalisation
- being unable to communicate
- having to depend on others
- social and educational exclusion.

ACTIVITY 6.2 Components of a local children's clinical network

- NHS Direct
- ambulance service
- primary care provision (including general practice and out-of-hours services and walk-in centres)
- community pharmacy
- accident and emergency/minor injuries units
- a base unit, providing children and young people's inpatient services and training and support to the other components and can support one or more local units
- local units – in some areas, these local units may not provide a full inpatient paediatric service, but may provide a range of assessment and short interventions/treatments as determined by local need

- community children's nurses able to provide home-based assessment and care for acutely ill children, where appropriate
- children's community teams providing health and social care and family support
- specialist clinical networks that ensure the best expert advice is available 24 hours a day at local level
- other local health services that see children and young people
- managerial/administrative support
- formal links with education and social services.

ACTIVITY 6.3 BiPAP ventilation

Bilateral positive airways pressure. Bilateral positive airways pressure (BiPAP) is similar to a combination of pressure support and continuous positive airway pressure (CPAP). The person initiates all their breaths, but the ventilator provides pressure at the end of expiration as it does in CPAP and gives a 'top-up' to the inspiratory part of each breath as it does in pressure support. This means that the work of breathing is reduced at both ends of each breath and the airways are kept open.

ACTIVITY 6.4 Key goals in discharge planning

- To understand the local community and the range of services available to meet health, housing and social care needs.
- Ensure individuals (children and young people) and carers (parents and extended family members) are actively engaged in planning and delivering the care.
- The role of parents and other carers is recognised and their own rights for assessment and support acknowledged and met.
- Ensure effective communication between primary, secondary, social care, education and voluntary sector to focus care on meeting the needs of the individual child and their family.
- Agree, operate and performance-manage a joint discharge policy facilitating effective multi-disciplinary working at all levels and between organisations.
- Provide appropriate training for those undertaking care and co-ordinating roles.

- Begin preparations for discharge as early as possible, setting realistic timescales and targets.
- Develop an integrated discharge planning team to provide specialist discharge planning for the patient and other members of the multi-disciplinary team. This specialist support may need to be provided by a centre or area with previous experience of working with children with complex needs at home.
- Facilitate trial periods outside the hospital setting before any definitive decisions on longer-term care-package options are made.
- Funding decisions relating to NHS continuing care, social services and education provision should be made promptly so that discharge plans and eventual discharge are not delayed.

Source: adapted from DoH

ACTIVITY 6.5 Planning meeting invitees and their role/responsibilities

Professional/parent	Role
Parents	Expert parents
Medical paediatric consultant	Medical responsibility
Medical registrar	Up-to-date clinical input
Named ward children's nurse	Up-to-date nursing needs
Hospital clinical nurse specialist	Specialist nursing input
General practitioner	Medical responsibility
Social worker	Social care responsibilities

Professional/parent	Role
Nurse consultant community children's nursing	Nursing responsibility for community children's nurses
Child development team	Role of therapists and community paediatrician
Health visitor/school nurse	Named primary care practitioner
Complex care team coordinator /CCN	Coordinator of care packages
Hospital therapists, for example, play specialist, occupational therapist, physiotherapist, speech and language therapist	Advisory role in community and transfer

Source: Stephens (2005)

ACTIVITY 6.6

Physically: sleeplessness, domestic disruption, the negative impact on caregiver health; time spent undertaking nursing procedures.

Psychologically: emotionally exhausting, 24-hour vigilance, loss of privacy, disruption to family life, the stress of care giving; lack of time.

Financially: income reduction because one parent is obliged to stop working to give care; costs for travelling to clinics, providing additional heating; special equipment, food or clothes.

Social: restriction of schooling or social activities for both the child and their siblings.

ACTIVITY 6.7 List of equipment

- pulse oximetry
- portable BiPAP ventilator
- Shiley tracheostomy tube
- Swedish nose/humidification device
- Ambu Bag
- speech valves
- portable suction machine
- suction catheters and gloves
- oxygen mask
- non-invasive nasal CPAP
- tracheostomy tapes (Velcro).

ACTIVITY 6.8 SWOT analysis of a community children's nursing service

Strengths	<ul><li>A well-established CCN team to assess and plan nursing care.</li><li>Extensive knowledge within CCN team.</li><li>Able to critically examine own services.</li><li>A child development centre with children's therapy services on site.</li><li>Knowledge of the community from social, environmental, political, economic and cultural perspectives.</li><li>Links with social, education and voluntary sectors.</li><li>Children and families are key to the strategic planning of the PCT.</li><li>Each condition has a nurse specialist or clinical lead, i.e. asthma, oncology, preterm babies.</li></ul>
Weaknesses	<ul><li>Manpower resources.</li><li>Provision of a fragmented package of health and social care.</li><li>Limited resources for providing complete and comprehensive packages to meet the needs of families in respite care, sibling support and psychological support.</li><li>Limited respite care resources.</li><li>No training provided to statutory or voluntary services, i.e. social services and crossroads/home start, due to CCN workload.</li><li>Too many variants in commissioning within local PCTs.</li></ul>

Opportunities	• Review of skill mix and service criteria to provide a more focused service. • Closer networking with local PCTs in developing service level agreements. • Provision of collaborative training and clinical supervision between health, other statutory agencies and voluntary services. • Provision of a coordinated, collaborative package of care from health, social, education and voluntary sectors. • Development of a supportive culture for staff from a variety of professional backgrounds. • Improved networking and communication across health, social and educational boundaries.
Threats	• Decline of existing services within the CCN team. • Impact of CCN reduced service provision on acute children's ward and A&E services. • Difficulties convincing commissioners of the need to invest in existing services. • Emotional fatigue of team members. • Moral and ethical implications of developing a service with short-term investment.

Source: adapted from Hughes and Horsburgh (2002)

ACTIVITY 6.9 Types of short-break service

Non-residential short-break services

Non-residential services may include support workers enabling disabled children to participate in community-based activities or volunteers supporting disabled children in befriending schemes.

Shared care family-based short breaks

Foster carers are recruited to have a disabled child stay with them on a regular basis: breaks can be a few hours, overnight stays, weekends or longer periods. A key aspect of this service is partnership with parents and the development of an effective working relationship between the foster carer and the family.

Residential short-break services

Residential breaks are the best option for some children, but this needs to be in settings as much like an ordinary home as possible, with specialist equipment unobtrusively available to maximise independence. Only small numbers of children or young people will stay at any one time, creating the feeling of a sleepover. While parents and siblings have a break from caring, disabled children and young people can enjoy new activities, experiences and a wider social network, helping them to develop social and life skills and enjoy independence from their families.

SELECTED REFERENCES

Appierto, L., Cori, M., Binnchi, R. et al. (2002). Home care for chronic respiratory failure in children: 15 years experience. *Paediatr Anaesth*, 12(4), 345–350.

Beresford, B., Williams, J. and Lawton, D. (2003). Community equipment: use and needs of disabled children and their families. University of York, Social Policy Research Unit: **http://www.york.ac.uk/inst/spru/pubs/pdf/equip.pdf**.

Board R. (2004). Father stress during a child's critical care hospitalization. *J Pediatr Health Care*, 18, 244–249.

Board, R. and Ryan-Wenger, N. (2000). State of the science on parental stress and family functioning in pediatric intensive care units. *Am J Crit Care*, 9, 106–124.

Board R. and Ryan-Wenger, N. (2002). Long-term effects of pediatric intensive care unit hospitalization on families with young children. *Heart Lung*, 31, 53–66.

Boosfield, B. and O'Toole, M. (2000) Technology-dependent children: transition from hospital to home. *Paediatric Nursing*, 2(6) 20–22.

Carlin, J. (2005). *Including me: managing complex health needs in schools and early years settings*. Council for Disabled Children, Department for Education and Skills: London.

Carlin, J. (2010). *Guidelines on the discharge from hospital of children and young people with high support needs*. Council for Disabled Children, Department of Health: London.

Carnevale, F.A., Alexander, E., Davis, M., Rennick, J., and Troini, R. (2006). With ventilator-assisted children at home, daily living with distress and enrichment: the moral experience of families. *Pediatrics*, 117, 48–60.

Carter, B. and Coad, J. (2009). *Community children's nursing in England: an appreciative review of CCNs in England*. University of Central Lancashire and Children's Nursing Research Unit: Lancaster.

Colville, G. (2008). The psychological impact on children of admission to intensive care. *Pediatric Clinics of North America*, 55, 605–616.

Colville, G. and Cream, P. (2009). Post-traumatic growth in parents after a child's admission to intensive care: maybe Nietzsche was right? *Intensive Care Medicine*, 35, 919–923.

Colville, G.A. and Gracey, D. (2006). Mothers' recollections of the pediatric intensive care unit: associations with psychopathology and views on follow up. *Intensive Critical Care Nursing*, 22, 49–55.

Crawford, N. and Powell, C. (2004). Paediatric high-dependency care. *Current Paediatrics*, 14, 197–201.

Darvill, J., Harrington, A. and Donovan, J. (2009). Caring for ventilated children at home – the child's Perspective. *Neonatal, Paediatric and Child Health Nursing*, 12(3), 9–13.

Davies B., Steele, R., Collins, J.B., Cook, and Smith S. (2004). The impact on families of respite care in a children's hospice program. *Journal of Palliative Care*, 20, 277–286.

Deatrick, J.A., Thibodeaux, A.G., Mooney, K., Schmus, C., Pollack, R. and Davey, B.H. (2006). Family management style framework: a new tool with potential to assess families who have children with brain tumours. *Journal of Pediatric Oncology Nursing*, 23, 19–27.

Department for Children, Schools and Families (DCSF) (2008). *Aiming high for disabled children: transforming services for disabled children and their families*, DCSF Publications: Nottingham.

Department for Education (DfE) (2010). Support and aspiration: a new approach to special educational needs and disability. Progress and next steps. Framework for the Assessment of Children in Need and their Families. Stationery Office: London.

Department for Education and Skills (DfES) (2003). *Every child matters* (Green Paper). Stationery Office: London.

Department for Education and Skills (DfES). (2007). *Aiming high for disabled children: better support for families*. Stationery Office: London.

Department of Health (DoH) (1996). *Child health in the community: a guide to good practice*. HMSO: London.

Department of Health (DoH) (1997). *House of Commons select committee health services for children and young people in the community – home and school*. Stationery Office: London.

Department of Health (DoH) (2000a). *Framework for the assessment of children in need and their families*. Stationery Office: London.

Department of Health (DoH) (2000b). *Assessing children in need and their families: practice guidance*. Stationery Office: London.

Department of Health (DoH) (2001). *High-dependency care for children: report of an expert advisory group*. Department of Health: London.

Department of Health (DoH). (2003a). *Getting the right start: National Service Framework for children. Emerging findings.* Stationery Office: London.

Department of Health (DoH) (2003b). *Children and young people's strategy*. Department of Health: London.

Department of Health. (DoH) (2004). National Service Framework for children, young people and maternity services. Core Standards. Stationery Office: London.

Department of Health. (DoH) (2007). *Making it better: for children and young people*. Stationery Office: London.

Department of Health (DoH) (2008). *Better care: better lives*. Stationery Office: London.

Department of Health (DoH) (2009a). *Securing better health for children and young people through world class commissioning: A guide to support delivery of Healthy lives, brighter futures: The strategy for children and young people's health*. Department of Health: London.

Department of Health (DoH) (2009b). *Healthy lives, brighter futures. The strategy for children and young people's health.* HMSODH: London.

Department of Health (DoH) (2009c). *Transforming community services: enabling new patterns of provision.* Department of Health: London.

Department of Health (DoH) 2010. *National Framework for children and young people's continuing care*. Stationery Office: London.

Department of Health and Department for Education and Skills (DoH and DfES) (2003). *Together from the start – practical guidance for professionals working with disabled children (birth to third birthday) and their families*. DoH/DfES: London.

Draper, E., Hobson, R., Lamming, C., McShane, P., Norman, L., Parslow, R. and Skinner, S. (2011). *Annual report of the paediatric intensive care audit network: January 2008 – December 2010*. Paediatric Intensive Care Audit Network (PICANet), University of Leeds: Leeds.

Dybwik, K., Nielsen, E. and Brinchmann, B. (2011). Home mechanical ventilation and specialised health care in the community: between a rock and a hard place. *Health Services Research*, 11, 115.

Eaton, N. (2008). 'I don't know how we coped before': a study of respite care for children in the home and hospice. *Journal of Clinical Nursing*, 17, 3196–3204.

Edwards, E., O'Toole, M. and Wallis, C. (2004). Sending children home on tracheostomy dependent ventilation: pitfalls and outcomes. *Arch Dis Child*, 89, 251–255.

Elston, S. and Thornes, R. (2002). Children's nursing workforce: a report to the Royal College of Paediatrics and Child Health: **www.rcpch.ac.uk/doc.aspx?id Resource=2186**

Emond, A. and Eaton, N. (2004). Supporting children with complex health care needs and their families – an overview of the research agenda. *Child Care, Health and Development*, 30, 195–199.

Fradd, E. (1994). Whose responsibility? *Nurse Times*, 90(6), 34–36.

Glendinning, C. and Kirk, S., with Guiffridda, A. and Lawton, D. (1999) *The community-based care of technology-dependent children in the UK: definitions, numbers and costs.* Research Report Commissioned by the Social Care Group at the Department of Health. National Primary Care Research and Development Centre, University of Manchester: Manchester.

Glendinning, C., Kirk, S., Guiffrida, A. and Lawton, D. (2001). Technology-dependent children in the community: definitions, numbers and costs. *Child Care, Health and Development*. 27(4), 321–334.

Haines, C. and Wolstenholme, M. (2000) Family support in paediatric intensive care. In C. Williams, and J. Asquith (eds) *Paediatric intensive care nursing*. Churchill Livingstone: London.

Hall, B. and Hill, D. (1996). *The child with a disability*, 2nd edn. Blackwell Science: Oxford.

Heaton, J. et al. (2003). *Technology and time: home care regimes and technology dependent children. Final report. (ESRC/MRC innovative health technology research programme)*. Social Policy Research Unit, University of York.

Heaton, J., Noyes, J., Sloper, P. and Shah, R. (2005). Families' experiences of caring for technology-dependent children: a temporal perspective. *Health & Social Care in the Community*, 13(5), 441–450.

Hewitt-Taylor, J. (2003). Children who require long-term ventilation: staff education and training. *Intensive Critical Care Nursing*, 20, 93–102.

Hewitt-Taylor, J. (2005). Caring for children with complex and continuing health needs. *Nursing Standard*, 19(42), 41–47.

Hewitt-Taylor, J. (2007). *Children with complex and continuing health needs*. Jessica Kingsley Publishers: London.

Hughes, J. and Horsburgh, J. (2002). The role of the community children's nurse: the perspective of a practitioner and an educator. *Current Paediatrics*, 12(5), 425–430.

Jardine, E. and Wallis, C. (1998) Core guidelines for the discharge home of the child on long-term assisted ventilation in the United Kingdom. UK Working Party on Paediatric Long-Term Ventilation. *Thorax*, 53, 762–767.

Jardine, E., O'Toole, M. and Paton, J.Y. (1999). Current status of long-term ventilation of children in the United Kingdom: questionnaire survey. *British Medical Journal*, 318, 295–299.

Kirk, S. (1998). Families' experiences of caring at home for a technology-dependent child: a review of the literature. *Child Care, Health and Development*, 24(2), 101–114.

Kirk, S. (2001). Negotiating lay and professional roles in the care of children with complex health care needs. *Journal of Advanced Nursing*, 34(5), 593–602.

Kirk, S. (2008). A profile of technology-assisted children and young people in northwest England. *Paediatric Nursing*, 20(9), 18–20.

Kirk, S. (2010). How children and young people construct and negotiate living with medical technology. *Social Science & Medicine*, 71, 1796–1803.

Kirk, S. and Glendinning, C. (2002). Supporting 'expert' parents – professional support and families caring for a child with complex health care needs in the community. *International Journal of Nursing Studies*, 39, 625–635.

Kirk, S. and Glendinning, C. (2004). Developing services to support parents caring for a technology dependent child at home. *Child Care, Health and Development*, 30(3) 209–218.

Kirk, S., Glendinning, C. and Callery, P. (2005). Parent or nurse? The experience of being the parent of a technology-dependent child. *Journal of Advanced Nursing*, 51(5), 456–464.

Laverty, H. and Reet, M. (2001). *Planning care for children in respite settings*. Jessica Kingsley Publishers: London.

Lenehan, C., Morrison, J. and Stanley, J. (2004). *The dignity of risk. A practical handbook for professionals working with disabled children and their families*. National Children's Bureau; Council for Disabled Children: London.

Lewis, M. (2004). Establishing a service: a whole population approach. *Child Care, Health and Development*, 30(3), 221–229.

Lewis, M. and Noyes, J. (2007). Risk management and clinical governance for complex home-based health care. *Paediatric Nursing*, 19(6), 23–28.

Lewis, M. and Pontin, D. (2008). Caseload management in community children's nursing. *Nursing Children and Young People Journal*, 20(3), 18–22.

Lindahl, B. and Lindblad, B. (2011). Family members' experiences of everyday life when a child is dependent on a ventilator: a metasynthesis study. *Journal of Family Nursing*, 17(2), 241–269.

Ludvigsen, A. and Morrison, J. (2003). *Breathing space: community support of children on long-term ventilation – summary*. Barnardo's: London.

McConkey, R. (2008). *Developing services for children and young people with complex physical healthcare needs: 5. Proposals for the development of short-break (respite) provision*. Report for the Department of Health, Social Services and Public Safety. Institute of Nursing, University of Ulster: Belfast.

McConkey, R. and Truesdale, M. (2000). *Evaluation of Beechfield services: overnight breaks and domiciliary support services for families and children with learning disabilities*. University of Ulster/EHSSB: Belfast.

McConkey, R., Truesdale, M. and Conliffe, C. (2004). The features of short-break residential services valued by families who have children with multiple disabilities. *Journal of Social Work*, 4, 61–75.

MacDonald, H. and Callery, P. (2004). Different meanings of respite: a study of parents, nurses and social workers caring for children with complex needs. *Child Care Health Dev*, 30(3), 279–288.

Margolan, H., Fraser, J. and Lenton, S. (2004). Parental experience of services when their child requires long-term ventilation. Implications for commissioning and providing services. *Child Care, Health and Development*, 30(3), 257–264.

Meates, M. (1997). Ambulatory paediatrics – making a difference. *Archives of Disease in Childhood*, 76, 468–476.

Ministry of Health (MoH) (1959) *The welfare of children in hospital: report of the committee. (The Platt Report)*. Ministry of Health: London.

Murphy, J. (2008). Medically stable children in PicU: better at home. *Paediatric Nursing*, 20(1), 14–16.

Noyes, J. (2000a). Enabling young 'ventilator dependent' people to express their views and experiences of their care in hospital. *Journal of Advanced Nursing*, 31(5), 1206–1215.

Noyes, J. (2000b). Ventilator-dependent children who spend prolonged periods of time in intensive care units where they no longer have a medical need or want to be there. *Journal of Clinical Nursing*, 9(5), 774–783.

Noyes J. (2002). Barriers that delay children and young people who are dependent on mechanical ventilators from being discharged from hospital. *Journal of Clinical Nursing*, 11(1), 2–11.

Noyes, J. (2006a). Health and quality of life of ventilator-dependent children. *Journal of Advanced Nursing*, 56(4), 392–403.

Noyes, J. (2006b). Resource use and service costs for ventilator dependent children and young people in the UK. *Health and Social Care in the Community*, 14(6), 508–522.

Noyes, J. and Lewis, M. (2005a). *From hospital to home. Guidance on discharge management and community support for children using long-term ventilation*. Barnardo's: London.

Noyes, J. and Lewis, M. (2005b). *Care pathway for the discharge and support of children requiring long-term ventilation in the community: National Service Framework for Children, Young People and Maternity Services.* Department of Health: London.

Noyes, J. and Lewis M. (2007). Compiling, costing and funding complex packages of home based health care. *Paediatric Nursing*, 19(5), 28–32.

Noyes, J., Hartman, H., Samuels, M., and Southall, D. (1999). The experiences and views of parents who care for ventilator-dependent children. *Journal of Clinical Nursing*, 8(4), 440–450.

O'Brien, M.E. (2001). Living in a house of cards: family experiences with long-term childhood technology dependence. *Journal of Pediatric Nursing*, 16, 13–22.

O'Brien, L.M., Holbrook, C.R., Vanderlaan, M., Amiel, J. and Gozal, D. (2005). Autonomic function in children with congenital central hypoventilation syndrome and their families. *Chest*, 128, 2478–2484.

O'Brien M. and Wegner, C. (2002). Rearing the child who is technology-dependent: perceptions of parents and home care nurses. *Journal of the Society of Pediatric Nursing*, 7(1), 7–15.

Olsen, R. and Maslin-Prothero, P. (2001) Dilemmas in the provision of own home respite support for parents of young children with complex needs: evidence from an evaluation. *Journal of Advanced Nursing*, 34(5), 603–610.

O'Rourke, A. (2005). Minimising clinical risk. *Current Paediatrics*, 15, 466–472.

Pontin, D. and Lewis, M. (2008). Managing the caseload: a qualitative action research study exploring how community children's nurses deliver services to children living with life-limiting, life-threatening, and chronic conditions. *Journal for Specialist in Pediatric Nursing* 13(1) 26–35.

Prilleltensky, L. and Nelson, G (2000). Promoting child and family wellness: priorities for psychological and social interventions, *Journal of Community and Applied Social Psychology*, 10(2), 85–105.

Ratliffe, C.E. (2002). Stress in families with medically fragile children. *Issues in Comprehensive Pediatric Nursing*, 25, 167–188.

Reeves, E. (2006) Parents' experiences of negotiating care for their technology-dependent child. *Journal of Child Health Care.* 10(3), 228–239.

Rehm, R.S., Bradley, J.F. (2005). Normalization in families raising a child who is medically fragile/technology dependent and developmentally delayed. *Qualitative Health Research*, 15(6), 807–820.

Royal College of Nursing (RCN) (2009). A position statement – preparing nurses to care for children at home and community settings. RCN: London. **www.rcn.org.uk/data/assets/pdf_file/0008/234836/Preparing_nurses_to_care_for_children_at_home_and_community_settings.pdf**

Ruby, B., Daly, J., Douglas, S., Montenegro, D., Song R. and Dyer, A. (1995). Patient outcomes of the chronically ill: special care vs. intensive care unit. *Nursing Research*, 44, 324–331.

Sarvey, S. (2008). Living with a machine: the experience of the child who is ventilator dependent. *Issues in Mental Health Nursing*, 29(2), 179–196.

Sidey, A. and Widdas, D. (2005). *Textbook of Community Children's Nursing*, 2nd edn. Elsevier: Kidlington.

Sloper, P. and Beresford, B. (2006). Families with disabled children. *British Medical Journal*, 333, 928–929.

Smith, J., Williams, J. and Gibbin, K. (2003). Children with a tracheostomy: experience of their carers in school. *Child Care, Health and Development*, 29(4), 291–296.

Spiers, G., Gridley, K., Cusworth, L., Mukherjee, S., Parker, G., Heaton, J., Atkin, K., Birks, Y., Lowson, K. and Wright, D. (2012). Understanding care closer to home for ill children and young people. *Nursing Children and Young People*, 24(5), 29–34.

Taylor, J. (2000). Partnership in the community and hospital: a comparison. *Paediatric Nurse*, 12(5), 28–30.

Taylor, I., Sharland, E. and Whiting, R. (2008). Building capacity for the children's workforce: findings from the knowledge review of the higher education response. *Learning in Health and Social Care*, 7, 184–197.

Thompson, D., Whitmarsh, J., Southern, L., Brewster, S. and Emira, M. (2009). *Access the leisure activities: the perceptions of children and young people with Autistic Spectrum Disorder or ADHD and their parents/carers.* Centre for Developmental & Applied Research in Education, University of Wolverhampton: Wolverhampton.

Toly, V., Musil, C. and Carl, J. (2012). A longitudinal study of families with technology-dependent children. *Research in Nursing & Health*, 35, 40–54.

Trang, H., Dehan, M., Beaufils, F., Zaccaria, I., Amiel, J., Gaultier, C. and the French CCHS Working Group (2005). The French congenital central hypoventilation syndrome registry. General data, phenotype, and genotype. *Chest*, 127, 72–79.

United Nations (UN) (1989). UN Convention on the Rights of the Child. UN: Geneva.

Valentine, F. and Lowes, L. (2007). *Nursing care of children and young people with chronic illness.* Blackwell Publishing: Oxford.

Wallis, C., Paton, J., Beaton, S. and Jardine, E. (2011). Children on long-term ventilatory support: 10 years of progress. *Arch Dis Child*, 96, 998–1002.

Wang, K. and Barnard, A. (2004). Technology-dependent children and their families: a review. *Journal of Advanced Nursing*, 45(1), 36–46.

Wang, K. and Barnard, A. (2008). Caregivers' experiences at home with a ventilator-dependent child. *Qualitative Health Research*, 18(4), 501–508.

Weese-Mayer, D.E., Rand, C.M., Berry-Kravis, E.M., Jennings, L.J., Loghmanee, D.A., Patwari, P.P. and Ceccherini, I. (2009). Congenital central hypoventilation syndrome from past to future: model for translational and transitional autonomic medicine. *Pediatric Pulmonology*, 44, 521–535.

Whiting, M. (1997) Community children's nursing: a bright future? *Paed Nurse*, 9(4), 6–8.

Wilson, S. et al. (1998) Absolute involvement: the experience of mothers of ventilator-dependent children. *Health and Social Care in the Community*, 6(4), 224–233.

Yangzi, N.M., Rosenberg, M.W. and McKeever, P. (2006). Getting out of the house: the challenges mothers face when their children have long-term care needs. *Health Social Care Community*, 15(1): 45–55.

CHAPTER 7
Caring for Children and Young People in the Medical Setting

Carolyn Seeman

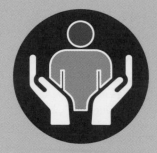
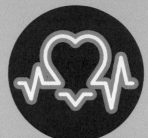
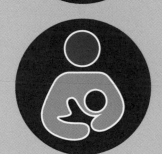

LEARNING OUTCOMES

On completion of this chapter, the reader will be able to:

- Consider the importance of a holistic approach to care through collaboration with the family and MDT.
- Explore the more common interventions of care required for children in a medical setting.
- Understand the appropriate practice required for IV sites and IV infusion.
- Investigate the importance of skin integrity and monitoring.
- Reflect on the pain management required for the child with medical needs.
- Explore the rationale for evidence-based infection control.

TALKING POINT

There was a TV police drama that was well known in the 1980s. The police team would gather for a briefing and these words of wisdom would be the last words of advice to them: 'Hey, let's be careful out there.' (Sergeant Phil Esterhaus, *Hill Street Blues*) (1981)

INTRODUCTION

At times it can feel like this when entering the children's acute medical ward following handover, due to the variety, complexity and sometimes unpredictability of the work that lies ahead. The essence of children's medical nursing is that of holism, considering that the children are usually admitted unexpectedly, have suddenly fallen ill and a trip to the doctor or the emergency department has meant a referral to the children's ward. Children and young people usually arrive with significant others, parents, siblings, grandparents or carers. Most children in today's society live busy, full and active lives and in confining them to hospital, there is always a danger of shrinking their world considerably. It is recognised that where possible children and young people should be in hospital for the shortest stay possible (DoH 2004) and then only if absolutely necessary.

Because of this key aim children who are inpatients should receive well-planned treatment and regular reviews to ensure that they can return to families and their lives as soon as is safe. Along with the members of the interprofessional team, children's nurses are pivotal in ensuring the delivery of high-quality, holistic care. This chapter will, with the use of a case study allow insight into some of the care issues within the children's medical ward, highlighting some of the key aspects of care that may be encountered. It has to be acknowledged that, in many hospitals, children's wards combine the care of children with medical needs and surgical needs in one area. This is cost effective in relation to management of staff and also has the added benefit of producing nurses who have skills which are transferrable in any setting.

CASE STUDY 7.1 Jonathan has infected atopic eczema

Jonathan is a 3-year-old who has been admitted to the children's ward with infected atopic eczema. He is accompanied by his mother who is a lone parent and lives with her mother and father (Jonathan's grandparents). Jonathan has commenced on a course of IV antibiotics and IV fluids and is slowly improving and taking more interest in his surroundings. He is on analgesia to manage his pain and is being nursed in a side room.

WHAT IS ECZEMA?

The NICE guidelines for the management of atopic eczema (2007a) state that 15 to 20 per cent of school aged children suffer from atopic eczema, a common inflammatory skin condition. Atopic refers to a hereditary tendency for allergy. Add to this the number of younger children who may also have presentation of this condition before school age, and it is clear that the likelihood of meeting a child who has eczema is high for all children's nurses (see Figure 7.1).

Symptoms can range from mildly dry, flaky skin and itching to red, raw and broken lesions. It is not known the exact cause of eczema, however, it is strongly linked to family history, irritants and environmental factors and typically a child has episodic flare-ups (flares) of the disease that can prove very disruptive for the child and for the family (NICE 2007a; Lawton 2008; Ayliffe 2009). It is often not considered to be a 'serious' childhood condition, however, it is vital for children's nurses to be able to assess holistically the impact of such a condition on all aspects of life. All professionals need to consider a holistic approach to care and, in addition to caring for the skin, must assess the other aspects that may have impact on the condition of the child and family. Table 7.1 demonstrates some of these factors, as well as illustrating the varying severity of the condition.

From the pictures and descriptions it can be seen that there is potential for a seemingly mild area of eczema to develop and

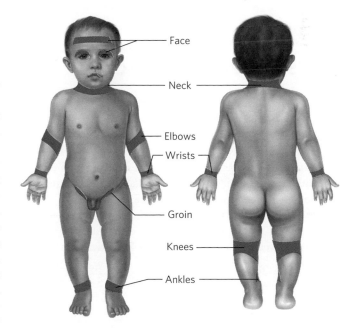

Figure 7.1 Common sites for eczema to occur in

become more serious. In particular, it is the excessive scratching that creates the most potential for skin damage and thus infection.

Table 7.1 Eczema and quality of life and psychosocial well-being

Skin/physical severity		Impact on quality of life and psychosocial well-being	
Clear	Normal skin, no evidence of active atopic eczema	None	No impact on quality of life
Mild	Areas of dry skin, infrequent itching (with or without small areas of redness)	Mild	Little impact on everyday activities, sleep and psychosocial well-being
Moderate	Areas of dry skin, frequent itching, redness (with or without excoriation and localised skin thickening)	Moderate	Moderate impact on everyday activities and psychosocial well-being, frequently disturbed sleep
Severe	Widespread areas of dry skin, incessant itching, redness (with or without excoriation, extensive skin thickening, bleeding, oozing, cracking and alteration of pigmentation)	Severe	Severe limitation of everyday activities and psychosocial functioning, nightly loss of sleep

Source: adapted from NICE (2007a)

ACTIVITY 7.1

Using Table 7.1 to help you, consider all the aspects of care for Jonathan as he enters the ward.

Think about Jonathan and his family. What impacts may eczema have on the family both before admission and as a result of his admission? List these impacts.

HOLISTIC APPROACH TO CARE

The concept of holism in relation to nursing is difficult to define, however Kozier et al. (2008) consider this to involve the nurse and the carer recognising the relationship between all the parts that make the whole. It is clear that the effects of being an inpatient on the child are significant and suffering from eczema presents ongoing issues for the child. Lawton (2008) quotes a child on how it feels to have eczema (see Voices 7.1).

For Jonathan, both the physical effects of the illness and the psychological effects of eczema must be considered. Hawkins (2005) reviewed a wealth of literature and found six key themes:

- quality of life
- sleep problems
- itching
- psychological problems
- maternal anxiety
- education.

Camfferam et al. (2010) concluded that children with eczema had an overall poorer quality of life and, in particular, poorer sleep patterns. It is vital to recognise the impact of this on Jonathan and his family. You may have already identified some of the key issues (from Activity 7.1). Recognition of need is only the first part of the nursing process and it is the planning and implementation that is sometimes the challenge for nurses, particularly in the medical ward.

The key issues for Jonathan will be addressed to demonstrate how this holistic approach can be managed:

- **physical treatment:** venepuncture, IV fluid management, skin care, infection control, administration of medicines, pain management, pyrexia management, nutrition
- **psychological issues:** isolation, therapeutic play, developmental concerns (regression)
- **social concerns:** parental stress, involvement of grandparents, potential safeguarding issues
- **interprofessional involvement:** GP, health visitor, social worker, nursery workers, CCN team.

VOICES 7.1 A child's viewpoint on having eczema

'I cry a lot and I can't go swimming and it hurts the eczema on my legs when I run and I don't feel like wearing nice clothes.

Also I feel tired in the morning because I don't get much sleep.'

PHYSICAL TREATMENT

Primary Assessment

It is vital that Jonathan receives an accurate and comprehensive physical assessment in order that care can be planned. This involves an assessment of airway, breathing, circulation, disability and exposure/environment (ABCDE assessment) (APLS 2005).

Jonathan's vital observations are as shown in Table 7.2.

ACTIVITY 7.2 Assessment for Jonathan's physical status

From the description of the assessment for Jonathan's physical status (Table 7.2), consider your priority of care and what your course of actions and interventions would be.

Pain Management

Pain management is an element of medical nursing that is sometimes overlooked. Pain is often more immediately considered on a surgical ward where pain is a reality following a surgical procedure and thus it is factored into the care more specifically. It is of equal importance within a medical setting where the result of illness and at times the interventions and procedures to manage the condition can lead a child to have significant pain. A core skill for children's nurses is that they are familiar with the assessment of pain and appropriate effective treatment of pain, either through the administration of medication or non-therapeutic methods. Dawber (2008) go as far as suggesting that nurses have a moral obligation to deliver effective pain relief and that pain assessment is the first step in managing pain. There are many pain assessment tools available to assist nurses in assessing children's pain and these are explored in other chapters in this volume.

However, it is very important that nurses acknowledge that every child who is admitted to a medical ward has the potential to be in discomfort or pain and this has to be addressed. A guideline produced by the RCN in 2009 contains suggested pain assessment tools that are validated for children and young people of a variety of ages and abilities. These tools are primarily reliant on behavioural cues and self-reporting and although the term 'physiological tools' is identified, as yet there is no validated or recognised tool that measures pain using physiological cues, even though we know that pain can lead to altered physiological responses (Fisher and Morton 1998).

ACTIVITY 7.3 Pain assessment tools

What pain assessment tools are you familiar with?

Imagine that you have been asked to introduce an easy-to-use and reliable pain assessment tool to the children's medical ward. Take a look at the RCN chart (Figure 7.2) that identifies a range of assessment tools. Select one or two and consider which of these would be most suitable for use for a 3-year-old such as Jonathan.

List the limitations and ease of use to justify your choices.

Pain Management

For Jonathan, the breakdown of his skin will be causing considerable topical pain and there may also be pain from the systemic infection. These will be considered in turn.

Table 7.2 Primary assessment

Airway	Jonathan has a patent airway. He is talking to mum and there are no unusual airway sounds (stridor) or signs of upper airway obstruction (tracheal tug)
Breathing	Jonathan has got a raised respiratory rate of 40 breaths per minute. He has mild intercostal recession only and no wheezing. He is able to hold a conversation with mum. His SaO_2 is 98% in room air
Circulation	Jonathan has a raised heart rate of 150 and appears flushed in the face (although it is hard to tell with the eczema). His feet and hands are cool to touch and his central capillary refill is 2 seconds
Disability	Jonathan is alert, although very miserable and agitated due to pain and itching
Exposure/environment	Jonathan has eczema on most of his face, trunk, arms and legs. You note that his back has large lesions that are broken, weeping and in some places the skin is peeling. On his legs and arms, there are other isolated areas where the skin is broken. His face is red and the skin is raised on his cheeks. Temperature is 39.7°, weight 18 kg.

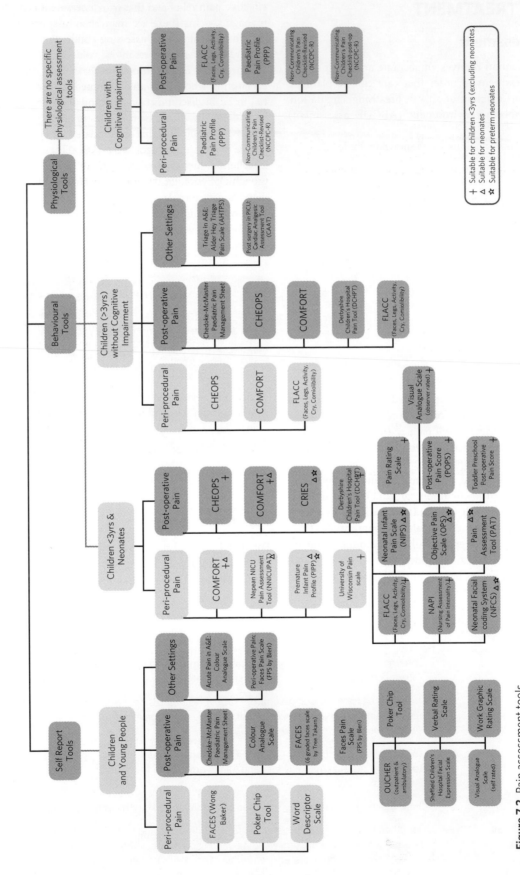

Figure 7.2 Pain assessment tools

Source: RCN (2009)

Topical Pain

Due to the irritation caused by the eczema, Jonathan has been feeling very itchy and uncomfortable. This often causes constant scratching which subsequently damages the skin, opening the way for skin flora to enter into the soft tissues. Due to the rich blood supply to the skin, any infection can enter into the systemic blood supply and in severe cases can cause an overwhelming septicaemia (see Figure 7.3).

Thus, reducing topical itching can reduce the risk of developing breakdown of the skin. Interestingly the issue of pain is not addressed specifically in the NICE (2007a) eczema guidelines. Within the guidelines there is much discussion in relation to treatment options, however due to the individual nature of each child and their responses to the allergens which cause eczema, effective pain management will also require the same individualised approach

A 'stepped approach' for the treatment is included in the guidelines (see Figure 7.4) which demonstrates the care pathway for children with atopic eczema.

For Jonathan, the use of emollients will be the first line of treatment, both for pain relief and skin protection. Emollients are moisturising products that act by providing the skin with a barrier, forming a film that prevents loss of moisture (Dawber 2008). Emollients are the firstline treatment for the local areas of inflammation and key to preventing the further breakdown of the skin (Lancaster 2009). These emollients are often used to replace soap for skin cleansing and it is recommended that

where possible 'leave-on' emollients should be used (although, in some cases, even these may cause irritation for some children). It has been shown that soap products can act as irritants to the skin and thus should be avoided (NICE 2007a). It is pertinent for nurses to consider that in some cases the application of emollients themselves can be very painful for children and while they ultimately offer some relief, systemic pain relief before application is essential. Peters (2005) found that some common emollients may cause further stinging and that specific application methods were important in pain reduction, ensuring that products are applied in the direction of hair growth and that the friction of rubbing is avoided as this will increase heat on the skin and potentially increase irritation. Once topical emollients have been applied, more inflamed areas are treated with corticosteroid creams (such as hydrocortisone). This must be prescribed and applied sparingly, using less potent concentrations on more delicate skin areas such as the face and around the eyes (Ayliffe 2009). As these topical treatments can have side-effects of skin atrophy it is recommended by NICE (2007a) that these preparations are for short-term use only.

As Jonathan has severe eczema, areas of his skin will be broken and sore so it may be that application of these steroid creams is not appropriate or possible without causing further damage. Oral steroids may be effective for Jonathan and also an antihistamine preparation orally in order to help with inflammation reduction. The antihistamine may also have a sleep-inducing effect. In addition minimal handling will be required, as will constant monitoring of his pain. In a case of very infected eczema such as this addressing the underlying infection will be the priority.

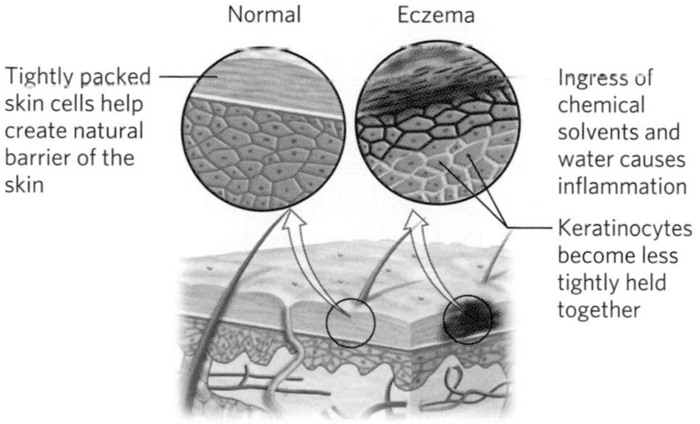

Systemic Management of Pain

Prior to any intervention it is vital that Jonathan should undergo a pain assessment and most importantly, have that assessment acted on. Following the WHO analgesia ladder (WHO 2012) and the BNF for children (2009) pharmacological interventions will assist in promoting quality care for Jonathan as well as non-pharmacological interventions (see Figure 7.5).

Following this framework, Jonathan should have his pain managed effectively. There is no excuse for ignoring or minimalising the discomfort of having broken, sore and infected skin. It is easy to consider that children with eczema are just 'itchy' or 'irritated'; however, the condition often results in pain.

Non-Pharmacological Therapy

In addition to the pharmacological treatment of pain, the use of non-pharmacological methods of pain management should always be considered. Twycross (2007) identified that children's nurses do not always employ basic distractions for children during painful procedures so, while it may appear obvious to use these techniques for interventions such as venepuncture, there is value in using the same techniques alongside pharmacological sources, for pain relief. Remember, however, that non-pharmacological therapy will not necessarily take away pain. It

Figure 7.3 What eczema 'looks like'

Normal   Eczema

Tightly packed skin cells help create natural barrier of the skin

Ingress of chemical solvents and water causes inflammation

Keratinocytes become less tightly held together

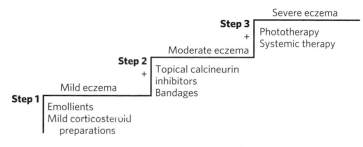

Figure 7.4 Stepped approach for eczema treatment

Severe eczema

Step 3
+
Phototherapy
Systemic therapy

Moderate eczema

Step 2
+
Topical calcineurin inhibitors
Bandages

Mild eczema

Step 1
Emollients
Mild corticosteroid preparations

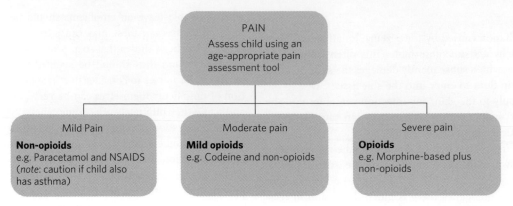

Figure 7.5 The WHO analgesia ladder

may however reduce the awareness and perception of the pain for the child, increasing the overall sense of well-being (Murray 2004).

To Swab or Not to Swab: the Practice Dilemma

As Jonathan has infected eczema there may be some discharge from the eczema sites. The majority of infection is caused through the staphylococcal aureus bacteria, which commonly colonises the skin of individuals with eczema and this is known to respond well to broad spectrum antibiotics such as flucloxacillin (National Eczema Society 2008). Therefore routine swabbing for microscopic bacterial culture is usually not necessary. If the child is not responding to the broad-spectrum antibiotics or has repeated infections then a swab to check for sensitivity is recommended (NICE 2007a). Gill (2006) suggests that nurses need to familiarise themselves with the clinical presentation of infected lesions as this can be a more reliable way to identify the micro-organism responsible. It is important not to forget that there are other organisms such as streptococci and herpes simplex but visual identification will help to determine these.

Pyrexia Management

Nursing a child like Jonathan with a raised temperature (pyrexia) 39.7°C is a common occurrence on a children's medical ward. Pyrexia occurs as the body's natural response to attack whether it is viral, bacterial or fungal in nature. It must always be remembered that fever, too, has a purpose. It can hamper the growth of some organisms and act as an accelerator for a body's immune response (Sidwell and Thomson 2011). Many children who present with a fever have minor infections (often viral) and this is recognised as 'to be expected' during early childhood. There is however, a lot of anxiety for parents as it is often difficult to identify why the child is pyrexial and distinguish between more or less serious causes (NICE 2007a).

Caring for the Child who is Pyrexial

Looking after a child who has a high temperature is challenging, mainly due to the fact that the child is likely to be suffering from the accompanying discomfort. The child may complain of a headache, shivering or feeling hot, muscle aches and generally feels miserable. Therefore the main aim of care is to promote comfort for the child or young person and relieve symptoms. This can be achieved through a combination of physical cooling and pharmacological cooling. It should be recognised that often the most distress and anxiety comes from parents, who remain concerned by the potential of the child having a febrile convulsion or be suffering from a serious illness (such as meningitis). Crocetti et al. (2001) describe this as 'fever phobia' and this remains common within practice settings and the community at large. To reduce this fear, it is important that medical professionals understand the mechanisms of fever and manage appropriately to instil confidence in management for parents in the future.

Recognising Pyrexia

It is important that the nurse can accurately record a temperature. It may seem obvious however there are several methods that can be used, each of which has advantages and disadvantages as well as variations in accuracy (see Figure 7.6).

The guidelines also suggest that the chemical dot thermometers are not recommended if multiple recordings are necessary but may be helpful for parents who are recording temperatures at home. In addition, forehead scanning thermometers are unreliable and not appropriate for use in the hospital.

Assessing the Severity of the Pyrexia

As a healthcare professional, it is important that the assessment of a child with fever is approached in the same way as any other assessment, using a holistic approach. As this will be a common response to illness and infection the incidence of fever alone

RESEARCH NOTE 7.1 Studies on the effects of raised body temperature (Waugh and Grant 2006; Broom 2007; Sidwell and Thomson 2010)

Positive effects of pyrexia	Negative effects of pyrexia
1 An increase in body temperature causes an inflammatory reaction to begin within the body, which, in turn, attracts the white blood cells (leucocytes) to launch an attack on the invading organisms. These macrophages engulf the organisms and release protein substances which in turn mediate with the immune system. Through a complex release of these protein cells (endogenous pyrogens) the hypothalamus, which, among other functions regulates temperature, responds by raising the core body temperature It must be recognised that fever is a beneficial mechanism for fighting infection	1 Febrile convulsions can occur as a secondary response to fever and is common in 2–4% of children under the age of 5. The cause remains unknown although there appears to be a link between the developing brain and the rate and level at which the temperature rises A febrile convulsion is distressing for all who witness this as well as having negative consequences physiologically (explored later)
2 Metabolism is increased (10% for every one degree of increase), stimulating the immune system and increasing the rate of tissue repair	2 An increase in metabolic demand on the body during a rise in temperature can be significant. For example, the heart rate increases, respiratory rate increases. If a child already has prolonged pyrexia or an underlying condition (e.g. cardiac/metabolic condition) this can prove potentially serious
3 There is also metabolic adjustment in relation to a reduction of free glucose in the circulation, in effect 'starving' the alien micro-organisms. The increase in overall temperature inhibits and arrests the survival of some micro-organisms, particularly viral organisms	3 Psychological effects on the child and family with a fever can be significant. The child will be miserable, uncooperative, confused and lethargic Parents will be concerned in relation to the potential for a serious illness (such as meningitis) and even of death
	4 Albeit rarely, cell destruction and death can occur if temperature is very high and prolonged

does not indicate the seriousness of the fever. Moreover, it is vital that staff engage in communication with the parents to be able to assess the nature and seriousness of the condition and, as always, the ABCDE assessment is essential. The guidelines also suggest a colour-coded risk assessment, which is useful for staff to use alongside other routine observations. It may well also be useful for parents to see this for reassurance (see Table 7.3).

Medication (Pharmacological)

Drugs that have the effect of reducing body temperature are known as antipyretics. **Paracetamol** is commonly used as an antipyretic. This can be given orally or rectally, which can be an advantage, particularly if a child is unable to tolerate fluids for any reason. It should be noted that although rectal administration can be useful in some circumstances, the rate of effectiveness

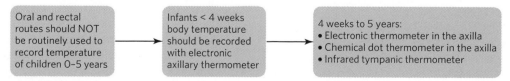

Figure 7.6 Recording tools for temperature
Source: NICE (2007a)

Table 7.3 Feverish illness in children: risk assessment guidelines

	Green – low risk	Amber – intermediate risk	Red – high risk
Colour	• Normal colour of skin, lips and tongue	• Pallor reported by parent/carer	• Pale/mottled/ashen/blue
Activity	• Responds normally to social cues • Content/smiles • Stays awake or awakens quickly • Strong normal cry/not crying	• Not responding normally to social cues • Wakes only with prolonged stimulation • Decreased activity • No smile	• No response to social cues • Appears ill to a healthcare professional • Unable to rouse or if roused does not stay awake • Weak, high-pitched or continuous cry
Respiratory		• Nasal flaring • Tachypnoea: RR > 50 breaths/minute age 6–12 months RR > 40 breaths/minute age > 12 months • Oxygen saturation M 95% in air • Crackles	• Grunting • Tachypnoea: RR > 60 breaths/minute • Moderate or severe chest indrawing
Hydration	• Normal skin and eyes • Moist mucous membranes	• Dry mucous membrane • Poor feeding in infants • CRT U 3 seconds • Reduced urine output	• Reduced skin turgor
Other	• None of the amber or red symptoms or signs	• Fever for U 5 days	• Age 0–3 months, temperature U 38°C • Age 3–6 months, temperature U 39°C
		• Swelling of a limb or joint • Non-weight bearing/not using an extremity	• Non-blanching rash • Bulging fontanelle • Neck stiffness • Status epilepticus • Focal neurological signs • Focal seizures
		• A new lump > 2 cm	• Bile-stained vomiting

Source: NICE (2007b)

Note: CRT, capillary refill time; RR, respiratory rate

PRACTICAL GUIDELINES 7.1

Physical cooling can be achieved in several ways:

- Undress the child – light clothing only, such as underwear and cover with a light cotton sheet or blanket. It is common for children to complain of feeling cold so comfort has to be considered.
- Put socks on child – as their feet may be cold.
- The room environment should be cooled – this can be achieved by ensuring a circulation of air by opening a window or using a fan.

- Care must be taken not to have cooling air directly on the child's skin or cooling the skin through tepid sponging – this may cause shivering, which, in turn, may cause an increase in temperature (Mohammed 2006; Hay et al. 2008; NICE 2007b; Hay et al. 2009). Overall there is no evidence to suggest that the practice of tepid sponging has any effect on reducing temperature (Watts et al. 2003).
- Encourage cool, oral fluids as able to tolerate – consider that the child may need intravenous fluids.

on pyrexia may be delayed with peak plasma level in the blood being longer than oral administration (30 to 90 minutes). Therapeutic doses must be administered in line with British National Formulary (BNF) and prescribed. While paracetamol is relatively safe to use, renal and hepatic (liver) toxicity can result if overdosing occurs. It must be noted that the symptoms of overdose are not always apparent for 4 to 6 days and that children who have a febrile illness are at higher risk of liver impairment (BNF 2009). In the healthy child, paracetamol is a relatively safe drug when given within the recommended dosage and side-effects are rare (Paul et al. 2011). It is also possible to administer paracetamol intravenously, which may be considered if the child has a cannula sited and is unable to tolerate fluids.

Ibuprofen is the other most commonly used antipyretic for children. Ibuprofen has the additional property of having an anti-inflammatory quality. Ibruprofen must be used with caution with some groups of individuals such as those with renal or cardiac impairment, active or previous gastrointestinal bleeds or those with a hypersensitivity to non-steroidal anti-inflammatory drugs (NSAIDs). It also may carry a risk for the exacerbation of asthma (Paul et al. 2011). As children with atopic eczema are more likely to have asthma this is not always an appropriate medication for pyrexia. Recent studies reflected in the NICE guidance (2007b) suggest that either paracetamol or ibuprofen is equally effective in reducing temperature in most cases, but should not be given at the same time. The guidance suggests that alternating the medication can be administered if one or other of the drugs is not managing the pyrexia.

Febrile Convulsions

There is one effect of a raised temperature that causes concern among parents and carers of younger children. Febrile

---

ACTIVITY 7.5 Research that contradicts guidance in regards to antipyretics

http://news.bbc.co.uk/1/hi/health/7592585.stm: This link identifies research that contradicts the guidance.

'Children were randomised to receive paracetamol plus ibuprofen, just paracetamol, or just ibuprofen. Over a 24-hour period, children given both medicines experienced 4.4 hours less time with fever than those given just paracetamol and 2.5 hours less time with fever than those just given ibuprofen.'

Consider the impact that this may have for parents of children with a fever.

---

convulsions (sometimes referred to by parents as 'fever fits') are common in around 3 per cent of children between the ages of 6 months to around 6 years of age (Broom 2007). When it is clear that the seizure is the result of a fever, it does not follow that the child will go on to develop epilepsy in the future, however, this is a concern for parents. It is difficult to determine the certainty of this not happening as many factors contribute to the onset of non-febrile seizures and epilepsy (Vestergaard et al. 2007). Therefore, it is likely that all children's nurses will have experience of caring for a child who is having a febrile seizure, has had one, or is at risk of having a seizure. A febrile seizure usually presents as a generalised seizure and the majority of these are self-limiting, lasting up to 5 minutes in duration. Febrile convulsions must be managed as any other seizure as the risks remain as with any convulsion, that of airway obstruction, hypoxia and, if prolonged, lasting neurological damage. Therefore it is important to remain calm and supportive during the seizure, particularly if this is a sudden occurrence when parents are ill prepared.

PRACTICAL GUIDELINES 7.2

For the successful management of a seizure, you must ensure that the child is safe from the environment, using pillows or blankets to protect from hard objects (e.g. cot sides). If safe to do so (for self and child) place the child on his side to allow for natural drainage of oral secretions:

- Note the time of onset.
- Observe nature of seizure such as arm and leg movements, eye movements (focal) or noises.
- Observe airway and breathing: if there appears to be difficulty in breathing or maintaining oxygenation, then commence 15l of oxygen via an oxygen mask with reservoir bag.
- Oral suctioning may be necessary if there are excessive secretions or vomit during seizure.

- Call for help and ensure the child is not left alone. A bag and valve mask device should be accessible if needed.
- If the seizure continues for 3 minutes, consider administration of anticonvulsant, which must be prescribed, following guidelines for local hospital policy.
- Post-seizure, the child should be placed in the recovery position and monitored until neurologically recovered. As the child may often sleep following a seizure, it is important that neurological assessment (Glasgow Coma scale) be carried out until the child is no longer fitting.
- Note that some anticonvulsants can cause a sedating response and changes to pupil reactions (e.g. diazepam).
- Treat pyrexia if this has not already been addressed.
- Give full explanation and reassurance to parents throughout.

Review of the Case Study for Further Interventions for Pyrexia

As Jonathan has a temperature of 39.7° the administration of paracetamol as an antipyretic as well as an analgesic will be appropriate and important, as this will not only address the pain and discomfort he will be feeling, but also the added effects of a raised temperature on the skin. There is also the risk of a febrile convulsion for Jonathan, so close observation and assessment of his overall condition is essential. It is also pertinent to ask for any history of seizures although this needs to be communicated sensitively with parents so that they are not unduly alarmed.

Management of Venepuncture

Once Jonathan has settled and had his pain and pyrexia managed, it is important to actively treat the infected eczema with a systemic treatment of intravenous antibiotics. In order to facilitate this, Jonathan will need to have an intravenous cannula inserted and blood taken. This is known as venepuncture and is a common intervention on a children's medical ward although considered only when absolutely necessary, due to the invasive and distressing nature for young children (Tak and van Bon 2006). For Jonathan, this is a necessary procedure. Due to his increased temperature (an indication of systemic disease) and clinical presentation of inflamed, weeping lesions it is likely that intravenous antibiotics will be necessary. At the very least a blood sample will indicate the presence of infection via a full blood count (FBC) and also sample for blood cultures. It is important that at the time of cannulation these samples are obtained to reduce the need for further venepuncture. Some oral medications are as well absorbed as intravenous medication so it may be that, if this is the case and the child can tolerate it, oral medication is the preference.

With the development of children's rights (Human Rights Act 1998; Children Act 1989; UN Convention on the Rights of the Child 1989), the issue of restraining children in order to carry out interventions must be a primary consideration for children's nurses, in order to uphold the child's right to participate and be involved in their care. Within the medical setting, there are many occasions on which restraint is required as, due to the age and stage of development, fully cooperative subjects may be an impossibility. Despite the hard work of all members of the healthcare team it must be recognised that, in line with a nurse's duty of care (NMC 2008), every intervention that is undertaken must be in the best interests of the child as well as promoting and protecting the rights of children. This conflict can prove to be a difficult aspect of working as a children's nurse and there will inevitably be times when staff feel uncomfortable when expected to restrain children (Lambrenos and McArthur 2003). The Royal College of Nursing (RCN) has produced a set of guidelines (RCN 2010). The document uses terms such as 'therapeutic holding' in situations where it is considered in the child's best interests to have a procedure completed quickly and effectively. All procedures should be carried out with the consent of the child and in very young children, full collaboration with parents (including explanation) is an essential principle.

PRACTICAL GUIDELINES 7.3

The process for obtaining consent will vary from simple situations such as assistance with dressing, when a question 'shall I help you' would suffice if the child is able to understand, to complex situations where a considerable amount of information would be needed to support decision making. See Department of Health, Social Services and Public Safety (Wales 2003, page 3) Seeking consent: working with children (**http://www.dhsspsni.gov.uk/consent-guidepart2.pdf**).

Jonathan is 3 years old and due to his age and stage of development, the presence of his mother will be paramount during venepuncture. Good preparation is vital for all concerned. Mahoney et al. 2010 identified that the approach and attitude of the adult present at venepuncture has a powerful effect on a child's ability to cope. Therefore it is essential to communicate with Jonathan's parent, explaining explicitly the reason why the procedure is necessary, how long it will take and whether the parent is willing to be present. Giving plenty of time to allow the parent to ask questions and have full understanding of the procedure and reasons why it is necessary will be good practice in obtaining informed consent. While the involvement of parents is often assumed to be the best thing for the child, the nurse must take into account the parent's ability to cope with the procedure. Although Jonathan is young, he will have some understanding of what is going to happen but this will be limited to his age and stage of development. At 3 years of age Jonathan will have some language but will certainly have developed the ability to express verbally his wishes. It is likely he will know the word 'no' for most attempts to engage with him about his treatment and care, but this could be driven by fear of the unknown and lack of understanding. In this case, it is in his best interests to have the treatment; however, the child must still be involved in how any procedures are carried out.

ACTIVITY 7.6

What would your approach be to preparing Jonathan and his family for this and any other procedure?

What are some of the choices that you could give to Jonathan?

What toys or aids could you use to distract and/or explain what is going to happen?

Duff (2003) considers that children and young people should be given permission to cry and respond verbally rather than always being told to 'be brave'. This is one way of valuing the reactions and responses of children, thus demonstrating the ability to acknowledge their discomfort, having the knock on effect of a more cooperative child. Holistic assessment is essential prior to commencement of the procedure and in doing this the nurse is able to act in Jonathan's best interests. Venepuncture for smaller children cannot be rushed so having sufficient time to perform this should also be taken into consideration.

PRACTICAL GUIDELINES 7.4

Preparation for venepuncture should include:

- preparation of child and parent/carer through explanation and information
- preparation of equipment and environment (away from bedside)
- skin preparation through use of topical anaesthetic creams (such as Ametop or Emla cream)
- ensuring that sites are appropriate for insertion of cannula, the aim being to select a vein that is clearly visible. It is important to consider dominant hand not being used unless absolutely necessary and in any case consider position of cannula for maximum viability and longevity (Chalk et al. 2010)

- input from play specialist to work with child; may be able to employ the use of distraction
- discussing/demonstrating the positioning of child when undergoing the procedure, making sure parent is comfortable and aware of what is expected of them; following guidelines for safe holding (RCN 2010)
- ensuring that the person carrying out the venepuncture is clear that frequent unsuccessful attempts are unacceptable so agree on an attempt limit and time limit to minimise distress for all concerned.

Note that, due to Jonathan's eczema, the application of topical anaesthetic cream may not be possible, as the cream or the occlusive dressing could become an irritant. Ethyl chloride spray might be suitable (as it acts as a skin refrigerant) but do not use on broken skin. If none of the preparations is suitable, it will be very important to promote a calm, controlled environment to gain intravenous access. When faced with an emergency cannulation, it may not be possible to have the time for prolonged preparation or topical anaesthesia, however all the above should be considered.

RESEARCH NOTE 7.2 Association between parents' and healthcare professional's behaviour and children's coping and distress during venepuncture (Mahoney et al. 2010)

The aim of this research was to explore the verbal interactions that healthcare professionals and carers displayed during venepuncture for children. This was UK based and was carried out in an outpatient department. The hypothesis of the research was that there was a correlation between adult and child distress as well as adult and child coping. Anxiety levels were monitored before the procedure and the procedure was then video-recorded in order to capture vocalisations. These vocalisations were then categorised. One of the interesting conclusions of this research was that the healthcarer's behaviour affected children's coping more strongly than that of parents. So it is important that children's nurses are calm, controlled and aware of the anxieties of both the child and the parent during cannulation and venepuncture.

Care of the Intravenous Cannula

Caring for any child who has an intravenous cannula in place is an important part of the role of the nurse. Cannulation is the insertion of a plastic tube into a vein in order to facilitate the removal of blood and administration of fluids/medication and poor management of this site can be potentially life threatening. The position of the cannula is crucial in reducing the risk of dislodging the device, with staff being careful to avoid sites such as veins over bony prominences, veins in areas of flexion or infected sites or over broken skin (Chalk et al. 2010). Jonathan may have large areas of broken skin and therefore the cannulation sites may be limited, which means that maintaining a patent cannula is even more important. In smaller children, the anatomical structure of the veins can sometimes result in veins that are difficult to locate due to the covering of connective tissue (Gabriel 2008).

Once in place the cannula must be secured by a sterile dressing (Nicol et al. 2008) although the site of cannula entry must be visible for monitoring of the site (McCann 2003; Lavery and Ingram 2006). The use of a bandage and the need to splint the site may be necessary. It must be remembered that the splint should be commercially produced, fit for purpose and of single use only. In 1996 four babies died of serious fungal infection in a neonatal unit and this was attributed to infection introduced by the wooden tongue depressors that were used as improvised splints to secure cannulae (Mitchell et al. 1996).

Careful monitoring of the cannulation site is essential and is primarily visual. In recent years there has been the development of visual assessment tools to assist nurses to maintain safe practice. Phlebitis is swelling or inflammation of the vein. For children and young people (particularly nonverbal children) it can be difficult to assess for this, due to the psychological effects of cannulation associated with fear and distress of the actual procedure and the circumstances surrounding this. However, this is all the more reason why staff should be extremely vigilant in observing cannulation sites. The RCN (2005) produced guidelines for managing intravenous infusions and within this document included Jackson's example (1998, cited in NMC 2007) (see Figure 7.7).

Administration of Intravenous Antibiotics

Within children's nursing it is preferable that, where possible, medications are administered orally; however, a holistic assessment will assist the staff in deciding the best route of administration. The NMC (2007) guidance on the safe administration of medicines clearly states that practitioners must assess the patient and administer medication via the most appropriate route. In addition, the guidance also emphasises that if intravenous administration is chosen as the best route, the site must

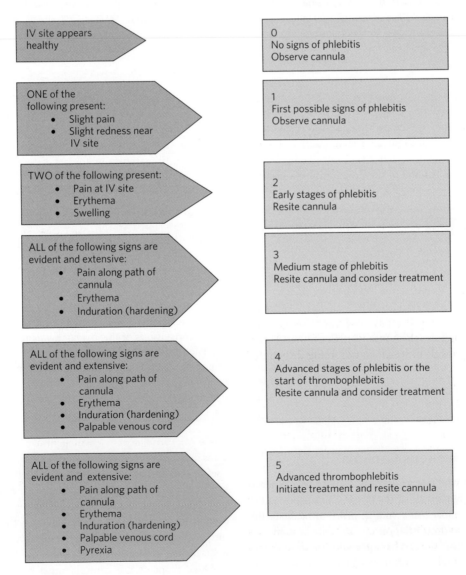

Figure 7.7 Phlebitis scale at IV sites

be closely monitored throughout the administration process. In reviewing the case study, Jonathan has received pain relief, had a cannula inserted, and commenced on IV antibiotics. Maintenance fluids may also be indicated for Jonathan.

Fluid Maintenance

Assessment of dehydration is a major consideration for the sick child or young person who resides on a medical ward. There are several factors to consider in relation to fluid management as their physiology differs from adults. These are:

- Body surface is proportionally greater in children.
- The proportion of weight that consists of fluid is greater.
- In children, the majority of fluid is found in the extracellular compartment (plasma, lymph, interstitial fluid and connective tissue).

As a result of this differing distribution, the child who is unwell is particularly vulnerable to fluid loss and its effects, so fluid balance must be considered for every child, as it can easily become overlooked. Consider Jonathan for a moment in relation to fluid loss. Jonathan has a developing infection and a raised temperature. Due to the body's response to infection there will be an increase in his metabolic rate. This will increase his respiratory rate and effort. He may not be eating or drinking as much as necessary to cope with the extra demands on his body and may have an increase in sweating or be miserable and crying. This extra fluid loss is known as 'insensible' fluid loss.

Insensible fluid loss refers to the loss of fluid from skin (perspiration), respiratory system, tears and water excreted through the digestive system and bowels. It is difficult to identify exactly how much is lost, however, depending on the symptoms and condition of the child, this can be considerable. So a child who is upset and crying excessively can lose a considerable amount of fluid. As the infected eczema has broken the surface of the skin, there is no protection for moisture loss, creating another surface for fluid to escape. Additional therapies such as oxygen therapy also have a further 'drying' effect to the mucous membranes. The consequences of one or more of these factors may result in Jonathan becoming dehydrated over time.

Fluid management charts must be completed throughout care and all input and output monitored. The nurse can involve the family and the child in recording this, although ultimately it is the responsibility of the nurse to act on the information and address any deficits. Children should be encouraged to drink what they can, through whichever method they can. Some younger children may regress to using a bottle or beaker when unwell and this is acceptable if it reduces the risk of having to have further intervention intravenously. For young children, it may be necessary to weigh nappies or consider providing a potty to improve the accuracy of output and for all children, regardless of age or development, privacy and dignity should always be promoted.

Note that the recording abbreviation of 'PU' or 'passed urine' is not a sufficiently accurate recording if the child is not drinking well. More accurate measurements are required to achieve a more exact reading. This may mean the use of a potty or nappy in younger children, but once again, this needs to be discussed and explained to the child and the family. For the older child, a bedpan or bottle may be appropriate but it may be possible to let the child use the bathroom – but place a commode for the child to use.

Calculation of Maintenance Fluids

Dehydration levels are commonly classified as mild, moderate or severe (see Table 7.4).

For children who are showing signs of moderate to severe dehydration (e.g. more than 5 per cent fluid loss) intravenous maintenance fluids are indicated and in addition there may be the need for bolus resuscitation and replacement of percentage loss. Table 7.5 contains an easy formula for calculating intravenous maintenance fluids.

Table 7.4 Dehydration levels

Dehydration levels	Signs
Mild	5% loss of body weight
	Mildly dry mucous membranes
	Mildly decreased urine output
	Increased sensation of thirst
Moderate	5–9% loss of body weight
	Increased heart rate (tachycardia)
	Sunken eyes, poor tear production
	Decreased urine output
	Restless or lethargy
Severe	> 10% loss of body weight
	Absence of urine output (oliguria < 1 ml urine/kg/hour)
	Lethargy or loss of consciousness
	Low blood pressure

Table 7.5 Formula for calculating intravenous fluids

Body weight (kg)	Formula
<10 kgs	100 mls/kg/day
11–20 kgs	1000 mls + 50 mls/kg over 10kgs
>20 kgs	1000 mls + 20 mls/kg over 20kgs

Source: Howe et al. (2010)

PRACTICAL GUIDELINES 7.5

Based on this formula, for Jonathan (18 kgs), the maintenance fluid requirements would be as follows:

- 1000 mls + 400 mls (8 kgs × 50) = 1400 mls /day
- 1400/24 (hrs) = 58.3 mls rounded down to 58 mls /hour

Fluid input and output should be recorded on an hourly basis when receiving intravenous fluids and also when it is suspected that fluid balance is deteriorating.

ACTIVITY 7.7

Isobel weighs 35 kgs and needs to have maintenance fluids.

Calculate her hourly rate.

Skin Integrity

Maintaining skin integrity is an important and sometimes overlooked skill of the children's nurse. Skin cleaning is at the very heart of this process and the act of bathing a child or infant during admission gives a natural opportunity for the nurse to assess the skin for any breakdown. In health, children and young people's skin provides a natural barrier, repelling water and micro-organisms as well as preventing water and electrolyte loss from the body. So, it follows that when unwell, there is the potential for this mechanism to be interrupted and thus cause the child to become more vulnerable. This can be due to injury, breakdown of skin due to poor blood supply or, as in the case of Jonathan, atopic eczema. Therefore preserving the integrity of the skin is of utmost importance when considering the holistic approach to care.

This can be achieved in several ways with routine daily hygiene being central. While parents are primary participants in care, the nurse has a responsibility to ensure that parents are well educated in some of the risk factors should skin integrity become compromised. Damaged skin anywhere is more likely to become an entry point for infection so removal of dirt and good moisturising is the key to healthy skin. Take care with using cleansers that may cause irritation (such as soap-based products) as they can cause the skin to become dry and flaky, increasing the risk of cracking (Keeton 2010). If parents are carrying out the hygiene routine for the child then it is essential that clear and frequent communication is maintained with the nurse to ensure that accurate monitoring and if necessary treatment, is instigated.

Infection Control on a Medical Ward

To fully understand and appreciate the concept of infection control the chain of infection and all the conditions have to be in place for the chain to progress. If this can be broken, the spread of infection can be controlled.

The chain of infection consists of:

- a micro-organism
- a source
- a susceptible host
- a portal of entry
- a means of transmission.

Imagine this another way . . . a burglar (**micro-organism**), has opportunistically walked through an estate of very affluent houses (**source**). The night is dark, the occupants are out (**susceptible host**) and the back window is open (**portal**). The burglar finds a ladder in the garden shed (**means of transmission**) and climbs in the window. Once in the house, he makes himself at home, makes a mess, writes on the wall and enjoys the contents of the fridge and decides to become a resident.

Sources of infection on the ward can be kept to a minimum in several ways. A clean environment and hand washing are proven to be the most effective means of minimising the risk of micro-organisms developing in the ward setting (RCN 2012; see also Health and Social Care Act 2008). It is not possible to totally eliminate micro-organisms through cleaning of equipment and environment; however, this is effective in reducing the risk. Carducci et al. (2010) suggests that eliminating viral organisms is particularly challenging within modern hospital environments and this is borne out with the increase of infections such as norovirus or human rotavirus. The spread of micro-organisms is dependent on a mode of transport. This can take several forms such as direct contact or indirect contact.

Direct contact suggests passing an infection from one person to another, whereas indirect contact is through a contaminated object that comes into contact with the host.

Indirect contact through droplet and airborne infections are potentially more difficult to manage. Often these are spread through sneezing, coughing or talking with particles of residue containing micro-organisms being deposited with the host. Each airbourne particle is smaller, remaining suspended in the air for longer and is inhaled. Within wards, there are often laminar air flow rooms that are designed to filter the room air, reducing the risk of airbourne contaminates.

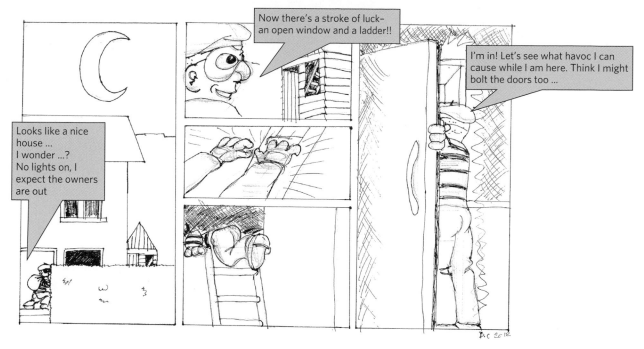

Chain of infection as burglary
Source: Collier (2012)

All children on a medical ward who are unwell take the role of susceptible host so therefore it is clear that all efforts to protect them from healthcare associated infections (HAI) should be in place. Young children have particularly immature immune systems and therefore are vulnerable. The Healthcare Protection Agency acts to protect the UK public health by seeking to assist and advise agencies such as the NHS, local authorities and emergency services, to name a few.

Infection Control in the Medical Setting

Due to the very nature of the medical setting, it is an environment that will undoubtedly have children and young people who are being treated for a variety of illnesses and infections. In an ideal NHS children's ward, it may be considered best to have only single rooms for children and their families to reduce the risk of the spread of infection; however, this is impractical both economically and physically. In 2009 the National Audit Office (NAO) found that many practitioners considered the lack of isolation facilities (56 per cent) and ward design (59 per cent) to be a significant factor. For children, the use of the side room or isolation room is not entirely conducive to a warm and inviting ward environment as children and their parents value the company and support of other families during hospitalisation. This must be balanced against the cost of longer admissions, more need for resources, longer recovery time and the negative effects of hospitalisation on the child and family. However, there are times when

the risk to others and the child or young person has to override this and there are strict guidelines that must be followed to prevent the spread of infection. Risk assessment is considered to be a key element of being a nurse and many clinical decisions must be taken following such a judgement. Within the area of infection prevention, there are many guidelines to assist nurses in ensuring that patients are not put at a higher risk than is necessary when they have to be admitted to the hospital environment.

Standard Precautions

Standard precautions relate to basic safe practices that should be used when working with **all patients** and not just those who may have an infection or who may be at risk of developing an infection. Consideration of these few simple and yet essential skills will undoubtedly protect the safety of patients.

There are six elements of standard precautions:

- hand hygiene
- appropriate use of gloves and aprons
- precautions with blood and body fluids
- use of correct disinfectants
- aseptic technique
- correct disposal of equipment (including linen, dressings, sharps etc.) (see Figure 7.8).

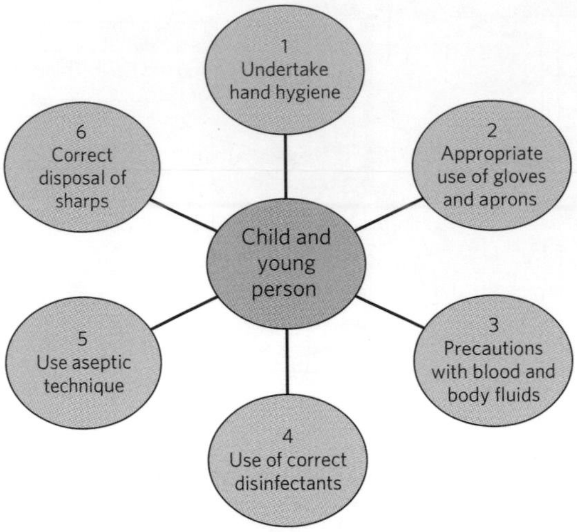

1
Undertake hand hygiene – prior to every direct contact with patient, skin, food, devices or dressings

2
Appropriate use of gloves and aprons – when direct contact with mucous membranes, bodily fluids, broken skin or invasive procedures. Consider aprons when risk of clothing being contaminated

3
Precautions with blood or body fluids – protection of self and risk of contamination for others when dealing with all bodily fluids e.g. blood, saliva, sweat, vomit, faeces and breast milk

4
Use of correct disinfectant – refer to the local trust policy for cleaning procedures

5
Use aseptic technique – reduce risk by following asepsis and non-touch technique where possible

6
Correct disposal of sharps – follow and adhere to local trust policy

Figure 7.8 Principles of standard protection

TYPES OF ISOLATION

Essentially there are two categories of isolation that are required for infections.

Source Isolation

Sometimes known as barrier nursing, this is necessary to prevent the transmission of micro-organisms from one patient to another. The decision to place a patient in a source isolation side room is made by considering assessment of the risk to others. Consider how the infection is transmitted, the age of the child and the availability of side rooms in some areas. All trusts will have specific policies for isolation of parents and also an infection control team who advise and recommend.

Protective Isolation

This resolves to do exactly as it says, protect the patient himself from other infection sources. It may be that a child is immune suppressed or compromised and is susceptible to infections. In cases like this, a common and seemingly innocuous infection (such as viral cold) may result in a more serious outcome. Children who may be at risk are those undertaking any therapy that may lower their resistance to infection, such as chemotherapy and large doses of steroids.

Because of the nature of isolating children, there needs to be clear and honest communication with parents and children to explain the rationale behind placing a child in a side room. In particular, the principles of standard precautions must be enforced by all involved in care, including parents and visitors. If these precautions are not undertaken, then there is little value in being in an isolation room at all.

ACTIVITY 7.8 True or false?

Give rationale for your answers. You need to be able to explain your decisions:

1 'Jonathan must be placed in a side room.'
2 'Gloves and aprons should be worn when doing anything for Jonathan.'
3 'All crockery and cutlery for Jonathan must be disposable.'
4 'A specific nurse must be assigned to care for Jonathan and no one else can do so.'

It must be remembered that staphylococcus aureus is an opportunistic pathogen and poses a serious threat to the very sickest patients. In 2001 the Department of Health commissioned the production of EPIC (evidence-based practice in infection control), which initially gave broad guidelines for infection control. This was updated in 2007 to include further information targeted to prevent healthcare-acquired infections through the correct care of medical devices that can introduce infection. This was known as EPIC2 (Pratt et al. 2007).

THE INTERPROFESSIONAL TEAM ON THE MEDICAL WARD

As with all areas of healthcare the quality of outcomes is reliant on the strength of the whole team. Section 7 of the National Service Framework for children, young people and maternity services (DoH 2004) particularly identifies the care of children and young people in the hospital setting and Section 2 considers that parents are assisted to a good quality of information, services and support throughout their stay. There are some specific concepts that need to be incorporated into care alongside the need for day-to-day communication between healthcare professionals in the ward setting. The children's medical ward has an array of professionals who work alongside one another and with children and their families. A care experience that is disjointed is confusing and fails to meet the holistic needs of the child. However, where team work abounds care can positively move forward towards the ultimate aim of children being well provided for. Every member of the team has a part to contribute and a unique ingredient to bring. It is often the children's nurse who draws it all together over the span of the day and night.

PRACTICAL GUIDELINES 7.6

Family-centred care (Chapter 1) centred on the particular needs of Jonathan is essential. Jonathan's mother is a lone parent but lives with her mother and father. This means that there are several main carers for Jonathan. Early on the nurse will need to establish the boundaries for information giving, ensuring that mum is aware of Jonathan's progress, changes in treatment and future plans. This will need to be well planned.

PRACTICAL GUIDELINES 7.7

Play is essential, not only to keep Jonathan occupied, but also to address his developmental needs. Jonathan is of an age when play is his work, how his learning takes place. Play specialists should be introduced to Jonathan early on in his stay, not only for therapeutic reasons (to assist with interventions) but for developmental and adjustment to the new and strange surroundings. It must be remembered that, as part of the interprofessional team, the play specialist has a part to play in continuing a child's developmental progress as well as supporting the whole family.

PRACTICAL GUIDELINES 7.8

All parents and carers should receive up-to-date information and education. This will be important for Jonathan's mum and potentially grandparents; however, it must be remembered that his mother maintains parental responsibility and as such all decision making in relation to care. For this reason, the channels of communication, individual to Jonathan and his family, must be established early on in the admission. Integrated communication relies on each member of the healthcare team working by the same standards and any breakdown in the chain of communication can affect outcomes.

Burzotta and Noble (2011) identify that nurses specifically have a unique role to play in promoting holistic care, including the observation that good communication between professionals relies on each individual sharing the same vision and goal for the ultimate outcome (see Figure 7.9). This can be difficult at some times within a children's ward when time is precious, staff are busy and perceptions of what is most important can be so very different. Parents can also be concerned with work commitments, other siblings, travelling issues and the surge of emotions that follow a child being unwell and admitted to hospital.

To be functioning as a member of an interprofessional team, each member must firstly be willing to communicate with others and have developed skilful communication. Many

Family support

GP, health visitor, practice nurses

Community children's nurses

Paediatrician

Play specialist

Figure 7.9 Nurse's role in promoting holistic care

RESEARCH NOTE 7.3 Student approaches to learning in a clinical interprofessional context (Hylin 2011)

This study considered the evaluation of IPE (interprofessional education) by a group of healthcare students (40 occupational therapists, 85 medical students, 52 physiotherapy students and 192 student nurses). The information was collected via a questionnaire.

The study considered the students' learning approach and how this related to their attitude to the importance of IPE. The results demonstrated that all the students thought that IPE was helpful and in particular when they were able to 'rehearse' through an 'interprofessional training ward'. There are points of learning from this, that rehearsal and interaction are effective in improving confidence in communication.

---

individuals consider that their skills of communication are 'good' but what is meant by that? Hammick et al. (2009) consider the additional attribute to be one who is aware of the needs of those you are working with, taking into account their unique knowledge and skills also. Within the medical setting managing care is reliant on good teamship, which is not just a case of one person giving instruction and the other carrying out the care. There is a multiplicity of factors that impinge on the effectiveness of that communication, such as the time and timing of exchange can have an impact, as well as hierarchy, power and mode of delivery. Take for example a doctor assessing a child and writing a plan of care to be implemented by a nurse without verbally communicating. Written documentation may be sufficient and appropriate for some instructions but if the action needs to be implemented with urgency then this may be ineffective.

ACTIVITY 7.9

Dr Watts has inserted the cannula for Jonathan and has written the following instructions in the notes: 'Jonathan requires a chest X-ray to rule out chest infection.'

However, Dr Watts has not verbalised this and on the ward round it comes to light that this investigation has not happened. Dr Watts is furious and the consultant is not happy and angry with the nursing staff.

What has been the key cause for this event?

What underlying factors have contributed to this event?

CASE STUDY REVIEW 7.1

Jonathan has been admitted to the ward and had the following interventions and care:

- Pain relief – Jonathan has had regular pain assessment using an age-appropriate tool.
- Antipyretic management has been undertaken.
- Venepuncture and cannulation occurred to support administration of antibiotics.
- Jonathan has been nursed in a side room with standard isolation in place as he has open, infected wounds and is particularly distressed due to his sore, excoriated skin. When there is no further exudation from the wounds, then Jonathan may leave the room; however, implementation of all standard precautions are still necessary (e.g. good hand washing).
- Fluid assessment and commencement of intravenous maintenance fluids continued throughout his stay.
- Intravenous antibiotics were administered as prescribed.
- Emollients and topical medication to eczema lesions was undertaken as prescribed.
- Monitoring of skin integrity and pressure areas occurred at regular intervals.
- All these interventions will be evaluated and any changes reported to the interprofessional team.

SUMMARY OF KEY LEARNING

This chapter has identified, through application to the care of Jonathan, just a few of the aspects of caring for children on a medical ward. Every day the nurse will be faced with many differing families, illnesses, conditions and interactions. In some ways the medical ward is the very heart of children's nursing, offering the opportunity to assess, plan, implement and evaluate care, all with collaboration with family and other professionals.

FURTHER RESOURCES

http://www.hpa.org.uk/HPAwebHome/: this website provides information in relation to current developments in the health of the nation; it includes access to evidence-based practice documentation that supports the advice. There are particular sections that refer to healthcare associated infections.

ANSWERS TO ACTIVITIES

ACTIVITY 7.1

Using Table 7.1 to help you, consider all the aspects of care for Jonathan as he enters the ward.

Think about Jonathan and his family. What impacts may eczema have on the family both before admission and as a result of his admission? List these impacts.

Suggested responses: anxiety for mum, child and family due to sudden admission.

Mum may feel she has not been able to manage this at home and may feel guilty about this, feeling she has caused this deterioration.

This may be especially evident as mum works full time (as she is a lone parent) and perhaps Jonathan is cared for at nursery or by grandparents.

The grandparents may feel some responsibility.

Sudden admission can cause turmoil for family.

There may be work-related issues or concern that it may not be possible for a carer to stay with the child.

Provision for alternative carer may have to be arranged and staff should understand this.

Grandparents will also need support as it is not known how old they are and whether they are actively involved in care.

Loss of sleep resulting in a tired family!

Jonathan may be in pain that has not been controlled so it may take some time to address this.

Fear of the unknown for all family and Jonathan, in particular.

Wounds – may be bleeding and weeping. Skin may be cracked particularly around joints, making movement difficult.

Psychologically, Jonathan may be miserable, lethargic and tired, due to pyrexia and unfamiliarity with surroundings.

ACTIVITY 7.2 Assessment for Jonathan's physical status

From the description of the assessment for Jonathan's physical status (Table 7.2), consider your priority of care and what your course of actions and interventions would be.

- **Physical treatment:** venepuncture, IV fluid management, skin care, infection control, administration of medicines,

pain management, pyrexia management, nutrition.
- **Psychological issues:** isolation, therapeutic play developmental concerns (regression).
- **Social concerns:** parental stress, involvement of grandparents, potential safeguarding issues.

ACTIVITY 7.3 Pain assessment tools

What pain assessment tools are you familiar with?

Imagine that you have been asked to introduce an easy-to-use and reliable pain assessment tool to the children's medical ward. Take a look at the RCN chart (Figure 7.3) that identifies

a range of assessment tools. Select one or two and consider which of these would be most suitable for use for a 3-year-old such as Jonathan.

List the limitations and ease of use to justify your choices.

ACTIVITY 7.4

During admission, list the non-pharmacological interventions you could use to help Jonathan cope with the pain.

Distraction – use of toys, games, DVDs and reading books, bubbles.

Consider using basic guided imagery with parental involvement, e.g. telling a story and asking for child's input.

Simple breathing and relaxation techniques.

Physical comfort and cuddling from mum/carer

Ensure presence of a familiar toy/comforter.

ACTIVITY 7.5 Research that contradicts guidance in regards to antipyretics

Parents may be confused on misinformation; they will need

reassurance and information on the best evidence-based practice.

ACTIVITY 7.6

What would your approach be to preparing Jonathan and his family for this and any other procedure?

What are some of the choices that you could give to Jonathan?

What toys or aids could you use to distract and/or explain what is going to happen?

Explain the rationale to Jonathan's mum and discuss how Jonathan can best understand what will happen.

Ask mum what her previous experience is of venepuncture and if Jonathan has any previous experience of this.

Decide with mum who will be present with Jonathan during the procedure and if so what her role will be.

Ensure that where possible the procedure is not carried out at the bedside so that Jonathan can see his bed space as a 'safe' environment.

Explain that some restraint may be necessary.

Explain that venepuncture attempts will be limited and what this number will be.

Introduce the person who will be carrying out the procedure

and involve them in preparation (for example, looking at possible venepuncture sites to ensure as few attempts as possible and correct positioning of the topical analgesia).

Consider play therapy with play specialist if possible.

Use toys to show Jonathan what will happen, using age-appropriate language that is jargon free. Take care not to instil more anxiety by using words such as needle or stinging.

Make full use of topical analgesics as well as ensuring that systemic analgesics are up to date and effective.

Choices:
- Ask Jonathan how he would like to be positioned for the procedure, for example on mummy's lap/on the couch with mum close by/ with granddad etc.
- Involve Jonathan in the application of the topical analgesic or the removal of the plasters.
- Ask Jonathan to choose a 'treat' to have after the procedure (sticker or small toy).

ACTIVITY 7.7

Isobel weighs 35 kgs and needs to have maintenance fluids.

Calculate her hourly rate:

ACTIVITY 7.8 True or false?

Give rationale for your answers. You need to be able to explain your decisions.

1 'Jonathan must be placed in a side room.' True
2 'Gloves and aprons should be worn when doing anything for Jonathan.' True

3 'All crockery and cutlery for Jonathan must be disposable.' False
4 'A specific nurse must be assigned to care for Jonathan and no one else can do so.' True

ACTIVITY 7.9

Dr Watts has inserted the cannula for Jonathan and has written the following instructions in the notes: 'Jonathan requires a chest X-ray to rule out chest infection.'

However, Dr Watts has not verbalised this and on the ward round it comes to light that this investigation has not happened. Dr Watts is furious and the consultant is not happy and angry with the nursing staff.

What has been the key cause for this event?

What underlying factors have contributed to this event?

There has been no integrated communication and a breakdown in the chain of communication that affects outcomes.

Poor communication skills between the team members both verbally and via documentation.

Lack of professional respect across professionals.

Losing focus on the child being the centre of the care.

SELECTED REFERENCES

Advanced Life Support Group (APLS) (2005) *Advanced paediatric life support: the practical approach,* 4th edn. BMJ: London.

Ayliffe, V. (2009) Clinical features and management of atopic eczema in children. *Paediatric Nursing,* 21, 35–43.

British National Formulary (2009) *BNF for children.* BNF: London.

Broom, M. (2007) Physiology of fever. *Paediatric nursing,* 19(6), 40–44.

Burzotta, L. and Noble, H. (2011) The dimensions of inter-professional practice. *British Journal of Nursing,* 20(5), 310–315.

Camfferam, D., Kennedy, J., Gold, M., Martin, J., Winwood, P. and Lushington, K. (2010) Eczema, sleep and behaviour in children. *Journal of Clinical Sleep Medicine,* 6(6),

Carducci, A., Verani, M., Lombardi, R., Casini, B. and Privitera, G. (2010) Environmental survey to assess viral contamination of air and surfaces in hospital settings. *Journal of Hospital Infection,* 77, 242–247.

Chalk, S., Harvey, J., Watson, N. and Kelsey, J. (2010) Venesection, cannulation and the care of children requiring intravenous infusion, in A. Glasper, M. Aylott and C. Battrick (eds) (2010) *Developing practical skills for nursing children and young people.* Hodder Arnold: London.

Crocetti, M., Moghbeli, N. and Serwint, J. (2001) Fever phobia revisited: have parental misconceptions about fever changed in 20 years? *Pediatrics,* 107(6), 1241.

Dawber, S. (2008) Management of paediatric-onset atopic eczema. *Nurse Prescribing,* 6(5).

Department of Health (DoH) (2004) National Service Framework for children, young people and maternity services: **http://www.dh.gov.uk/en/Publicationsandstatistics/Publications/PublicationsPolicyAndGuidance/DH_4089100**

Duff, A. (2003) Incorporating psychological approaches into routine venepuncture. *Archives of Diseases in Childhood,* 88, 931–937.

Fisher, S. and Morton, N. (1998) Pain prevention and management in children, in N. Morton (ed.) *Acute paediatric pain management: a practical guide.* WB Saunders: London.

Gabriel, J. (2008) Infusion therapy part one: minimising the risks. *Nursing Standard,* 22(31), 58–60.

Garland, L. and Kenny, G. (2006) Family nursing and the management of pain in children. *Paediatric Nursing,* 18(6), 18–20.

Gill, S. (2006) An overview of atopic eczema in children: a significant disease. *British Journal of Nursing,* 15(9).

Gimbler-Berglund, I., Ljusegren, G. and Enskar, K. (2008) Factors influencing pain management in children. *Paediatric Nursing,* 20(10), 21–24.

Hammick, M., Freeth, D., Copperman, J. and Goodsman, D. (2009) *Being interprofessional*. Cambridge University Press: London.

Hands, C. (2010) Evaluating venepuncture practice on a general children's ward. *Paediatric Nursing*, 22(2).

Hawkins, C. (2005) The effects of atopic eczema on children and their families: a review. *Paediatric Nursing*, 17(6).

Hay, A., Redmond, N., Costelloe, C., Montgomery, A., Fletcher, M., Hollinghurst, S. and Peters, T. (2009) Paracetamol and Ibruprofen for the treatment of fever in children: the PITCH randomised controlled trial. *Health Technology Assessment*, 13(27).

Howe, R., Forbes, D. and Baker, C. (2010) Providing optimum nutrition and hydration, in A. Glasper, M. Aylott and C. Battrick (eds) (2010) *Developing practical skills for nursing children and young people*. Hodder Arnold: London.

Hylin, U. (2011) 'Student' approaches to learning in clinical interprofessional context. *Medical Teacher*, 33, e204–e210.

Keeton, D. (2010) *Skin health care*, in A. Glasper, M. Aylott and C. Battrick (eds) (2010) *Developing practical skills for nursing children and young people*. Hodder Arnold: London.

Kozier, B., Erb, G., Berman, A., Snyder, S., Lake, R. and Harvey, S. (2008) *Fundamentals of nursing: concepts, process and practice*. Pearson: Harlow.

Lambrenos, K. and McArthur, E. (2003) Introducing a clinical holding policy. *Paediatric Nursing*, 15(4), 30–33.

Lancaster, W. (2009) Atopic eczema in infants and children. *Community Practitioner*, 82(7).

Lavery, I. and Ingram, P. (2006) Prevention of infection in peripheral intravenous devices. *Nursing Standard*, 20(49).

Lawton, S. (2008) Management of atopic eczema in children. *Practice Nursing*, 19(6).

McCann, B. (2003) Securing peripheral cannulae: evaluation of a new dressing. *Paediatric Nursing*, 15(5).

McIntosh, N. (2010) Intravenous therapy, in E. Trigg, and T. Mohammed, (eds) (2006) *Practices in children's nursing. Guidelines for Hospital and community*, 2nd edn. Elsevier: London.

Mahoney, L., Ayers, S. and Seddon, P. (2010) The association between parents' and healthcare professionals' behaviour and children's coping and distress during venepuncture. *Journal of Pediatric Psychology*, 35(9), 985–995.

Melhuish, S. and Payne, H. (2006) Nurses' attitudes to pain management during routine venepuncture in young children. *Paediatric Nursing*, 18(2), 20–23.

Mitchell, S., Gray, J., Morgan, M., Hocking, M. and Durbin, G. (1996) Nosocomial infection with Rhizopus microsporus in preterm infants: association with wooden tongue depressors. *The Lancet*, 348(9025), 441–443.

Murray, G. (2004) Managing acute pain in children. *World of Irish Nursing*, 12(11), 35–37.

National Audit Office (2009) The prevention, management and control of healthcare-associated infections (HCAI) in hospitals: **http://www.nao.org.uk/**

National Eczema Society (2008) Infection and eczema: **http://www.eczema.org/Factsheet_Infection_and_Eczema.pdf**

National Institute for Clinical Excellence (NICE) (2007a) *Atopic eczema in children. Management of atopic eczema in children from birth up to the age of 12 years*. RCOG Publications: London. (Available at **http://www.nice.org.uk/nicemedia/pdf/CG057FullGuideline.pdf**.)

National Institute for Clinical Excellence (NICE) (2007b) Feverish illness in children. Assessment and initial management in children younger than 5years. NICE guideline 47: **http://www.nice.org.uk/nicemedia/pdf/CG47NICEGuideline.pdf**

National Medical Council (NMC) (2007) Guidance on the safe administration of medicines. **http://www.nmc-uk.org/Documents/Standards/nmcStandardsForMedicinesManagementBooklet.pdf**

National Medical Council (NMC) (2008) *The code: standards of conduct, performance and ethics for nurses and midwives*. NMC: London. (Available at **http://www.nmc-uk.org/Documents/Standards/The-code-A4-20100406.pdf**.)

Nicol, M., Bavin, C., Cronin, P. and Rawlings-Anderson, K. (2008) *Essential nursing skills*, 3rd edn. Mosby, Elsevier: London.

Noonan, C., Quigley, S. and Curley, M. (2006) Skin integrity in hospitalized infants and children: a prevalence survey. *Journal of Pediatric Nursing*, 21(6),

Paul, F., Jones, M.C., Hendry, C. and Adair, P.M. (2007) The quality of written information for parents regarding the management of a febrile convulsion: a randomized controlled trial. *Journal of Clinical Nursing*, 16(12), 2308–2322.

Paul, S., Prosad, Mayhew, J. and Mee, A. (2011) Safe management and prescribing for fever in children. *Nurse Prescribing*, 9(11), 539–544.

Peters, J. (2005) Exploring the use of emollient therapy in dermatological nursing. *British Journal Community Nursing*, 11(5).

Pratt, R., Pellowe, C., Wilson, J., Loveday, H., Harper, P., Jones, S., McDougall, C. and Wilcox, M. (2007) epic2. National evidence guidelines for preventing healthcare associated infections in NHS hospitals in England: **http://microtrainees.bham.ac.uk/lib/exe/fetch.php?media=epic2_20-_2021aug06_20final_20draft_20for_20consultation.pdf**

Purssell, E. (2002) Treating fever in children: paracetamol or ibuprofen? *British Journal of Community Nursing*, 7(6), 316–320.

Royal College of Nursing (RCN) (2005) *RCN standards for infusion therapy*. RCN: London.

Royal College of Nursing (RCN) (2008) *Caring for children and young people with atopic eczema: Guidance for nurses*. RCN: London.

Royal College of Nursing (RCN) (2010) *Restrictive physical intervention therapeutic holding for children and young people. Guidance for nurses*. RCN: London. (Available at **http://www.rcn.org.uk/—data/assets/pdf_file/0016/312613/003573.pdf**.)

Royal College of Nursing (RCN) (2012) Wipe it out. Essential practice for infection prevention and control. Guidance for nursing staff: **http://www.rcn.org.uk/—data/assets/pdf_file/0008/427832/004166.pdf**

Sidwell, R. and Thomson, M. (2011) *Easy paediatrics*. Hodder Arnold: London.

Tak, J.H. and van Bon, W. (2006) Pain- and distress-reducing interventions for venepuncture in children. *Child Care, Health & Development*, 32(3), 257–268.

Twycross, A. (2007) Children's nurse's post-operative pain management practices: an observational study. *International Journal of Nursing Studies*, 44(6), 869–881.

Vestergaard, M., Pedersen, C., Sidenius, P., Olsen, J. and Christensen, J. (2007) The long-term risk of epilepsy after febrile seizures in susceptible subgroups. *American Journal of Epidemiology*, 165(8), 911–918.

Walsh, A.M., et al. (2005) Fever management: paediatric nurses' knowledge, attitudes and influencing factors. *Journal of Advanced Nursing*, 49(5), 453–464.

Watts, R., Robertson, J. and Thomas, G. (2003) Nursing management of fever in children: a systematic review. *International Journal of Nursing Practice*, 9(1), S1–8.

Willock, J., et al. (2004) Peripheral venepuncture in infants and children. *Nursing Standard*, 18(27), 43.

Willock, J., Baharestani, M.M. and Anthony, D. (2009) The development of the Glamorgan paediatric pressure ulcer risk assessment scale. *Journal of Wound Care*, 18(1), pp.17–21.

World Health Organization (WHO) (2012) Pain relief ladder: **http://www.who.int/cancer/palliative/painladder/en/**

CHAPTER 8
Caring for Children and Young People in the Surgical Setting

Chris Thurston

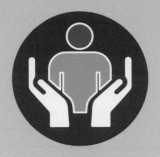
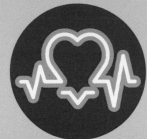
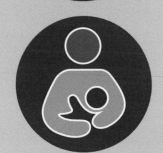

LEARNING OUTCOMES

On completion of this chapter, the reader will be able to:

- Explore why accidents and injuries may occur in children and young people.
- Reflect on assessment with children, young people and families when challenges to LOC and pain are present.
- Plan and implement surgical care for orthopaedic conditions.
- Investigate legal and professional themes around consent to surgical treatment.
- Discuss the effectiveness of surgical nursing care interventions for perioperative orthopaedic care management.

TALKING POINT

Road accidents: the Department of Transport estimates that the average cost per seriously injured casualty on the roads is £178,160 and that the average cost per fatality is £1,585,510.

In 2009, 2,671 children were killed or seriously injured on the road – that's seven children every day. The number of children dying on the roads is decreasing year on year, but there is still some way to go. In 2009, 81 under-16s were killed on the roads.

http://www.makingthelink.net/tools/costs-child-accidents

INTRODUCTION

This chapter will discuss the occurrence of accidents and injuries and the effects of surgery on the child or young person highlighting how good assessment and planning is vital in helping professionals to develop individualised planning, resulting in optimum quality of care and swift post-operative recovery. The approach will acknowledge the challenges faced by staff in surgical settings and encourage the reader to develop suitable strategies to aid in delivery of perioperative care. The specific needs and care required for general and orthopaedic surgery will also be highlighted.

This chapter will enable an understanding of the nursing support required for a young person following a road traffic accident (RTA). The rapidly changing symptoms following injuries and the interventions required means that every health practitioner working with children and young people like James have to develop the capacity to undertake rapid assessments and interventions within the surgical settings. To start the healing process for James (from the case study in the chapter) with his health needs following the RTA. An exploration of the accident and the need for consent will offer explanations of the process required to care for a young person following accident or injury. This includes an acknowledgement of the effects of physical pain on the healing process for the young person. There will also be a focused exploration of assessment, planning, implementation and evaluation of care in a surgical setting.

CASE STUDY 8.1 James on a children's ward following an accident

James is 14 years old and has been admitted to the children's ward following an accident on his bicycle. He had to brake abruptly as a car stopped in front of him and he went over the top of his handlebars. The fall has left him with a head injury, a deep cut to his left arm (1" long) and a left fractured tibia and fibula.

He was on the way to school at the time and now needs consent to go to theatre for a closed manipulation of the simple fracture and suturing of the cut. The interprofessional team is also worried about his head injuries as he is confused.

Gillham and Thomson wrote in 1996: 'The word "accident" denotes chance occurrences but research has revealed that accidents do not happen at random. Most of them are preventable' (Gillham and Thomson 1996, page 12).

Consider the following:

- Each year, over 1,000,000 children under the age of 18 are taken to A&E because of accidents in the home.
- A lot of children get treated at home by their GP as a result of home accidents.
- Boys are more at risk than girls.
- Choking, suffocation and strangulation also cause a significant number of deaths.
- Minor accidents are generally viewed as an inevitable part of growing up.

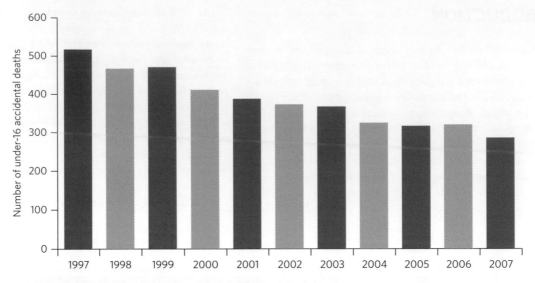

Figure 8.1 Accidental deaths among the under-16s
Source: ONS Mortality Division and the General Register Office for Scotland and Great Britain

- Accidents accounted for 18.3 per cent of deaths among boys and 12.8 per cent of deaths among girls.
- Land transport accidents were ranked third for both boys and girls (see Figure 8.1).

There does appear to be a clear link between age, gender and social class when exploring accidents and injuries both at home and RTAs. When exploring information on accidents in children and young people it is worth noting that while the amount of deaths has reduced it is still significant. Deacon et al. in their study on road traffic collisions and casualties in the northwest of England (2011) confirm this stating that hospital admission rates for RTAs is almost double when the child lives in an area of deprivation.

ACTIVITY 8.1

Why do children have accidents?

List all the reasons why, in your opinion, children and young people have injuries and accidents.

RESEARCH NOTE 8.1 Accident and emergency attendances in England, 2009–2010

Road traffic accidents are the most significant cause of unintentional injury for young people. In 2010 just under 20,000 0 to 15 year-olds were injured on roads in Great Britain, 2500 of whom were killed or seriously injured. Although this represents a two-thirds reduction in the numbers killed or seriously injured compared to the mid-1990s, there are still substantial inequities: young people living in the most deprived areas are three times more likely to be hit by a car than those in the least deprived wards; and, overall, children and young people whose parents have never worked or are long-term unemployed are 13 times more likely to die from unintentional injury. Young males accounted for 58% of all injury-related admissions (**http://www.hesonline .nhs.uk/Ease/servlet/ContentServer?siteID=1937&categ oryID=1502**). See Table 8.1 for data on admission to a children's ward.

Table 8.1 Comparison of routine and emergency surgical admission

Routine	Emergency
Planned	Unplanned
Allows time for child and family to reflect on the admission	No time for child and family to reflect on the admission
Establish therapeutic relationship at pre-admission	Therapeutic relationship must develop quickly after admission
Reduced level of stress as information that is specific to the operation is given before admission	Increased levels of stress and anxiety for patient and carer as information may be general
Exploration of all treatment options	Quick decisions due to accident, injury or illness
Commenced physical and psychological preparation	Very little time for physical and psychological preparation
Long-term outcomes usually known	Outcomes not often known until post-operation
Any underlying condition usually known	Underlying condition may not be known
Usually appropriately qualified personnel to undertake interventions	Could be junior staff at weekends or during the night undertaking interventions
Pre and post-op care organised	Pre and post-op care may be disjointed
Time spent in achieving informed consent	May not be time for all explanations to be given

HOSPITALISATION

This is a potentially stressful event for both the child and parent; when the admission is planned, information can be used to decide on the intervention required and follow-up care. However, when an emergency admission occurs the timescale of interventions may be very short, so it is therefore important that children's nurses take time to explain things to the child using appropriate information. When a child or young person is admitted to a children's ward she should expect to quickly and efficiently receive care and treatment and be treated with dignity at all times. Chapter 1 explored the relationship the nurse is required to develop with the child and her family and also explored the communication and approach required when dealing with the younger child. This age-appropriate communication is vital when the admission is an emergency, and James

is also confused, in pain and requiring surgery. Interventions and care needs to be age appropriate and the care needs to be given by appropriately qualified staff. All professionals, nursing and medical, need to introduce themselves to James and explain what interventions and investigations need to be undertaken. This is more difficult for James as consent is also required if he is to have his fracture manipulated in theatre.

Initial Information about James

height: 160 cm
weight: 90 kg
head circumference: within normal limits
investigations: X-rays of skull and leg were undertaken in A&E; while the skull was intact his left leg has a # tibia and fibula (see Table 8.2).

Table 8.2 Initial assessment of James on admission to the children's ward

Airway	No problems
Breathing	Breathing was a little fast (26 respirations/min), but oxygen saturation was normal (99%)
Circulation	Observations of blood pressure, pulse volume, capillary refill, cardiac rhythm were within normal limits, his heart rate was a little fast at 84
Disability	Neuromuscular observations: Observation of the left leg – the limb remains pink and warm, slightly swollen, with James having some pins and needles Level of consciousness (LOC): Both pupils had an equal reaction, however consciousness level was inconsistent and James was unable to remember what had happened and where he was
Exposure/Environment	Temperature 37.5°C. James was in pain, although a pain score was inconsistent for James due to varying LOC James has an inch-long laceration through both skin and muscle

Head Injury Overview

'Head injury is defined as any trauma to the head, other than superficial injuries to the face' (NICE 2007).

Following the initial assessment there is a need to decide what interventions are undertaken for James; first, there needs to be a balance between pain relief and support for the head injury; while it is necessary for James to be free from pain it is also a priority to ensure that his LOC is not compromised. Most head injuries are mild and not associated with brain injury or long-term complications. A mild headache, nausea and dizziness are common, especially during the first few hours after the injury. If James is nauseous or has vomited, clear liquids (water or squash) could be offered, as long as theatre is not imminent. Very rarely, children with more significant injuries may develop serious complications (e.g. brain injury or bleeding around the brain). Signs and symptoms of head injuries may include scalp swelling, loss of consciousness, headache, vomiting, seizures

and concussion. This is the rationale for undertaking regular neurological observations on James, and why being taken to theatre will need to be delayed until the interprofessional team can be confident that the risk of further complications of the head injury is significantly reduced.

It is necessary to observe James closely for 4 to 6 hours after the accident, with frequency of observation in keeping with current evidence-based practice (every 15 minutes for at least the first hour): due to the fractured lower leg and the requirement of an operation the observations will continue on the children's ward. Before James is able to undergo surgical interventions it is important to ensure that he does not develop any other symptoms. If no further symptoms occur, then he can be prepared for theatre. Children who are well more than 12 hours after a head injury have a low risk of brain injury that requires surgical intervention. James needs to have his fracture manipulated and it is therefore appropriate to assess when he will be physically fit for the anaesthetic.

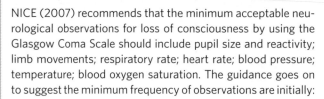

PRACTICAL GUIDELINES 8.1

NICE (2007) recommends that the minimum acceptable neurological observations for loss of consciousness by using the Glasgow Coma Scale should include pupil size and reactivity; limb movements; respiratory rate; heart rate; blood pressure; temperature; blood oxygen saturation. The guidance goes on to suggest the minimum frequency of observations are initially:

- half-hourly until GCS equal to 15 has been achieved
- then half-hourly for 2 hours

- then 1 hourly for 4 hours
- then 2 hourly thereafter.

If James's score lowers at any time then the nurse should increase the frequency again and inform the medical team (see Table 8.3 for the GCS).

PRACTICAL GUIDELINES 8.2

Observation of infants and young children under 5 years is always a difficult exercise and therefore should only be performed in units with staff experienced in the observation of infants and young children with a head injury. Infants and young children may be observed in normal paediatric observation settings, as long as staff have the appropriate experience (NICE 2007).

When observing James for his LOC, there is a need to assess three main areas:

- **Pupil reaction:** eyes need to open spontaneously and the pupils need to be checked for reaction to light: the best response is for both pupils to be equal in size and response (score 4). If the pupil reactions becomes increasingly sluggish or do not respond (commonly called fixed and dilated) then this needs to be reported and the observations need to be increased in frequency.

- **Verbal response:** the ability to verbally interact and have a sensible conversation if old enough is the best response (score 5). If the language becomes confused and the person is or becomes disoriented and does not respond to speech then this needs to be reported and the observations need to be increased in frequency.
- **Motor response:** the ability to move normally and follow command if old enough is the best response (score 6). If movement is only to localise pain or no response at all then this needs to be reported and the observations need to be increased in frequency.

Table 8.3 Glasgow Coma Scale (GCS) for infants, children and adults

	Infant < 1 yr	Child 1–4yrs	Age 4–Adult
EYES			
4	Open	Open	Open
3	To voice	To voice	To voice
2	To pain	To pain	To pain
1	No response	No response	No response
VERBAL			
5	Coos, babbles	Oriented, speaks, interacts, social	Oriented and alert
4	Irritable cry, consolable	Confused speech, disoriented, consolable	Disoriented
3	Cries persistently to pain	Inappropriate words, inconsolable	Nonsensical speech
2	Moans to pain	Incomprehensible, agitated	Moans, unintelligible
1	No response	No response	No response
MOTOR			
6	Normal, spontaneous movement	Normal, spontaneous movement	Follows commands
5	Withdraws to touch	Localizes pain	Localizes pain
4	Withdraws to pain	Withdraws to pain	Withdraws to pain
3	Decorticate flexion	Decorticate flexion	Decorticate flexion
2	Decerebrate extension	Decerebrate extension	Decerebrate extension
1	No response	No response	No response

Source: **http://i.ehow.com/images/a02/5k/7b/status-using-glasgow-coma-scale-800X800.jpg**

PAIN

This section will focus on acute pain (Chapter 14 explores chronic pain in more detail). While no one wants to feel pain, it has its uses: it stops a person from undertaking activities which could lead to short- or long-term injury and is therefore a defence mechanism used by the body to restrict risky physical behaviours.

Life Without Pain

Figure 8.2 shows a child's fingers, which became injured due to the child's lack of pain sensation (congenital insensitivity to pain).

However, many assumptions and myths have developed over time in regards to how children and especially babies react to pain (Table 8.4).

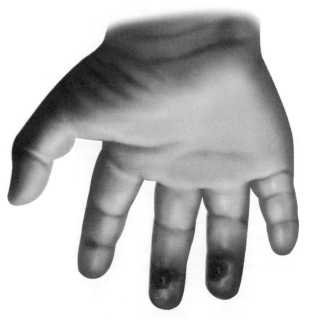

Figure 8.2 Injury due to congenital insensitivity to pain

Table 8.4 Pain myths and assumptions

Myth	Truth
Newborn infants and babies feel less pain than older children and adults	Pain receptors (although immature) are present at birth and therefore pain is felt in a similar way in pain centres in the brain regardless of age
Children will always tell you when they are in pain	There may be a fear of painful interventions (such as injections), which leads to the denial of pain
Children in pain cannot sleep	Sleep may be used as distraction or caused by exhaustion
Children in pain will restrict their movements	Movement and play may be used as distraction
Assessment of pain is inaccurate in non-verbalising children	A number of assessment tools have been developed for non-verbalising children
Pain medication should reduce rather than relieve pain	Appropriate analgesia should always be administered to relieve pain as this aids healing, and encourages earlier post-operative movement
Children have a greater risk of becoming addicted to opioids	There is no evidence to back up this myth therefore appropriate analgesia should be given and evaluated at regular intervals

ACTIVITY 8.2

List the factors that influence experience for children and young people.

however, the most important factor to remember is that every baby, child or young person has a unique perception related to the condition or injury they have, their life experiences and whether or not the pain, or indeed, fear of pain, is a regular occurrence.

The letter from Chloe highlights the individual experience for children in regards to pain (see Figure 8.3). Pain is more than a physical sensation; there are emotional, cultural and gender issues that may influence how James or any other individual may feel pain and also react. Many definitions have been given,

ACTIVITY 8.3

List the words you use to describe the experience of pain.

RESEARCH NOTE 8.2 Recognition and assessment of acute pain in children (RCN 2009)

A number of professional groups, including children's nurses, paediatric anaesthetists and the British Pain Society, worked together to compile an analytical review of studies around recognition and assessment of acute pain. This is a revision of a previous guideline using evidence-based analysis to offer guidelines for health staff for recognising and assessing pain. The study explored and evaluated 41 assessment tools, highlighting their use with different age groups, setting and amount of training required. The study concluded that: 'Children vary greatly in their cognitive and emotional development, medical condition, response to painful interventions and

to the experience of pain, as well as in their personal preferences for care. Health professionals and parents have a responsibility to learn the language of child pain expression, to listen carefully to children's self-reports of pain and to attend to behavioural cues. The detection of children's pain can be improved by strategies to facilitate their expression of pain in ways that are appropriate to their cognitive development, and that can be understood by the adults caring for them' (RCN 2009, page 9) (see Table 8.5). Therefore, use of the most appropriate tool can enhance patient care and encourage recovery.

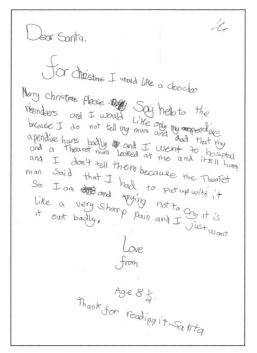

Figure 8.3 A child wish for Santa to take her pain away

PRACTICAL GUIDELINES 8.3

James needs to be supported both for his LOC and his pain due to his head injury and fracture; therefore, pain medication (analgesia) needs to be prescribed appropriately.

When undertaking James's regular observations, pain assessment should always be included.

For James to have successful pain management the results of the assessment should be used to plan and implement care both for his head injury and his fractured tibia and fibula (Figure 8.4).

Plans need to be compiled for James in regards to the analgesia required and the route of entry post-operatively.

Pain assessment for James should be seen as an ongoing process that continues when he is discharged and therefore his parents need to have the resources and information to learn the approach in hospital and to continue this at home.

A pain nurse specialist should be a member of James's MDT and involved in any situation requiring more challenging interventions such as pain relief for head injury and surgical interventions.

Table 8.5 Recognition and assessment of acute pain in children

Recommendation 1	Be vigilant for any indication of pain
Recommendation 2	Children's self-report of their pain, where possible, is the preferred approach
Recommendation 3	If pain is suspected or anticipated, use a validated pain assessment tool No tool can be recommended for pain assessment in all children and across all contexts
Recommendation 4	Assess, record, and re-evaluate pain at regular intervals Be aware that language, ethnicity and cultural factors may affect the presentation of pain

Source: RCN (2009)

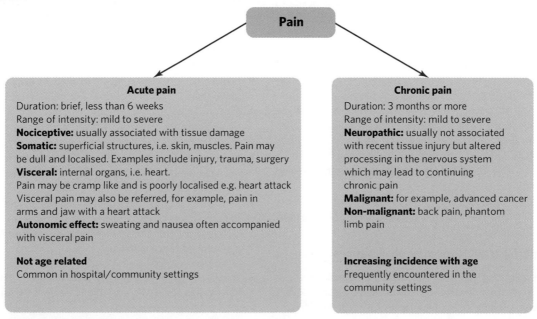

Figure 8.4 Main types of pain
Source: Seeman (2012)

ASSESSMENT TOOLS

Self-reporting tools work very well for children such as James who are over 3 years of age who can vocalise and include number scales, faces, colours and poker chips.

Behavioural tools can be used for children with and without cognitive disabilities of all age and include CHEOPS, FLACC, COMFORT and PPP.

BONES OF THE BODY

Figure 8.5 shows the major bones in the human body.

The lower legs consist of the tibia and the fibula.

Tibia (Shin Bone)

The tibia articulates with the femur (upper leg) and the talus (ankle) and measures about one-fourth to one-fifth of the length of the body. This bone carries all the body's weight. It is the main bone of the lower leg.

Fibula

Although this bone runs alongside the tibia, it carries little weight. Rather, it acts as a stabiliser. It articulates with the tibia and the talus. Its lower end is the bone that sticks out on the outside of the ankle. The fibula can be found on the outside of the lower leg (O'Rahilly et al. 2008) (Figure 8.6).

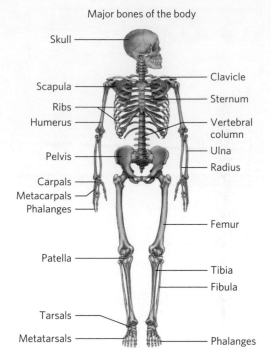

Major bones of the body

Figure 8.5 Major bones of the body

PRACTICAL GUIDELINES 8.4

Neuromuscular observations should examine the colour, warmth, sensation and movement of the limb; if any of the assessments highlight an area of concern then this needs to be recorded and monitored and, if necessary, reported to the medical team. The most extreme complication is compartment syndrome, in which the nerves in the limb can become damaged and, if not observed early, may lead to amputation of the affected limb. Neurovascular observations must be analysed in conjunction with knowledge of the injury and other observations as documented. The observations should be used in reference to one another and not as individual points of concern. Both limbs should be assessed simultaneously, although it is only required that the injured or affected limb be recorded. The observations should occur both pre- and post-operation.

Explanation appropriate to James's age and condition must be given. The family should have the need for the observations explained to them.

How to perform neurovascular observations

- Colour, warmth, swelling, ooze – visually assess James's naked foot comparing this with the uninjured foot checking for colour, swelling. Check for warmth with superficial touch.

- Pulse and capillary refill – Check James's foot for presence and magnitude of pulses distal from the injured area and venous return (capillary refill). Capillary refill should be measured by pressing on the digit for 5 seconds, then counting the seconds until the digit returns to its usual colour, normally taking less than 2 seconds.
- Pain score – pain score should be done in conjunction with movement.
- Movement when limb is restricted – because James's movements are restricted by a temporary cast, the digits should still be flexed and extended.
- Movement while child is asleep – when James is asleep, full movement of the limbs should be carried out passively and documented.
- Sensation – all touchable or visible surfaces (including between digits) should be checked for presence and type of sensation. This should preferably be done with James's eyes closed or not watching.

All these assessments should be recorded and repeated every half an hour to begin with and should be undertaken alongside the neurological observations.

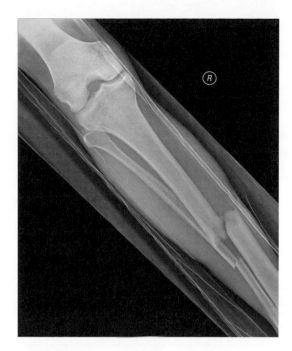

Figure 8.6 X-ray of fractured tibia and fibula

PRESSURE AREA CARE FOR CHILDREN AND YOUNG PEOPLE

Pressure area care needs to be considered when caring for children and young people such as James on a general children's ward. The prevalence of pressure ulcers may appear to be less likely to develop in younger people, sometimes only being considered for those who are seriously ill children or are less mobile due to orthopaedic conditions or injuries; however, this is not necessarily the case. Noonan et al. (2006) carried out an audit relating to the skin integrity of a group of children within a children's hospital (252 in total). While the limitation of sample size was acknowledged, one of the key findings was that the risk of developing pressure areas for children is strongly linked to where the sores may develop (see Figure 8.7). For children and young people, the places in which sores occur is the main difference from adult patients. The risk comes from interventions that are part of their treatment, such as IV infusions, nasogastric tubes, saturation monitors, as well as more 'obvious' sites such as bony prominences, sacral area and heels.

In recent years there have been assessment tools that have been specifically designed for children and young people (Waterlow, cited by Anthony et al. 2007). Willock et al. (2009) developed the Glamorgan Paediatric Pressure Ulcer Risk Assessment Scale in response to this (see Figure 8.8). The scale was developed based on the knowledge that children and young people encounter different factors that predispose them to developing pressure areas than adults. Primarily, pressure ulcers develop as a result of medical devices becoming an obstruction to the blood supply to an area of skin (such as the nasal passages following use of oxygen nasal cannula). While James has open wounds that may need dressing, if he lies in one position for too long, there is a risk that his already compromised skin could be further damaged; the assessment will ensure that areas of his skin that may cause concern will be regularly relieved of pressure.

As well as pressure area care, James also needs support for the laceration on his arm.

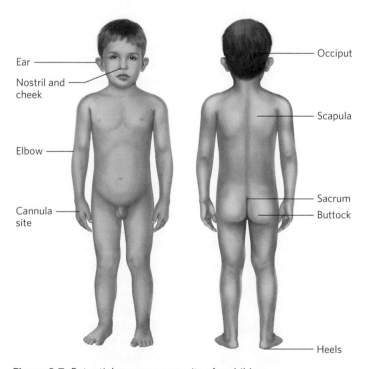

Figure 8.7 Potential pressure area sites for children

Child name		DOB	Admission date						
Risk Factor *(If data such as serum albumin or haemoglobin is not available, write NK – not known and score 0)*	Score	**Date and time of assessments** **(reassess at least daily and every time condition changes)**							
Child cannot be moved without great difficulty or deterioration in condition / under general anaesthetic >2 hours	20								
Unable to change his/her position without assistance /cannot control body movement	15								
Some mobility, but reduced for age	10								
Normal mobility for age	0								
Equipment / objects / hard surface pressing or rubbing on skin	15								
Significant anaemia (Hb <9g/dl)	1								
Persistent pyrexia (temperature > 38.0ºC for more than 4 hours)	1								
Poor peripheral perfusion (cold extremities/ capillary refill > 2 seconds / cool mottled skin)	1								
Inadequate nutrition/PYMS score >2 (discuss with dietician if in doubt)	2								
Low serum albumin (< 35g/l)	1								
Incontinence (inappropriate for age)	1								
Total score									
Action Taken (Yes or no – Ensure plan of care is implemented / reviewed for all identified areas of concern)									
Signature									

Risk score	Category	Suggested action
10+	At risk	Inspect skin at least twice a day. Relieve pressure by helping/ encouraging the child to move at least every 2 hours. Use a size and weight appropriate pressure redistribution surface for sitting on &/or sleeping on if necessary.
15+	High risk	Inspect skin with each repositioning. Reposition child / equipment/ devices at least every 2 hours. Relieve pressure before any skin discolouration develops. Use a size and weight appropriate pressure redistribution surface for sitting on &/or sleeping on.
20+	Very high risk	Inspect skin at least hourly if condition allows. Move or turn if possible, before skin becomes discoloured (refer to EUPAP grade 1). Ensure equipment / objects are not pressing on the skin. Consider using specialised pressure relieving equipment. Refer to local guidelines/protocol if available, if not contact / refer to TVN.

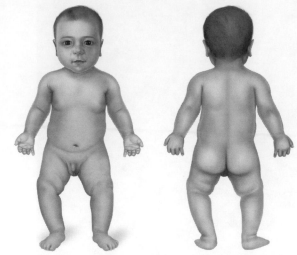

Using numbers, indicate on the diagram above any discoloured areas or pressure ulcers, then using the box below describe the lesion, the date it was first observed and the outcome (resolved or not resolved) on resolution, completion of this form, transfer or discharge (whichever comes first).

Lesion number	Date lesion first observed	Brief description of lesion (also document in child's nursing record)	Outcome (resolved/not resolved)	Date of reassessment

Figure 8.8 Glamorgan Paediatric Pressure Ulcer Risk Assessment Scale
Source: Willock et al. (2009)

TYPES OF WOUND

- **Lacerations:** injury where skin and sometimes muscle tissue is cut or torn, these can be superficial or deep.
- **Abrasions:** injury where the top layer of tissue is removed, as seen with first-degree burns: when skin loss is extensive there is an increased risk of infection.
- **Contusions:** injuries resulting from a forceful blow to the skin and soft tissue, however, leaving the outer layer of skin intact.
- **Avulsions:** injuries where a section of tissue is torn off, either partially or in total. A total avulsion means that the tissue is completely torn from the body with no point of attachment.

Source: adapted from Zinn.

As James has a deep laceration, this will also be sutured when he is in theatre.

Preoperative Assessment

Once the medical team is satisfied that James is physically fit for surgery including having a stable LOC, then safe preoperative care is required to minimise, eliminate or accommodate any risks of surgery or anaesthesia to James and to reduce the risk of perioperative illness or death. Appropriate nursing practice includes a preoperative check list which is required to collate information about James including allergies and medical history and whether he has a history of any reactions to surgical interventions. Preoperative assessment is more than deciding the medical fitness of James; it is also assessing his physical, psychological and social circumstances. Part of the process is to check when he last ate or drank, to inform him and his family about the procedure, and to gain informed consent.

The preoperative checklist for James should include:

- consent form signed by a parent
- knowledge of any allergies
- James's weight in kg
- most recent observations
- site marked for surgery
- care pathway specific for orthopaedic surgery
- NBM (safe fasting time for James)
- checking James's notes and documentation
- checking James's X-rays and any other relevant information
- whether James had a pre-med
- whether James has a correct ID band
- whether James has had all jewellery removed
- whether James has been checked for loose teeth
- safe transfer to theatre
- detailed handover of James.

Consent

Consent is the agreement by a patient or parent/guardian that an intervention or treatment may be undertaken.

There are three types of consent:

- **Oral consent:** when requested the patient voices their consent to treatment: 'Yes, you may undertake my observations.' Or the patient requests care: 'Could I have help with my skin care?'
- **Implied consent:** when the patient cooperates with an intervention: the nurse offers a nebuliser to the patient and he places it over his own nose and mouth.
- **Written consent:** an approved written form details the intervention as discussed between patient and doctor and signed: the surgeon explains to James and his parents the surgical procedure and both parties sign the consent for orthopaedic surgery form.

Gaining consent for a surgical intervention is a legal requirement and should be child-centred to ensure that James and his family understand the procedure and if there are any available alternatives: alongside this the postoperative care is explained and the risk of complications. The consent form would be signed for James by his parents as he is under the age of 16 and the surgeon also signs. There could be a number of issues for James. If he needed to go to theatre before his parents arrived at the hospital, the surgeon would need to assess the urgency of the intervention; if it was felt that James was in mortal danger then his health would override the need for consent:

A life-threatening emergency may arise when consultation with either a person with parental responsibility or the court is impossible, or the person with parental responsibility refuses consent despite such emergency treatment appearing to be in the best interests of the child. In such cases the courts have stated that doubt should be resolved in favour of the preservation of life, and it will be acceptable to undertake treatment to preserve life or prevent serious damage to health. (DoH 2009, page 39)

James is 14 years old and for some interventions he could be said to be competent, in that he is able to consent to treatment or interventions himself, however, this is not always consistent and James needs to feel supported in the process. Gillick competence is an approach used to assess decision making in young people where they have had the opportunity due to their experiences to gather knowledge, information and have the ability to reflect on the different interventions that are being offered; this is often acknowledged for young people who have a long-term health condition (Hayhoe 2008). Clinical policies on consent should also include what to do when there is disagreement between a competent young person and their parent. However, there is a requirement to ensure that **situation dependency** is taken into consideration. While the young person may be competent to make a decision about some elements of his treatment, each situation needs to be treated on an individual basis so that the young person is still supported and informed at the appropriate level.

ACTIVITY 8.4

List the interventions that you would encourage James to take control over.

List the interventions that you think should be professional or parent led.

RESEARCH NOTE 8.3 Preoperative fasting in adults and children (RCN 2005)

This systematic review explored the studies to investigate how long patients should be nil by mouth before and after general anaesthesia and what food and fluids can and should not be permitted. While the review explores both adult and children, this research note will focus on outcomes for children under 18 years of age. Some additional clinical questions relevant to the development of the guideline were also included. It is seen from the recommendations that water and other clear fluids may be taken up to 2 hours before induction for elective surgery in healthy infants and children and enhances the child's well-being. The amount of oral fluids does not appear to have an impact on gastric volume. Therefore, children may have unlimited amounts of water and other clear fluid up to 2 hours before induction of anaesthesia. Clear drinks can be offered to healthy infants and children when they are fully awake, but may need to be withheld if there are any other medical issues.

Safe Transfer to Theatre

Once the checklist is complete, James needs to be safely transferred to theatre. Younger children are often transported to theatre in toy cars or an adapted trolley or are able to walk to reduce the level of anxiety. However, as James is older and immobilised he will be transported on his bed to reduce the amount of movement to his leg. A children's nurse is required to escort James to theatre so that a safe transfer into the anaesthetic room can occur. This involves not only going through the checklist with the theatre staff but also ensures that James has a clear explanation of the operation. James may also wish for one of his parents to accompany him.

Anaesthetic Room

In the past parents were refused permission to enter the anaesthetic room with their child. On the whole, most parents wish to be with their children and the child is more settled because of their presence. The experience for children going to theatre is stressful for both the child and parent. If all the professionals involved work as a team then that stress is kept to a minimum. While parental presence can be seen as a challenge from some anaesthetists, the AAGBI (2010, page 21) confirm that: 'Parents should be invited to accompany the child at induction of anaesthesia and his/her role in the induction room discussed.' For James, this could be beneficial as he may be frightened and still a little confused due to his head injury. The children's nurse should stay with James and his parent so that they can take the parent back to the ward and offer support and information.

Theatre

James is going for a closed manipulation of his simple displaced fracture and this is the typical approach for reducing common fractures. The reduction for James as with most children is carried out under general anaesthesia, but local anaesthesia may sometimes be used. The surgeon holds the bone fragments through the skin, adjusting the fragments to achieve as natural a position as possible. The limb is then encased in plaster of Paris (PoP) to hold the leg in alignment until the bone heals. The laceration will also be sutured, as the cut was very deep and the muscle will need to be sutured as well as the adipose and skin.

Recovery Room

Once the surgery is complete James is taken to the recovery room to wake up. The AAGBI (2010) recommends that as soon as the child is awake the parents should called; James's parents could then stay with him until he is fit to return to the ward. When the children's nurse comes to collect James she needs to check that James's condition postoperatively is stable and that he is breathing unaided without any effort before returning to the ward. The circulation to the toes also needs to be assessed for colour, warmth and sensation. The nursing staff in recovery should give a detailed handover, including the outcome of the surgery and the medication prescribed for James. The postoperative care prescribed by the surgeon may also be highlighted in James's medical notes. This should include pain management, care of the fractured limb and care of the sutured laceration.

Postoperative Care

Once James returns to the ward it is important to resume the neuromuscular observations every hour for a least 24 hours after the operation and offer pain relief following assessment of pain. When James is sufficiently awake he can be offered clear fluids and if he does not feel nauseous within a couple of hours he can have something to eat. Care should be taken to ensure that any changes in LOC are also monitored, as James is still recovering from the head injury and arm laceration.

Postoperative observations may include:

- blood pressure: normal range < 101–149 mmhg systolic
- pulse (rate, rhythm and amplitude): 51–100 bpm
- respiration rate (rate, depth, effort, pattern): 9–14 rpm
- peripheral oxygen saturation: > 95%
- temperature: 36.1–37.9°C
- neurological observations: score 12–15
- neuromuscular observations: limb warm and pink with good movement of toes and good sensation.

Source: adapted from Royal Marsden Hospital (2011)

Procedure for Wound Care

James will need to have his sutured laceration monitored and, when necessary, the dressing will need to be changed and finally the sutures removed.

Aseptic Technique

1. Wounds must not be touched with dirty hands and aseptic procedure used.
2. Explain to James what is going to happen.
3. Wash and dry hands.
4. Lay up a trolley with a sterile wound dressing pack.
5. The pack should have:

   - gallipots or an indented plastic tray
   - low-linting swabs and/or medical foam
   - disposable forceps
   - gloves
   - sterile field
   - disposable bag
   - fluids for cleaning and/or irrigation
   - hypoallergenic tape
   - appropriate dressing.

6. Remove old dressing and inspect the wound.
7. If wound clean and dry, then just replace the dressing.
8. If wound seems inflamed or has any leaking fluid, the wound needs cleaning.
9. Wash hands thoroughly, dry hands and wear sterile gloves.
10. Clean the wound with gauze using 0.9% sodium chloride.
11. Wipe the wound site as dry as possible.
12. Cover the wound if indicated.
13. Discard all dirty dressings in a clinical waste bag.
14. Wash and dry hands.

Removal of sutures is usually performed between 7 and 10 days post-insertion, but this depends on where the wound is and whether it has healed. Following the same routine as above, once the wound is exposed, good practice is to remove every other suture or staple, with the rest removed if the incision remains securely closed. If any sign of suture line separation is evident during the removal process, the remaining sutures are left in place and reported to the medical team.

Mobilisation

Once James is fully awake and has been given pain relief it is important to encourage him to mobilise. The children's nurse needs to work with the physiotherapist to support James to learn to use crutches and be able to walk up and down stairs. Early weight-bearing exercises with a broken leg may shorten the time spent in the hospital as well, resulting in a faster recovery period and cost-saving healthcare; however, each orthopaedic surgeon has his own regime and it is the nurse's role to work with the interprofessional team to use evidence-based practice to support James in his recovery.

PRACTICAL GUIDELINES 8.5

Now that James's leg is in plaster, he needs to keep his leg raised on a pillow for the first 12 hours and rest. This will help any swelling to go down. He needs to continue to do this for another 12 hours if the cast still feels tight. James must not get the plaster cast wet. This will weaken it and the bone will no longer be properly supported. James can use a plastic bag to cover up the cast when he has a bath or shower. James needs to be informed not to poke anything underneath it. This could cause a nasty sore.

More Plaster Cast Tips

- Don't let any small objects fall inside the cast, as they could irritate.
- Don't try to alter the length or position of the cast.
- Don't lift anything heavy until the cast has been removed.
- Use crutches as advised by the health professional.

Plaster Cast Problems

James should go to A&E (accident and emergency) if:

- The plaster cast still feels too tight after keeping it elevated for 24 hours.
- The toes on the affected limb feel swollen, tingly, painful (even after taking painkillers) or become numb.
- The toes turn blue or white.
- The cast feels too loose.
- The cast is broken or cracked.
- The skin underneath or around the edge of your cast feels sore.
- There is an unpleasant smell or discharge coming from the cast (adapted from NHS Choices, available at: **http://www .nhs.uk/chq/Pages/2543.aspx?CategoryID=72&SubCate goryID=721.**)

THE BONE-HEALING PROCESS

Many individuals in the UK break bones with millions of fractures occurring every year. Fractures happen in all age groups, but the young, especially boys, and old are the most susceptible. Teenagers have more risk of fracture due to their increasing level of activity and bone growth due to puberty (**physioroom.com**).

Immediate Healing Following the Fracture

For the first 5 days the area around the fracture, which has a rich blood supply, becomes swollen and bruised: this leads to inflammation around the fracture fragments forming a haematoma (see Figure 8.9).

Once the haematoma is formed cells called osteoclasts work to remove the dead bone cells. This clot or haematoma is the first bridge between the bone fragments, within the clot cells called fibroblasts, join together to begin the granulation process between 4 and 10 days after the fracture occurs. This leads to the development of a soft callus (see Figure 8.10).

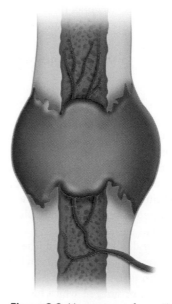

Figure 8.9 Haematoma formation

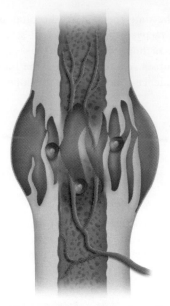

Figure 8.10 Soft callus formation

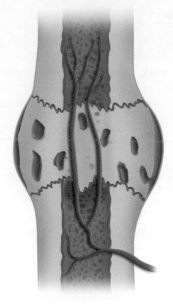

Figure 8.11 Hard callus formation

Four Days to Three Weeks Following Fracture

In the granulation tissue, cartilage and fibrocartilage begin to form. This is a spongy material that lies between the two fracture fragments, although it is weak to external stresses for at least 6 weeks. Therefore, there should not be very much movement of the fracture fragments. Following James's discharge he will attend a fracture clinic where the orthopaedic team will ensure there is not too much movement at the fracture site by doing repeat X-rays and making sure that the broken bone remains immobilised with the plaster cast.

After 2 or 3 weeks, while still fragile, the soft callus becomes stable enough at the fracture site for new blood vessels to begin forming and for osteoblasts (bone-building cells) to begin laying down what is called 'woven bone'. This is the first permanent bone contact between the two fracture fragments.

From 3 Weeks to 12 Weeks Following the Fracture

From 3 weeks the process begins with the cartilage of the soft callus turning into woven bone. This usually goes on for 6 and 12 weeks; this is affected by the area on the skeleton and the type of fracture it is (6 weeks for the upper body and 12 weeks for the lower body and legs). It is a more complicated process to form the hard callus and it is supported by the release of minerals including calcium and phosphate into the cartilage; this turns into a bridge of hard callus over the fracture (see Figure 8.11).

Fracture union is said to have occurred when the hard callus has formed at the former fracture site and can be seen on X-ray. When an X-ray confirms the hard callus is present, then gentle weight bearing can be encouraged, which helps the bone to lay down more bone tissue.

Bone Remodelling

The body will typically lay down more hard callus than is needed to repair the fracture, and the site looks enlarged when viewed on X-ray. Bone remodelling begins once the fracture has knitted and may progress for several years (see Figure 8.12).

Over time, the bone is returned to a more typical shape. The osteoblasts and osteoclasts grow and model the bone and this can be affected by exercise, and the more weight bearing exercises the better. When the fracture healing process is finished, typically the bone will be as strong as it was originally.

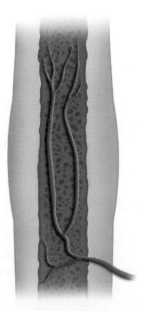

Figure 8.12 Bone remodelling

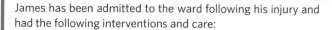

CASE STUDY REVIEW 8.1

James has been admitted to the ward following his injury and had the following interventions and care:

- James has had regular pain assessment and relief using an age-appropriate tool.
- Management of his head injury has been undertaken.

- James had surgery to realign the fracture.
- The laceration has been sutured.
- Monitoring of skin integrity and pressure areas occurred at regular intervals.
- All these interventions will be evaluated and any changes reported to the interprofessional team.

SUMMARY OF KEY LEARNING

This chapter has identified, through the care of James, just a few of the aspects of caring for children on a surgical ward including neurological and neuromuscular observations and preparation for theatre. Pressure area care was explored along with pain and wound management. It is important to assess, plan, implement and evaluate care for James in collaboration with family and other professionals. It is also important to offer information and advice on discharge so that James and his parents can care for his plaster at home. James will be in the plaster cast for 8 weeks and will need to attend the OPD to have the progress of healing assessed. Once the hard callus has been formed, James will be encouraged to weight bear, then following X-ray confirmation that the bone is healed, the plaster will be removed.

FURTHER RESOURCES

HES is the national statistical data warehouse for England of the care provided by NHS hospitals and for NHS hospital patients treated elsewhere. HES is the data source for a wide range of healthcare analysis for the NHS, government and many other organisations and individuals: **http://www.Hesonline.Nhs.Uk/**

Ease/Servlet/Contentserver?Siteid=1937
IASP definition of pain: **http://www.Iasp-Pain.Org/Terms-P.Html**
American Pain Society definition of addiction: **http://Www.Ampainsoc.Org/Advocacy/Opioids2.Htm**
Pain guidelines: **www.Rcn.Org.Uk/Childrenspainguideline**
Aseptic technique images: **http://www.cetl.org.uk/learning/print/aseptic-dressing-print.pdf**

ANSWERS TO ACTIVITIES

ACTIVITY 8.1

Children and young people have accidents, for example, due to:

- their sex
- their age
- social and geographical factors
- environmental factors
- stages of development
- attitude
- behaviour aggressiveness and over–activity
- sight and sound
- handicap
- medical conditions.

ACTIVITY 8.2

Factors that influence experience for children and young people include:

- age
- gender
- understanding/cognition
- previous experience
- culture/belief
- psychological state
- environment
- parental influence.

ACTIVITY 8.3

Words you might use to describe the experience of pain include:

- sharp
- stabbing

- dull
- aching
- nagging
- pricking
- burning.

ACTIVITY 8.4

Interventions that you would encourage James to take control over include:

- when to have pain relief
- when to have hygiene care
- what to eat and drink
- where and when to mobilise
- who visits
- timing of observations.

Interventions that you think should be professional or parent led include:

- having prescribed medication
- having physical therapy
- having to mobilise
- requirement of observations.

SELECTED REFERENCES

AAGBI (2010) *Safety guideline: Pre-operative assessment and patient preparation: the role of the anaesthetist.* Association of Anaesthetists of Great Britain and Ireland: London.

Anthony, D., Parboteeah, S., Saleh, M. and Papanikolaou, P. (2008) Norton, Waterlow and Braden scores: a review of the literature and a comparison between the scores and clinical judgement. *J Clinical Nursing,* 17(5), 646–653.

Deacon, Perkins and Bellis (2011) Study on Road Traffic Collisions and Casualties in the North West of England.

Department of Health (DoH) (2009) Reference guide to consent for examination or treatment, 2nd edn. DoH: London.

Gillham, B. and Thomson, J.A. (eds) (1996) *Child safety: problem and prevention from preschool to adolescence.* Routledge: London.

Hayhoe, B. (2005) Clinical practice guidelines, perioperative fasting in adults and children. An RCN guideline for the multidisciplinary team.

National Institute for Clinical Excellence (NICE) (2007) Head injury: triage, assessment, investigation and early management of head injury in infants, children and adults: **http://guidance.nice.org.uk/cg4**

Noonan, C., Quigley, S. and Curley, M. (2006) Skin integrity in hospitalized infants and children: a prevalence survey. *Journal of Pediatric Nursing,* 21(6), 445–53.

ONS Mortality Division and the General Register Office for Scotland and Great Britain (2009) *Number of under 16 accidental deaths.*

O'Rahilly, R., Müller, F., Carpenter, S. and Swenson, R. (2008) *Basic human anatomy, a regional study of human structure.*

Royal College of Nursing (RCN) (2009) The recognition and assessment of acute pain in children: **www.rcn.org.uk/childrenspainguideline**

Royal Marsden Hospital (2011) *Manual of clinical nursing procedures,* 8th edn.

Seeman, C. (2012) *Lecture notes,* Anglia Ruskin University.

Willock, J., Baharestani, M. and Anthony, D. (2009) The development of the Glamorgan paediatric pressure ulcer risk assessment scale. *Journal of Wound Care,* 18, 17–21.

CHAPTER 9
Neonatal Nursing Care

Jacki Dopran (Oughton) and Sue Collier

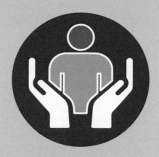

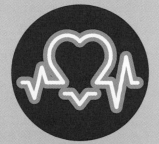

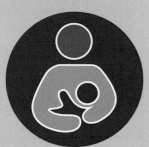

LEARNING OUTCOMES

On completion of this chapter, the reader will be able to:

- Critically explore the political drivers and professional values that impact on the ethos of neonatal nursing.
- Critically explore the environmental, developmental, social and cultural factors relating to the delivery of holistic and family-centred care to the infant and their family when special and/or transitional care is required.
- Critically reflect on nursing and medical interventions required for the appropriate management of the infant needing special and/or transitional care.
- Critically explore the delivery of evidence-based holistic care to the neonate and family when special and/or transitional care is needed.

TALKING POINT

'In England, there are approximately 54,000 preterm births every year – approximately 8.3% of the total number of live births.'

European Foundation for the Care of Newborn Infants (2009)

'Survival for births of 24 and 25 weeks has risen significantly between 1995 and 2006 ... Babies born at 26 weeks of gestation have higher survival still.'

EPIcure (2008)

'93% of preterm births occur after 28 weeks of gestation, but 6% occur between 22 and 27 weeks, and just under 1% occur before 22 weeks.'

Tommy's online

INTRODUCTION

The neonatal unit is a very different environment from any other unit or ward and the new parents may not have been expecting their new baby to be born early or to require neonatal services. Parents and their families can be experiencing a range of emotions and are possibly just trying to cope with this new and unexpected event. During the past two decades, neonatal care has changed dramatically, which has led to new developments in technology, improved understanding through research and changes to the organisation of neonatal care nationally. This adds further mystification to the care of the preterm baby and potentially adds to the stresses the parents are already experiencing.

There are three main points of focus for parents: dealing with the stressors of seeing their baby lying among all the technology sustaining life; feelings of loss and grief about the curtailment of the pregnancy and their baby's position and learning to trust the healthcare professionals to facilitate the building of a therapeutic relationship. Family-centred care seeks to involve a partnership with the whole family unit to enable them to understand the needs of their baby, the care and management of their baby and the rationale for care interventions and strategies.

The purpose of this chapter is to explore key themes of care in relation to a baby who is born before the expected date of delivery. To this end, the chapter uses Jacob as a focus. This chapter will seek to explore key themes related to neonatal nursing and explores what is the practice of neonatal nursing.

CASE STUDY 9.1

Jacob, the first child of Ellie-Mae and Lloyd, was born unexpectedly at 33 weeks' gestation. Jacob was successfully resuscitated and initially required some support to breathe via a nasal CPAP system. Jacob is being nursed in an incubator and is receiving some ambient oxygen. Jacob is receiving nutrition via a nasogastric feeding tube and has early signs of physiological jaundice.

Janice and Karen are experienced nurses who have worked on the neonatal unit for several years and are both respected members of the neonatal team. Ellie-Mae and Lloyd are happy that their son is 'doing well' but have nothing prepared for his arrival. Ellie-Mae was meant to finish work at 34 weeks of pregnancy and had planned to go 'baby shopping' at that point. Jacob is currently in a stable condition and is feeding well. The mum is finding travelling 30 miles each day to the hospital challenging. A discharge planning meeting has taken place and it has been decided that Jacob could be discharged.

PROFESSIONAL VALUES AND COLLABORATIVE WORKING

Neonatal Networks

A network is the term used in healthcare when services that deliver the same speciality work together in a collaborative way and across traditional healthcare boundaries to deliver care and improve outcomes for patients (see Figure 9.1). National Service Frameworks for children (NSF) define networks as:

> Linked groups of professionals and organisations from primary, secondary and tertiary care, working in a co-ordinated manner, unconstructed by existing and professional [organisational] boundaries, to ensure equitable provision of high-quality, clinically effective services. (Department of Health 2004)

There is a variety of types of network in England, including pathology, cancer, cardiac, burns, children's and neonatal specialities. A fully functional network predominantly provides benefits for the patient, their families and the professionals, by utilising skills, services, knowledge and experience. Neonatal or perinatal networks were put in place across England from 2002 onwards following an in-depth review of neonatal care (Department of Health 2003).

During the late 1990s the number of babies being born preterm or sick was rising in the United Kingdom (UK) (Department of Health 2003). The number of cots and services that were able to support these babies did not match the demand.

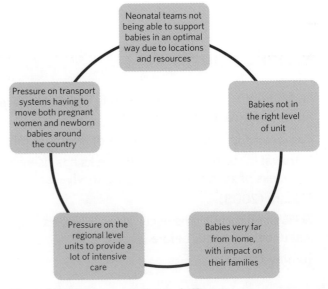

Figure 9.1 Why are networks needed?

It was clear from the work that was done looking at the movements of women and babies around the country that there was no clear system or pathway for the neonatal care group and this meant that many transfers of babies were taking place that could have been avoided if there were better systems in place. In order to create workable systems for neonatal care, network formation began. Working in networks holds many benefits. The Royal College of Paediatrics and Child Health (RCPCH 2012) has recently published a guide on how to implement clinical networks, which details the benefits and possible pitfalls of networking, but the key message is that networks are sustainable and positive systems for neonatal care.

How Neonatal Care Works

Neonatal care has traditionally been split into categories or 'levels' of care. These levels apply to the type of care and the type of neonatal unit that provides care. This approach to neonatal care has been defined and led by the British Association of Perinatal Medicine (BAPM) (RCPCH 2012) (see Table 9.1). This association sets the standards and recommendations for neonatal care in the UK and is a key association for driving forward safe high-quality medical and nursing care for all neonatal patients and their families (see Table 9.2).

Before the networks were established there were some pathways for hospitals to contact one another when they needed a neonatal cot or management support for a sick baby, which their unit did not have the resources, experience or staff provision to support. Some Level 3 services had been working with a regional focus for many years.

Staffing

BAPM (2001) set standards for the numbers and type of staff who should work in neonatal units. Nursing staff are referred to as being qualified in speciality (QIS) when they have undertaken a period of postgraduate study in neonatal care: this can be study at diploma or degree level. QIS nurses should be looking after the babies that are at care Levels 1 and 2, ITU and HD care. Therefore it is recommended that all nursing teams should have 70 per cent of the team who are QIS. In the UK, another very important problem for neonatal services is that there are insufficient nurses who are QIS across the country to look after all the babies who are being born preterm or sick (Ashworth and Evans 2003; Milligan et al. 2008).

Table 9.1 Care levels

Type of care	Level of care
Intensive care or ITU	Level 1
High dependency or HD	Level 2
Special care or SC	Level 3

Source: BAPM (2001)

PRACTICAL GUIDELINES 9.1

BAPM set out ratios of nurse staffing to babies (RCPCH 2012):

- ITU baby = 1:1 nursing care
- HD baby = 1:2 nursing care
- SC baby = 1:4 nursing care

- shift leader does not have babies allocated to her for direct care.

Table 9.2 Types of neonatal unit

Level of unit	What the unit can provide	DoH toolkit terminology for the unit
Level 3 NICU Regional unit: will take babies from other services	All types of ITU, HD and SC care, long term or short term, complex medical and in some units surgical care	Neonatal intensive care units (NICUs)
Level 2 NICU Local unit: supports babies whose mothers have booked to have their baby in the hospital where the unit is	All types of care, but only short-term ITU care	Local neonatal units (LNUs)
Level 1 Special care baby unit (SCBU)	Mainly HD and SC, with stabilisation of ITU care for transfer to a Level 1 or 2 unit	Special care units (SCUs)

Source: BAPM (2001)

Medical staffing also has clear standards recommended by BAPM including dedicated consultant cover for Level 3 neonatal units and a rota of doctors to support the work that is needed (BAPM 2001). At times there are also difficulties with covering medical rotas, due to shortages of specially trained neonatal doctors. Before the neonatal networks were formed the described structures were in place in some services, but the correct ratios of staffing have never been achieved across the country. This means that neonatal care is under significant pressure. Much work has been undertaken to highlight this situation and new ways of working have been designed to try and support proactive and effective workforce development and expansion (Ashworth and Evans 2003; Milligan et al. 2008).

Parents and Families Using Neonatal Services

The importance of parents and families being at the centre of the care of their baby is well researched. Within neonatal care a philosophy of care always includes parents and the wider family unit. Some of the issues in preterm and sick baby care are different to those in the general care of the child, predominantly because this new person has not had time to be imbedded into the family dynamics and their birth can herald a time of profound anxiety, stress and disruption for the family unit. Neonatal teams have a key and vital role in ensuring support is given to parents to bond and get to know their baby amid the high technology workings of an intensive care environment and the trauma of being separated from the 'normal' pathway of celebratory status of the birth.

VOICES 9.1 Collective parent voice

Throughout the formation of neonatal networks, parents have played a key role in advising, guiding and sharing their experiences. National organisations that support the families of preterm and sick babies have contributed widely to this work and in lobbying with a political approach to apply pressure for further central investment to drive up the standards and quality of care. This has given a voice to parents who are experiencing neonatal care (Bliss; Tommy's online).

A website that deals specifically with neonatal networks has been set up on which there is detailed information about pathways and function of the network, along with individual service information. The site has both parent and professional pages and was set up by the network leads in 2005. Within the parents' pages there are links to organisations and charities that can support parents through their journey in neonatal care (**http://www.neonatal.org.uk/ parents_pages**).

Forming the Networks

Following a national collection of information and data about activity levels and transfers, neonatal networks were defined and began to be formed. The key principle for networks is:

Each network ensures that every infant has access to the right level of care, with the right resources and that they are cared for by staff with the right skills (Gupta et al. 2006, page 1).

There are currently 24 neonatal networks in England. The networks cover defined geographical areas, taking into account the population of these areas and the number of births in each area. Within each network, there is a group of units working together. A typical small neonatal network structure is as shown in Figure 9.2.

The number of units that make up a network will vary depending on the number of births that are taking place in the geographical area. Some units may have two or three Level 3 units. Some of the Level 3 units will provide surgical care for neonates. Sometimes there will not be a surgical Level 3 in a

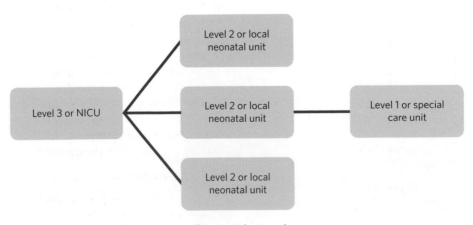

Figure 9.2 Structure of a typical small neonatal network

North Central London
North East London
North West London
South East London
South West London

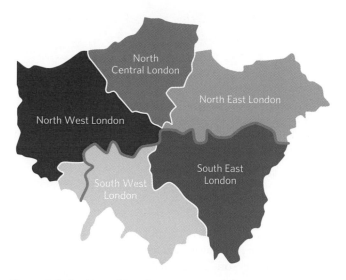

Figure 9.3 Position of North East London network

network and in this configuration a special pathway across networks will be agreed to support this management and care.

In London, there are currently five neonatal networks. The North East London network has the highest number of births (see Figure 9.3).

The hospitals in the North East London network that support the delivery of neonatal care are made up of nine units – this is a large network (see Figure 9.4).

At the time the networks were formed pathways of care were then set up and each of the units in the network will follow these. The aim of the pathways is for 95 per cent of the activity in the network to remain within the network units. Some babies will need to go to a specialised hospital for very specific management and as not all networks can provide this, there will be some activity that goes out of the networks.

Pathway of Care

This is a basic network pathway for one baby. Pathways can be basic or more complex with some babies moving to several hospitals for their neonatal care (see Figure 9.5).

x2 Level 3 or NICUs x1 providing surgery
Level 2 or local neonatal unit
Level 2 or local neonatal unit
Level 1 or special care unit
Level 2 or local neonatal unit
Level 2 or local neonatal unit
Level 2 or local neonatal unit
Level 2 or local neonatal unit

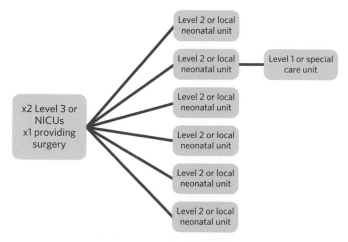

Figure 9.4 Structure of the North East London network

Baby Peter is born in a level 2 unit, his home unit; he needs ITU care that will be long term
The level 2 unit talk with their network level 3 units and there is a cot for Baby Peter at the level 3 unit
Baby Peter is transferred with his mother to the network level 3 unit where he has ITU care
Baby Peter has done well and is now at HD care level; his mother is at home and comes to visit him in the level 3 unit every day, but has to travel some way to do this.
Baby Peter is now ready to go back or be repatriated with his home unit
Baby Peter returns to his 'home' unit for his HD and SC. His parents can visit him more easily and play a bigger part in his care
Baby Peter is now ready to go home
Baby Peter is transferred home and the neonatal community nurses from his home unit visit him at home to support the family with his ongoing care needs

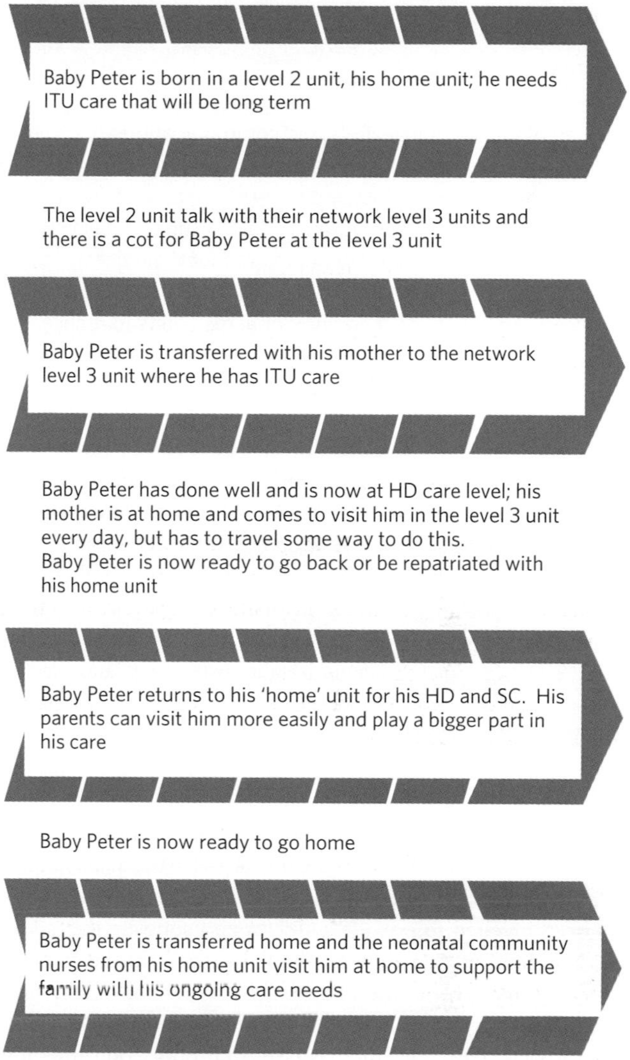

Figure 9.5 A basic pathway of care

Functions of Networks

As networks have developed, the work that is undertaken in them has expanded to include professionals working together in a positive and productive way to produce many benefits. The network generally has a management team to lead and coordinate the functions. There will also be a lead clinician, lead nurse and sometimes educators; these professionals will often also work in units that are within the network, therefore allowing them to be able to have a good operational comprehension of what is actually happening in the units. This supports work being undertaken in subgroups that allow many developments to take place: often other members of the multidisciplinary team will join the subgroups to widen the expertise in the work that is being done. Examples of network working are shown in Table 9.3.

Transferring Babies

Transfer of neonates requires a specific skill set and knowledge as well as a dedicated approach. In the UK, there are many neonatal transport teams. These teams have been set up over the past

Table 9.3 Examples of network working

- Clinical guidelines and policies
- Agree pathways and designated care delivery
- Parent information leaflets and communication
- Expanding and sharing of good practice
- Sharing of risk incidents and governance approaches to allow wider learning and development
- Clinical placements for nursing staff to support development
- Setting up of dedicated neonatal transport services
- Production of parent information to allow seamless care across the network
- Procurement of some equipment across units to reduce cost and standardisation of equipment used
- Looking at activity data to see the reality and effectiveness of pathways

10 years to make sure the right care can be delivered when moving infants. The transfer teams often work across network boundaries; the geographical areas that they cover will vary and are driven by distances. For example, in the London networks, the distances are short but there is a high density of activity. In more rural settings, for example Yorkshire, the transfer distance and placement of units is much wider and therefore greater time is spent in travel between units. The transport teams undertake emergency and elective work. The elective work is focused around returning or repatriation of babies to their home units (Fenton and Leslie 2011).

Activity Data

These are good-quality data that show the overall picture of movements of babies and the care that is given: the quality of that care is paramount. During the network developments much time has been invested to provide a system and software that allows this high level of data collection. The data inform the commissioner's teams, which fund and ensure governance of networks; these teams are known as specialist commissioners. The neonatal approach across England has been to produce outcomes and quality indicators from extensive data collection. Project groups and data assessment units specific to neonatal care have been set up to support this work. Every unit will have a team that focuses on a daily basis on ensuring all data and information regarding the baby are entered into the data system (National Neonatal Audit Program (NNAP) Neonatal Data Analysis Unit).

Progression of Neonatal Care and Standards

In 2008 the Department of Health (DoH) commissioned work to be undertaken looking at how standards and recommendations were being achieved in neonatal care, as it was clear that the networks had considerably improved the care delivery, but there were still problems in regard to resources, staffing, workforce development and support of families through the neonatal pathways (House of Commons Select Committee 2008). This work was informed by a report from the National Audit Office (2007) and this report initiated a House of Commons Select Committee report, which drew conclusions and made recommendations of how to move forward with improving neonatal care (NNAP).

The House of Commons Select Committee reached the following key conclusions and recommendations:

- demand for neonatal services and the impact of health inequality on prematurity and neonatal mortality
- progress in networking neonatal services and its impact on capacity
- recruiting, retaining and training the staff required to deliver an effective service
- improving the understanding of costs and the financial management of neonatal services (House of Commons Select Committee 2008).

From these recommendations, working groups were set up with lead professionals from across England working together. The key areas of service delivery were redefined and expanded; the importance of support for families was included as paramount in this work. The aim of the toolkit work is to create more equity, better compliance with standards and therefore increase the quality of care and outcomes. The toolkit has key principles for care with indicators for compliance that units have to demonstrate they are meeting or working towards. The funding of neonatal care is then linked to this compliance (Department of Health 2009). The National Institute for Clinical Excellence (2010) has taken the principles of the toolkit and embedded them into a 'quality standards' document that further supports the quality of care and parity across the country. BAPM was very involved with this work and, following the toolkit publication, it reviewed and redefined its categories of care during 2011.

Networks in 2012

With the reforms in healthcare and changes in organisation and commissioning of the NHS, changes to neonatal networks are pending at the time of writing. The professionals within the neonatal networks are working hard to ensure the work invested in the past 10 years is maintained and further enhanced. The clinical pathways that have developed are robust, improving patient outcomes and the positive benefits are clear (Gale et al. 2011).

Care Bundles

Care bundles are a tool that can be used in healthcare to support improvements in outcomes. Originally designed by intensive care teams, the aim of a care bundle is to produce a set of interventions that are research based, and best practice that, when implemented, will support the progress of care and positive outcome. In order for a care bundle to be effective, the interventions must be carefully followed, point by point, with a recordable approach that allows a demonstration that the full process of care has been completed.

Care Bundles in Neonatal Care

During the past few years there has been increasing interest in the use of a care bundle approach in neonatal care. Key aspects of care or conditions that have been found to be productive to risk events and patient harm have driven forward the use of this approach. The National Patient Safety Agency (NPSA), which deals specifically with patient safety, has featured neonatal care bundles in its national alerting system and in a series of 'signals' (NPSA n.d.), which provide a sharing approach of work that is being undertaken in different services in England. The formation of neonatal or perinatal networks has provided an excellent arena for care bundle approaches and an open culture of shared learning across organisations and traditional boundaries (see Practical Guidelines 9.2).

Neonatal Practice

Patient safety in neonatal care is a high priority for all neonatal units (Department of Health 2010). The vulnerable patient group presents challenges that are unique to the care environment. Key areas in which care bundles have been utilised are:

- avoidance of intravenous extravasations
- infection control
- drug administration

- specific neonatal disease: necrotising enterocolitis (NEC)
- extravasation of neonates.

Drug Administration

Through national reporting and learning systems that have been set up by the NPSA, it was identified that there were frequent and repeated reports of drug incidents with dosing and administration of the antibiotic gentamicin.

Gentamicin is a broad-spectrum antibiotic that requires very specific administration and dosing criteria according to the gestational age of the baby in order to avoid harmful toxicity levels building up. During courses of the antibiotic, blood levels are monitored after set doses have been given; the results of the levels of the drug in the blood will then allow the correct dose to be given.

The NPSA issued an alert, via their own national alert system, that advised all neonatal and paediatric services of a care bundle approach to support safety in administration of the drug (see Figure 9.6). NPSA monitoring systems follow the alert release to ensure that hospitals are compliant to the alerts and warnings that the systems have highlighted.

Network Approaches

Using the existing structure of a neonatal network has become an effective way to support neonatal care across a region. A demonstration of this innovative approach can been seen where a regional approach to the gentamicin care bundle was taken. These include avoidance of overinfusion of intravenous fluids and intravenous cannula care.

PRACTICAL GUIDELINES 9.2

While working at Luton and Dunstable Hospital, Oughton (2010) developed a neonatal care bundle for intravenous cannula care, a high-impact intervention that aims to reduce the incidence of peripheral intravenous cannula infections and extravasations. The care bundle consists of 10 elements including:

- hand hygiene
- insertion and site choice

- dressing
- use of appropriate infusion devices.

An audit tool was also designed to accompany the care bundle. The care bundle also has an accompanying audit tool that can be used to audit compliance with the care bundle.

Summarising of care bundle interventions or components is important in order to disseminate and imbed in practice across large nursing and medical teams. In Level 3 neonatal units, it is not unusual to see teams of over 150 people and ensuring the messages of good practice across a team of this size is challenging. One approach taken to support this is the production of laminated 'tools' or 'flash cards', which provide the interventions of the care bundle. These tools are then supported with an available full version of the care bundle.

Compliance to Care Bundles

Monitoring compliance, improved outcomes and a measurable demonstration of a reduction of risk events and patient harm

is a vital part of care bundle use. Audit tools to accompany the care bundle are essential and allow regular feedback to the team of progress and improvement in outcome.

Management of Clinical Risk in Neonatal Care

Patient safety in healthcare should form part of daily working and care delivery. Creating a culture of patient safety awareness and use of systems to ensure this premise is interfaced into daily care delivery supports outcomes for patients in all care environments. In the NICU, there is an essential need to ensure that robust systems are in place to protect the patients. Neonatal care is described as a speciality where there are some of the highest risks of errors or incidents causing harm to the patient (Gray and Goldmann 2004).

Alert

Patient Safety Alert

NPSA/2010/PSA001
09 February 2010

NHS
National Patient Safety Agency

National Reporting and Learning Service

Safer use of intravenous gentamicin for neonates

Patient safety incidents have been reported involving administration of gentamicin at the incorrect time, prescribing errors and issues relating to blood level monitoring.

Gentamicin is a broad spectrum aminoglycoside antibiotic that is widely used as the first choice antibiotic for the treatment of neonatal infection.

An NPSA telephone survey of 180 neonatal units in England carried out in 2007 indicated that 89 per cent (166) used gentamicin. Side effects of gentamicin administration can include vestibular and auditory damage, and nephrotoxicity. In addition, gentamicin has a narrow therapeutic range which necessitates its administration within an accurate timing regime, as well as regular monitoring of blood serum concentrations[1].

Patient safety incidents

A review of neonatal medication incidents reported to the Reporting and Learning System (RLS) between April 2008 and April 2009, identified 507 patient safety incidents relating to the use of intravenous gentamicin – 15 per cent of all reported neonatal medication incidents.

Analysis of these incidents highlighted that in 36 per cent of cases (182 incidents) the reason for the incident related to administration of the medicine at the incorrect time. In 24 per cent (124 incidents) of cases there had been a prescribing error, and in 17 per cent (86 incidents) there were issues relating to gentamicin blood level monitoring.

Ninety-six per cent (483) of incidents reported to the RLS resulted in no harm or low harm, and four per cent (23 incidents) were reported as causing moderate harm. However, it should be noted that the incidence of long-term hearing or renal damage as a result of gentamicin toxicity may not be apparent until some time after discharge from the neonatal unit, and therefore may not be captured in incident reports.

Supporting information

Further information and support materials to implement this guidance are available from **www.nrls.npsa.nhs.uk/alerts**

Further information

E: **gentamicin@npsa.nhs.uk**
T: 020 7927 9500

Action for the NHS

NHS organisations, clinical directors and those responsible for the provision of neonatal services should ensure that by **9 February 2011:**

1. a local neonatal gentamicin protocol is available that clarifies the initial dose and frequency of administration, blood level monitoring requirements, and arrangements for subsequent dosing adjustments based on these blood levels;

2. local policies and procedures are developed or revised to state that intravenous gentamicin should be administered to neonates using a care bundle[2] incorporating the following four elements:

   • When prescribing gentamicin, the 24-hour clock format should be used and the unused time slots in the prescription administration record blocked out at the time of prescribing to prevent wrong time dosing.

   • Interruptions during the preparation and administration of gentamicin should be minimised by the wearing of a disposable coloured apron by staff to indicate that they should not be disturbed.

   • A double-checking prompt should be used during the preparation and administration of gentamicin[3].

   • The prescribed dose of gentamicin should be given within one hour of the prescribed time.

3. neonatal units implement this care bundle using small cycles of change with a sample group of patients[4];

4. compliance with the care bundle is measured daily for each patient in the sample group until full compliance for all patients receiving gentamicin is achieved;

5. all staff involved in the prescribing and administration of intravenous gentamicin are provided with training relating to its use. This should include education regarding the interpretation and management of gentamicin blood levels including actions to be taken in relation to dose or frequency following a blood level result[5].

1 Paediatric Formulary Committee. *British National Formulary for Children 2009*. London: BMJ Publishing Group, Royal Pharmaceutical Society of Great Britain, and RCPCH Publications; 2009.
2 A care bundle is a number of evidence-based practices, generally three to five, relating to a disease or care process that when undertaken collectively and consistently for a particular patient group offers a structured way of improving the processes of care and patient outcomes.
3 Double-checking prompt is available to download as a word document from the supporting materials.
4 As outlined in the supporting tool 'A guide to help you implement the neonatal gentamicin care bundle'.
5 Support for this is provided in the PowerPoint presentation and frequently asked questions of the supporting materials.

Figure 9.6 NPSA hazard notice

Working in a neonatal unit requires the nurse to have a good comprehension of these risks, which in general focus around the size, instability and immaturity of the patient group. A drug error where an overdose is given can have a far more serious outcome in a neonate than in any other type of patient. Therefore systems that support patient safety are in place to avoid incidents taking place. Reporting of incidents is the first step in this protective approach.

Human Behaviour

Much work has been produced that examines the way in which people behave when they make a mistake or are involved in an error. The consequence of errors in healthcare is well researched and published and all nurses should ensure they have a clear understanding of risks to patients and how these risks can be managed by using a systems approach and positive learning from events that take place. Over recent years risk management has developed and expanded to support safety in healthcare (Reason 2000) (see Practical Guidelines 9.3).

Reactions and Behaviour

How these two nurses now behave on discovery of this error is vital for the outcome for the baby and for future learning for the team. As this is an underdose, there is no direct risk of harm to the baby, but over time this outcome will change if the correct drug dose is not in place. In the unit in which the nurses work, all staff are encouraged to report incidents. The nurses both feel terrible that this error has occurred and they are aware of the importance of reporting, so they stop the infusion device, call the senior nurse on duty and a process of risk management has then begun that will allow the nurses to act within their NMC Code (2008), share the learning from this event and ensure the patient is safe

The two nurses in this example are confident in their team approach for managing incidents and although they feel very anxious about the incident they do not have a fear of being blamed or reprimanded, rather they have an awareness that they will be supported to reflect, learn and share this learning across the team in a positive manner. This approach demonstrates a

---

PRACTICAL GUIDELINES 9.3

Nurses Janice and Karen are checking a complex medication that requires many stages of preparation and administration for a neonate:

- Checking the prescription of the drug for correct dose, volume, rate of administration, frequency and interactions.
- Complex calculation of the drug to ensure the correct imperial quantities, dilution, rate of administration over several hours, via an infusion device.
- Checking the patient to ensure they are identifiable by their name, DOB and cot location.
- During this process, there are clear steps that should be followed. Nurse Janice has calculated and checked the dose and rate of administration. Just as the drug is to be drawn up, an alarm on one of the monitors in the nursery sounds and Nurse Karen leaves the checking process to respond to the needs of the baby whose vital signs are outside normal range. Nurse Janice decided to carry on and draw up the medication. Without a second checker,

this is in breech of the unit policy for medication administration.
- Nurse Karen then returns to the checking process; she had not calculated the drug or watched the preparation and drawing up process, but as there are many medications to be checked, she accepts the syringe contents and goes with Nurse Janice to the cot side to set up the infusion pump and run the drug via this pump.
- Once the bedside check, done as per the unit policy, is complete, Nurse Janice returns to the checking work surface to dispose of the equipment used to prepare and administer the drug. Nurse Janice notices that there is too much of the medication left in the ampoule from which it was drawn up and recognises that the volume in the syringe that is infusing to the baby is incorrect. She alerts Nurse Karen to this situation and both nurses recognise that a drug error has occurred.

---

culture of openness in the way that the hospital works and the quality of care that the organisation is delivering to its patients.

Reason and Vincent (2010) have both written extensively about human behaviours and factors in incidents and errors both within our healthcare system and in other high-risk industries. Human beings make mistakes; not getting everything right all the time is what makes us humans. It is how the nurse learns and responds to mistakes that is the key factor in risk management. By reporting and learning, it is clear that there can be a reduction of incidents; recognising that to some degree there

will always be mistakes when humans are undertaking high-risk practices in itself supports avoidance of errors.

Reporting Culture

Most hospitals have software systems that allow staff to report incidents or errors that occur. Reporting is the first step to learning. Communication and understanding how an incident occurred is an important part of the risk management process. Looking at the example of the two nurses, Janice and Karen, it is clear there was no intent to harm the patient. The intensive care unit is a pressurised and demanding environment but the process and policy for drug administration was not followed and this is the root cause of the drug error. Policies and practices are in place to support patient safety and both these nurses can now clearly see how moving outside policy can lead to incidents.

Sharing incidents with a wider team is a demonstration of mature risk management culture, where the approach of the team is to grasp the opportunity to learn from others' misadventures with a positive approach: avoidance of recrimination is important in this communication and neonatal teams are in general very good at working within this strategy.

CASE STUDY REVIEW 9.1 Systems and staff competence

At 33 weeks' gestation, it is unlikely that Jacob would have been transferred to a network NICU. In terms of neonatal care, Jacob's care is considered to be 'straightforward' and could be managed in the local neonatal unit.

It is likely that Jacob would have required antibiotics and it may be that as gentamicin is a broad-spectrum antibiotic this may have been prescribed. Janice and Karen, the nurses who have been involved in caring for Jacob, should have been able competently to follow policy and procedure when administering medication. There would have been clear policies in place, yet Janice and Karen have perhaps become complacent as their trust in one another developed and have slipped into 'bad

habits' which could impact on the care of Jacob and the other babies. It is important that the neonatal unit is as safe as possible. Risk assessment and risk assessment tools facilitate decision making and the recording process.

It is clear that systems are in place to ensure that the neonatal costs are managed according to need (see Table 9.4). Ellie-Mae and Lloyd would be unaware of the structure of the neonatal network but would be aware of the care Jacob receives. Care should be of a high quality, evidence based and safe. In the future, Ellie-Mae and Lloyd may wish to add to the collaborative voice to support Bliss and other charities to help advocate the needs of preterm babies (see Table 9.5).

Table 9.4 Timeline of neonatal policy drivers

1967	Abortion law changes
1993	UNICEF baby-friendly initiative
1995	EPIcure 1: a European wide project for epilepsy to develop new therapeutic strategies
2001	BAPM Guidelines
2007	NAO: *Caring for Vulnerable Babies* Reorganisation of neonatal services in England
2008	House of Commons Select Committee
2008	POPPY (*Parents of Premature Babies Project – Your needs*, a 3-year research project to identify effective interventions for communication, information and support)
2008	EPIcure 2
2009	Department of Health: Toolkit for High Quality Neonatal Care
2010	NICE: Quality Standards for Neonatal Care
2010	NICE: Neonatal Jaundice
2011	BAPM Guidelines
ongoing	Neonatal Data Analysis Unit (NDAU)
ongoing	National Neonatal Audit Programme
[List is not exhaustive.]	

Table 9.5 Defining a neonate

Neonate	A baby from birth to day 27
Preterm	A baby born before the 37th week of gestation
Post-term	A baby born during or after the 42nd week of gestation
Small for gestational age (SGA)	A baby weight that is < 10% of the population for gestational age
Appropriate for gestation age (AGA)	A baby weight that meets expectations
Large for gestational age (LGA)	A baby weighing more than expected
Low birth weight (LBW)	A baby weighing less than 2.5 kgs at birth
Very low birth weight (VLBW)	A baby weighing less than 1.5 kgs at birth
Extremely low birth weight (ELBW)	A baby weighing less than 1 kg at birth

NEONATAL ENVIRONMENTS

Pre-Birth and Biological Environments

During pregnancy, the 'baby's world' is a familiar dark womb, where the baby has become used to hearing muffled sounds from the 'outside world' through the mother's abdomen and uterine wall. The baby is also familiar with the comforting sounds of the mother's body systems such as the heart beat. The baby is surrounded by gentle water, which both supports her and aids movement to achieve the right position; and the baby's temperature is maintained at appropriate levels by the supporting network of the mother's body systems. In order to use the mother's body systems, the baby's own circulatory system is organised for this to occur; this is known as the fetal circulation (see Figure 9.7). Having some insight into fetal circulation and changes to the circulatory system at birth facilitates understanding why resuscitation may be challenging.

Fetal Circulation

The fetal circulation is a separate blood circulation from the maternal circulation and the only point of contact is at the placenta. The fetus only has the placenta to supply all its oxygen needs. The fetal circulation is organised so that the organs have the correct oxygen supply for their function or development needs.

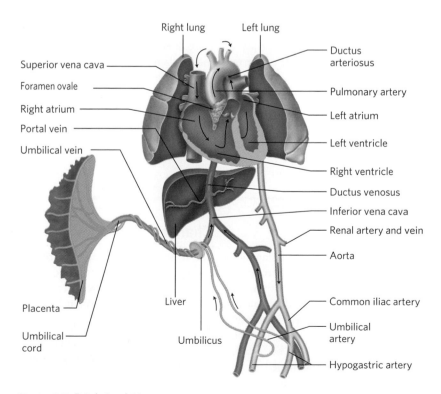

Figure 9.7 Fetal circulation

The organs that need a good oxygen supply include:

- heart – fetal heart is active throughout fetal life
- brain – preparing for post-uterine life
- kidneys – supplies amniotic fluid
- liver.

The organs that receive a restricted oxygen supply:

- gut
- lungs.

The structures of the fetal circulation are in place to direct the flow of blood to oxygenate the organs that need a good supply of oxygen.

The Ductus Venosus

The liver is the first organ on the path of the umbilical vein moving oxygenated blood away from the placenta and up to the heart. It allows sufficient blood to go to the liver for healthy growth and function but the remainder of the blood passes by the liver and onto the heart.

Foramen Ovale

The foramen ovale provides an open route between the two atria of the heart. The oxygenated blood arriving at the heart mixes with deoxygenated blood flowing back through the fetal venous system. Most blood returning to the heart will be pushed through the foramen ovale. Blood flows to left ventricle then to the aorta.

Ductus Arteriosus

Blood that has been pumped into the right ventricle will continue into the pulmonary artery towards the lungs. The lungs are vasoconstricted and require a reduced blood supply; therefore the remaining blood needs an alternative route. The ductus arteriosus provides the channel through which blood can flow to the aorta and avoid the lungs.

Fetal Lungs

The lungs are not functioning during fetal life but have to prepare to work efficiently immediately following birth. The blood vessels that supply the lungs are vasoconstricted, only allowing sufficient blood for healthy growth and development. The fetal lungs produce lung fluid for healthy growth and preparation for expansion following birth. The alveolar cells manufacture surfactant which allows air to enter the alveoli of the lungs following birth. The foetus makes breathing movements in uterine life.

Kidneys

The renal artery supplying the kidneys is partially vasoconstricted but supplies sufficient blood to produce sufficient urine for correct volume of amniotic fluid.

CASE STUDY REVIEW 9.2 Pre-birth and biological environments

At 33 weeks' gestation, it is likely that Jacob's internal systems have enabled him to grow, receiving appropriate support from Ellie-Mae's body to maintain an adequate oxygen supply. In uterine life, Jacob would have received nutrients to facilitate growth and development. Jacob's uterine world enables him to exist in a supportive environment (see Table 9.7).

Maternity care advocates participation in routine pre-birth screening. Ellie-Mae would have been invited to attend for screening:

- confirmation that Jacob had four chambers in the heart
- growth estimation
- abnormality screening.

The scenario does not give insight into whether Ellie-Mae had prepared her body for pregnancy by taking folic acid supplements. As Jacob is the first child of Ellie-Mae and Lloyd, it is assumed that there would have been great excitement related to the pregnancy and that Lloyd would have attended the scans. There is sometimes the opportunity for photographs of the scan to be purchased. If this were the case, then Ellie-Mae and Lloyd would be able to share early images of their baby with friends and family.

Birthing and Biological Environments

At birth, the 'baby's world' changes and becomes an unfamiliar place. The delivery suite is very bright to facilitate appropriate care to mother and baby. The baby is no longer bathing in water and is often placed on a hard surface to facilitate effective resuscitation of the newborn and then rubbed vigorously with a towel. The interprofessional team will have prepared the physical environment to respond to the needs of the baby, each of them possessing up-to-date knowledge and honed skills. While all this is occurring in the outside world, changes are occurring within the baby.

Changes that Follow the First Breath

The reason for all the changes reflect that the baby has to get its oxygen supply from inspired air, and all organs and systems need a good supply of oxygen in order to function. The changes to the lung following birth include:

- the removal of lung fluid
- the inflation of the lungs during the first inflation breaths
- the alveoli become patent to receive inspired air.

There is vasodilation of the pulmonary blood vessels to receive oxygen for circulation and removal of carbon dioxide.

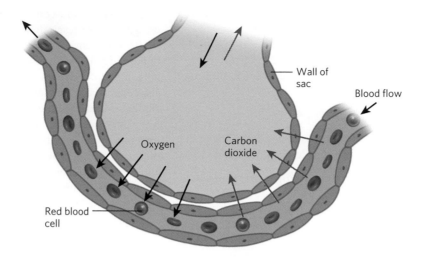

Figure 9.8 Alveoli

How the removal of lung fluid is achieved is still uncertain. The traditional view of drainage coming from the head down, with vaginal birth providing gravity and helping chest compression, is being challenged. Research suggests that nearly all lung fluid is removed through the sodium channels of the alveolar cells. Activation of these channels is through steroids, oxygen and catecholamines.

Initiation of First Breath

There are a number of theories surrounding the first breath; the following are thought to have some influence on the initiation of the first breath:

- startle from cold environment
- breath initiated by hypoxic state
- breath initiated by increase in circulating carbon dioxide
- mechanical recoil of chest muscles
- removal of lung fluid creating space and negative pressure in the lung.

The Alveoli

The alveoli become patent to receive inspired air. Increased air pressure within the alveoli occurs from increased volumes of inspired air. Oxygen and carbon dioxide move through the alveoli walls. Nitrogen in air remains in the alveolus and creates a gas pressure that holds the alveolar walls open. Surfactant reduces the surface tension of water, enabling water molecules to position themselves over the inside walls of the alveoli (see Figure 9.8).

Pulmonary Blood Vessels

Vasodilation of the pulmonary blood vessels occurs. The blood vessels of the newborn lungs dilate to increase capillary blood flow and exchange of oxygen and carbon dioxide. Endothelium-derived nitric oxide (EDNO) is produced by the lung tissues. It is the presence of EDNO in the lung epithelium that initiates the action of vasodilators such as acetylcholine, bradykinin and histamine (see Glossary). The increased air in the alveoli seems to stimulate this action.

Control of respiration

The rate at which air enters the alveoli should match the demands of the body exactly. Normal breathing is regulated by the respiratory centre in the pons and medulla of the brain (see Figure 9.9).

Air passes down the trachea, into the bronchi, bronchioles and enters the alveoli. Gaseous exchange takes place at the alveoli. The inspired air enters the alveolus. The inspired air has a higher oxygen partial pressure than the circulating blood (see blood gases). The oxygen moves by passing down diffusion gradients. Oxygen diffuses through the alveolar wall and passes through the wall of the capillary blood vessel, and then passes through the plasma and becomes attached to the haemoglobin of the red blood cells.

The Heart

At birth the placenta is removed by the cord being clamped and cut. The rise in oxygen causes the constricted blood vessels to dilate. The ductus venosus, foramen ovale and ductus arteriosus are no longer needed to divert the blood away from vasoconstricted organs. There is enough oxygen to supply all organs.

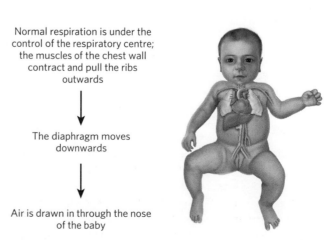

Normal respiration is under the control of the respiratory centre; the muscles of the chest wall contract and pull the ribs outwards

↓

The diaphragm moves downwards

↓

Air is drawn in through the nose of the baby

Figure 9.9 Normal respiration

The Ductus Venosus

- No blood supply from the placenta.
- Liver has own blood supply through hepatic arteries.
- Pressure in the venous return to the heart through the vena cava is reduced.

Foramen Ovale

The foramen ovale is a flap of skin positioned according to the pressure of blood flowing over it or holding it in position:

- Pressure of blood from venous return right atrium becomes low.
- The pressure of blood flowing back from the now functioning lungs becomes high.

Ductus Arteriosus

The ductus arteriosus remains open during fetal life because the low oxygen values allow prostaglandins to be active in the walls of the duct:

- With the first breath, there is a rise in blood oxygen and the increase in oxygen knocks out the prostaglandin activity. The walls of the ductus venosus collapse.
- In the end, the baby's lungs expand, with a full blood supply and are able to provide all the oxygen that is necessary for the baby's survival. The heart is in normal cardiac cycle and all organs and systems fully perfused with blood.

Assessments at birth

At birth, the interprofessional team will assess the condition of the baby in order to plan and implement appropriate care. There are several assessment tools that may be used during this process (see Table 9.6). One of the assessment tools that aid assessment during neonatal resuscitation is the Apgar score.

> **ACTIVITY 9.1** Neonatal resuscitation guidelines
>
> Access the neonatal resuscitation guidelines (**http://www.resus.org.uk/pages/nls.pdf**). Consider the differences in this algorithm to that for infants.

The Apgar score considers and rates the baby's condition using heart rate, respiration, muscle tone, reflexes and colour.

The experiences of the family are important as birth is an important milestone in life. The full-term birth occurs at a given point at 38 to 42 weeks and the mother will have made personal choices in relation to planned pain relief, planned birth, normal labour and safe birthing. The mother and baby are separated from one another, but they remain together to 'get to know each other' and begin the bonding and attachment process. The mother takes her baby home at a planned time following birth and the baby is incorporated into the society in which the family lives. It is a time of celebrating the birth of the new baby and the safe delivery of the mother. The family are given a new social position because of the birth.

In the case of a sick or preterm baby, the birth occurs at no particular time and can be from 24 to 37 weeks gestational age. The pain comes as an unexpected shock and the birth plans for labour are potentially not completed. The birth is less safe and the baby may be taken away from the mother for care and management. The attachment between the mother and baby is interrupted by separation. Social recognition of the birth is not expected, parents may be greeted with 'what a shame' or 'I am sorry to hear that' rather than the elated congratulations. There may be a long delay before the baby goes home, and the mother goes home without the baby. There is either no celebration or a delayed celebration to mark the baby's entry into the world. Being unprepared causes stress to the mother and requires the support of family and friends (see Chapter 1). This also means the incorporation of this baby into its wider family and society is potentially flawed.

Neonatal Environments

The neonatal unit environment continues to be a bright, noisy environment with alarms ringing to herald the baby in need of some assistance. Every effort is taken to minimise the level of noise within the neonatal unit as noise can have a profound effect on the baby. The neonatal staff try to minimise the hard environment of the incubator and cots with soft linen and the provision of 'boundaries' to aid positioning and increase the sense of security in the baby. The variable temperatures are more controllable with the use of thermostatic controls. Every effort is made to consider skin integrity and a range of strategies facilitate this.

Table 9.6 Apgar score

Sign	Score 0	Score 1	Score 2
Heart rate	0	< 100	> 100
Respiration	Absent	Gasping or irregular	Regular or crying lustily
Muscle tone	Limp	Diminished or normal with no movements	Normal or active movements
Reflexes	Nil	Grimace	Cough
Colour	White	Blue	Pink

CASE STUDY REVIEW 9.3 Birthing and biological environments

Being prepared for all eventualities would have enabled the interprofessional team to be responsive to any condition Jacob presented with. It is evident that the interprofessional team had undertaken routine checks in preparation for Jacob's arrival. It is likely that Jacob would have been transported to the neonatal unit in a portable incubator to maintain his temperature.

Jacob's circulatory system made the switch to ex-uterine life, but the scenario does not provide insight into the Apgar score or whether Jacob required any resuscitation. Transition from uterine life to the outside world would have initiated some changes to Jacob's world (see Table 9.7).

Ellie-Mae would need to be offered emotional and physical support due to tiredness following the birth of Jacob and will be anxious about Jacob's early arrival. Further stresses and anxieties will be associated with the immediate time following birth until either a cry is heard or there is confirmation that Jacob is breathing and the interprofessional team confirms a plan of action.

Lloyd will be concerned for Ellie-Mae and concerned for Jacob prompting levels of stress and anxiety. Lloyd may also be concerned how he may approach the situation if Jacob's arrival had presented an unsuccessful resuscitation. Both Ellie-Mae and Lloyd will need further information as they may have limited prior knowledge of preterm infants that may have come through media portrayal. Seeing the technology in the delivery suite and neonatal unit would also be daunting.

The extended family may also be anxious about Jacob's arrival and may have only limited insight into preterm births. The extended family will be a good support for Ellie-Mae and Lloyd providing that there are positive relationships between them.

Babies are admitted to the neonatal unit for a range of reasons, which include: being vulnerable and at risk of deterioration; being preterm (under 37 completed weeks gestational age); having a congenital abnormality and requiring further support and management; or on their way to foster care. The babies receive expert medical and nursing care to support the body systems until the baby is able to support the systems unaided. Care is based on assessment of needs. The essential philosophies for care within the neonatal unit are family-centred care, environmental care and developmental care (see Table 9.7).

Neonatal Health Issues

Neonatal health issues are varied and result in different lengths of stay which are appropriate to their diagnosis or condition. There are five groups of admissions to the neonatal unit:

1. Planned: predicted admissions identified through obstetric and midwifery assessments
2. Emergency: unplanned admissions as a consequence of birthing process or maternal health issues

Table 9.7 Environmental experiences of the baby

Womb	Delivery suite	Neonatal unit	Neonatal unit adaptations
Dark	Bright	Bright	Cycled lighting Incubator covers
Muffled sounds	Noisy	Noisy	Noise control strategies policed by neonatal staff
Comforting sounds	Alarms	Alarms	Parents' voices able to be heard by family-centred care
Gentle water	Hard environment	Hard environment	Adaptations to hard environment by introducing soft boundaries and nesting informed by developmental care
Right position	Needs positioning	Needs positioning	Extremities be brought into the midline with developmental care strategies
Temperature right	Temperature variable	Temperature variable	Ambient temperature and incubator temperatures controlled by neonatal staff to maintain neutral thermal environment

3. Unforeseen: pregnancy and prebirth screening have not identified conditions or congenital abnormalities requiring specialist care
4. Transfer: admission where the baby is to be transferred for specialist care in a network neonatal unit
5. Social: admissions where there may be a social reason such as on the way to fostering or safeguarding reasons.

There are a variety of reasons or conditions that require the knowledge and expertise of neonatal staff. Reasons can be seen in two categories: those frequently occurring and requiring care and management in a local neonatal unit, and those that occur less frequently but may require higher levels of care and expertise (see Tables 9.1, 9.2, 9.7 and 9.8).

Table 9.8 Examples of neonatal health issues

	Frequent health issues requiring care and management in local neonatal unit	Less frequent health issues requiring care and management in network neonatal unit
Respiratory system	Transient tachypnoea of the newborn Respiratory distress syndrome Mild meconium inhalation Drug-induced respiratory depression Birth asphyxia (may also affect other systems)	Congenital diaphragmatic hernia Choanal atresia Tracheo-oesophageal fistula Severe meconium inhalation Drug-induced respiratory depression Birth asphyxia (may also affect other systems)
Gastrointestinal	Necrotising enterocolitis	Oesophageal atresia Imperforate anus Meconium ileus Gastroschisis Exomphalos Necrotising enterocolitis
Renal system	Acute renal failure Chronic renal failure Some congenital abnormalities	Acute renal failure Chronic renal failure Congenital abnormalities
Cardiac system	Cardiac failure Ventricular septal defect Patent ductus arteriosus	Cardiac failure Tetralogy of Fallot Triscuspid atresia Coarctation of the aorta Transposition of the great vessels Ventricular septal defect Patent ductus arteriosus
Blood	Jaundice ABO incompatibility Rhesus incompatibility	Jaundice ABO incompatibility Rhesus incompatibility
Nervous system	Birth trauma Intracranial haemorrhage Maternal recreational drug misuse in pregnancy	Birth trauma Structural deformities such as spina bifida Intracranial haemorrhage Maternal recreational drug misuse in pregnancy
Infection control	Neonatal septicaemia Thrush Conjunctivitis Omphalitis HIV	Neonatal septicaemia Thrush Conjunctivitis Omphalitis HIV

MAINTAINING SAFE ENVIRONMENTS

Neutral Thermal Environment

It is important that the baby remains in a neutral thermal environmental temperature that does not cause the baby to raise his metabolic rate to maintain haemostasis. Oxygen is consumed when keeping a baby warm or when the baby's temperature is elevated. The neutral thermal environment is responsive to the baby's care needs in terms of whether the baby is being cared for in an incubator, open incubator/radiant warmer or cot (see Figure 9.10). It may be related to maturity and his ability to maintain his temperature within normal parameters.

Temperature Control

Heat Loss

Preterm infants can lose heat because they have a small body with a large surface area. There are four ways in which the baby can lose heat:

- conduction: baby laid on cold surface
- convection: baby is cooled by the air currents circulating the body
- evaporation: baby loses heat due to evaporation of water on the skin
- radiation: baby loses heat by radiation onto nearby objects.

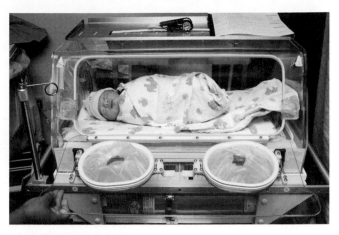

Figure 9.10 Radiant warmer with manikin

Heat Production

In the first weeks of life, the baby can produce heat by a process of non-shivering thermogenesis and by burning brown adipose tissue. There are enzymes that get within the fat and have the capacity to rapidly convert the fat into heat and energy. Thermogenesis can be affected by medication, hypoglycaemia and other conditions (see Figure 9.11).

Heat Conservation

Babies born at term will naturally conserve heat by being in a tightly flexed position, also referred to as the fetal position. However, babies who are born preterm or who are sick appear

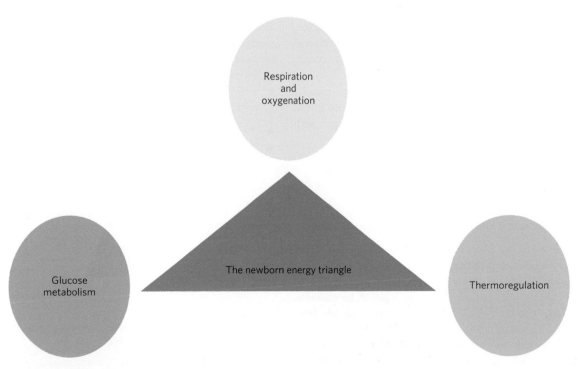

Figure 9.11 The newborn energy triangle

to lose muscle tone and lay supine in a 'frog-like' position that maximises heat loss. In adults, skin vasoconstriction conserves heat yet, in the baby, it is far less effective. As a baby's head has the largest surface area, neonatal staff use hats to aid heat conservation.

Respiration and Oxygenation

Following birth and the first breath, the baby now needs to establish a regular breathing pattern to maintain oxygenation. The baby's respiratory centre becomes the control of his breathing. Lung fluid clears and the alveoli of the lungs open and prepare to receive inspired air. Normal respiration is under the control of the respiratory centre; the muscles of the chest wall contract and pull the ribs outwards. The diaphragm moves downwards and air is drawn in through the nose of the baby. Air passes down the trachea, into the bronchi, bronchioles and enters the alveoli. The alveolus provides the fine membrane connection with the capillary blood vessels of the lung that allows oxygen to pass from inspired air to the blood and carbon dioxide to pass from the blood into the alveoli for expiration. To allow this gaseous exchange the alveoli must remain open and ready to receive inspired air. To do this it needs a surfactant. To maintain surfactant production, **glucose and oxygen** are required.

Glucose Metabolism

The next point of the triangle is glucose metabolism. Babies are born with glucose circulating in their blood that has come across the placenta from their mother and stores of liver glycogen that they can convert into glucose and put out into the blood circulation if glucose gets low. Birth is an energetic business and the process of birth needs energy, as do the changes that take place following birth. Being a baby is a far more energetic process being than a fetus. The baby is born with glucose, stored liver glycogen to convert to glucose and additional stores of lactate to use for anaerobic metabolism if oxygen becomes short.

The goal of nursing neonates is to achieve a blood glucose balance. Healthy babies are born with sufficient glucose to use with oxygen and the ability to breathe in sufficient oxygen with fuels that produce energy without using oxygen.

Problems can occur when the baby:

- is born with deficient glucose stores
- does not take in adequate amounts of glucose to replace glucose used
- uses up glucose at a more rapid rate during post-birth life.

If available glucose becomes low, the baby begins to utilise other sources of energy, for example, lactate or breakdown of fats and proteins for use as glucose. This is effective but some sources of energy will eventually become depleted, for example, lactate. The by-products of gluconeogenesis are acidic and have the potential for contributing to a metabolic acidosis.

As available glucose becomes depleted, the energy to power cells will become less. The available energy to power the muscles

of respiration becomes less active affecting the ability of the baby to inspire oxygen. As a result of this the baby becomes hypoxic and requires the administration of oxygen.

Without glucose and oxygen to supply fuels to energise cells, the cells will become less active. The baby becomes lethargic. The baby will utilise its energy reserves to maintain physiological balance such as activating the immune system. The baby will have less energy to use to keep warm and will become hypothermic and will require intervention to achieve a **neutral thermal environment** (see Figure 9.12).

Effects of Cold Stress 1

The baby responds by increasing the metabolic rate of cells. This increases the rate of oxygen consumption. This causes an increase in the respiration rate. There becomes insufficient oxygen available for both heat production and the increased rate of respirations. This results in the baby becoming hypoxic. The baby starts to use anaerobic methods for energy production and lactic acid is produced. This leads to lowering of body pH and a metabolic acidosis. The acidosis causes pulmonary vasoconstriction which increases the hypoxia and results in respiratory distress.

Effects of Cold Stress 2

There is an increased cell metabolism to generate heat, leading to an increased need for glucose to fuel increased metabolism. Liver glycogen stores are emptied to support this increased need for glucose. Depleted glycogen stores become unable to support a normal blood glucose value which results in **hypoglycaemia** (see Figure 9.13).

Effects of Cold Stress 3

Brown adipose tissue is used to produce heat by non-shivering thermogenesis. The metabolism of brown adipose tissue generates release of fatty acids. The increase of fatty acids causes a fall in body pH as a metabolic acidosis. The baby increases respiratory effort in an attempt to expire carbon dioxide to regain pH balance. The need for oxygen rises to support:

- the increased respiratory effort
- the heat generation from brown fat.

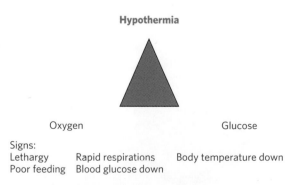

Hypothermia

Oxygen   Glucose

Signs:
Lethargy   Rapid respirations   Body temperature down
Poor feeding   Blood glucose down

Figure 9.12 Energy triangle: hypothermia

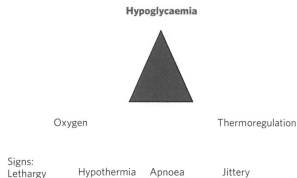

Hypoglycaemia

Oxygen   Thermoregulation

Signs:
Lethargy   Hypothermia   Apnoea   Jittery
Poor feeding   Drowsy   Coma (if untreated)

Figure 9.13 Energy triangle: hypoglycaemia

The amount of oxygen available for surfactant production is reduced which results in respiratory distress. The signs of respiratory distress include increased rate of respirations, nasal flaring, sternal recession, grunting, apnoea and cyanosis (see Figure 9.14).

Caring for a neonate requires interventions that support homeostasis within three key parameters: oxygen, respiration and a neutral thermal environment to avoid thermogenesis. It is possible to begin at any point of the energy triangle to see the relationship for newborn physiology: respiration and oxygenation; thermoregulation, and glucose metabolism to see that there is an inseparable relationship. The reason for this is that oxygen and glucose enter cells to produce ATP energy molecules, which create the energy needed for every cell to fulfil its function.

The role of the nurse is to plan the care of the baby in order to prevent or minimise causes of deterioration in the baby and to optimise the health and wellbeing of the baby by implementing evidenced-based care (see Table 9.x and Research Note 9.1).

Components of the Arterial Blood Gases

Interpreting blood gases and taking appropriate action subsequently requires knowledge and experience. In many trust organisations,

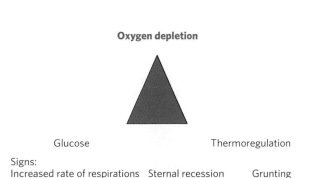

Oxygen depletion

Glucose   Thermoregulation

Signs:
Increased rate of respirations Sternal recession   Grunting
Apnoea   Cyanosis   Nasal flaring

Figure 9.14 Energy triangle: oxygen depletion

there are identified personnel to undertake this important task. This is because the blood sample would be taken from an indwelling catheter. Without these skills, it is inappropriate to attempt to obtain a blood sample or change ventilator settings, yet it may be interesting to have an insight into why the arterial blood test can aid diagnosis and help determine a certain management of care. In order to interpret and read arterial blood gases there needs to be an understanding of the concept of **pH**, the measurement of acidity or alkalinity, as it is an essential measurement as part of blood gases to evaluate the degree of acidity or alkalinity of the body. This is because the degree of acidity or alkalinity of a liquid or substance is measured by pH (potential hydrogen). As the level of a solution becomes more acidic or less alkaline, the pH falls (hydrogen ion concentration rises). The opposite happens when solutions become less acidic or more alkaline.

Enzymes are extremely vital components in our body as they ultimately control chemical reactions that happen in our body and any change or imbalance in the acidity or alkalinity in the blood will affect how enzymes work or function. Electrolytes will move in and out of cells to try and maintain electrolyte balance. This causes electrolyte imbalance. The neutral level of pH is accepted as 7.0. The pH is important as the blood has a normal pH range of 7.35 to 7.45 and is therefore slightly alkaline, which is quite specific. For the purposes of pH assessment in the blood, the language used would be:

a pH measurement below 7.35 = acidosis
a pH measurement above 7.45 = alkalosis.

Blood Gas Measurement

There are other terms used when interpreting an arterial blood gas sample (ABG):

- acid/base balance
- PO_2 – partial pressure of oxygen
- O_2 sat – oxygen saturation value
- PCO_2 – partial pressure of carbon dioxide
- pH – hydrogen ion concentration
- HCO_3 – bicarbonate
- base deficit
- base excess.

pH and Hydrogen Ion Concentration

About 90 per cent of plasma, the fluid part of blood, is made up of water (see Figure 9.15). When CO_2 enters the blood from cells, it mixes with water to become carbonic acid. It then goes through another transformation stage to become **bicarbonate** and **hydrogen ions (H+ions)** and then back into CO_2 to be allowed to be expelled by the lungs.

pH and Bicarbonate

Hydrogen ions are acid and bicarbonate is alkaline. For blood to be pH 7.4 the balance must be: hydrogen ions 1:20 bicarbonate. A raised hydrogen ion level means the blood becomes acidotic. A raised bicarbonate level means the blood becomes alkaline.

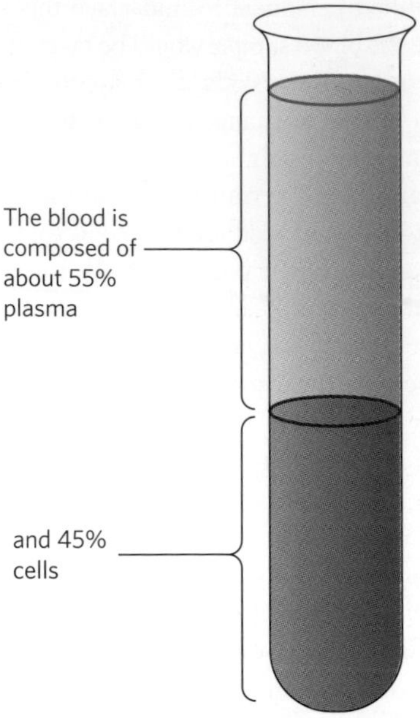

Figure 9.15 Blood components

A decreased hydrogen ion level means the blood becomes alkaline. Decreased bicarbonate levels means the blood becomes acid.

Raised hydrodgen ions means the blood becomes acidotic. Hydrogen ions are generated from carbon dioxide changing as it travels in blood. If carbon dioxide is prevented from being expired, this means the hydrogen ions will increase resulting in a respiratory acidosis.

A raised bicarbonate level means the blood becomes alkaline. Bicarbonate is excreted through the kidney. If the kidneys are not working, blood bicarbonate is raised. The bicarbonate will increase resulting in a metabolic alkalosis.

Alternatively, there can be a decrease in hydrogen ions, then the blood becomes alkaline. If too much carbon dioxide is being breathed out, the circulating hydrogen ions will decrease. If hydrogen ions increase, this will result in a respiratory alkalosis.

Decreased bicarbonate level means the blood becomes acid. If the kidneys excrete too much bicarbonate this results in a metabolic acidosis.

Other sources of acids:

- ketones from protein breakdown
- lactic acid from anaerobic metabolism
- fatty acids from fat breakdown
- these acids are metabolised by the liver
- if they are in excess in the blood, they will produce a metabolic acidosis.

Base Deficit/Base Excess

Buffers have the ability to accept hydrogen ions and therefore decrease the volume of hydrogen ions circulating in the blood. Once sited on a buffer, the hydrogen ion is no longer part of the acid/base balance mechanism. Due to the cancellation effect it has on hydrogen ions, bicarbonate is regarded as a buffer. Buffers that have sites to accept hydrogen (H+) ions are:

- red blood cells
- plasma proteins
- phosphates.

The number of sites available on these buffers is limited. By estimating the numbers of red blood cells, plasma proteins and phosphates in the blood and the number of receptor sites each carries for hydrogen ions, a calculation can be made to assess the number of buffer sites there are (see Table 9.9). As hydrogen ions rise, the buffer sites accept hydrogen ions to reduce the acidosis. As buffer sites fill, a base deficit occurs as fewer buffer sites are available. As hydrogen ions fall, the buffer sites expel hydrogen ions to reduce the alkalosis. As buffer sites empty, a base excess occurs as more buffer sites are available.

ACTIVITY 9.2 Arterial blood gas (ABG)

tic-tac-toe examples
Access arterial blood gas (ABG) tic-tac-toe examples (**http://www.youtube.com/watch?v=_OpvyEIIFj8**).

Table 9.9 Normal arterial blood gas values for children and neonates

	Infant/child values	Neonatal values
pH	7.35–7.45	7.3–7.4
PCO$_2$ (kPa)	4.5–6.0 (35–45 mmHg)	4.6.–6.0 (35–45 mmHg)
PO$_2$ (kPa)	10–13 (75–100 mmHg)	7.3–12 (55–90 mmHg)
Bicarbonate (mmol/l)	22–26	18–25
Base (mmol/l)	2 to +2	4 to +4

CASE STUDY REVIEW 9.4 Maintaining a safe environment

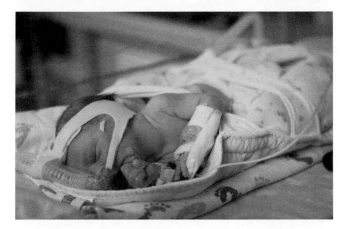

Figure 9.16 A baby on nasal CPAP through infant flow driver

From the moment of birth, interprofessional teamwork is required to enable Jacob's body system to remain in optimal condition and maintain homeostasis. Jacob will need support to maintain temperature within acceptable boundaries. Blood gases would have been taken and, responding to the results, the treatment of nasal CPAP was implemented. Nasal CPAP through an infant flow driver can cause pressure to the delicate tissues around the nose and cheeks and strategies for dealing with this would have been incorporated into his care plan (see Figure 9.16).

For Jacob, it is clear that glucose, oxygen and temperature can have an effect on one another and will be considered in care planning.

At 33 weeks' gestation, Jacob may have fairly mature lungs which have produced an adequate level of surfactant to enable his lungs to expand. Surfactant helps relieve surface tension in the lungs. Had Jacob been born earlier, he may have required the administration of artificial surfactant.

Ellie-Mae and Lloyd will require explanations from the neonatal team to understand the reasons why Jacob needs technological support. They will also need to come to terms with the machinery supporting Jacob. Even though every attempt is made to maintain comfort, safety and high-quality care, Jacob will be receiving unpleasant stimuli through his clinically necessary treatment. Jacob needs Ellie-Mae and Lloyd to provide love and positive, pleasant stimuli to support him. Ellie-Mae and Lloyd will require support from the neonatal team to begin this process as they may be feeling as if they cannot even touch Jacob.

DEVELOPMENTAL CARE

Developmental care is the umbrella term for a collection of strategies that enable the staff to facilitate the parent attachment bonding process. The baby will let the staff know when it is the right time to provide care interventions by displaying approach cues. Equally, the baby can guide staff when to avoid approaching him by displaying stress signals. Over time, the neonatal team working with neonates learn to interpret the approach cues and avoidance cues indicated by the baby.

Baby Cues

Over the past 30 years, neonatal staff have become aware of the ability of the baby to communicate physiological parameters through the work of a number of authors (including Brazelton 1973, 1995; Als 1982; Lissauer and Fanaroff 2006). Understanding these communication methods facilitates a further dimension to caring for the baby (see Table 9.10).

Baby Body Language

In addition to the physiological signs, the neonatal team have become more understanding of the baby's ability to communicate using facial expression, thanks to the work of many long-term contributors (Brazelton 1961; Als 1982; Sparshott 1997; Warren and Bond 2010) (see Figure 9.17).

Baby Stress Signals

The topic of infant stress signals has also been explored in the literature and, as have indications to access the stress signals the

Table 9.10 Infant cues by body systems

	Approach behaviour	Avoidance behaviour
Autonomic	Regular, gentle breathing	Breathing irregular, fast and laboured
	Healthy pink colouring	Pale, dusky, flushed or mottled
	Comfortable digestion	Straining, gagging or vomiting
Motor	Smooth, varied movement	Jerky, disorganised movement
	Softly flexed posture	Extended or flat posture
	Modulated muscle tone	Flaccid or stiff tone
State	Restful sleep	Restless sleep
	Periodic sleep/wake pattern	Diffuse, disorganised state
	Quiet alertness	Frequent state changes
Attention	Sustained, focused alertness	Glazed, strained hyper-alert look
Self-regulation	Self-calming	Inconsolable
	Socially responsive	Shut down

baby uses to gain help and support (see Figure 9.18). Brazelton was among the earlier writers to recognise that babies could be 'active participants and social partners' during caregiving (Boxwell 2000).

PAIN AND ASSESSMENT TOOLS

It is a human right to be pain free; however, pain in children is an under-recognised problem around the world (International Association for the Study of Pain 2005). It is not surprising that there has been a wealth of research to ensure that babies receive appropriate pain relief (see Table 9.11).

Having recognised the baby's signals of distress, it would be unethical for the neonatal team to ignore her. In order to assess the severity of pain, it is useful to use a pain assessment tool. Two of the most commonly used tools with the preterm baby are CRIES and FLACC, which are both mnemonics for the parameters being assessed for indicators of pain (see Figures 9.19 and 9.20). It is evident that these recognise the physiological parameters, baby cues and body language.

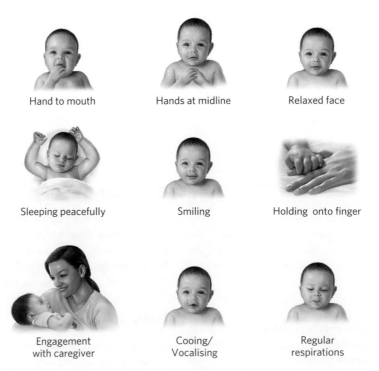

Hand to mouth   Hands at midline   Relaxed face

Sleeping peacefully   Smiling   Holding onto finger

Engagement with caregiver   Cooing/Vocalising   Regular respirations

Figure 9.17 Baby cues and body language

Infant stress signals

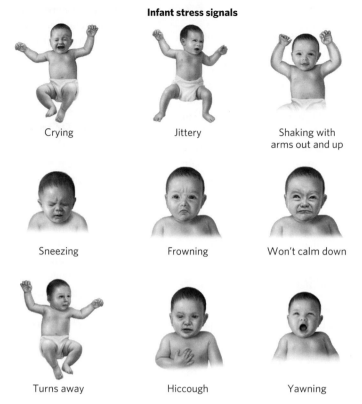

Crying	Jittery	Shaking with arms out and up
Sneezing	Frowning	Won't calm down
Turns away	Hiccough	Yawning

Figure 9.18 Infant stress signals

Table 9.11 Recognition of pain and distress in the newborn

Physiological changes	Abrupt change in skin colour
	Increase or decrease in heart and blood pressure
	Tachypnoea
	Apnoeic episodes
	Fall in oxygen saturation value
	Startle response
	Yawning
	Hiccoughing
	Gagging
	Vomiting
Body	Flaccidity
	Hypertonicity
	Splaying of fingers and toes
	Hand over face
	Arm extension
Facial expression	Facial grimace
	Frown
	Tongue thrust
	Facial twitches
	Averted glaze
	Low level alertness
	Eyes closed
State	Crying and fussing
	Abrupt change to sleep or wake state

Pain Management

Pharmacological methods of pain relief with the use of analgesia are available and are used from birth using medications such as fentanyl, morphine and diamorphine. However, research into dosages and timings may not be entirely evidence based, meaning that dosage is to some degree a 'guestimate'. At the other end of the medication spectrum is the use of sucrose for analgesia properties. Stevens et al. (2004) undertook a systematic review of 44 studies and concluded that sucrose in varying doses decreased physiological and behavioural pain indicators when undergoing heel prick or venepuncture procedures. Other studies report on similar effects with breast milk or non-nutritive sucking. Whichever medication or other substance is used as analgesia, it is important to reassess its effectiveness in addition to the initial assessment.

Monitoring and Deterioration

The needs of the neonatal patient determine the amount of monitoring that would be required. The use of monitoring equipment can be noisy and cause the baby stress. The purpose of monitoring is to continually assess the vital signs and detect early signs of deterioration. These are generally recorded at intervals in the

baby's care plan according to guidance from the NMC (2009). For some time children's nursing has been using early warning tools. The development of a neonatal early warning tool may facilitate earlier detection of deterioration and, together with the SBAR system, may result in timely reviews and interventions (see Chapter 1 and Research Note 9.1).

CARE ENVIRONMENT

The types of noise a neonate hears changes from being in the uterus and hearing soothing, rhythmic sounds of the mother's heartbeat. The baby has become accustomed to and wants to hear the one mother voice that they recognise from being in the womb, yet this is 'lost' among the other rhythmic, often painful sounds, from medical devices and their alarms. Muffled sounds of conversational voices become much louder with professionals trying to sustain life through interventions and professional conversations.

At birth, noises present themselves in two ways: pitch/frequency and loudness/decibels (Boxwell 2010). The sounds present in a more exacerbated form than those the baby hears in the uterus and these become a source of distress for the baby. The baby is not able to habituate or self-console and this can then compound her stress levels (Brazelton 1973, 1995;

Date/time						
Crying – Characteristic cry of pain is high pitched 0 - No cry or cry that is not high pitched 1 - Cry high pitched but baby is easily consolable 2 - Cry high pitched but baby is inconsolable						
Requires O$_2$ for SaO$_2$ < 95% – Babies experiencing pain manifest decreased oxygenation. Consider other causes of hypoxaemia, e.g., oversedation, atelectasis, pneumothorax 0 - No oxygen required 1 - < 30% oxygen required 2 - > 30% oxygen required						
Increased vital signs (BP* and HR*) – take BP last as this may awaken child making other assessments difficult 0 - Both HR and BP unchanged or less than baseline 1 - HR or BP increased but increase is < 20% of baseline 2 - HR or BP is increased > 20% over baseline						
Expression – The facial expression most often associated with pain is a grimace. A grimace may be characterised by brow lowering, eyes squeezed shut, deepening naso-labial furrow, or open lips and mouth 0 - No grimace present 1 - Grimace alone is present 2 - Grimace and non-cry vocalisation grunt is present						
Sleepless – Scores based on the infant's state during the hour preceding this recorded score 0 - Child has been continuously asleep 1 - Child has awakened at frequent intervals 2 - Child has been awake constantly						
Total score						

Figure 9.19 CRIES

	Date/time						
Face 0 – No particular expression or smile 1 – Occasional grimace or frown, withdrawn, disinterested 2 – Frequent to constant quivering chin, clenched jaw							
Legs 0 – Normal position or relaxed 1 – Uneasy, restless, tense 2 – Kicking or legs drawn up							
Activity 0 – Lying quietly, normal position, moves easily 1 – Squirming, shifting back and forth, tense 2 – Arched, rigid or jerking							
Cry 0 – No cry (awake or asleep) 1 – Moans or whimpers; occasional complaint 2 – Crying steadily, screams or sobs, frequent complaints							
Consolability 0 – Content, relaxed 1 – Reassured by occasional touching, hugging or being talked to, distractible 2 – Difficult to console or comfort							
Total score							

Figure 9.20 FLACC

RESEARCH NOTE 9.1   Development of a neonatal early warning tool (Roland et al. 2010)

Early warning tools have been accepted in both adult and children's nursing as a means of identifying early indicators of potential acute deterioration and subsequent transfer babies. The early warning tool is based on physiological observations that trigger a medical review. It is a way of quantifying the baby's condition in a succinct and meaningful way. As far as the authors are aware there is no other similar neonatal warning tool. The early warning tool was used with three risk factor groups.

Prenatal:
- pathological cardiograph
- scalp pH < 7
- group B strep risk
- prolonged rupture of membranes (maternal).

Perinatal:
- thick meconium
- venous cord pH 7.1
- ventilatory support > 3 mins
- five min Apgar < 8.

Postnatal:
- grunting
- abnormal movements
- any ongoing concerns
- at the request of reviewing medical or neonatal staff.

There were two studies undertaken. Parameters drawn from key texts and there was some degree of success using the tool. A retrospective review of observations of babies were audited from NNU to compare key observations with proposed early warning tool criteria to determine whether assessment against these criteria could have altered management. A prospective study of babies at risk at a network neonatal intensive care unit was used. The tool was developed as risk stratification measures and used a 'traffic light' presentation to the chart, however budgetary restraints compromised the traffic light coding by use of grey scale. The authors indicate that more work was needed and that the tool did prompt earlier review of those demonstrating signs of deterioration.

Als 1982). Philbin and Evans (2006) also identify that noise levels should be controlled to provide freedom from intrusive noise and protect the baby's sleep. It is vital that neonatal staff develop awareness in minimising noise levels from day-to-day activities. Darcy et al. (2007) recommend that neonatal staff advocate for decreased noise levels (see Figures 9.x and 9.21).

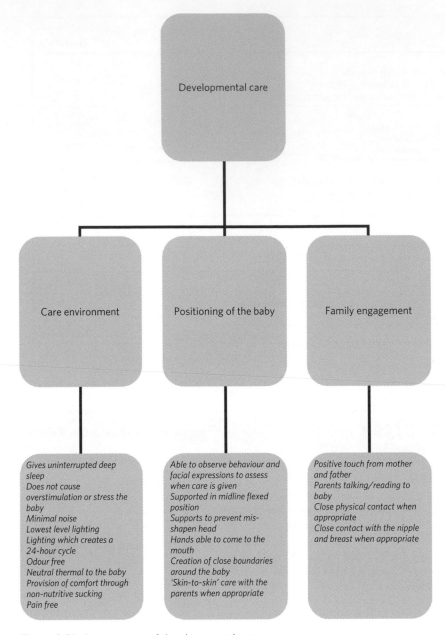

Figure 9.21 Components of developmental care

Light

In the womb, the baby is in a dark environment and at birth this changes and becomes extremely bright because of the need for a safe delivery and assessment of the baby (see Table 9.7). Box-well (2010) highlights that preterm infants are unable to block out stimulation, yet there needs to be a balance with adequate lighting to safely observe, monitor and safely intervene for care. Incubator covers help facilitate more control in the management of light.

Touch

In the womb, the baby is bathed in warm fluid creating a gentle environment: this is replaced with hard, painful, stress invoking touches (see Table 9.7). This situation can be exacerbated by

careless touch from misplaced lancets or misplaced tubing becoming entwined in the baby's environment. These interventions are not the mother's touch and positive touch from the mother is very important in comforting the baby. Preterm babies do not always find touch a pleasant stimulus and to the end minimal handling is employed as a principle of care. Human nature finds it a challenge to observe this process and attempts should be made to arrange care interventions around the work of other health professionals.

Infection Control

Infection control is a key principle in maintaining a safe environment for preterm infants due to their immature immune systems. It is crucial that all steps are taken to comply with infection control policies and guidelines and reduce the risk of infection. Preterm babies are also at risk of infection from the mother and the care environment.

POSITIONING OF THE BABY

Positioning

Before birth, the baby's position is maintained in a tight space where there is little room for movement. After birth, neonatal staff need to facilitate the neonate in maintaining a flexed position. This can be done by placing boundaries around the baby that enable the baby to self-comfort. Boundaries can also be used to support equipment around the baby (see Table 9.7 and Figures 9.22, 9.23 and 9.24).

Family Engagement

Each mother has a unique smell, which the baby will begin to recognize as an important caregiver, therefore it essential that there is positive touch from mother and father to make contrast to the unpleasant stimuli of care interventions and unpleasant experiences around the mouth and nose through forms of ventilatory support. Parents should also be encouraged to engage in talking/reading to the baby and having close physical contact when appropriate (see Table 9.7 and Figure 9.21). Communicating with the preverbal baby and engaging the family in normative play activities provides stimulation for the baby. Parents can also be taught how to use distraction techniques for procedures such as X-ray or phlebotomy.

Parents can communicate with their baby through skin-to-skin care. This will also enable parents the opportunity for natural conversations and singing nursery rhymes, which they may have been naturally engaging with if their baby had been born at term. Kenner and McGrath (2004) suggest that smooth communication between parent and baby serves to maintain parental competence in care and protection for their baby, and additionally the baby learns to build trust and regulate his emotions. McFadyen (1994) highlights that babies can 'actively contribute' and 'initiate interactions' and respond to contacts made with them thus encouraging reciprocal bonding and attachment. Skin-to-skin contact through holding the baby close to a parent's chest in 'kangaroo care' and positive touch of infant massage will facilitate opportunities for bonding and

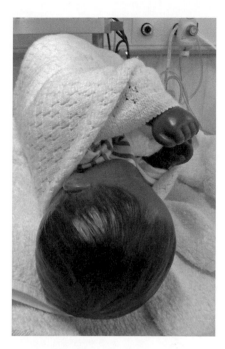

Figure 9.23 Manikin from skills labs showing position for self-consolation

attachment (see Figure 9.24). Containment is placing a hand on the baby's crown and/or rump so he feels secure. All aspects of developmental care can be included when planning care to facilitate on going care and management (see Figure 9.25).

ACTIVITY 9.3 Kangaroo care

Watch the YouTube clip of a premature baby, born much earlier than Jacob and note key points (**http://www.youtube.com/watch?feature=endscreen&v=jYann2Wnoac&NR=1**).

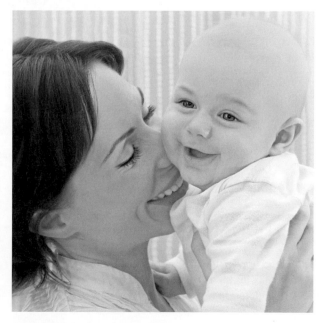

Figure 9.24 Kangaroo care

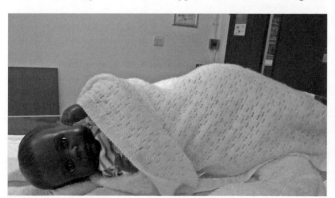

Figure 9.22 Demonstrating swaddling using a manikin

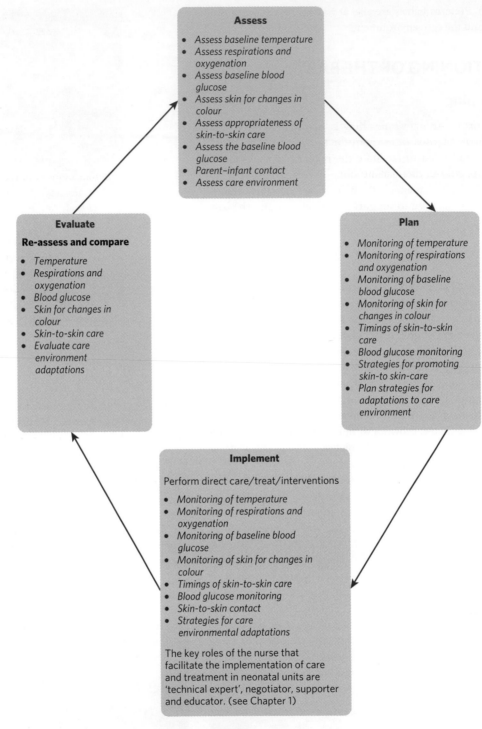

Figure 9.25 Nursing/clinical process for Jacob

NUTRITIONAL MANAGEMENT

When babies are unable to feed due to their prematurity and respiratory status then the doctors may prescribe total parenteral nutrition (TPN) until the baby can receive enteral feeding.

Breastfeeding is recommended for the preterm baby and mothers are encouraged to express their breast milk. There is thirst-quenching milk, the foremilk, and hind milk, which satisfies hunger. The WHO baby-friendly initiative (2011) promotes breastfeeding strategies in hospital. Mothers will want to do the best for their baby but the choice to breastfeed should be made by them with informed consent and not through coercion.

ACTIVITY 9.4 Breastfeeding

Breastfeeding is recommended for all babies and has particular benefits for preterm babies. Watch the YouTube clip and make a list of the benefits of breastfeeding for preterm infants (**http://www.youtube.com/watch?v=w4 GKpxEvfWk&feature=relmfu**).

Tube Feeding

Due to prematurity, the baby may not be able to suckle from a breast or bottle and may require feeding via a nasogastric tube. Although this looks a simple task, there are some complex issues related to the procedure such a placing the tube, testing position prior to feeding and risk of aspiration into the lungs should the tube become misplaced. Parents can be taught to tube feed their baby in the organisation's policies permit and follow a planned programme of teaching.

Cup Feeding

Due to breastfeeding using different mouth movements to suck from the breast than through artificial feeding, cup feeding is a recommended strategy as babies move on to more independent feeding. Babies need to be in a well-supported upright position with the cup being placed to the lips. The baby will use the tongue

---

ACTIVITY 9.5 Cup feeding

Watch the YouTube clip following the link and then list the instruction points for cup feeding (**http://www.youtube.com/watch?v=fXatck_YTLg**).

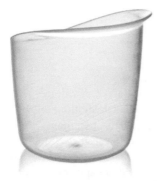

Figure 9.26 Cup

to 'lap' the milk. The cups have been designed with rounded edges to protect the delicate gums of the baby (see Figure 9.26).

Jaundice

Physiological Jaundice

Thurlby (2007) identifies that all babies undergo changes within the blood, leading to the breakdown of bilirubin and that this can affect 40 to 50 per cent of term infants and approximately 80 per cent of preterm babies. This is because, in uterine life, the fetus has a higher number of red blood cells to facilitate the transport of oxygen through the fetal circulation to the tissues. Red cells have a lifespan of approximately 120 days, yet, in the fetus, the red blood cells have a shorter lifespan of 80 to 100 days and the cells that need to be destroyed (Brophy and Barrow 2006). The oxygen is transported around the body in the haemoglobin part of the red blood cell.

Physiological jaundice typically appears on the third day after birth and refers to natural cause and process blood cells' lifecycle. Jaundice means 'yellow', therefore, one of the early signs babies with physiological jaundice can display is a yellow colouration to the skin and, in some cases, it can also affect the sclera of the eyes (Moules and Ramsay 2008). This is due to higher levels of bilirubin in the bloodstream (hyperbilirubinaemia). After birth, the baby has more red blood cells than are required by the body and the red blood cells are broken down. As the red blood cells break down, the haemoglobin breaks down into haemoglobin. The haem part contains iron and is stored by the body or used to make more red blood cells and the globin part is a protein that can be used by the body. The unconjugated (indirect) bilirubin needs albumin-binding sites and is in an insoluble state.

The unconjugated bilirubin is transported to the liver for a detoxification process or for unconjugating on albumin-binding sites carried in the plasma (Brophy and Barrow 2006). In the liver, the action of glycoronyl transferase changes the bilirubin into conjugated (direct) bilirubin with glucoronide acid (Thurlby 2008; Williamson and Crozier 2008). The conjugated (direct) bilirubin glucoronide can then be transferred into the bile. Following the detoxification process, the conjugated (direct) bilirubin gluconoride can be excreted in faeces as stercobilin or excreted in urine as urobilinogen (Skinner 2008; Williamson and Crozier 2008) (see Figure 9.27). There may be insufficient binding sites to cope with the unconjugated bilirubin, therefore alternative storage needs to be found in the skin (Brophy and Barrow 2006). There is, however, limited capacity in the skin for unconjugated bilirubin storage. If the liver is unable to metabolise the bilirubin, it can become free flowing and is able to pass the blood–brain barrier, causing a rare condition called kernicterus.

Physiological jaundice can be delayed or overloaded due to:

● mechanisms to facilitate the metabolism of bilirubin
● passing meconium
● prematurity
● underlying condition or disease.

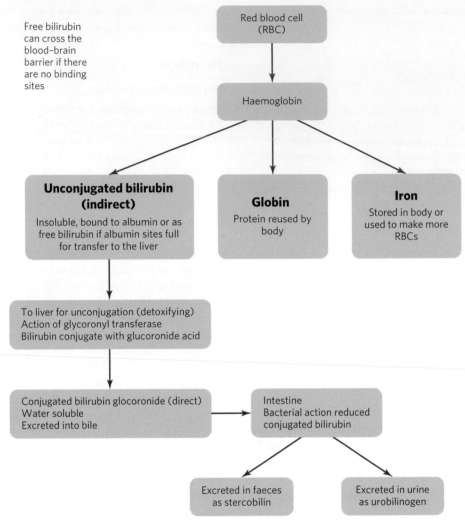

Free bilirubin can cross the blood–brain barrier if there are no binding sites

Red blood cell (RBC)

Haemoglobin

Unconjugated bilirubin (indirect)
Insoluble, bound to albumin or as free bilirubin if albumin sites full for transfer to the liver

Globin
Protein reused by body

Iron
Stored in body or used to make more RBCs

To liver for unconjugation (detoxifying)
Action of glycoronyl transferase
Bilirubin conjugate with glucoronide acid

Conjugated bilirubin glocoronide (direct)
Water soluble
Excreted into bile

Intestine
Bacterial action reduced conjugated bilirubin

Excreted in faeces as stercobilin

Excreted in urine as urobilinogen

Figure 9.27 Red cell breakdown
Source: adapted from Thurlby (2007), Moules and Ramsay (2008) and Williamson and Crozier (2008)

PRACTICAL GUIDELINES 9.4

Taking capillary blood for serum bilirubin assay will estimate the levels of bilirubin present in the blood and will prompt decisions about the management of the baby presenting with jaundice. It is crucial that blood sampling occurs from particular areas of the foot in order to protect the underlying structures and to prevent complications such as osteomyelitis from introducing infection from the lancet to the calcanous bone (see Figure 9.28).

Care and Management of Physiological Jaundice

It is usually the first appearance of a yellowish colouration of the skin that prompts thoughts about the presence of physiological jaundice. The timing of the first appearance of the condition will alert healthcare professionals to other potential causes. Family history and history of the birth may also give insight into any increased risk for the neonate.

The aim of the treatment is to prevent kernicterus and monitor the levels of bilirubin over a period of time. The baby will require an adequate intake of calories and may require additional water to prevent dehydration. Bilirubin is also light soluble, therefore, using light treatments to help maintain serum bilirubin within safe levels is useful. Phototherapy continues to be an effective treatment. Being nursed under lights will mean being nursed with a nappy on and no other clothes. Strong lights can damage the baby's eyes and therefore, it is crucial to ensure the baby wears eye protection to prevent retinal damage.

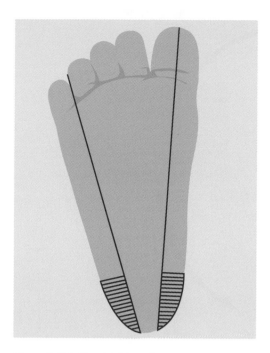

Figure 9.28 Blood-taking sites

(NICE 2010). Occasionally, babies require phototherapy from more than one source, which could be two conventional phototherapy units or a combination of conventional phototherapy and fibre optic phototherapy (NICE 2010). While an essential treatment, phototherapy can look intrusive and give the impression that the baby is uncomfortable. Phototherapy can also cause the baby to develop some spots due to local histamine response (Watson 2007). Phototherapy can also cause loose green stools, which is due to decrease of bowel transit time. Extra fluids may be required to compensate for insensible water loss. This may cause the mother to feel anxious, therefore, it is important to give the parents explanations of the condition and the treatment. The serum bilirubin levels usually return to acceptable tolerances requiring no further treatment by day 10 or 11 although it may be a fraction sooner (Figures 9.29 and 9.30).

If the serum bilirubin continues to rise above acceptable limits an exchange blood transfusion may be required. NICE (2010) describes this procedure which involves slowly removing the baby's blood and replacing it with fresh donor blood. This is not considered to be a regular treatment option as most babies respond to the earlier steps.

Pathological Jaundice

There are many other causes of jaundice, which can arise from high levels of bilirubin production, poor bilirubin metabolism, poor excretion of conjugated bilirubin and breast milk jaundice.

Being nursed without clothing on means that the baby is at risk of an unstable temperature and careful monitoring of the baby's temperature is required. Phototherapy treatment should continue until the serum bilirubin levels are below the treatment line in accordance with operation policies and guidelines

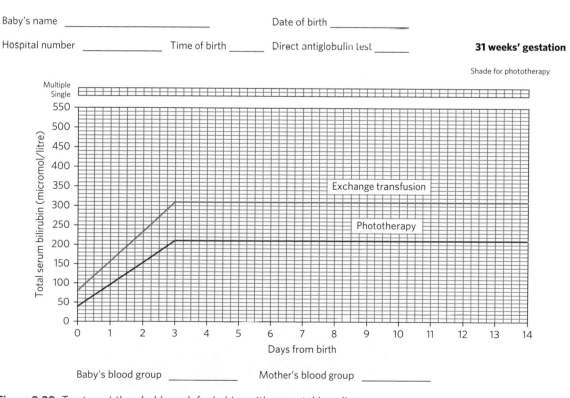

Figure 9.29 Treatment threshold graph for babies with neonatal jaundice
Source: NICE (2010)

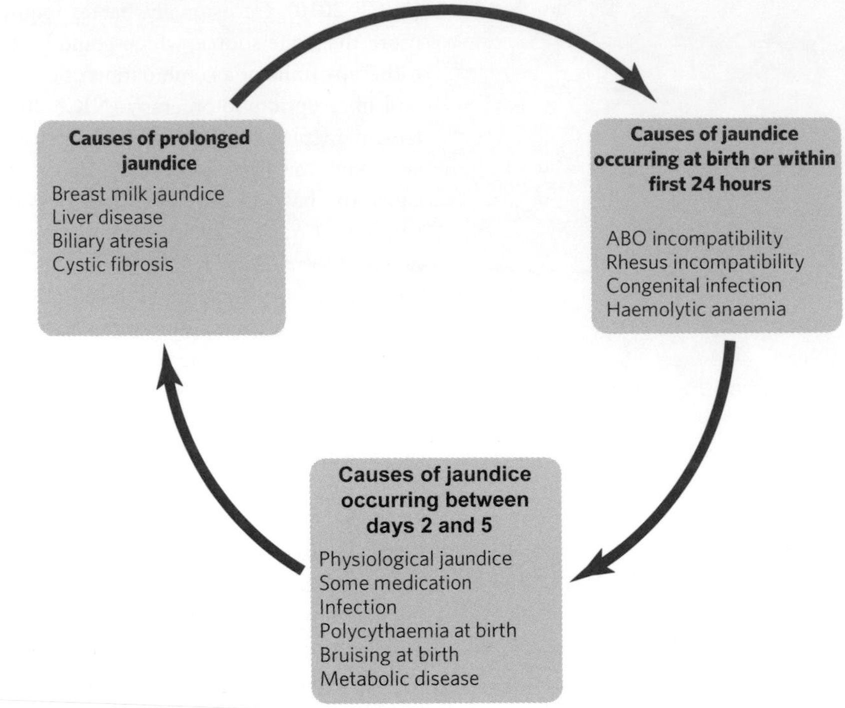

Causes of prolonged jaundice

Breast milk jaundice
Liver disease
Biliary atresia
Cystic fibrosis

Causes of jaundice occurring at birth or within first 24 hours

ABO incompatibility
Rhesus incompatibility
Congenital infection
Haemolytic anaemia

Causes of jaundice occurring between days 2 and 5

Physiological jaundice
Some medication
Infection
Polycythaemia at birth
Bruising at birth
Metabolic disease

Figure 9.30 Timeline of jaundice

Parents/baby

Medical and nursing staff

Unit and trust organisation

Figure 9.31 POPPY model of family at the centre of care

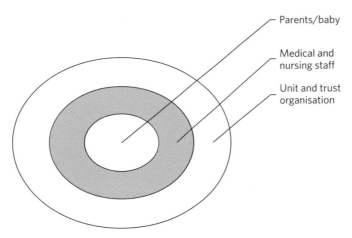

	In the hours after birth	Participating in adaptations to nursing their baby	Managing increasing care activities as the baby's condition improves	
Nurse led	Involvement	Participation	Partnership	Parent/child led
Nurse led	Nurse led	Nurse led	Equal status	Parent/child led

Figure 9.32 Interprofessional levels of family-centred care

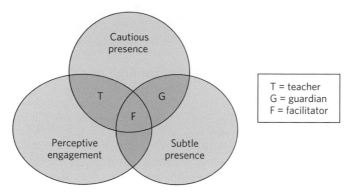

Figure 9.33 Model of negotiated partnership

Family-Centred Care

There is no one single definition of family-centred care and over 60 years many authors have considered ways of defining its meaning. Family-centred care has produced debates related to the need for further concerted research or has opened debates whether child-centred care should reframe ideas (Chapter 1). The POPPY Report identifies a parent pathway (see Figure 9.31) that identifies parents and the single unit at the centre of care and medical and nursing staff surrounding it. In a third layer, the unit and trust organisation surround the other two layers.

Family-centred care is seen as beginning prebirth and continuing through to home care if required. There are similarities between the model arising from the POPPY Report and the ideas of Smith et al. (2010, page 72) related to interprofessional levels of family-centred care (see Figure 9.32). It could be seen that both models work in conjunction with the other as dependency on the neonatal team decreases and the family takes a more active role in choices in the baby's care.

Research into family-centred care has explored the needs of both parents. Fathers need to bond with their baby as well as the mother (see Research Notes 9.2 and 9.3). Fegran et al. (2008) highlighted that a large proportion of literature focuses on the connections between mother and child, seeing the fathers' role as 'supportive and peripheral', and undertook research to consider the views of both fathers and mothers. The results from the research indicated that premature birth had created

---

RESEARCH NOTE 9.2 POPPY steering Group (2009)

POPPY was a collaborative 3-year research project that focused on effective interventions for communication, information and support. The report is divided into two parts: a summary of the findings from three linked research studies; and the model of family-centred care developed from the POPPY Project, which drew from the research findings and practical indicators for family-centred care. It is not possible to give an overview of this lengthy research report here, but we would recommend accessing the report for personal reading. Instead, this consideration focuses on one section related to family-centred care issues of communication, support and within the neonatal unit throughout the baby and parents journey through their neonatal experiences and journey.

Prenatal considerations

If a high-risk pregnancy is diagnosed, the recommendations are related to providing information to parents: in order for the parents to be able to prepare, they should be offered a tour of the neonatal unit.

1. Provide information on 'a day-at-a-time basis' –
   - prioritise information order
   - staff to be sensitive to behavioural cues
   - infant development and behaviour
   - caring for the baby.
2. Supporting parents with –
   - kangaroo care
   - baby massage
   - breastfeeding.
3. Introduce individualised development and care programmes.
4. Set up and refer to support groups.
5. Improving communication –
   - recording or providing parents with written information of consultations with doctors.
6. Offer stress education programmes.
7. Teach parents –
   - behavioural cues
   - development.
8. Discharge planning programme.
9. Structured homecare programme.

RESEARCH NOTE 9.3

Developing nurse–parent relationships in the NICU through negotiated partnership

(Reis et al. 2010)

The team explored parents' experience and satisfaction with care in the neonatal intensive care unit. The qualitative design used an interpretive descriptive method in a tertiary-level care 69-bed NICU. There were 10 parents (nine mothers and one father) who were interviewed. Parents were interviewed in person or via telephone, either following or close to discharge. Interviews were recorded, transcribed and then analysed using an evolving coding guide. All parents indicated that the relationship they developed with the bedside nurse was the most significant factor affecting their satisfaction with their NICU experience; all parents described nursing actions of perceptive engagement, cautious guidance and subtle presence, which facilitated the development of this relationship. Further analysis of the data revealed that parents portrayed nurses in an ideal nurse–parent interaction as fulfilling the roles of teacher, guardian and facilitator. Developing a collaborative and effective nurse–parent relationship is the most significant factor affecting parent's satisfaction with their NICU experience. Providing nursing care in a manner that optimises consistency and continuity of care facilitates the ability of both parties to develop this relationship.

ACTIVITY 9.6 Teaching planning

Imagine that Jacob was requiring more respiratory support from low-flow oxygen via nasal cannulae. Consider formulating a teaching programme considering all aspects of Jacob's care, which Ellie-Mae and Lloyd would need in order for this to occur.

a feeling of powerlessness for the mother with immediate feelings of being surreal and strange; the fathers experience birth as a shock but are ready to immediately engage with parenting (Fegran et al. 2008).

Family-centred care should be negotiated and put forward as a model of negotiated partnership. There are three overlapping elements: (1) cautious guidance; (2) subtle presence; and (3) perceptive engagement. There are also three roles of guardian, facilitator and teacher. When all these parts come together negotiated partnership is achieved (see Figure 9.33).

NEONATAL SCREENING

Babies who are born early may require oxygen to maintain adequate respiration. Oxygen is carefully monitored to ensure that oxygen delivery is according to the baby's needs. There may be a locally managed screening programme. Babies who have retinopathy of the newborn may be offered treatment according to the stage and progression of the damage.

Neonatal Blood Spot Screening

Early detection of long-term conditions that require lifestyle change will have a positive effect on any child's life, particularly if adjustments can be made to improve outcomes. The National Health Service (n.d. (a)) offers a screening programme to detect long-term conditions. In order for the blood spot screening to be effective, crucial timeframes must be adhered to. The blood spot screening programme provides an opportunity to screen all babies for five long-term conditions:

- phenylketonuria
- cystic fibrosis
- sickle cell disorders
- hypothyroidism
- medium chain acyl–CoA dehydrogenase deficiency (MCADD).

Newborn Hearing Screening

The National Health Service (n.d. (b)) provides newborn hearing screening for the early detection of hearing deficits. Hearing screening occurs in the first few weeks of life. Hearing deficits may impact on the development of the child. Early detection will lead to early treatment, care and management.

LONG-TERM OUTCOMES OF NEONATAL CARE

The long-term outcome for neonatal care is a baby who is in optimum health, going home with her family who will care for her as they would care for their children who did not need care in a neonatal unit. As excellent as the care and management may be for a preterm baby, there are potential long-term problems that can arise (see Table 9.12).

Table 9.12 Long-term problems: EPIcure 2

Cerebral palsy	20% chance of cerebral palsy compared with two to four per 1000 births
	Majority of the children with cerebral palsy have mild associated disability and attend mainstream school; 7% have severe associated problems
Learning difficulties	Two in three children require additional help at school
	Two in eight children will go to a special school
Behaviour problems	One in four children has behavioural problems: inattention seems a common problem
	Some children display autism-like symptoms, which is different from those who were not born prematurely
Chest problems	Extremely premature children have more respiratory and asthma related-issues than their peers. It is challenging for the lungs to reach full development
Growth	Growth is slower up to 6 years and height and weight catch up over later childhood
	Puberty is reached at same time as peers

CASE STUDY REVIEW 9.5 Family experiences throughout the neonatal journey

Ellie-Mae and Lloyd will have received support from the neonatal staff to enable them to begin to bond with Jacob. Parent–child attachment is crucial in establishing a relationship between them and that relationship will be pivotal throughout childhood. In addition to the care of Jacob, the needs of his parents must also be considered through the ethos of family-centred care and partnership. In order to achieve this, Ellie-Mae and Lloyd need to be in a position in which they have:

- established a therapeutic relationship with the neonatal staff

- bonded with Jacob
- begun to be involved with Jacob's care
- begun to feel empowered to participate in care
- felt able to negotiate which parts of care.

In time, Ellie-Mae and Lloyd may wish to share their experiences with other people such as service users locally or become involved with a charity such as Bliss or Tommy's to share their experiences with a larger and wider service user forum.

SUMMARY OF KEY LEARNING

The delivery of high-quality care is affected by the way in which neonatal care is organised and managed. The education and training of staff will facilitate the delivery of evidence-based care. There is a deficit of qualified nurses in the neonatal speciality, yet the specialism strives for quality care delivery and improving outcomes for babies requiring special, high-dependency, intensive or specialist care. Political systems are also in place to ensure that neonatal patients receive safe, evidence-based care through the work of NICE, National Patient Safety, MHRA and neonatal networks. Research is ongoing and researchers study all aspects of care. Research can be time and labour intensive, which adds to the cost. Research could be ad hoc and repetitive, yet there is clear evidence in the EPIcure 2 and POPPY studies that there has been a collaborative approach to neonatal research. Research has also taken place that acknowledges issues for the neonate and separate research that acknowledges the issues for parents.

FURTHER RESOURCES

Neonatal outcomes: **https://www.npeu.ox.ac.uk/neonatalnetwork**; **http://www.epicure.ac.uk/overview/survival/**

Bliss: **http://www.bliss.org.uk/**

Sands: **http://www.uk-sands.org/**

Tommy's: **http://www.uk-sands.org/**

Genetic screening: **http://www.geneticseducation.nhs.uk/about-us/resources.aspx**

Neonatal screening: **http://newbornbloodspot.screening.nhs.uk/bloodspotfilm**;**http://www.screening.nhs.uk/screening\#fileid7942**

Neonatal resuscitation: **http://www.resus.org.uk/pages/GL2010.pdf\#search=neonatal**

ANSWERS TO ACTIVITIES

ACTIVITY 9.1   Neonatal resuscitation guidelines

Access the neonatal resuscitation guidelines. Consider the differences in this algorithm to that for infants (see Figure 9.34).

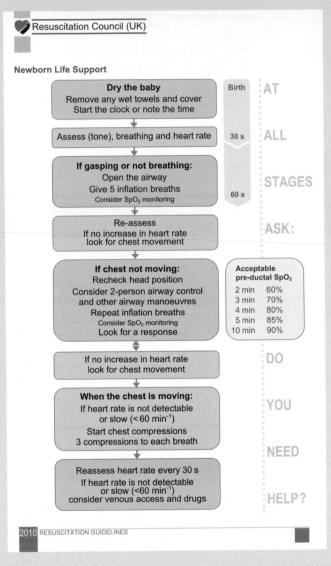

Figure 9.34   Neonatal resuscitation guidelines

ACTIVITY 9.2   Arterial blood gas (ABG) tic-tac-toe examples

Access arterial blood gas (ABG) tic-tac-toe examples (**http://www.youtube.com/watch?v=_OpvyEllFj8**).

The clip takes the viewer through interpretation of blood gas using a tic-tac-toe (naughts and crosses) system to determine if the results are acid, neutral or base (acidotic, normal or alkaline).

Acid	Base
7.35 = acidosis	7.45 = alkalosis

ACTIVITY 9.3 Kangaroo care

Watch the YouTube clip of a premature baby, born much earlier than Jacob and note key points (**http://www.youtube.com/watch?feature=endscreen&v=jYann2Wnoac&NR=1**)
Good explanations to mum
Hand hygiene

Reassurance
Positioning
Mum likes the closeness with her baby

ACTIVITY 9.4

Sit baby upright.
Support baby well.
Place a towel around the baby.
Place cup to lower lip.

Tip until the milk touches the tongue.
Do not pour.
Baby will control the flow of the milk.
Baby will decide when meal is completed.

ACTIVITY 9.5 Cup feeding

Watch the YouTube clip following the link and then list the instruction points for cup feeding (**http://www.youtube.com/watch?v=fXatck_YTLg**).
Sit baby upright
Support baby well
Place a towel around the baby

Place cup to lower lip
Tip until the milk touches the tongue
Do not pour
Baby will control the flow of the milk
Baby will decide when meal is completed

ACTIVITY 9.6 Teaching planning

Imagine that Jacob was requiring more respiratory support from low-flow oxygen via nasal cannulae. Consider formulating a teaching programme considering all aspects of Jacob's care, which Ellie-Mae and Lloyd would need in order for this to occur.
Basic life support resuscitation teaching

Suctioning
Applying pulse oximetry for night time use occasionally
Replacing oxygen cylinders
Danger of oxygen in the home
Contact insurers regarding oxygen in the home
Contact fire brigade

SELECTED REFERENCES

Armstrong, E.K., Ball, A.L. and Leatherbarrow, J. (2012) Constructing a programme of change to improve the provision of family-centred developmental care on a neonatal unit. *Infant*, 8(3), 86–90.

Ashworth, C. and Evans, J. (2003) Recruitment and retention in neonatal care – a collaborative solution to everybody's problem? The North West Neonatal Induction Programme. *Journal of Neonatal Nursing* 9(5), 168–172.

Barrett, D.H. (2003) Acid base balance and interpretation of blood gas results: **http://www,nda.ox.ac.uk/wfsa/html/u1602 01.htm**

Berg, A., Chavez, C. and Serpanos, Y. (2010) Monitoring noise levels in a tertiary neonatal intensive care unit: **http://web.ebscohost.com/ehost**

Bliss (n.d.) **www.bliss.org.uk**

Boxwell, G. (2010) *Neonatal intensive care nursing*. Routledge: London.

Boyd, C.A., Quigley, M.A. and Brockleurst, P. (2007) Donor breast milk versus infant formula for preterm infants: systematic review and meta-analysis: *Archive Diseases in Child Fetal Neonatal Ed*, 92, F169–F175.

Brazelton, T.B. (1995) *Neonatal behavioral assessment scale*, 3rd edn. MacKieth Press: London.

British Association of Perinatal Medicine (BAPM) (2001) *Standards for hospitals providing neonatal intensive and high-dependency care*, 2nd edn: **www.bapm.org**

British Association for Perinatal Medicine (BAPM) (2010) *Standards for hospitals providing neonatal intensive and high dependency care and categories of babies requiring neonatal care*, 2nd edn.

British Association of Perinatal Medicine (BAPM) (2011) Categories of care: **www.bapm.org**.

British Association of Perinatal Medicine (BAPM) (n.d.) **www.bapm.org/networks_info**

Cameron, J. and Cox, H. (1989) *Interpreting blood gas results*. London Hospital School of Midwifery: London.

Cooper, N. (2004) Acute care-arterial blood gases. *Student BMJ*, 12, March.

Darcy, A.E., Hancock, L.E., Ware, E.J. and Davies, J. (2007) Descriptive study of noise in the neonatal intensive care unit ambient levels and perceptions of contributing factors. *Advances in Neonatal Care*, 8(5S), S16–S26.

Davies, J. and Hassell, L. (2007) *Children in intensive care*, 2nd edn. Churchill Livingstone: London.

Department of Health (DoH) (2003) Neonatal intensive care services: report of the Department of Health expert working group – consultation. DOH: London.

Department of Health (DoH) (2004) National Service Framework for children, young people and maternity services. HMSO: London.

Department of Health (DoH) (2009) Toolkit for high-quality neonatal services. HMSO: London.

Department of Health (DoH) (2010) Essence of care, 2010: benchmarks for safety. TSO: Norwich.

Drage, S. and Wilkinson, D. (2001) Acid base balance. *Pharmacology*, 13,

Fegran, L., Helseth, S. and Solveig, M. (2008) A comparison of mothers' and fathers' experiences of the attachment process in a neonatal intensive care unit. *Journal of Clinical Nursing*, 17, 810–816.

Fenton, A. and Leslie, A. (2011) The state of neonatal transport services in the UK. *Arch Dis Child Fetal Neonatal Ed.*

Franck, L., Cox, S., Allen, A. and Winter, I. (2005) Measuring neonatal intensive care unit-related parental stress. *Journal of Advanced Nursing*, 49(6), 608–615.

Gale, C., Santhakumaran, S., Nagarajan, S., Statnikov, Y., Modi, N. and the Neonatal Data Analysis Unit and the Medicines for Neonates Investigator Group (2012) Impact of managed clinical networks on NHS specialist neonatal services in England: population based study. *BMJ*, 3(344).

Glasper, E.A., Mcewing, G. and Richardson, J. (2007) *Oxford handbook of children and young people's nursing*. Oxford University Press: Oxford.

Gray, J. and Goldmann, A. (2004) Medication errors in the neonatal intensive care unit: special patients, unique issues. *Perspective, Arch Dis Child Fetal Ed*, 89, F472–F473.

Gupta, M. et al. (2006) Regionalization of neonatal intensive care: past, present and future. *Neonatology*, 1(7).

House of Commons Select Committee (2012) 26th report: **http://www.publications.parliament.uk/pa/cm200708/cmselect/cmpubacc/390/39002.htm**

International Association for the Study of Pain (2005) Children's pain matters! Priority on pain in infants, children, and adolescents: a position statement from the special interest group: **http://iasp-pain.org/sigs.html**

Johnson, S., Fawke, J., Hennessy, E., Rowell, V., Thomas, S., Wolke, D. and Marlow, N. (2009) Neurodevelopmental disability through 11 years of age in children born before 26 weeks of gestation: **http://pediatrics.aappublications.org/content/124/2/e249.full.pdf+html**

Kenner, C. and McGrath, J. (2004) *Developmental care of newborns and infants: a guide for health professionals*. Mosby: St. Louis, IL.

Lissauer, T. and Fanaroff, A. (2006) *Neonatology at a glance*. Wiley: Chichester.

Lynch, F. (2009) Arterial blood gas analysis: implications for nursing. *Paediatric Nursing*.

McFadyen, A. (1994) *Special care babies and their developing relationships*. Routledge: London.

Marlow, N. and Gill, B. (2007) Establishing neonatal networks: the reality. *Archives of Diseases in Childhood – Fetal and Neonatal Edition*, 92, F137–F142.

Milligan, D.W., Carruthers, P., Mackley, B., Ward Platt, M.P., Collingwood, Y., Wooler, L., Gibbons, J., Draper, E. and Manktelow, B.N. (2008) Nursing workload in UK tertiary neonatal units. *Archives of Diseases in Childhood*, 93(12), 1059–1064.

National Audit Office (2007) *Caring for vulnerable babies: the reorganisation of neonatal services in England*. NAO: London.

National Health Service (NHS) (n.d. (a)) Blood spot screening programme: **http://newbornbloodspot.screening.nhs.uk/**

National Health Service (NHS) (n.d. (b)) Newborn hearing screening programme, **http://hearing.screening.nhs.uk/5million**

National Institute for Clinical Excellence (NICE) (2009) Neonatal jaundice CG98: **http://guidance.nice.org.uk/CG98/Guidance/pdf/English**

National Institute for Clinical Excellence (NICE) (2010) Quality standards for neonatal care: **http://www.nice.org.uk/media/17A/A8/SpecialistNeonatalQualityStandardRevisedOct10.pdf**

Nursing and Midwifery Council (NMC) (2009) *Record keeping guidance for nurses and midwives*. NMC: London.

Oughton, J. (2010) Extravasation of neonates revisited, National Patient Safety Agency: signals: **http://www.nrls.npsa.nhs.uk/resources/type/signals/?entryid45=66756**

Philbin, M.K. and Evans, J.B. (2006) Standards for the acoustic environment of the newborn ICU. *Journal of Perinatology*, 26, S27–S30.

POPPY Steering Group (2009) *Family-centred care in neonatal units. A summary of research results and recommendations from the POPPY Project*. NCT: London.

Reason, J. (2000) Human error: models and management, *BMJ*, 320.

Reis, M.D., Rempel, G.R., Brady-Fryer, S.D. and Van Arde, J. (2010) Developing nurse/parent relationships in the NICU through negotiated partnership. *JOGNN, AWHONN*, 39(6), 675–683.

Robertson, N.R.C. (1993) A manual of neonatal intensive care, 3rd edn. Hodder & Stoughton: London.

Roland, D., Madar, J. and Connolly, G. (2010) The newborn early warning (NEW) system: development of an at-risk infant intervention system. *Infant*, 6(4), 116–120.

Royal College of Paediatrics and Child Health (RCPCH) (2012) Bringing networks to life: an RCPCH guide to implementing clinical networks: **www.rcpch.ac.uk/.../Bringing%20Networks%20to%20Life**

Royal College of Paediatrics and Child Health (RCPCH) (n.d.) National neonatal audit program: **www.rcpch.ac.uk/child-health/standards...nnap/national-neonatal**

Skinner, S. (2008) Care of the sick and preterm newborn, in T. Moules and J. Ramsay (eds) (2008) *The textbook of children's and young people's nursing*, 2nd edn. Blackwell Publishing: Oxford.

Smith, L., Coleman, V. and Bradshaw, M. (2010) *Child and family-centred healthcare: concept, theory and practice*. Palgrave: Basingstoke.

Sparshott, M. (1997) *Pain, distress and the newborn infant.* Blackwell Science: Oxford.

Stevens, B., Yamada, J. and Ohlsson, A. (2004) Sucrose for analgesia in newborn infants undergoing painful procedures. *Cochrane Database of Systematic Reviews*, 3.

Taddio, A., Shah, V., Atenafu, E. and Katz, J. (2009) Influence of repeated painful procedures and sucrose analgesia in the development of hyperalgesia in newborn infants. *International Association for the study of Pain*, 43–48.

Tommy's (n.d.) **http://www.epicure.ac.uk/overview/survival/**

Vincent, C. (2010) *Patient safety*, 2nd edn. Wiley-Blackwell: Chichester.

Williamsom, A. and Crozier, K. (2008) *Neontal care: a textbook for student midwives and nurses*. Reflect Press: Exeter.

Woodrow, P. (2004) Arterial blood gas analysis. *Nursing Standard*, 18(21), 45–52.

World Health Organization (WHO) (2010) The worldwide incidence of preterm birth: a systematic review of maternal mortality and morbidity: **http://www.who.int/bulletin/volumes/88/1/08-062554/en/index.html**

World Health Organization (WHO) (2011) Exclusive breastfeeding for six months best for babies everywhere: **http://www.euro.who.int/en/what-we-do/health-topics/Life-stages/child-and-adolescent-health/news/news/2011/01/exclusive-breastfeeding-for-six-months-best-for-babies-everywhere**

CHAPTER 10
Emergency Care of Children and Young People

Carolyn Seeman and Joanne Outridge

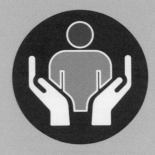
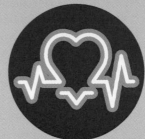
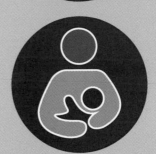

LEARNING OUTCOMES

On completion of this chapter, the reader will be able to:

- Discuss the use of a structured approach to assessing children and young people with emergency care needs.
- Outline the appropriate interventions in managing the care needs of the deteriorating child or young person.
- Identify key individuals involved in the care of the child or young person who presents with emergency care needs, recognising the importance of communication throughout the patient's journey.
- Analyse the impact that acute/stressful situations may have on the family of a child or young person who is receiving emergency care.

TALKING POINT

In reality, how many of these standards are met in the emergency setting where children are admitted? Standards for Children and Young People in Emergency Care Settings:

- Initial clinical assessment occurs within 15 minutes of arrival.
- At least one clinical cubicle or trolley space is designated for use by children for every 5,000 annual child attendances.
- Emergency departments seeing more than 16,000 children a year employ a consultant with sub-speciality training in paediatric emergency medicine.
- All staff in emergency care settings are able to access child protection advice 24 hours a day from a paediatrician with child protection expertise.
- All emergency departments receiving children have a lead registered children's nurse and sufficient registered children's nurses to provide one per shift.

(Continued)

TALKING POINT (CONTINUED)

- Emergency clinicians with responsibility for the care of children and young people receive training in how to assess and manage their mental health needs and support their family/carers.
- Regional critical care networks are in place to develop protocols to stabilise and transfer children to specialist centres.
- Injury surveillance data is collected and accessible as appropriate.
- All emergency care attendances by children and young people are notified to the primary care team (GP and school nurse/health visitor).

Standards for Children and Young People in Emergency Care Settings Developed by the Intercollegiate Committee for Standards for Children and Young People in Emergency Care Settings (2012)

www.rcpch.ac.uk/emergencycare

INTRODUCTION

Waking up from a nightmare, heart pounding, sweating profusely and dreading the forthcoming shift on the children's ward. As you make that strong cup of coffee you recall your dream. You are called into the cubicle, your mentor is shouting instructions at you in a language you do not understand and a woman is pulling your uniform, begging you to 'do something'! But your feet appear to be glued to the floor.

Recognise the scenario? It is very common to feel concern that, when faced with an emergency situation, you will not know exactly what to do. However, understanding the care of the child who requires emergency care and intervention is crucially important for all children's nurses. Within contemporary society sick children are no longer only nursed in the hospital setting but their care spans the primary, secondary and tertiary centres within the healthcare environment (and all the spaces in between!). Therefore it is imperative that children's nurses have the right skills and tools for the job and are able to respond in an appropriate manner when a child or young person requires emergency care.

For many healthcare professionals, children are often perceived as being more challenging to manage in an emergency due to the very nature of being a child (Davies 2011). However,

once these challenges are faced and understood, it becomes clear that a systematic approach to assessment, timely intervention and good communication with appropriate professionals will assist all those caring for children to deliver effective care and management for patients who are deteriorating or who need immediate intervention. The assessment processes will be discussed in more detail further on. This chapter aims to equip nurses with the essential tools that are required to enable safe and sound assessments and initiate interventions to care for these sick children. The aim is to explore some of the objectives using a case study approach, following the journey of a child assisting identification of the factors to consider when caring for any child who may deteriorate.

EMERGENCY SETTINGS

Where do emergencies occur? Often it is assumed that these are only within the hospital setting, however, when caring for children and young people the only certainty is that they can be unpredictable. Figure 10.1 illustrates the variety of settings in which emergencies can occur and in which children's nurses may care for these children and young people specifically.

CASE STUDY 10.1 William has an upper respiratory tract infection

William is 6 months old and lives with his mother, father and 7-year-old sister, Sophie. William has had symptoms of an upper respiratory tract infection for the last 3 days and Mum attends the GP surgery as William has been off his feeds and seems to be 'struggling' to breathe.

The GP refers William to the emergency department of the local district general hospital for further assessment and

William is admitted to the children's ward for supplementary oxygen and support with his feeding.

After 2 days as an inpatient, William deteriorates and suffers from a respiratory arrest. Following this, William requires mechanical ventilation and is transferred to a paediatric intensive care unit in a tertiary centre over 30 miles away.

Child or
young person

Primary
setting

Secondary
setting

Tertiary
setting

Figure 10.1 Where emergencies occur

When a child becomes seriously unwell within any of these settings, the management and the optimum outcome of care is dependent on all involved working closely together to form the complete picture of care. From birth to adulthood, children and young people are surrounded by carers and professionals, all of whom have a responsibility to ensure that the health needs of that individual are met (see Figure 10.2). The moment a baby arrives home from hospital, has her first immunisation, takes a first step and starts school, she is reliant on others to understand her needs. Throughout these first few years a child will come into contact with an array of professionals (as well as her parents), all of whom have a duty to ensure the child reaches her full health potential. All of this requires specific skills of observation, interpretation and communication. These are progressive skills and as such failure at any stage will affect the next.

It would be useful to consider an example: a child is observed to be unwell by their parent who interprets this as being concerning enough to seek help from a professional such as the GP. This concern has to be communicated to the GP who then has to observe the child, interpret the findings and communicate back to the parent or refer on. If referral takes place, then the

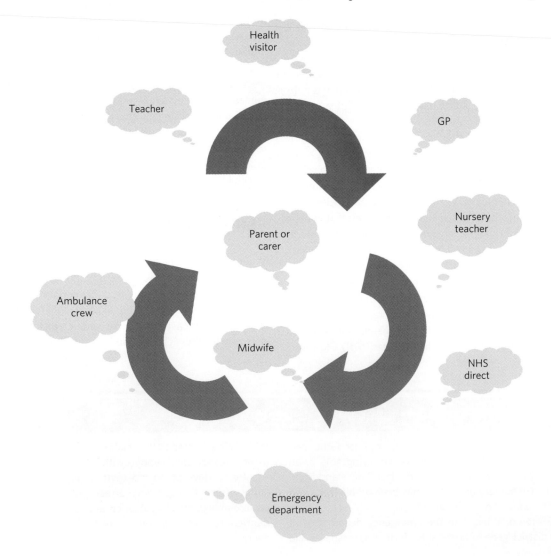

Figure 10.2 Common childhood contacts

observation and interpretation will need to be communicated accurately to the next professional. This is a continuous cycle; however, many voices and collaborations may have the potential to confuse the true picture. Therefore one of the key elements of becoming confident in caring for a child who is potentially becoming unwell is being able to focus on the child and communicate concerns confidently using a structured approach.

Within healthcare, children may often be seen as merely smaller versions of adults, however, this is not the case and as such their needs when seriously unwell are often of concern to professionals involved in their care. Harnden et al. (2009) considered the quality of primary care and noted that while there was a considerable amount of good practice at this level, avoidable factors were still present. This is supported by the Department of Health (DoH 2001) expert advisory group, which reported on high dependency care provision for children and young people. Within this report it is clear that children who are seriously ill or have the potential to become seriously ill, are cared for in places other than paediatric specialist areas and intensive care areas (see Figure 10.3). The local district general hospital will often be caring for children who fulfil the

categories described in the report and arguably some of these children will already have had contact with other professionals before reaching secondary care centres. Good communication and care from appropriately trained staff even within the primary sector will assist seamless care (Evans 2008).

Therefore it is imperative that children's nurses are aware of the role of each sector and professional group in an attempt to ensure a high quality of care delivery and more positive outcomes for children and young people.

It would be easy to assume that children who have high dependency needs are only found in designated high dependency areas of a hospital, however if the categories described by the DoH (2001) are explored in more detail it is clear that these children may present in any setting, even if they are in the first stages of illness. There have been several high-profile cases of situations where a delay in recognition of the seriousness of illness has resulted in loss of life.

Consider the following case as reported in a national newspaper (Hull 2010): **http://www.dailymail.co.uk/news /article-1258705/Boy-11-dies-asthma-attack-left-die-school-corridor.html**.

Medical Policies 'Inadequate'

MORE than one million British school-children – around one in ten – are affected by asthma.

Schools are supposed to have policies in place to ensure children with medical conditions receive proper treatment.

But Asthma UK a support group, says policies in too many schools are inadequate.

It is also demanding better training for teachers in handling asthma, both on teacher training courses and in schools themselves.

Training in dealing with pupils' asthma attacks should become a compulsory part of courses, it says.

Asthma UK also says the Government should make it mandatory for schools to have a clear policy on asthma, which would spell out schedules for staff training to

ensure teachers are aware of procedures to follow in the event of an attack.

It is currently recommended only that schools have a specific asthma policy.

In the wake of 11-year-old Sam Linton's death, Neil Churchill, chief executive of Asthma UK, said: 'This tragic event reinforces the urgent need for mandatory asthma training as part of teacher training, including ongoing assessment, and we will be pursuing this vital requirement with Governments across the UK.

'It also highlights how important it is that every school takes asthma seriously and has in place policies and procedures to deal with students with asthma.

'Schools should be safe environments and parents and carers should be able to feel confident leaving children with asthma in their care.'

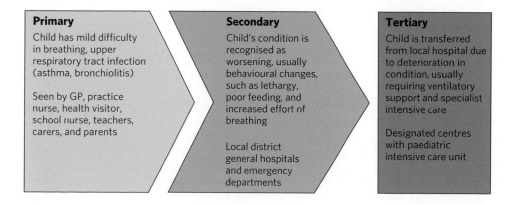

Figure 10.3 Primary, secondary and tertiary settings – example of child with respiratory problems

Although children with high dependency needs will eventually be placed within secondary and/or tertiary settings, all begin the journey at different stages demonstrating that potentially these children can be encountered both in the community as well as in hospitals (see Table 10.1).

In addition to the guidelines and policies available to inform management there is also firm evidence that early recognition of children who have serious illness or injury can improve outcomes. One of the key findings in the confidential enquiry into maternal and child health (CEMACH 2008) starkly entitled 'Why children die' was that of a failure of staff (both in the primary and the hospital setting) to recognise and act on the standards of care that would help this early detection of ensuing illness or deterioration of condition. Included in this were suggestions that staff failed to take sufficient care to observe and anticipate complications. Children's nurses are often those who deliver care regularly and consistently and need to take the responsibility to initiate, facilitate and at times coordinate

Table 10.1 High-dependency care and implications for primary, secondary and tertiary settings

Child or young person with	Potential in primary setting	Potential in secondary setting	Potential in tertiary setting
Prolonged seizure < 1 hour	Child seen within home or in remote rural areas Consider potential non-recognition of seizure or frequent shorter seizures with little respite in between episodes (possibly child with known seizure disorder)	May present in emergency department (ED) and/or on a general children's ward Consider the management of seizure, utilising all protocols and guidelines to prevent deterioration and development of status	Usually transferred when seizures are uncontrollable and/or child may need ventilatory support Neurological conditions or injury may result in complex and specialist intervention
Circulatory instability due to hypovolaemia resulting in the need for intravenous fluid resuscitation of > 10 mls/kg and < 30 mls/kg	This would begin in the community , for example childhood gastroenteritis	May present to ED following prolonged illness, such as diaorrhea and vomiting where parents or carers have been unable to manage oral rehydration Inpatients should be monitored with accurate fluid balance monitoring	Cardiac failure due to severe shock which has resulted in potential multi-organ failure May be septic, hypovolaemic, cardiogenic or neurogenic
Diabetic ketoacidosis with drowsiness	This could be encountered by GP, school teacher, community health carer in the primary setting	Usually presents in ED and is transferred to children's ward Child or young person will present with severe dehydration, altered blood gases and altered conscious level	Transferrred when stabilisation is not progressing and if child has altered physiology that is affecting ventilation and fluid management, resulting in multi-organ failure
Recurrent apnoeas	This presentation could be seen at GP surgery, by visiting midwife or health visitor/CCN who will need to recognise potential significance of this symptom	Any child on ward may develop apnoeic episodes as a result of impending deterioration or disease process, e.g. baby with whooping cough (pertussis) or any child who has had prolonged respiratory distress	Transferral required when apnoeic episodes are not resolving and the child requires ventilatory support
Upper airway obstruction – close observation	Children may present with croup or acute tonsillitis at the GP surgery/practice nurse	Child may be admitted for IV antibiotics or oxygen therapy as a result of continued illness, swelling and respiratory distress Important to observe for physiological effects of prolonged increased respiratory effort	Transferred for ventilatory support May require other circulatory support due to effects of prolonged respiratory compensation

Child or young person with	Potential in primary setting	Potential in secondary setting	Potential in tertiary setting
Asthma on IV drugs or hourly nebulisers	An acute asthma attack can be potentially life threatening A child may present at school, nursery or to the GP surgery/walk-in centres	Child may present to the ED and children's ward with moderate to severe respiratory distress Medications to treat asthma may have side-effects that can affect other systems (such as tachycardia) Close monitoring for signs that the child is beginning to decompensate and tire	Transferred for ventilatory support May require other circulatory support due to effects of prolonged respiratory compensation
Bone marrow transplant/severe neutropenia	Many children who are receiving oncology treatments are cared for primarily in the community While there is usually a direct admission policy through shared care, GP/CCN will be involved in the care and should be able to identify significant neutropenia and act appropriately	Child may be febrile and neutropenic due to their treatment. This can result in the child being at risk of developing severe sepsis and becoming very unwell Will need observation and interventions to prevent multi-system failure	Transferred for ventilatory and circulatory support and follow-up with shared care centre

Source: DoH (2001)

care for a child who is not improving, is causing concern or who presents with potentially life threatening symptoms or injuries.

PRIMARY CARE

William is initially seen in the primary setting by the GP (general practitioner). Within the primary setting there are a number of professionals who may potentially observe and assess a child long before a children's nurse. The Kennedy Review (DoH 2010) raised the issue that the UK death rate remains above that of the rest of the European Union and that, despite the volume of children who access primary care, there is still a lot of uncertainty in assessment and diagnosis that could go some way to proving this. In addition children attend pre-school nurseries, schools, after-school clubs, voluntary and leisure activities, which opens even more widely the context where other professionals and carers may engage with holistic care, including physical need. Therefore inability to adequately assess a child at any stage can contribute to an emergency situation and the individual who has the first point of contact with a child is significant in determining the final outcome (Cooper 2011; Pearson et al. 2011). Furthermore, it is not only recognising the illness but anticipating and recognising potential complications that are so important (Pearson et al. 2011). From

this we can conclude that training and developing overall good assessment is the key to improving outcomes within the primary care setting. This will be the first contact that William will have had with a healthcare professional so it is imperative that the assessment that the GP makes will accurately assess his need for referral. It may be that William has already had some contact with the telephone assessment team through NHS Direct. This service has been accessible in some areas of the UK since 1998 (Stewart et al. 2006). NHS Direct was a UK government initiative, healthcare telephone triage service that began operating in 1998 and there has been an increase in the number of families who access this form of advice (Aitken et al. 2003).

NHS Direct offers advice and support through discussion with a registered nurse aided by a computer program that links to what is described as 'algorithmic rules' by Smith (2010). In some ways, the algorithm acts as a systematic approach in assessing the urgency of the child's (or adult's) condition. In the early days of NHS Direct there were incidences when children were inappropriately or inaccurately assessed due to the system using adult-based parameters (Hall 2003). However, it could be argued that the assessment skill is more about the ability of the nurse and the parent/carer to adequately communicate than any other limitation. For example, the nurse must ask the most pertinent questions to gain knowledge to build the mental picture of the child and thus assess the condition. All this is reliant on the parent/carer being able to communicate and translate the mental picture of the child they have before them. This is seen by some to be problematic at times with some risk of an incorrect assessment (Hall 2003). Monaghan et al. (2003) carried out a study that considered NHS Direct in relation to assessment of children, identifying that 40 per cent of calls related to children. One of the conclusions from this was that this percentage should be reflected in the staffing with 40 per cent being specifically trained to deal with calls regarding child-specific concerns.

Assessing Children and Young People

Whoever is assessing William will need to have sufficient tools to be able to make an effective and reliable assessment. This applies whenever and wherever a child is being assessed but in particular it must be remembered that all children who are sick have the potential to deteriorate if subtle signs are not addressed early. There are some 'golden rules' to remember when considering any health professional's involvement in caring for children and young people. Most important of these is the individual's ability to thoroughly assess the child. In settings in which the admission is planned and thus the encounter is also planned, the assessment may appear to be less structured due to more time allocation. However, the very term 'emergency' implies that a quick response is necessary and time to respond may be limited. Having a very structured approach to assessment is vital in ensuring that every area is addressed and interventions are timely, reducing the risk of missing vital information that may lead to further damage (ALSG 2005). In fact, damage limitation may be the overriding factor in some cases when decisions made prior to emergency care settings (hospital) may not have been conducted using a structured approach.

The Resuscitation Council and the Advanced Life Support Group lead the way in formalising a structured approach to assessment and this is currently the basis of assessment of the seriously ill child within the UK healthcare system. One of the most structured approaches that is used across all settings is the ABCDE (Figure 10.4) assessment (Resuscitation Council 2010) and acts as a tool for all professionals who care for children.

While Table 10.2 provides a structured approach to assessing the acutely unwell child, this should be considered along with local PEWS (paediatric early warning scoring) systems and hospital guidelines for assessing children. Every child must also have his weight measured or estimated. Consider the safety of yourself and others and use of personal protective equipment.

During the physical assessment of William a systematic approach will aid the GP in giving a thorough and complete handover to the secondary receiving unit. When assessing any child it is important that the normal anatomy and physiology of each body system is understood as this will help in determining the severity of illness and therefore the risk of deterioration. The part of the child's body affected by the presenting complaint will have its normal functions disrupted, and this can lead to predictable signs and symptoms once the normal structure and function is understood. As discussed earlier when looking at the role of NHS Direct, this leads to a logical, algorithmic approach, ensuring that any treatment or management follows best practice guidelines, whether the setting is primary, secondary or tertiary. The ABCDE approach provides a quick assessment of the respiratory, circulatory, and neurological systems and any immediate environmental concerns.

Thorough assessment at the initial stages will provide vital information in addressing the emergency needs for William. As he progresses through the healthcare system he arrives at the secondary centre (usually a children's ward or assessment unit). Verbal and written communication between the referrer and the receiver can be crucial in aiding the health professionals to provide seamless care for William; it is vital that all health professionals 'speak the same language' and communicate clearly. However the importance of reassessment using the same ABCDE approach at this stage cannot be underestimated as the transition time from primary to secondary care may have an effect on the status of the child on arrival. Following his arrival on the ward it is clear that William will be requiring some urgent interventions to address the physical needs that the assessment has revealed:

- Respiratory compensation (A and B assessment) – indicated by increased rate and effort of breathing.
- Circulatory compensation (C assessment) – indicated by increased heart rate.
- Altered conscious level – indicated by increased sleeping, behaviour changes.

Airway

Breathing

Circulation

Disability

Environment/exposure

Figure 10.4 ABCDE assessment tool

ACTIVITY 10.1

What key questions would the GP need to ask William's mother in order to gain a relevant history for assessment?

Based on the information you have been given, what do you consider to be the major factors in the GP's decision to refer William to the local hospital?

What are the potential factors that may have distracted the GP from making a referral?

Table 10.2 Structured approach to assessment of infants (0–1 year) and children (1 year–puberty)

	Infant and child	Observation	Action	Other considerations
Airway	Patency	Is the infant crying/vocalising appropriately for age/able to speak? Can you hear any airway noises that indicate struggling – such as stridor or grunting? Can you see any tracheal tug? Is there any obvious obstruction? How is the child positioned?	Ensure the airway is clear and remove obstruction if visible and safe to do so Ensure the child/infant is in correct position to maximise air entry	Try and keep child/infant as calm as possible to prevent stress which could result in further obstruction Sitting upright on a parent's lap may meet both calming and positioning needs
Breathing	Effort and efficacy	Look, listen and feel *Effort* – Can you see chest rising and falling? Can you see recession, intercostal/sternal, or increased work of breathing? Is there nasal flaring? What is the respiratory rate and is it within recommended parameters? *Efficacy* – Can you hear breath sounds such as wheezing (expiratory) or stridor (inspiratory) or gasping? Auscultation – can you hear breath sounds? Feel for symmetry of chest movement.	Give high flow oxygen (15 l/min via mask with reservoir bag) as soon as possible when respiratory distress is evident or circulatory assessment shows inadequate perfusion (consider hospital policy, as oxygen needs to be prescribed) Monitor oxygenation of haemoglobin with pulse oximeter (SaO_2)	Neonatal issues – the lungs develop up to and beyond birth. Neonates, ex-premature babies and those with chronic respiratory disease may have altered 'normal' ranges Consider capillary blood gas to measure plasma carbon dioxide levels (pCO_2) and oxygenation of plasma (pO_2) Increased respiratory rate with recession and respiratory acidosis is respiratory in origin: without recession and with metabolic acidosis is likely to be circulatory in origin
Circulation	Assess for effective perfusion	Look, listen and feel *Look* – Is the child pale? (Remember to consult with parent/carer as to usual 'well' skin colour and consider ethnic origin) *Listen* – Assess heart rate and sounds using a stethoscope *Feel* – Can you feel a pulse? Is it regular? Strong or weak? Check peripheral and central	Administer oxygen as above if ineffective perfusion (to maximise pO_2) Consider IV access and employ fluid resuscitation as per guidelines (usually 20 mls/kg normal saline 0.9%) Local guidelines may suggest 10 mls/kg followed by a further 10 mls/kg	Environmental temperature Is there a difference between central and peripheral capillary refill – look for a line of demarcation.

(Continued)

	Infant and child	Observation	Action	Other considerations
		Is there any difference in strength? What is the pulse rate and is it within recommended parameters? Assess a baseline blood pressure – is it within normal limits? Does the child feel cold peripherally? What is the capillary refill time? > 2 secs? Check centrally for accuracy Ask for history of urine output	Attach cardiac monitoring to check for sinus rhythm Check that manual pulse rate matches heart rate on monitor Capillary blood gas to check pH levels and bicarbonate levels (HCO_3) – is there evidence of metabolic acidosis? Strict input and output chart	Poor perfusion means poor delivery of oxygen to the peripheries; administer oxygen until capillary refill is less than 2 seconds, with a heart rate within normal limits and SaO_2 > 93% Assist in taking blood for U&Es, FBC, CRP Once oxygen and fluids have been administered as per guidelines, if assessment is still showing observations outside of normal limits, consider inotropic support
Disability	Assess for alertness and conscious level	Rapid assessment using the AVPU scale Alert *Voice responsive* *Pain responsive* *Unresponsive* Even if child is alert, consider if there are signs of drowsiness or lethargy Is there any differing of behaviour from usual? What about feeding? Is the child sleeping a lot? In and out of sleep? Is the child showing unusual posturing?	If less than 'alert', or there is any other reasons for concern over consciousness level (e.g. head injury, diabetes), perform a full GCS Repeat a minimum of hourly until stable Consider other reasons for reduced level of consciousness: check blood glucose level; check SaO_2 /pO_2; check pCO_2	Age and stage of development Known developmental delay or known disability/ communication difficulties Pain/fear may affect response Are there any other neurological problems, e.g. seizures? If consciousness is reduced, consider positioning to maintain airway
Environment	What other factors may be affecting the child?	Has the child a raised temperature? Are there any signs of a rash? Has the child been exposed to any extremes of temperature for any length of time? Has the child experienced any psychological factors that may be affecting responses? Could the child have ingested a poison? Are there any safeguarding issues?	Normalise the child's temperature; warm or cool to normal limits Use antipyretics as prescribed if there are underlying respiratory or circulatory problems Observe for signs of infection Assist in taking bloods for CRP (C-reactive protein) and culture and administration of antibiotics as prescribed Barrier nurse the child if infection control is an issue	Is there a history of febrile convulsions? Do not warm too quickly if severely hypothermic; risks of reperfusion injury In case of any marks on the skin (rash or bruises), the child's whole body should be assessed and careful documentation as to the appearance of the marks, size, and location Dipstick urine – collect sample for microscopy, culture and sensitivity if any abnormality

	Infant and child	Observation	Action	Other considerations
Family	Assess the family status	Is the primary carer with the child? What is the current family dynamic? Are there any safeguarding concerns? Who has legal parental responsibility? Consider using CWILTED tool (see Figure 10.5)	Consider the child and family's wish to be involved in care – negotiate and document their wishes Communicate your assessment and the planned interventions	Do parents wish to be resident? What are the child's views?
Fluids	Maintain hydration and blood glucose levels	Can the child eat and drink? Are there any indications for remaining nil by mouth? Assess hydration state; urine output, skin turgor, mucus membranes, tears Are IV maintenance fluids needed?	Ensure that the child and family know the safety reasons why the child may be nil by mouth Maintain strict input and output chart Administer IV fluids as prescribed; care of IV site as per hospital policy	Consider blood glucose level Dipstick urine Check calculation of IV fluids based on child's weight, the disease process and prescription

Source: Resuscitation Council (2010) and RCN (2011)

Paediatric Early Warning Scores

In the last few years there has been an increasing awareness of the need to strive for early identification of those children who are at risk of deterioration. This has resulted in the development of tools to help with assessment, commonly known as paediatric early warning scoring systems (PEWS). These have been developed to help all staff in the interprofessional team identify when a child is deteriorating or is at risk of deterioration. The tools themselves measure against vital signs, resulting in a score that identifies severity of condition. Currently there are several systems under development, but no single tool is used universally and very few have yet been validated (Monaghan 2005; Haines et al. 2006). Much of the research into the effectiveness of the tools has been conducted in the adult arena as good assessment of adults has been a topic of concern for many years (McArthur-Rouse 2001).

Secondary Care

As William moves through into the hospital setting, it is vital that the consistent management of his care is continued. This will be a stressful, difficult time for the whole family and all staff will need to be aware of this. In this instance, William first meets the local hospital through the emergency department and although this is the second part of his journey, for most families this is the point at which there is a realisation of the potential for serious illness.

Care of Children and Young People in the Accident and Emergency Department (A&E)

The National Service Framework gives guidance for all children who are cared for in any hospital and any setting. Within the UK, 20 per cent of the population who attend A&E are children

---

RESEARCH NOTE 10.1 Use of a paediatric early warning system in emergency departments (Adshead and Thomson 2009)

This paper reviews and evaluates the introduction of a paediatric early warning system in a district general emergency department, where adult nurses care for and assess children and young people. The paper contains a short literature review and describes the positive effect of the addition of the tool: adult nurses feeling more empowered and confident in their abilities and actions (see Table 10.3).

Table 10.3 Example of a paediatric early warning tool

	0	1	2	3	Score
Behaviour	Playing/appropriate	Sleeping	Irritable	**Lethargic/ confused** **Reduced response to pain**	
Cardiovascular	Pink or capillary refill 1–2 seconds	Pale or capillary refill 3 seconds	Grey or capillary refill 4 seconds Tachycardia of 20 above normal rate	**Grey and mottled or capillary refill 5 seconds or above** **Tachycardia of 30 above normal rate or bradycardia**	
Respiratory	Within normal parameters, no recession or tracheal tug	> 10 above normal parameters, using accessory muscles, 30+% FiO2 or 4+ litres/min	> 20 above normal parameters recessing, tracheal tug, 40+% FiO2 or 6+ litres/min	**5 below normal parameters with sternal recession, tracheal tug or grunting** **50% FiO2 or 8+ litres/min**	

Score 2 extra for 1/4 hourly nebulisers or persistent vomiting following surgery

Source: Monaghan (2005)

PRACTICAL GUIDELINES 10.1

Any tools, including PEWS, are only as good as the assessor, so while they are useful for confirming and communicating concerns in relation to children and young people, the need for thorough assessment is still crucial for all children's nurses and any professional who cares for children. Tume and Bullock (2004) consider that these tools are still reliant on the skills of the individuals who are carrying out the assessment.

There may also be ambiguity between assessors; different assessors may score differently when examining the same child, depending on interpretation of qualitative aspects such as 'mottled' and 'lethargic'.

Within primary care, the use of early warning tools may be of benefit, considering the number of professionals who have contact with children during and prior to their admission.

and young people and as such the workforce should be proportionate to this percentage. The NSFCYPMS (DoH 2004) recommends that in all areas where children and young people are cared for there should be staff trained in life support but that in A&E, staff should have recognised advanced life-support training. In addition, staff should be trained in paediatric airway management and venous access. This recommendation is now a decade old and not the first recognition that children and young people have specific physical and holistic care needs. The RCN has also produced numerous guidelines for healthcare workers who care for children and, within these, the emphasis is on children being cared for in appropriate settings and by appropriately trained staff (RCN 1999). In 2011 the RCN produced the paper 'Health care service standards in caring for neonates, children and young people', which yet again gave guidelines for managers in relation to the presence of dedicated children's nurses in all areas where children are cared for, including the

emergency department and the operating department. The reality is that, over these years, this has not been consistently implemented across the UK.

This is recognised to be an issue and within the NSFCYPMS (DoH 2004) it is suggested that, where this is not possible, there are contingency plans when children become seriously unwell. It also states that children may become ill 'suddenly and unpredictably' (DoH 2003). There are several specific assessment tools that are used within the emergency department. Included in this are triage systems such as the Manchester triage system and the now commonly used CWILTED system (Figure 10.5). While these are essential to ensure a system for assessment and a family-centred approach, these should be used in conjunction with the ABCDE tool of assessment. Willis (2001) does suggest that while the CWILTED tool is most often used to assess accidents, it was found to be helpful for assessing medical conditions too.

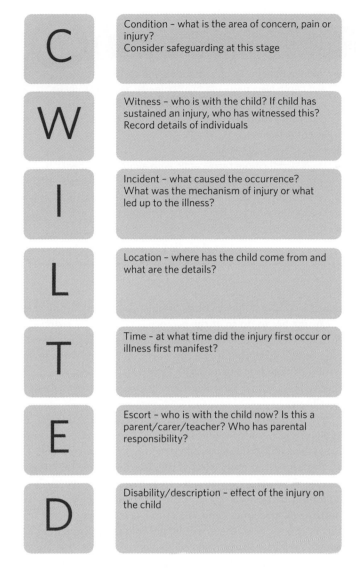

Figure 10.5 The CWILTED tool
Source: Adapted from Willis (2001)

The Manchester Triage System (MTS) (see Activity 10.3) is a further assessment tool that is commonly used in the emergency department although many authors feel that alone it does not replace the ability for good clinical assessment (Mackway-Jones 2012; Newell and Smith 2012). Van Veen et al. (2008) carried out research to consider the validity of this and concluded that the MTS is moderately valid for assessing children although positively, as children tend to be overtriaged.

For William, this referral may initially be seen as a routine occurrence, particularly for staff within the emergency department and yet again the emphasis for care is resting on accurate assessment of William's physical condition. Within the emergency department, whether there are children's nurses present or not, good systematic assessment is vital for accurate identification of the status of William's illness. The involvement of parents throughout the process is essential in assisting with this (Bentley 2005).

It is important here to discuss the stages of deterioration that occur when children become unwell. The body is capable of maintaining homeostasis through a system of mechanisms. Homeostasis is a state of equilibrium and is a fine balance, particularly in children and young people (see Figure 10.6). In the simplest of illustrations, when the temperature outside drops, a child also becomes cold, so, temporarily, the natural balance is altered. To restore the balance the child may feel shivery, which, in turn, raises the temperature, restoring the balance. For sick children and indeed adults, too, the mechanisms to restore normal balance are effective for a limited time in an attempt for normal function to be maintained. This is known as a period in which the child is compensating.

CASE STUDY REVIEW 10.1

On admission to the children's ward (through A&E and secondary care), William would have been treated with supplementary oxygen. This may have been high-flow oxygen initially, but now he is receiving 0.5 litre of oxygen via nasal cannulae to maintain saturations above 95%. He has had a nasogastric tube in place and is tolerating milk at 120mls/kg/day on a 4-hourly basis, taking what he can orally with the remainder being given via the tube.

The most recent handover is as follows:

- William is tolerating O_2 via nasal cannula and maintaining his SaO_2 at 95% although the oxygen has been increased to 0.75% over the last hour to achieve this.

- William has had an increased respiratory rate and depth also, particularly after feeds, and currently he has marked sternal recession, intercostal recession and a respiratory rate of 65 breaths per minute. He has vomited after the last feed.
- He is looking quite pale.
- He is slightly more tachycardic with a rate of 165 beats at rest although his capillary refill time is less than 2 seconds.
- Mum reports that he is wakeful and miserable and not consolable when he has bouts of coughing.
- His temperature is 36.8°C.

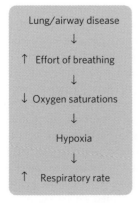

Figure 10.6 The fine balance of homeostasis

It is clear that William's natural physiological balance is altered due to his illness. His body is showing signs that compensatory mechanisms are beginning to manifest.

Compensation Mechanisms

This term can be applied to all the body systems and within children it is recognised that accurate assessment can often be impaired or delayed due to the child's ability to compensate well (see Figure 10.7). It is vitally important to acknowledge that if a child is compensating, there is clearly something that is causing her to do so. If the balance is not quickly redressed then the effects of this compensation may cause further physiological deterioration as she can only compensate for a finite period of time (see Figure 10.8). From this scenario, it is clear that William would have been in the compensatory stages of the illness.

What does the compensating child look like? Let us refer to William and his admission to the A&E department once again using the ABCDE framework to structure the consideration.

The airway is obstructed through either lung or airway disease. This could be due to bronchiolitis, asthma or any condition that affects breathing (mechanical factors such as underdeveloped lungs and structural defects may also have this effect). At first, there will be an increase in breathing as an attempt to increase oxygen demands and, at this stage, provided that the increased rate is effective, there will be no other signs of hypoxia (such as a reduction in oxygen saturation levels). However, over time, as the child tires and the metabolic demands increase, the levels of oxygen may begin to fall and the respiratory rate will climb. This will cause the cycle to continue.

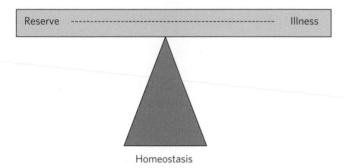

Figure 10.7 Ability to compensate

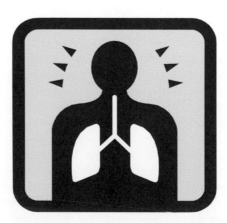

Figure 10.8 Compensated airway and breathing

Monitoring Oxygen Levels

The most accurate way to measure the level of oxygen delivery to an individual is through measuring oxygen levels in the blood. This is achieved through obtaining an arterial blood sample. However, on initial assessment this is an invasive procedure and in causing distress by performing venepuncture, extra demand is placed on the child, which can result in further increase in oxygen use. The use of an external saturation monitoring device is common practice in most clinical areas and is undoubtedly helpful as part of the assessment, although on its own does not always produce an accurate account of the severity of illness, particularly in the compensatory stage as, if all mechanisms of compensation are functioning well, levels of oxygen will not initially be affected.

Oxygen is carried in the blood in two ways, bound to haemoglobin and dissolved in the plasma (imagine plasma as the carrier fluid). Each haemoglobin molecule can carry up to four oxygen molecules and once these are bound together this forms oxyhaemoglobin (see Figure 10.9).

Only 1.5 per cent of oxygen is dissolved in the plasma so most of the oxygen is carried on the haemoglobin. As the blood flows through the body, haemoglobin collects carbon dioxide to be expired (given up).

While a child is in the compensatory state extra oxygen (through increased breathing) is being inhaled, increasing the chances of oxygen being taken on board. The pressure of oxygen in the blood is high, encouraging the binding of O_2 to the haemoglobin. This explains why at times children may have external saturation monitoring readings within normal limits (98 to 100 per cent) even though they are showing signs of respiratory distress. However, over time, as the child tires the pressure of oxygen may drop which means the binding

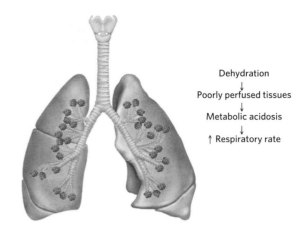

Figure 10.10 Respiratory distress due to non-respiratory origin

power to haemoglobin is reduced, therefore swift administration of oxygen will maintain pressure of oxygen, increase the binding power to haemoglobin and potentially prevent hypoxia. As oxygen uptake is reliant on haemoglobin, this is an important consideration. If the child has pronounced anaemia, the carrying potential in the blood is limited, causing breathlessness and hypoxia, but for a very different reason.

It is worth mentioning that respiratory distress can also occur due to non-respiratory origin and this can sometimes confuse the issue (see Figure 10.10). This is why accurate and thorough assessment is vital.

When a child becomes dehydrated there is a reduction in the blood volume (carrier for oxygen), reducing the delivery of oxygen to all cells in the body. This in turn alters the pH of the blood (see Chapter 9) and, as a result, the respiratory rate is increased to compensate. If there is doubt about the origin of the respiratory distress, this can be clarified through blood gas analysis; however, this should never delay the administration of oxygen.

Compensated Circulation

One of the first indicators that a child is entering a compensatory stage in relation to her ability to maintain circulation is that of an increase in heart rate. This is particularly notable in younger children, due to the physiology of the heart in early childhood. Cardiac output is determined by stroke volume × heart rate. However, in very young children the stroke volume is less, increasing as the child grows and develops. Therefore it follows that the heart rate increase is the young child's main mechanism for increasing output in response to stress, illness and demands on the heart. It must be remembered that the majority of hearts are young and healthy, although children compromised by congenital conditions or chronic illness may be less able to compensate in this way.

When assessing the pulse rate, also be careful to monitor the force of the pulse, noting the difference between peripheral and central pulses. The central pulses should always be stronger and

ACTIVITY 10.4

On transfer to the ward, William's transferring nurse reports that his oximetry readings show that his saturations are 99–100% in air. William has signs of respiratory distress and has a respiratory rate of 60.

Your mentor suggests that some oxygen therapy should be commenced but the nurse handing over the care feels this is unnecessary. What will you do and why?

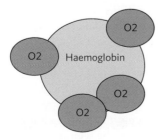

Figure 10.9 Oxyhaemoglobin

ACTIVITY 10.5

Demonstrate the position of key palpation points on Figure 10.11 and alongside identify which pulse points would be most suitable for a child and which for an infant.

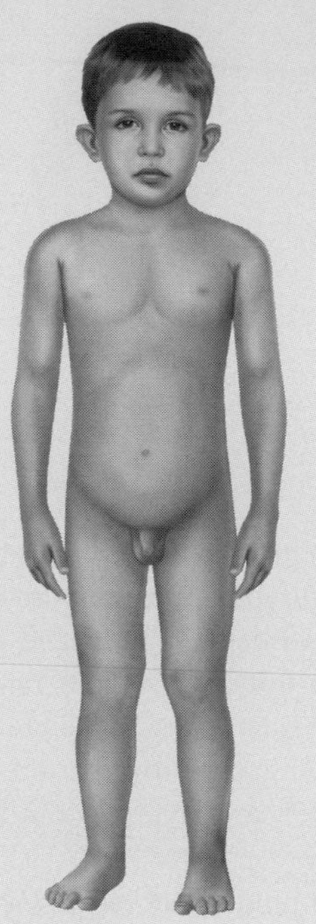

Figure 10.11 Key palpation and pulse points to be identified

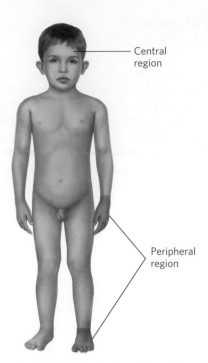

Central region

Peripheral region

Figure 10.12 Central capillary refill and peripheral capillary refill areas

Figure 10.12 locates central capillary refill and peripheral capillary refill areas. The differences between the responses can also indicate that the circulation is beginning to become compromised.

Owing to this ability to compensate, a child's blood pressure may not show signs of alteration, as initially the heart rate increase will 'hold' the blood pressure to a sufficient level to provide adequate perfusion of oxygen. It must be remembered that a low blood pressure may be indicative of a very seriously ill child as the compensating mechanisms begin to fail. A reduction in urine output is another indicator that the circulatory system is struggling due to reduced blood volume and therefore reduced oxygen to the renal system.

Compensated Disability

For some, the word 'disability' may be difficult to relate to. Consider this as the level at which the illness affects or 'disables' the child. As the breathing and circulation becomes compromised oxygen levels may fall. The brain requires a continuous supply of oxygen to function at the optimum level and interruptions in supply (even temporarily) may affect cognitive function and possibly mechanical control of other body systems. Think about when you are in a stuffy lecture theatre with very little air circulation and therefore some reduced oxygen supply. Gradually as people begin to be deprived of oxygen, they begin to yawn (an attempt to take in more oxygen) and become sleepy or, in extreme cases, lose consciousness. Apply this to the child who is unwell (such as William) and it can be seen that he may begin to have an alteration in his conscious level.

more forceful on palpation or auscultation (apex, carotid, femoral) owing to the size of these vessels and the position of the pulse points being more central. The peripheral pulses such as radial, brachial and temporal are positioned further from the heart in smaller vessels. When a child is in the compensatory stage the pulse will be raised. For William, he has a raised temperature, which will also increase metabolic rate and heart rate so this alone will not be an indication of compensation.

Capillary refill time is a further indication of the level of oxygen perfusion and can be indicative of a failing circulatory system. The capillary refill time is recorded by applying pressure to an area of skin, in effect occluding the capillaries for five seconds. While compressed the skin will blanch, but on release, the blood flow will return. In healthy circulation, this should respond in less than 2 seconds. If the circulation is rather more sluggish, the venous return will be similarly slower. Thus if the return time is longer, this may indicate circulatory insufficiency.

When recording the capillary refill, using a central area of the body is most reliable as peripheral areas (such as fingers and toes) may only indicate the outside temperature or reflect that the child is pyrexial, which causes vasoconstriction peripherally.

A – Alert

V – Voice responsive

P – Pain responsive

U – Unresponsive

Figure 10.13 AVPU assessment tool

Salati (2004) gives a useful illustration. He says that: 'If a child accepts a nasal cannula, she is probably too sick to care and needs more than low flow oxygen.' While this cannot be taken completely at face value (as the approach of the nurse may affect the compliance of the child), it can be a good measure of severity of illness.

The AVPU is a good tool for a quick assessment, however, if the child is less than voice responsive then a full neurological assessment must be commenced using the Glasgow Coma scale (see Figure 10.13).

When compensating, the child may be breathing more quickly, yawning or become slightly more drowsy. These signs are concerning, indicating that, for some reason, oxygen and therefore nutrients may not be reaching the brain. As compensatory methods begin to fail, the conscious level may further deteriorate, putting other systems at risk, such as the respiratory system and the airway in particular.

Compensated Exposure/Environment

Exposure or environment is an important area of assessment. Although it is last on the structured approach it is no less important in the overall assessment. Temperature is part of the assessment and, as we are aware, a raised or low temperature will significantly affect the presentation of a child. A child with a pyrexia may have cool peripheries (fingers and toes) which may affect capillary refill time, the conscious level and mood of the child, all of which may affect the parameters of the observations. Simply environmental elements such as the ambient temperature or the time the child has been exposed (due to undressing and examination) may have an impact on the previous assessments. Observing for abnormal rashes is also imperative at this stage as this could be an indication of serious illness or infection. Having this element at the end of the assessment ensures these issues are not ignored and safely reduces the risk of practitioners rationalising abnormal physiological responses.

PRACTICAL GUIDELINES 10.2

William has a temperature of 36.8°C during his admission, causing his heart rate and respiratory rate to increase, an expected response to fever. It would be pertinent to treat this fever, although it cannot be assumed that the temperature alone is causing the increase in respiratory and heart rate. Once the fever has reduced reassessment must be carried out. ABCDE assessment may reveal underlying causes, such as serious infection, in addition to the primary respiratory presentation.

ACTIVITY 10.6

Consider the following information and answer the questions.	Notes
Airway William has a patent airway although he has increased secretions, which results in coughing and some difficulty in clearing his airways Why is this of significant importance in the assessment?	
Breathing William already has increased respiratory effort and is described as 'struggling to breathe'. This will result in an increase in respiratory rate and effort. The amount of effort may be of significant importance. Why? During this initial compensatory stage, what actions would you take and why?	
Circulation William will have a raised heart rate. This indicates that his heart has to work harder to adequately perfuse all the cells of his body. What may be the reason for this increase in heart rate? During this initial compensatory stage, what actions would you take and why?	

(Continued)

Consider the following information and answer the questions.	Notes
Disability	
William may be miserable and irritable. At this age, communication and assessment may be difficult due to the age and stage of development. However, a good history, discussion with Mum and rapid assessment using the AVPU and PEWS tools may help. List some of the behaviours that William may demonstrate.	
During this initial compensatory stage, what actions would you take and why?	
This may be one of the most difficult assessments to achieve accurately.	
Environment	
William has been brought to yet another strange environment (having previously been to the GP). He will be disturbed by the sights and sounds. Considering these issues, what is the next step for assessing William?	
During this initial compensatory stage, what actions would you take and why?	

During the compensation stage in A&E William can begin to have access to the treatment that will potentially prevent deterioration and give supportive therapy to his condition. While it is likely that William may be suffering from bronchiolitis, the interventions and system of assessment will be appropriate for any child who has these symptoms and clinical presentation. Therefore it can be concluded that this skilled approach to assessment should provide the children's nurse with all the tools required for caring for the seriously ill child.

Decompensation

Decompensation occurs when the compensatory mechanisms fail and become ineffective. Resources are not infinite and, as the child tires and compensatory states linger, there is an increasing risk that deterioration will follow, resulting in the need for further intervention. The compensatory stage therefore is the stage at which potentially (depending on the underlying cause) the child's condition may be determined by the interventions and actions of the carers. Ignoring or underassessing severity or delaying appropriate treatment at this stage may have a detrimental affect. By the same token, appropriate and timely interventions may reduce the risk of deterioration.

Communication Factors

Aside from the treatment regimes and considerations for care for children and young people who are seriously unwell one of the major factors in health outcomes for children, parents and staff remains that of ensuring a sound method of communication. The communicators straddle the settings and involve a vast number of professionals and personnel, not forgetting the child also (see Figure 10.14). The importance of good communication at all levels will also highlight the opportunities for nurses to identify moments in care when an intervention can reduce the risk of deterioration and improve outcomes. It has to be acknowledged that each action at each stage of William's journey can have significant impact, either negatively or positively.

It is vital that William remains in the centre of the communication cycle, and that communication between the professionals

RESEARCH NOTE 10.2 Experience of trained nurses caring for critically ill patients within a general ward setting (Cox et al. 2006)

Although this work primarily relates to adult care, it contains an interesting insight into the feelings, thoughts, anxieties and needs of nursing staff when caring for seriously ill patients who are not in an intensive care area. Communication and interprofessional working as well as education are highlighted as areas for development.

and the family is consistent and ongoing to enable safe monitoring and appropriate care at all stages. Any breakdown in communication, poor communication or, at worst, failure to communicate at all could result in a slower response to William's ever changing condition.

ESCALATING CARE

As discussed previously, with any change in setting or new personnel caring for a child, it is vital to re-establish a baseline set of observations, and not just rely on the 'handover'. If William's condition indicates that he is requiring more support to assist his body in compensation, then he may be moved to a designated children's high dependency bed. This may be on a general children's ward, in a bay separated from the children's ward, but still managed by children's nurses, or linked to an intensive care unit in a tertiary centre.

High-dependency care describes care provided to a child who may require closer observation and monitoring than is usually available on an ordinary children's ward, although much of this care is already provided, with higher staffing

GP
A&E department
Triage nurse
Mother
WILLIAM
A&E staff
Ward staff
Accepting ward
Paediatrician

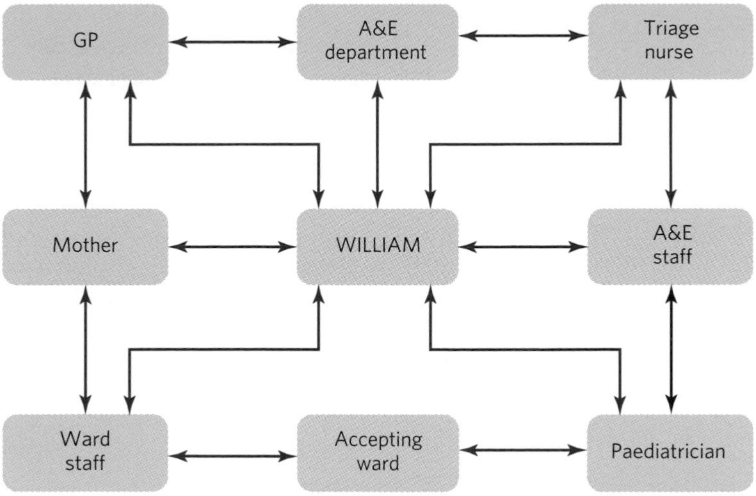

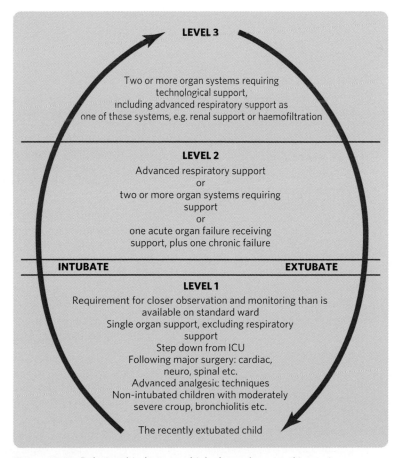

Figure 10.14 Key communicators in William's care

levels than usual, in such locations (DoH 1997). The document 'A framework for the future' was produced by the Department of Health in 1997, examining the provision of paediatric high-dependency and intensive care in the UK. Future working groups, and the National Service Framework were built on the information and recommendations from this report when writing on aspects related to high-dependency, retrieval, and intensive care. The relationship between high-dependency and intensive care in Figure 10.15 gives a good representation of escalation in care (DoH 1997, page 8).

LEVEL 3
Two or more organ systems requiring technological support, including advanced respiratory support as one of these systems, e.g. renal support or haemofiltration
LEVEL 2
Advanced respiratory support
or
two or more organ systems requiring support
or
one acute organ failure receiving support, plus one chronic failure
INTUBATE
EXTUBATE
LEVEL 1
Requirement for closer observation and monitoring than is available on standard ward
Single organ support, excluding respiratory support
Step down from ICU
Following major surgery: cardiac, neuro, spinal etc.
Advanced analgesic techniques
Non-intubated children with moderately severe croup, bronchiolitis etc.
The recently extubated child

Figure 10.15 Relationship between high-dependency and intensive care

High-Dependency Care

Level 1 care is considered to be high-dependency care, and according to the report, every district general hospital admitting children should be able to provide this level of care. This recognises how quickly the child can deteriorate, as every child who is unwell enough to be admitted to a children's ward has the potential to require high-dependency care. The child who requires high-dependency care is still in the compensatory part of the illness continuum, and it is hoped that, by supporting the child at this stage, decompensation will not happen. This should therefore reduce demands on paediatric intensive care beds and improve the quality of care provided to all children.

Physical assessment of the child requiring high-dependency and intensive care is exactly the same as the assessment depicted in Figure 10.4. However, the findings and actions following the assessment will be different according to the severity of the child's illness. The following section uses the assessment criteria in Table 10.4 to explain typical predicted findings and nursing management in a child requiring high dependency care. There are key differences observed in children who have a respiratory problem as their presenting complaint, and children who have other illnesses (see Table 10.5). Although management of each may be similar (or even the same) the predicted signs and symptoms which indicate decompensation will be different. It is therefore important to

Table 10.4 Additional issues specific to HD care

	Expected findings for HD care	**Potential management in HD Care**
Respiratory	The child who has a respiratory illness is likely to produce excess mucus. Therefore the nares become blocked Infants are obligate nose breathers, so this can lead to apnoeas Thick secretions may also block the upper airway	Suction to maintain patency of nares
Non-respiratory	Change in consciousness level will be the main concern when assessing ability to maintain own airway	Recovery position; insertion of Guedel airway

Table 10.5 Additional breathing issues specific to HD care

	Expected findings for HD care	**Potential management in HD Care**
Respiratory	*Effort* Increased respiratory rate Increased work of breathing (nasal flaring, tracheal tug, intercostals/subcostal recession, sternal recession) *Efficacy* May not have air entry to all lobes of the lungs (listen with stethoscope; feel with hands for equality of movement) May have added breath sounds (crackles, wheezes, stridor) Colour may be pale or cyanosed	Emergency management with 100% facemask oxygen. After this, oxygen must be prescribed, and will be given to keep the child's saturations above 92% All children who have a respiratory problem requiring high-dependency care, or those receiving oxygen, must be continuously monitored with a pulse oximeter. However, this only indicates the oxygen component on the haemoglobin; to measure carbon dioxide levels, or to measure oxygen dissolved in the plasma (pO_2), a blood gas must be taken Additional support, such as CPAP may also be given on a high-dependency unit
Non-respiratory	*Effort* Increased respiratory rate NO increased work of breathing *Efficacy* No added respiratory noises Colour may be pale or mottled	Emergency management with 100% facemask oxygen. This will be given until capillary refill and heart rate are within normal limits (following fluid administration) and then discontinued Blood gas will be done to assess acid–base balance. No expected change in pO_2 or pCO_2

understand exactly what information can be gained from your physical assessment.

Airway

The physiological response to a respiratory infection means that infants and young children are more likely to require high-dependency care due to respiratory infections than are older children and young people. The normal structural differences of a smaller airway (therefore swelling due to infection has greater impact on airway resistance) and fewer alveoli means that the infant and young child is more likely to reach the limits of compensation earlier and require high-dependency care earlier than the older child. This is the case for William in our scenario. Respiratory interventions range from suctioning to keep the airway clear and administration of oxygen and humidification (delivered in all settings), to CPAP (delivered in high-dependency and intensive care settings), to ventilation (delivered in intensive care settings).

Management of Oxygenation

One concept that is important to understand for all nurses caring for children requiring high-dependency care is the oxygen dissociation curve. By understanding this, you will be able to explain to colleagues and parents why administration of oxygen is important in the child who shows signs of respiratory compensation. Figure 10.16 shows a standard oxygen dissociation curve. On the vertical axis, values are given for saturated haemoglobin – 'sats' (SaO$_2$). On the horizontal axis, values are given for the oxygen dissolved in the plasma (PO$_2$).

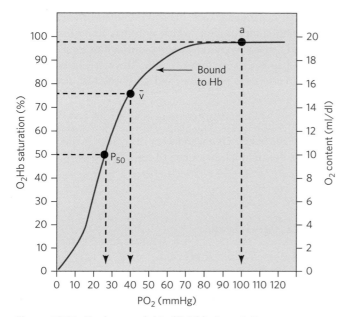

Figure 10.16 Oxyhaemoglobin (O$_2$Hb) dissociation curve

Note: Normal arterial PO$_2$ of 100 mmHg results in a saturation of 97% to 98%, a normal mixed venous PO$_2$ of 40 mmHg generates a saturation of 75%, and the P$_{50}$ point normally occurs when the PO$_2$ of 26.5 mmHg generates a saturation of 50%.

Oxygen passes through the alveolar membrane into the blood. Here, it dissolves in the plasma (fluid component of the blood), and also binds to the haemoglobin molecules. How many of the available haemoglobin molecules are filled or 'saturated' with oxygen is measured as a percentage, monitored on a pulse oximeter ('sats monitor'). Thus, if 97 per cent of the available haemoglobin molecules are filled with oxygen, 'sats' will measure at 97 per cent. However, remember, this is a percentage of the total available. Thus, if haemoglobin levels are 14 g/dl, there are twice as many molecules available (and therefore twice as much oxygen) as if levels were 7g/dl. However, saturations would still read at 97 per cent. Thus, saturation levels are only one component when considering oxygen carriage around the body.

Haemoglobin molecules can be viewed as 'carriers' of oxygen, merely a vehicle for transporting oxygen from A to B. It is the oxygen that is dissolved in the plasma that is in contact with the capillary walls, and therefore able to diffuse into cells. So the carriage of oxygen works thus:

- Oxygen passes from the alveoli into the pulmonary capillaries, where it dissolves in the plasma.
- Oxygen then passes from the plasma to the haemoglobin 'carriers'.
- This leaves some oxygen dissolved in the plasma (PO$_2$) and some on the haemoglobin (SaO$_2$).
- The blood gets to the target organs, where oxygen is needed.
- The oxygen leaves the plasma component (in contact with the cell walls). This drops the PO$_2$ values as the oxygen dissolved in the plasma is used.
- When the PO$_2$ reaches low enough levels (about 100 mmHg on oxygen dissociation curve), then it is 'replaced' by oxygen from the haemoglobin carrier. This ensures that there is always enough oxygen dissolved in the plasma and therefore enough oxygen in contact with the cell walls.
- However, the result of this is that the haemoglobin reserves are used, resulting in a drop in SaO$_2$ levels.

The clinical applications of this are:

- If the saturations monitored are below 94 per cent, this means that the blood oxygen chemistry is on the 'steep' part of the oxygen dissociation curve. Thus, a small use of oxygen from the plasma (PO$_2$) results in a large drop in haemoglobin saturations (SaO$_2$). Therefore, the child is at risk of exceeding her compensatory mechanisms (heading towards decompensation). In order to prevent this, we give oxygen to keep saturations above 92 per cent, allowing normal compensation to continue, but limiting the risks of decompensation.
- If circulation is poor, then there is limited blood reaching the peripheries (indicated by increased capillary refill time). This leads to the small amount of blood in the peripheries supplying oxygen for all the cells. This normal demand (or increased in the case of infection), with limited supply means that the PO$_2$ levels in this blood are used quickly. There is no problem with oxygen supply from

the lungs, thus monitored saturations are within normal limits. However, the decreased supply to cells means that the cells are still at risk of hypoxia. Therefore, oxygen will be delivered to the child to maximize their PO_2 in the shutdown peripheries. Once circulation has been restored (indicated by capillary refill less than 2 seconds and heart rate within normal limits for age), then oxygen administration can be discontinued.

Continuous Positive Airways Pressure (CPAP)

When a child has a primary respiratory illness, then the disease process may interfere with supply of air to the alveoli (due to oedema of some airways, and blockage of small airways with mucus), and the production of surfactant within the alveoli. These factors may lead to collapse of some of the small airways (atelectasis). Therefore, the first part of each inspiratory effort is needed to open these collapsed airways (think of blowing up a balloon – the first part to open the balloon is really difficult, it then becomes easier and, as the balloon reaches its maximum inflation, it becomes more difficult again – the lungs are exactly the same). This means that increased effort is seen. The result of reduced air entry is that oxygenation is poor (low SaO_2), and removal of carbon dioxide is poor (increased PCO_2, triggering increased respiratory rate). Delivery of oxygen will address the poor oxygenation, but it will not improve the CO_2 removal. If a pressure is delivered to the alveoli to keep them open, this will reduce the respiratory effort needed, and improve air supply to the alveoli, thus improving the removal of CO_2.

This pressure is provided by attaching a continuous flow of air to the child (oxygenated as required). This may be via a facemask or nasal prongs; in order to generate a pressure above normal air pressure, a tight seal will be required against the child's nose (in the case of prongs), or face (facemask). This is termed continuous positive airways pressure (CPAP), and is generated by specialist CPAP equipment. The advantages and disadvantages of using CPAP are summarised in Table 10.6.

The key disadvantage of reduced cardiac output can be understood as follows. During inspiration, the diaphragm moves downwards, and chest wall up and out, creating a negative pressure in the thoracic cavity. This causes air to be drawn into the lungs. However, the negative pressure also assists with the venous return from the body and head and neck back to

the right side of the heart. When administering CPAP, a continuous *positive* pressure is applied to the lungs, thus creating a less negative pressure during inspiration. This reduces the venous return back to the right side of the heart, thus reducing cardiac output. As we will see with other interventions, once you start supporting a child's normal physiology with abnormal interventions, this can then affect other body systems' abilities to compensate. For example, the child who is receiving CPAP will not be able to compensate for this reduced venous return if their circulatory system is already in compensation. Therefore, by introducing CPAP, they may become worse (circulatory decompensation) and require a bolus of fluid and these **fluids** will be considered as part of ongoing fluid management.

Additional circulation issues specific to HD care are displayed in Table 10.7.

Additional disability issues specific to HD care are displayed in Table 10.8.

Additional Environment Issues specific to HD care

One of the most common reasons for illness in children is infection. Normal physiological response to infection is to **raise the body temperature**. This inhibits the replication of viruses and bacteria and also accelerates healing (up to a point). When this happens, metabolic rate increases, leading to greater demand for oxygen and glucose. The oxygen dissociation curve shifts to the right, meaning that oxygen leaves the haemoglobin more easily, making extra oxygen available in the plasma to increase the supply to cells. **Respiratory rate increases** to make sure that the supply on the haemoglobin is constantly replenished. The oxygen and glucose are delivered at a faster rate by an **increased heart rate**, ensuring demand is met. This is all normal, and good, as it limits replication of the invading organism, and repairs damage. Why treat therefore?

In high-dependency care, the child is already showing signs of ongoing compensation, which only has finite limits. This increased demand on the respiratory and cardiovascular system may lead to earlier decompensation. Therefore, fever will be treated to minimize respiratory and cardiovascular demands.

Family

When a child requires high-dependency care, this places great stress on the family. Often, and as in the case of William in our scenario, the child has been unwell for a period of time before

Table 10.6 Advantages and disadvantages of CPAP

Advantages of CPAP	Disadvantages of CPAP
Increases functional residual capacity (the amount of air left in the alveoli at the end of expiration)	Increases intrathoracic pressure
Recruits atelectatic (collapsed) areas	Impedes venous return and cardiac output
Improves alveolar ventilation	Alveolar hyperinflation
Redistributes lung water	Air leaks (pneumothorax)
Maintains inspiratory muscles in a position of mechanical advantage (the 'balloon' effect)	Increases intracranial pressure
	Renal effects

Table 10.7 Additional circulation issues specific to HD care

	Expected findings for HD care	Potential management in HD care
Respiratory	Increased heart rate Prolonged capillary refill time (>2 seconds) Normal blood pressure – compensation continues	Capillary refill 2–3 seconds – administer **oxygen** as above in 'breathing'. Hypoxia may mean blood is redirected to central organs, thus reducing peripheral circulation
Non-respiratory	As respiratory above, plus: Strong central pulse, weaker peripheral pulses Reduced urine output Pale, mottled, cold peripherally Normal blood pressure or raised systolic	Oxygen will restore this If this does not work, or capillary refill > 3 seconds – administer oxygen and **fluids** In the case of ongoing deterioration, this may be IV fluid maintenance instead of oral fluids In the case of acute deterioration, a fluid bolus will be given. This is normally 20 mls/kg 0.9% normal saline (ALSG 2011) However, 10 mls/kg, reassess, then a further 10 mls/kg may be the preferred hospital policy to prevent fluid overload Attach the child to cardiac **monitoring** As the circulatory system compensates, blood is redirected to the central organs. This means that the kidneys receive less blood (reflected in poor urine output, hence strict **fluid balance**) However, the kidneys modify electrolyte balance as well as fluid balance, and deranged electrolytes can lead to cardiac arrythmias (hence also **take blood** for U&Es) A blood gas may also be taken to measure acid–base balance Part of high dependency care is the correction of fluid and electrolyte balance

he reaches the high dependency unit. Parents may well have had several sleepless nights, and anxious days, watching their child deteriorate. All of us, when tired and anxious, rarely present ourselves at our best. Taking in new information while reacting to bad news and perhaps dealing with other frustrations may all result in our normal reactions becoming impaired.

The fact that the parents have reached the limits of their ability to care for their child and now need medical help can lead to a sense of powerlessness. In addition, high-dependency care suggests that the child may not have survived if this care were not available and thus highlights their child's mortality, a frightening concept for any parent. However, some parents may see the converse: '*Thank goodness that someone is at last doing something*' is a common reaction and feel relief that now their child is safe. There may also be conflicts with other responsibilities. A hospitalised child may well have one parent with them and the other parent at work, or with siblings. However, in order to meet their own needs, both parents often feel that a child in high-dependency care is so vulnerable, that they both want to be present.

The increased monitoring, tests and equipment can be frightening for both the family and the child. As a rule, the nurse needs to ask herself: 'Why am I doing this, do I know what I am looking for, and if I find anything, what would I do about it?' There is no point in monitoring a child (or doing blood tests) just because you have the equipment. Consider the top-to-toe assessment first and only add in monitoring equipment when it is justified. This will help to minimise stress for

Table 10.8 Additional disability issues specific to HD care

	Expected findings for HD care	Potential management in HD care
Respiratory	AVPU should be part of routine assessment for all children	Assessment and documentation of AVPU with other observations
	For respiratory problems, confusion and agitation may be caused by rising PCO_2 levels, falling PO_2 levels, or reduced blood glucose levels	Less than 'Alert', or any reason for neurological pathologies, perform full GCS
		Check blood glucose levels
	Deterioration in consciousness should be anticipated and only follows compensatory mechanisms observed above and is thus preventable	Consider pain management early
	'P' or 'U' is an emergency situation	
Non-respiratory	Circulatory problems could reduce cerebral perfusion, reducing consciousness levels	
	Neurological involvement needs full GCS assessment a minimum of hourly (this includes head injuries, diabetic ketoacidosis, meningitis)	

the child and family. This increased equipment also takes up a lot of space, often where space is limited anyway. This may lead to the ideal of resident parents having a bed not being a reality and parents having to sleep in a chair, adding to their already sleep-deprived state.

In the Introduction, the nurse's feelings and stress at dealing with a child requiring high-dependency care was considered. Hold on to that feeling of confusion at equipment, terminology, 'expert' nursing practice and that slight rush of adrenaline. On repeated exposure to these children, do not become complacent; for each family, this is usually their first experience of high-dependency care and their feelings are magnified as this is their child in that bed.

Moving On from High-Dependency Care

As shown in Figure 10.15, Level 1, high–dependency care is usually defined by the fact that the child requires support of one body system, not including advanced respiratory support. The point at which a child moves to intensive care usually has intubation as the defining factor. Intubation is the insertion of an endotracheal (breathing) tube (ETT) into the trachea via the nose or mouth. This tube is then attached to a ventilator to support the child's respiratory system. This may be done because the child's respiratory system is no longer able to compensate. Alternatively, as we saw earlier in the ABCDE approach, if a child is requiring interventions for circulation or neurological issues, then interventions must already be in place to support the respiratory system. Thus, the child with meningococcal sepsis does not have a primary respiratory problem, but his circulation is receiving extensive support, and so breathing must also be supported.

The Department of Health (2001) stated that: 'All DGHs should be able to resuscitate, intubate and stabilise children prior to transfer, or provide care for a short period with support. It is hoped that, with a full physical assessment of the child, using knowledge based on normal physiology, the pathophysiology of the presenting complaint and evidence-based interventions, resuscitation situations can be avoided. However, children will still deteriorate and require stabilisation in district general hospitals prior to transfer to paediatric intensive care. This may be done in any high dependency area of the hospital; most frequently the paediatric high dependency theatres or adult intensive care. Once the child is intubated and stabilised, it is common practice for an intensive care nurse from the adult unit to manage the equipment and for a children's nurse to care for the child and family prior to transfer.

Retrieval

Retrieval refers to the movement of a child from a district general hospital to a tertiary centre with paediatric intensive care facilities. Due to the relatively small number of children needing intensive care, the high cost of the equipment and the staff training needed to care for these children, there are only a small number of paediatric intensive care units in the UK. Now that the aim is for children with high dependency needs to be cared for at district general hospitals, children have usually deteriorated to the point at which they need intubating prior to needing transfer to paediatric intensive care. Therefore, a specialist transport service is required. When working on a high dependency unit, it is necessary to understand what is expected by the retrieval team when preparing a child for transfer to a paediatric intensive care unit. Most regions will have a retrieval team whose remit also includes training at the district general hospitals to ensure that communication and the transfer process happens as smoothly as possible.

Paediatric Intensive Care

Paediatric intensive care is required where there is failure of two or more organs, or if the child requires advanced respiratory support. As discussed throughout this chapter, the approach to assessment will follow the ABCDE algorithm. Assessment of the child requiring intensive care is no different; it is the expected findings and management that will differ. The following sections discuss the main interventions seen in the majority of intensive care units for all children. It does not cover specific care for conditions such as heart surgery and traumatic brain injury, or management using extraordinary therapies such as haemofiltration, oscillation, or Extracorporcal Membrane Oxygen (ECMO). For more detailed discussion on paediatric intensive care nursing, see Asquith and Williams (2000).

Safety

As with all children, safety is the first assessment prior to the ABCDE assessment. Working oxygen (attached to a bag and mask as the child cannot self-ventilate in intensive care) and working suction are checked. The child must be wearing two name bands and these are checked against the notes. All IV lines and infusions should be labelled and lines checked to ensure they are secure and not bleeding (especially important in the case of arterial lines). A recent weight must also be recorded.

Airway

The majority of children in intensive care will have had an endotracheal tube (ETT) at some point to protect their airway and to enable mechanical ventilation. The diameter and length of the ETT will need to be clearly documented.

Breathing

Most children will have had their breathing supported with a ventilator at some point during their transfer or stay on paediatric intensive care. If a child has a primary respiratory problem, then a ventilator will be used to support their respiratory system when the child is no longer able to compensate. For the child whose problem is not respiratory in origin, the aim of ventilation is to rest, or manipulate the respiratory system. The effort required to breathe places demand for oxygen and glucose on the body; in addition, maintaining posture also requires oxygen and glucose. The critically ill child may receive sedation and muscle paralysis in order to minimize her oxygen and glucose requirements. This renders her unable to breathe, so she must be attached to the ventilator. For children with a head injury, their level of consciousness may mean that they are unable to maintain their own airway, and manipulation of CO_2 levels may be used to control cerebral blood flow.

Traditional ventilation works by delivering a positive pressure into the lungs and uses pressure from the ventilator via the ETT. The inspiratory cycle aims to open the lungs to ensure adequate diffusion of oxygen in and removal of CO_2. Oxygen is administered in concentrations similar to, or less than, required prior to intubation. The pressure delivered to open the lungs to the peak of inspiration is called the peak inspiratory pressure (or PIP). On expiration, the ventilator releases the peak pressure, allowing the elastic recoil of the chest to expel the air as happens in normal expiration. However, due to the presence of the ETT through the larynx, the normal pressure provided by the larynx and epiglottis is bypassed. This pressure normally retains the functional residual capacity of the lungs at the end of expiration. Therefore, a pressure needs to be in place to replace this. This is the positive end expiratory pressure (or PEEP) and has the same function as CPAP.

The nursing or medical staff controlling the ventilator set these pressures, as well as the rate of the ventilator and the inspiratory:expiratory ratio (how long is spent breathing in and how long is allowed for recoil of the lungs). They may also set the tidal volumes (how much air to be delivered with each breath). The manipulation of these figures depends on the values read on the blood gas. While the child is ventilated, he may or may not be breathing for himself in addition to the ventilated breaths. This depends on how unwell he is and if other body systems are also needing support. All children will need to be sedated and provided with pain relief due to the nature of this very invasive equipment. Assessment is exactly the same as earlier; however, the breathing that the child is doing will be documented separately to the breathing that the ventilator is doing.

Circulation

Due to the critical nature of the child's physical condition requiring intensive care, all children will be attached to a cardiac monitor and have a minimum of hourly blood pressure recordings. If a child is potentially unstable, then he will also have invasive blood pressure monitoring via an arterial line. This gives a continuous blood pressure reading in the format of a wave form and also allows for arterial blood gas sampling.

Positive pressure ventilation has an effect on venous return to the right side of the heart as described in the CPAP section; due to the increased PIP, this effect is even greater. Therefore, the body detects this as decreased circulating volume and thus causes the blood flow to the kidneys to be reduced. Therefore urine output will fall for the first 12 hours after intubation. However, the fluid is still in the body, placing the child at risk of circulatory overload. Therefore, all ventilated children will be on a reduced fluid maintenance (usually 70 per cent of normal).

As described earlier, assessment of reduced circulation (increased heart rate, prolonged capillary refill) will be treated by oxygen administration and fluid administration. It is recommended that only two boluses of 20 mls/kg NaCl 0.9 per cent (i.e., total 40 mls/kg) be given in the non-intubated child. If further fluid is needed, there is risk of pulmonary oedema; additionally, the child is extremely unwell if this is required. Therefore, intubation is recommended when 60 mls/kg is required. It is also likely that if the child is this unwell then their blood pressure will be affected, demonstrating signs of impending decompensation.

Once this fluid has been given, if the capillary refill and blood pressure are still demonstrating that the child's cardiac output is not meeting demand for oxygen and glucose, inotropic support may be initiated. Inotropes are drugs that support the cardiovascular system. They affect heart rate, contractility of the heart muscle and control blood vessel diameter. By constricting the peripheral blood vessels (as in the case of epinephrine) the blood is pushed back centrally to the vital organs, increasing venous return to the right side of the heart (preload). By vasodilating the peripheral blood vessels (as in the case of nitroprusside), it makes it easier for the blood to leave a weak heart (afterload). All of these help to maintain the cardiac output. However, inotropes have a very short half-life (they are metabolised quickly) and so need to be given by continuous intravenous infusion. In addition, the body becomes reliant on them, so they must be weaned slowly and also delivered via central access so that there is no risk of peripheral access 'tissuing' or becoming dislodged. Due to intense vasoconstriction caused by these drugs, peripheral access also has the added complication of causing necrosis of peripheral vessels requiring skin grafting. Therefore, intravenous inotropes are *always* delivered centrally. The immediate and intense effect on the cardiovascular system means that these are potentially very dangerous; therefore the child should be on continuous cardiac monitoring, with invasive blood pressure monitoring. The infusions should be checked by a nurse familiar with these drug calculations, and in a tamper-proof programmable infusion device.

Disability

All children will have a GCS performed hourly while in intensive care. However, their normal response will be altered due to the nature of the drugs that are being administered to sedate, provide pain relief and potentially paralyse them. Pain and sedation scoring will also be used to ensure that the child is kept as comfortable as possible. Children with head injuries require specific management in a neurological tertiary care centre. Key points to remember when transferring these children to a specialist centre are that they tend to be taken by the referring hospital rather than waiting for a retrieval team, as time is critical if neurosurgery is needed. They should not have any nasal tubes passed (ETT, suction, nasogastric tubes) in case of basal skull fracture and should have their cervical spine immobilised. They should not receive any infusions containing glucose as this will worsen cerebral oedema.

Environment

The discussion regarding fever management is the same for intensive care as for high-dependency care. Children in intensive care will often be immobile, and will need regular pressure relief and pressure area risk assessment completed. Skin assessment will be the same as earlier; however, the presenting condition may predispose them to skin breakdown. Meningococcal sepsis may cause areas of necrosis; use of inotropes causing severe vasoconstriction may also cause areas of necrosis, especially in pressure areas. Safeguarding issues will also cause specific management concerns.

Exposure to toxic substances, including self-harm, will lead to specialist management issues and perhaps liaison with other professionals including transplant teams. The child's inability to maintain her own hygiene needs will need to be addressed appropriate to her age. All ventilated children require regular eye and mouth care. They should also receive a wash daily and all secretions and blood spillages be promptly cleaned, both to minimise risk of infection and to maintain dignity and an acceptable appearance for their parents.

Fluids

Initially, fluids will be given intravenously while the child is stabilised, but he will be commenced on enteral feeds as soon as possible. This is to maintain his gut integrity, but also to provide calories for the increased metabolic demands of critical illness and to prevent catabolism.

Family

Many families with children in intensive care have shared with staff their main concerns. The key stressors can be divided into four areas: parental role alteration, the child, the environment and the staff (see Table 10.9).

In order to cope with these stressors, parental needs specific to intensive care can be divided into personal needs, information needs and support needs. Obviously, each individual will have her own unique needs under each of these headings, which must be fully assessed by the nurse caring for her child. We use ABCDE to assess the child; as yet there is no tool for assessing parental needs. Each of the concerns outlined in high-dependency care is also present in intensive care, along with the consideration that the tertiary centre may well be geographically removed from their usual place of residence, taking them away from their support systems.

Table 10.9 Key stressors for parent, child, the environment and staff

Parental role	Child	The environment	Staff
Loss of parenting role	Risk of mortality and morbidity	Machines that emit light, sound, heat	Use of jargon
Child's siblings	Uncertainty over outcome	Lack of privacy	Information inconsistent, unintelligible or insufficient
Depression	Altered appearance – tubes and wires	Busy staff	Behaviour – laughing, joking, talking too much or not enough
Financial concerns	Appears undressed, floppy, unresponsive	Other families	
	Parents of intubated children were more stressed by painful procedures; parents of non-intubated children were more stressed by behavioural and emotional responses		

CASE STUDY REVIEW 10.2

William has travelled on a long journey in only a few days. A child has undergone a transformation from a period of health to one of serious illness. His parents and sibling have been thrown into a sea of uncertainty and watched him be taken from their family home into the hostile environment of a PICU. The term 'life support' will imply the threat that William is in danger and grief processes will have been triggered. However, the future is positive. With rest and respiratory support, it is likely that, provided William has no underlying or developing complications, he will make a recovery and be discharged home soon.

SUMMARY OF KEY LEARNING

Whether a student nurse, a newly qualified children's nurse or an experienced nurse, the prospect of a child deteriorating or requiring increased interventions can be challenging for anyone. This chapter has attempted to give some insight into the importance of a structured approach to care and the difference that timely interventions can make to outcomes. Many situations of deterioration are not preventable but children will have better outcomes if symptoms are well managed as they present. The key to this is good assessment and reassessment, monitoring trends and making good use of all tools available for this purpose. Communicating with other members of the team may increase response times and there is need for urgent referral. Children's nurses can play a unique role in preventing deterioration due to their ability to develop strong relationships with the child, family and members of the multidisciplinary team. We cannot prevent children and young people from becoming unwell in all cases, however, having basic tools and good insight can only increase the possibilities of positive outcomes.

FURTHER RESOURCES

Colville, G., Orr, F. and Gracey, D. (2003) 'The worst journey of our lives': parents' experiences of a specialised paediatric retrieval service. *Intensive and Critical Care Nursing* 19(2), 103-108.

Tips for Quick Wins: Improving responses for children and young people requiring emergency or urgent care **http://www.dh.gov.uk/en/Publicationsandstatistics/Publications/PublicationsPolicyAndGuidance/DH_4112226**

Focus on emergency and urgent care pathway for children and young people: **http://www.institute.nhs.uk/quality_and_value/high_volume_care/focus_on%3A_emergency_and_urgent_care_pathway.html**

ANSWERS TO ACTIVITIES

ACTIVITY 10.1

What key questions would the GP need to ask William's mother in order to gain a relevant history for assessment?

When did the symptoms begin? Does William have a cough? Has William any known allergies?

How much fluid has William been able to take in the last 24 hours?

Has William had regular wet nappies today? Any vomiting or diarrhoea?

Does William have a fever?

Based on the information you have been given, what do you consider to be the major factors in the GP's decision to refer William to the local hospital?

William has increased respiratory effort, which has been worsening.

William may be too tired to feed, which is concerning and could indicate potential respiratory failure.

If he has reduced fluid intake and output then this would be a concerning sign of potential circulatory failure.

What are the potential factors that may have distracted the GP from making a referral?

The symptoms may coincide with other events, such as teething, immunisations, family cold.

William's Mum may underplay symptoms and feel she can manage him at home. This could be due to fear of admission.

GP may not recognise childhood behaviour from sick behaviour.

ACTIVITY 10.2

Participants: 17 600 children (aged <16) visiting an emergency department; this is a large sample size.

Over 13 months (university hospital) and seven months (teaching hospital); this enables the evaluation of computerised Manchester triage system for over a year and therefore was able to surmise that the triage of children with a medical problem or young patients (aged <1 year) was particularly difficult and the system should be specifically modified to cope with such cases.

The research was carried out in Emergency departments of a university hospital and a teaching hospital in the Netherlands, 2006–7; a comparison of the sample and conditions and the similarities and differences of the health services.

ACTIVITY 10.3

The Manchester triage tool categorises patients as to the urgency. Applying this system, identify the difference in interpretation that may occur. Look at the words in bold. What do these mean to you and how would you decide which category William can be placed in on arrival at the emergency department?

1	Requires immediate resuscitation	Patients who are in **immediate need** of treatment as a **life-preserving** measure
2	Very urgent	Patients who are seriously ill or injured but not in immediately **life-threatening** condition
3	Urgent	Patients who have **serious** illness but appear **stable**
		William would be placed in this category due to his age and the associated potential risks linked to respiratory disease. He may require immediate oxygen therapy as supportive treatment and if he is dehydrated he may need maintenance fluids or a fluid bolus.
4	Standard	**Standard** cases who are not in **immediate** danger
5	Non-urgent attention	Patient for whom condition is not considered **urgent** or **life threatening**

ACTIVITY 10.4

On transfer to the ward, William's transferring nurse reports that his oximetry readings show that his saturations are 99–100% in air. William has signs of respiratory distress and has a respiratory rate of 60.

Your mentor suggests that some oxygen therapy should be commenced but the nurse handing over the care feels this is unnecessary. What will you do and why?

William has signs of respiratory distress and although he is compensating he would benefit from oxygen therapy. It is wise to involve parents in delivery of oxygen as unduly upsetting William may increase distress and increase the demands on his respiratory rate; however, ignoring the clinical symptoms is not advisable. Consider low-flow oxygen via nasal cannula if tolerated or ask Mum to sit William with her and 'waft' 100% O_2 nearby so that William benefits from some oxygen to maximise each breath. This is not ideal but the nurse must weigh the risk of developing hypoxia should compensatory mechanisms fail.

ACTIVITY 10.5

Demonstrate the position of key palpation points and alongside identify which pulse points would be most suitable for a child or infant (Figure 10.17).

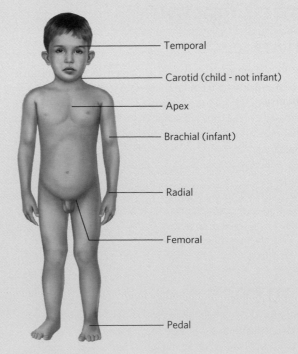

Temporal

Carotid (child - not infant)

Apex

Brachial (infant)

Radial

Femoral

Pedal

Figure 10.17

ACTIVITY 10.6

Consider the following information and answer the questions	Notes
Airway William has a patent airway although he has increased secretions, which results in coughing and some difficulty in clearing his airways. Why is this of significant importance in the assessment?	Coughing continuously may result in increased energy use – child tiring and potentially failing to maintain airway.
Breathing William already has increased respiratory effort and is described as 'struggling to breathe'. This will result in an increase in respiratory rate and effort. The amount of effort may be of significant importance. Why? During this initial compensatory stage, what actions would you take and why?	Young children will use valuable energy resources when breathing consistently at this high rate and effort. Over time this has a potential to alter excretion of CO_2. Oxygen saturation and administration of high-flow oxygen initially, reducing to nasal or facemask O_2 as saturations improve and respiratory effort/rate improves along with clinical appearance.
Circulation William will have a raised heart rate. This indicates that his heart has to work harder to adequately perfuse all the cells of his body. What may be the reason for this increase in heart rate? During this initial compensatory stage, what actions would you take and why?	Recognition of reduced oxygen intake and increased CO_2 due to difficulty in breathing resulting in heart compensating to maintain an adequate oxygen perfusion. Additionally William has reduced fluid intake, which will affect the circulating blood volume and therefore perfusion, as well as potential for reduction in energy supplies due to inability to feed. Continue O_2 therapy to maintain perfusion and reassess. Consider fluid intake and encourage oral hydration or IV cannulation and fluids. Closely monitor oral input and output.
Disability William may be miserable and irritable. At this age, communication and assessment may be difficult due to the age and stage of development. However, a good history, discussion with Mum and rapid assessment using the AVPU and PEWS tools may help. List some of the behaviours that William may demonstrate. During this initial compensatory stage, what actions would you take and why? This may be one of the most difficult assessments to achieve accurately.	Irritability and inconsolability, which may be transient during the compensatory stage. Increasing distress when separated from parent which may exacerbate physical symptoms further. May begin to show some signs of drowsiness and lethargy, which need to be assessed in light of usual routine. Reassess using AVPU scoring and discuss William's usual pattern of behaviour. An EWS may help. While it is important to be aware of factors that affect the alertness and sleep patterns of a 6-month-old, be wary of a child who is sleeping excessively. If bloods have been taken and cannula inserted record a blood glucose or perform a finger prick bedside glucose level.
Environment William has been brought to yet another strange environment (having previously been to the GP). He will be disturbed by the sights and sounds. Considering these issues, what is the next step for assessing William? During this initial compensatory stage, what actions would you take and why?	William will need to have his temperature recorded, be nursed in a warm environment and weighed, if possible. Opportunity to examine skin for rashes to check peripheral skin temperature. Safeguarding issues should also be considered during this intervention. Assess pain using an appropriate pain assessment tool.

SELECTED REFERENCES

Adshead, N. and Thomson, R. (2009) Use of a paediatric early warning system in emergency departments. *Emergency Nurse*, 17(1), 22–25.

Advanced Life Support Group (ALSG) (2005) *Advanced paediatric life support (APLS). The practical approach*, 4th edn. Blackwell Publishing: Oxford.

Advanced Life Support Group (ALSG) (2008) *Pre-hospital paediatric life support: a practical approach to out of hospital emergency care of the child*, 2nd edn. Blackwell Publishing: Oxford.

Advanced Life Support Group (2011) *Advanced paediatric life support: the practical approach (APLS)*, 5th ed. Wiley-Blackwell: Chichester.

Aitken, P., Birch, S., Cogman, G., Glasper, E. and Wiltshire, M. (2003) Quadrennial review of a paediatric emergency assessment unit. *British Journal of Nursing*, 12(4).

Asquith, J. and Williams, C. (2000) *Paediatric intensive care nursing*. Churchill Livingstone: London.

Bentley, J. (2005) Parents in accident and emergency: roles and concerns. *Accident and Emergency Nursing*, 13, 154–159.

Confidential Enquiry into Maternal and Child Health (CEMACH) (2008) *Why children die: a pilot study 2006. Children and young people's report*. CEMACH: London.

Cooper, N. (2011) Primary care for children: back to the future. *Education for Primary Care*, 22, 148–151.

Cox, H., James, J. and Hunt, J. (2006) The experience of trained nurses caring for critically ill patients within a general ward setting. *Intensive and Critical Care Nursing*, 22, 283–293.

Davies, F. (2011) Working with sick children. *British Journal of Health Care Assistants*, 5(7), 356–357.

Department of Health (DoH) (1997) Paediatric Intensive Care A framework for the future: Report from the National Coordinating Group on Paediatric intensive care to the Chief Executive of the NHS Executive.

Department of Health (DoH) (2001) High dependency care for children report of an expert advisory group for Department of Health 2001: **http://www.dh.gov.uk/en/Publicationsand-statistics/Publications/PublicationsPolicyAndGuidance/DH_4010058**

Department of Health (DoH) (2003) Getting the right start: National Service Framework for children. Standard for hospital services: **http://www.dh.gov.uk/en/Publicationsand-statistics/Publications/PublicationsPolicyAndGuidance/DH_4006182t**

Department of Health (DoH) (2004) National Service framework for children young people and maternity services. Core standards. DoH: London.

Department of Health (DoH) (2010) Getting it right for children and young people. Overcoming cultural barriers in the NHS in order to meet their needs. A review by Professor Sir Ian Kennedy: **http://www.dh.gov.uk/en/Publicationsand-statistics/Publications/PublicationsPolicyAndGuidance/DH_119445**

Evans, K. (2008) Improving paediatric emergency care. *Emergency Nurse*, 16(6), 14–15.

Haines, C., Perrott, M. and Weir, P. (2006) Promoting care for acutely ill children. Development and validation of a paediatric early warning tool. *Intensive and Critical Care Nursing*, 22, 73–81.

Hall, K. (2003) NHS Direct and children's A&E services: a case review. *Paediatric Nursing*, 15(5).

Harnden, A., Mayon-White, R. Mant, D. Kelly, D. and Pearson, G. (2009) Child deaths: confidential enquiry into the role and quality of UK primary care. *British Journal of General Practice*, 59(568), 819–824.

McArthur-Rouse, F. (2001) Critical care outreach services and early warning scoring systems: a review of the literature. *Journal of Advanced Nursing*, 36(5), 696–704.

Mackway-Jones, K. (2012) Manchester triage system: why, how and where?: **http://possibility.no/legevaktkonferan-sen2011/legevakt2011/wp-content/uploads/presentas-joner/Dag%202_Plenum_Manchester%20Triage%20System_Mackway-Jones.pdf**

Monaghan, A. (2005) Detecting and managing deterioration in children. *Paediatric Nursing*, 17(1).

Monaghan, R., Clifford, C. and McDonald, P. (2003) Seeking advice from NHS Direct on common childhood complaints: does it matter who answers the phone? *Journal of Advanced Nursing*, 42(2), 209–216.

Moorey, S. (2010) Unplanned hospital admission: supporting children, young people and their families. *Paediatric Nursing*, 22(10).

Newell, J. and Smith, P. (2012) Triage in the light of four hour targets. Results of a survey of current practice in Emergency departments in the UK: **http://www.rcn.org.uk/__data/assets/pdf_file/0014/232700/4.3.1_triage_in_light_of_four_hour_target.pdf**

Parshuram, C. et al. (2009) Development and initial validation of the bedside paediatric early warning system score. *Critical Care*, 13(4).

Pearson, G., Ward-Platt, M., Harnden, A. and Kelly, D. (2011) Why children die: avoidable factors associated with child deaths. *Archives of Diseases in Childhood*, 96, 927–931.

Resuscitation Council (2010) Guidelines, medical information and reports: **http://www.resus.org.uk/pages/mediMain.htm**

Royal College of Nursing (RCN) (1999) Guidance for clinical professionals and managers who are responsible for children's services in acute settings: **http://www.rcn.org.uk/__data/assets/pdf_file/0004/141673/001054.pdf**

Royal College of Nursing (RCN) (2011) Health care service standards in caring for neonates, children and young people: **http://www.rcn.org.uk/__data/assets/pdf_file/0010/378091/003823.pdf**

Salati, D. (2004) Caring for a sick child in a non paediatric setting. *Nursing*, 34(4).

Smith, S. (2010) Helping parents cope with crying babies: decision-making and interaction at NHS Direct. *Journal of Advanced Nursing*, 66(2), 381–391.

Stewart, B., Fairhurst, R., Markland, J. and Marzouk, O. (2006) Review of calls to NHS Direct related to attendance in the paediatric emergency department. *Emergency Medicine Journal*, 23, 911–923.

Tume, L. and Bullock, I. (2004) Early warning tools to identify children at risk of deterioration: a discussion. *Paediatric Nursing*, 16(8), 20–23.

van Veen, M., Steyerberg, E., Ruige, M., Van Meurs, A., Roukema, J., Van der Lei, J. and Moll, H. (2008) Manchester triage system in paediatric emergency care: prospective observational study. *British Medical Journal*, 337 (7673).

Wheeler, H. J. (2005) The importance of parental support when caring for the acutely ill child. *Nursing in Critical Care*, 10, 56–62.

Willis, M. (2001) CWILTED. *Emergency Nurse*, 8(9).

CHAPTER 11
The Challenges of Sexual Exploration for Young People

Susan Walker

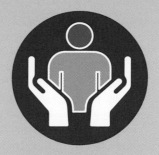

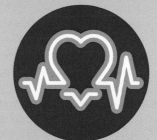

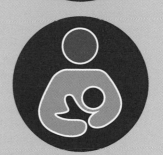

LEARNING OUTCOMES

On completion of this chapter, the reader will be able to:

- Talk about the main methods of contraception available in the UK.
- Describe and explain how each method of contraception works, what may make it fail, how often it may fail and the risks and benefits associated with it.
- Talk about the most common sexually transmitted diseases affecting young people in the UK and how these can be prevented.
- Understand the law regarding sexual practice and young people.
- Understand the social, cultural and political context in which young people explore their sexuality.
- Reflect on the ethical and professional challenges of caring for young people as they mature and explore their sexuality.
- Apply this knowledge in a non-judgemental and ethical manner, respecting the diverse views and experiences of young people and their families.

TALKING POINT

'Clear, understandable and up-to-date information for children, young people and their parents is provided through a variety of media and formats which are appropriate to the child's development and circumstances.'

However this does not appear to follow through in regards to sexual health, as the home and educational environment seem to play a greater part in the approach offered in relation to information and resources including contraception.

INTRODUCTION

The issue of young people and sexual behaviour is a complex one. It cannot simply be addressed within a biological context but involves social, ethical, cultural, religious and legal aspects. A health professional working with young people will inevitably encounter the issue of sexuality and must be equipped to deal with the subject compassionately and knowledgeably. Sexual desire, sexual behaviour, specific sexual practices and sexual orientation are highly charged areas of human existence and arouse strong emotions. This is particularly the case where young people are concerned because the gradual transition from childhood to adulthood is not clearly defined in mainstream 21st-century culture in the UK.

Sexual behaviour, in particular penetrative, heterosexual vaginal intercourse, is considered an adult behaviour by most people. However, the question of when a child becomes an adult and how young people should behave during the years between childhood and full adulthood are areas of contention. The question of when a child becomes an adult can be considered in social, legal, biological or religious frameworks, all of which provide contradictory answers to this question. A health professional working with young people who are exploring issues of sexuality must be aware of the different ways in which sexual behaviour can be 'framed' and thought about. These frameworks will be addressed later in this chapter.

Why are sex and sexuality, which are very private and personal aspects of a young person's life, matters for the health professional at all? The main reason is that sexual behaviour can have unintended and unwelcome consequences, i.e. unwanted pregnancy and sexually transmitted infection, which bring the young person within the remit of health service providers. By advising and guiding young people in matters of sexuality, a knowledgeable health professional may be able to help a young person avoid unwanted pregnancy or infection in the first place. Sexual exploitation of young people is also a subject that health professionals need to be aware of and have the skills to act appropriately if it is suspected. Safeguarding of young people is an important area of practice, which is dealt with in detail in Chapter 5.

This chapter will provide a basic knowledge of contraceptive methods, including emergency contraception, which will help when talking to young people. It will also provide a basic understanding of chlamydia, gonorrhoea, herpes simplex and genital warts, which will allow discussion of these infections with young people who may be at risk of acquiring them. The case studies guide through the issues that may arise in caring for a young person, as he or she matures and begins to explore sex and sexuality.

> ## ACTIVITY 11.1 Acting in Helen's best interests
>
> Consider the health and well being issues that arise as a result of Helen's diagnosis.
>
> What might you wish to do to ensure the best outcome for Helen?
>
> What anxieties might you have?
>
> What difficult legal or ethical situations might you find yourself in?

YOUNG PEOPLE AND SEXUALITY IN ITS LEGAL, SOCIAL, RELIGIOUS AND BIOLOGICAL CONTEXTS

When is a child no longer a child?

- Is it when he or she obtains a driving licence?
- Maybe when he or she can vote?
- Or perhaps a young person becomes an adult on completing puberty?
- Is a girl an adult when she has her first period?
- Or are children adults when sexual desire emerges?
- Maybe children are not full adults until they are in a position to live financially independently? (For more on independence, see Chapter 16.)

This question and the various answers suggested indicate how complex and nuanced our ideas are surrounding the line between adulthood and childhood. The boundary between childhood and adulthood can be viewed within differing frameworks. The idea of a 'framework' indicates that the context in which a question or idea is posed often influences how it is approached. Legal, sociological, biological and religious frameworks (to name but a few) construct and define the conditions of adulthood in different ways. In the 21st century in the UK, sexual interest, behaviour and activity are considered appropriate only for adults. For this reason, questions of when a child becomes an adult, and when it is lawful for a young person to engage in sexual activity, become

---

CASE STUDY 11.1 Helen's ectopic pregnancy

Helen is a 15-year-old girl who has been admitted to a surgical ward with suspected appendicitis. She was subsequently found to be pregnant with an ectopic pregnancy (i.e. a pregnancy that developed in the ovarian tube). Because of the delay in reaching the diagnosis, she suffered a rupture of her ovarian tube, lost large amounts of blood and nearly died.

Following emergency surgery she is making a slow but steady recovery.

On reading this chapter, consider how Helen might be cared for with regard to the issues raised by her pregnancy and the issues of sexuality it raises.

very important. For the child branch nurse, caring for a child or adolescent, questions regarding the appropriateness and lawfulness of sexual behaviour can become very troublesome.

Religious frameworks and definitions of adulthood are often concerned with when a child can accept for herself the religious responsibilities of her community. These include the moral and ethical responsibilities of the religion with regard to sexual practices. Religious frameworks can contain strong moral views concerning the timing of sexual expression in a young person's life course. For example, many religious teachings ban penetrative sexual activity unless within marriage.

Biological frameworks for defining adulthood focus on the physical changes of puberty and the biological preparedness for reproduction, in men and women.

Legal frameworks are concerned with when a person can accept full responsibility for wrongdoing or when a person can give consent.

Social frameworks more often define adulthood according to the role the person can assume in wider society. Financial independence, the ability to safely drive a car, completion of education and obtaining the right to vote are all markers of social adulthood (for more on the transition to adulthood, see Chapter 16).

To make matters more complicated these frameworks are influenced by one another. The law in many countries is heavily influenced by both religious belief systems and by later discoveries of biological science. Religious and social frameworks influence one another, so that religious practices, and the norms and expectations that derive from them, differ from country to country. All these influences, definitions and frameworks are in action when considering appropriate sexual expression and sexual behaviour in children and adolescents.

FRAMEWORKS WITHIN WHICH ADOLESCENT SEXUALITY CAN BE APPROACHED

Nurses must at all times act both within the law and in the best interests of their young patients. At times, acting in this way can go against prevailing social norms and expectations and occasionally against personally held or commonly accepted moral or religious beliefs. It is therefore helpful to understand the different frameworks in which sexual behaviour in young people and adolescents is defined and within which judgements must be made.

Biological Framework

Biological changes take place during puberty that prepare the male and female body for reproduction. It is important to note that sexual activity and reproductive activity are not identical. Many sexual activities, e.g. masturbation, will not lead to reproduction and can take place before the body of the child has developed capacities for reproduction. Nonetheless, the biological changes that take place at puberty produce an increase in sexual interest and behaviour in young people. In some societies and cultures, they are also taken as markers of a young person's transition into adulthood.

Physiological and Anatomical Changes at Puberty

Puberty refers to the time when young people develop secondary sexual characteristics that will eventually enable them to become full adults, capable of reproducing (see Figures 11.1, 11.2 and 11.3). Secondary sexual characteristics are, for girls, the enlargement of the breasts and hair growth in the axillae and pubic regions. For boys, secondary sexual characteristics include enlargement of the penis and testes, the deepening of the voice, hair growth in the axillae and pubic regions and beard growth. Both genders also undergo growth spurts and muscular and body fat changes. These changes are brought about by the stimulation of the ovaries and testes by substances released from the pituitary gland in the brain. The gonads (ovaries and testes) then produce oestrogen and testosterone in varying amounts, to bring about the changes just mentioned.

In boys and girls, the effects of hormonal changes in puberty eventually bring about maturation of the reproductive system. This results in menarche (the commencement of menstrual periods) and monthly ovulation in girls. For boys, the result is spermatogenesis (the production of sperm in the testes).

There is considerable variability and overlap in the ages when girls and boys enter and complete puberty. This makes it difficult

Stages of puberty

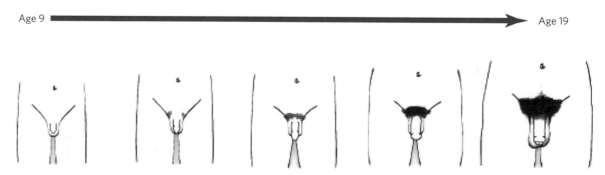

Age 9 ————————————————————————➤ Age 19

Figure 11.1 Stages of puberty in male

Stages of puberty

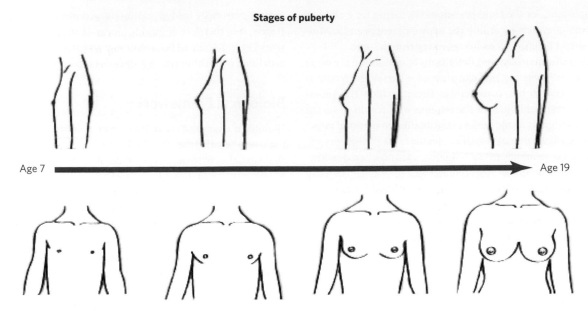

Figure 11.2 Stages of puberty in female breasts

to use age alone as an indicator of biological maturity. It also presents difficulties if biological maturity alone is considered the sole indicator of adult status. This is because if adulthood is judged solely using a biological framework, girls as young as 10 years old could be judged to be adult, because they have begun to menstruate and boys aged 15 years might still have prepubertal physical characteristics and would, therefore, be judged children.

Puberty brings about psychological changes, one of which is an interest in sex and increased sexual behaviour. If puberty occurs relatively early, a young person may have increased sexual interest at a time when legal and societal frameworks do not allow full expressions of sexual behaviour. The age of onset of puberty seems to have occurred at decreasing ages over the last 150 years (Okasha et al. 2001). This is thought to be due to improvements in nutrition. It has resulted in young people becoming sexually mature (and sexually interested) at a time when psychologically and socially they are not yet ready for the challenges of sexual relationships or reproduction. It is interesting to note, in this context, that one of the risk factors for early sexual intercourse in girls is early menarche. This is concerning since early sexual intercourse is associated with regret and with poor use of contraception (Wellings et al. 2001). This conundrum, of biological maturity at a time of social, emotional and legal immaturity, can present challenges for nurses caring for young people. This is further complicated by the fact that young people of the same calendar age can have differing biological ages and therefore exhibit variable sexual interest and activity.

Social Framework

Sex, sexuality and sexual activity are heavily influenced by social and cultural understandings of what is 'normal' behaviour. As stated in the introductory paragraph, sexual activity is thought of as an adult behaviour which is unacceptable for children. As a result, the social markers of adulthood deserve some thought. It is well commented on that a person in the UK may buy cigarettes at 16 years, drive a car at 17 years but must wait until he or she is 18 years old to purchase alcohol or to vote (see Chapter 16). These different age limits reflect a social judgement about when a person is sufficiently adult to carry out these activities either safely or with sufficient 'adult' judgement. The legal age of consent to sexual activity is set at 16 years because it reflects

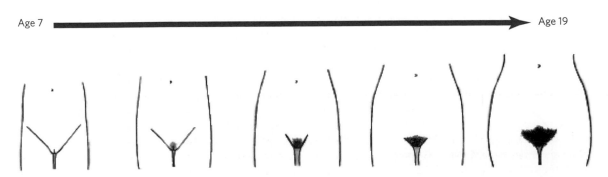

Figure 11.3 Stages of puberty in female pelvis

the social judgement of when a person is sufficiently mature to assume the risks and challenges of sexual activity. However, these social judgements change according to time and geography and according to other social factors. Early marriage and early sexual activity are the norm in some cultures. In earlier times in the UK, people married and were expected to produce children in their teenage years. Teenage pregnancy is generally held to be an undesirable social trend but this attitude is influenced by whether or not the birth occurs within marriage.

Social frameworks and, as a result, legal frameworks can change quite rapidly. Until recently in the UK a distinction was made between same-sex and opposite-sex partners, in terms of when a person was sufficiently adult to engage with the challenges of sexual behaviour. Recent changes in social framing of same-sex relationships led to this distinction being abolished in the recent Sexual Offences Act 2003. A health professional caring for young people, who are beginning to explore their sexual feeling, must be sensitive to the sometimes contradictory social attitudes towards sex and young people.

Religious and Moral Frameworks

In the UK, religious beliefs vary. As a result, religious opinions on when and how young people should express sexuality or engage in sexual behaviour also vary. The majority of UK citizens do not hold strong religious beliefs but sexual behaviour is an area in which ideas about morality and what is right and wrong are often expressed. Some of these opinions are influenced by pervasive religious teachings and attitudes, regardless of whether or not a person is personally committed to a religious faith. For those who do hold strong religious beliefs, these often have great influence over opinions regarding sexuality. In a multicultural and multifaith society like the UK, religious beliefs can provide an additional framework through which varying ideas of sex and the sexual behaviour of young people can be viewed. Religious belief is not required for a person to have a strong sense of what is morally acceptable or unacceptable and many

non-religious people have strong views on sex and sexuality. Thus young people and those who care for them must negotiate sexuality in an arena where differing religious and non-religious beliefs will provide different interpretations of what is acceptable in terms of sexual expression for young people.

Health professionals caring for young people should be aware of their own moral and religious views on sex and sexuality. They should also be sensitive to the diversity of moral and religious opinions that may be held by their patients and by the parents and guardians of their patients. It is not uncommon for young people to hold differing views to their parents regarding the rights and wrongs of sexual behaviour. This is a very sensitive area and one in which the child branch nurse must act to avoid discrimination and to treat patients with dignity and respect. It is also an area in which considerable tact and sensitivity may be required to meet the needs of young people in regard to sexual advice, while avoiding offending parents or guardians.

Legal Framework

The law regarding sexual offences became clarified in the UK when the Sexual Offences Act 2003 came into force. This aimed to update, clarify and consolidate previous legal acts. The 2003 Act states that a child may not legally consent to sexual activity until his 16th birthday. Sexual activity includes both heterosexual and homosexual activity. This makes sexual activity with a child under the age of 16 years a criminal offence. It is an offence to have sexual activity with a child under 16 regardless of the age of the other party. However, because the law is not intended to prosecute mutually consensual acts between teenagers of a similar age, it is not generally used to prosecute, for example, two 15 year olds who are sexual partners. There is an absolute limit to sexual activity with a young person, which is set at 13 years. Any sexual activity with a child below the age of 13 is statutory rape on the grounds that a child of that age cannot consent to the activity. A defendant cannot claim that he believed the child to be over 16 years (which can sometimes

CASE STUDY REVIEW 11.1

In this case, Helen is under the age of legal consent to sexual intercourse, so whoever her sexual partner was he was committing an offence. If this person was an adult then there are grounds for investigation by the police and prosecution under the Sexual Offences Act. It is in Helen's best interest to ascertain who her sexual partner was and how old. Given the possibility of a sexual offence having been committed, it is probably also in Helen's best interests for social services to be informed of what has happened. However, Helen is owed a duty of confidentiality concerning her medical details. The NMC gives clear guidance on maintaining and on breaking the confidentiality of an under age patient (NMC Guidance on Confidentiality 2012). In this case, because of the grave risk of sexual

exploitation, it is likely to be defensible to breach Helen's confidentiality by informing professionals beyond the healthcare team. These are actions that are undertaken only after discussion with senior colleagues.

It is important not to damage any trust built up with Helen. For this reason, it is best practice to inform a young person about his or her right to confidentiality, but also of the limits to that confidentiality. The young person must be aware that there will be occasions on which the duty to protect them by disclosing to an appropriate person some of the things they have disclosed will override the right to confidentiality. This is a difficult balance to achieve. It is also best practice to inform a young person and to try to obtain her permission, if breaching her confidentiality.

PRACTICAL GUIDELINES 11.1

NMC guidance on confidentiality includes the following:

- You must respect your patient's right to confidentiality.
- You must ensure that your patient is informed about how and why information is shared by those who will be providing their care.
- You must disclose information if you believe someone may be at risk of harm.

RESEARCH NOTE 11.1 Sexual behaviour in Britain: early heterosexual experience (Wellings et al. 2001)

Summary of findings:

- 30% of young women and 24% of young men reported that their first experience of sexual intercourse was when they were still under 16

- younger people were much less likely to use condoms at first intercourse
- nearly 10% of young women reported using no contraception at all at first intercourse.

be used to defend against a charge of sexual activity with a child aged between 13 and 15 years).

In addition, the Act made sexual activity within certain relationships illegal, if the younger party is under the age of 18 years. This is intended to protect young people where one party is in a position of trust for the other, e.g. a teacher and a student. (The Sexual Offences Act can be accessed online at **http://www.legislation.gov.uk/ukpga/2003/42/contents** to read it in more detail.) This very clear legal framework can sometimes present practical, legal and ethical difficulties for health professionals who work with children under the age of 16.

FRASER GUIDELINES

It is known that approximately 25 per cent of teenagers experience their first act of intercourse when still under 16 years of age (Wellings et al. 2001). These young people need access to advice on contraception and sexually transmitted infections and access to contraceptive methods and abortion. Fortunately, there exists guidance for health professionals regarding how to approach the issue of providing contraceptive advice and treatment, and advice

on sexual issues, to young people who are under the age of legal consent. These are known as the Fraser Guidelines, after Lord Fraser, who first set them out. These guidelines were developed after a series of legal challenges by a mother, regarding the rights of her daughters to receive confidential advice and treatment on contraception and sexual health matters.

The Sexual Offences Act 2003 also specifically protects health professionals who provide sexual health advice or treatment to young people from accusations of wrongdoing, if they can show that they were acting in the young person's best interests. The Act states that a person is not guilty of aiding, abetting or counselling a sexual offence against a child where they are acting for the purpose of protecting a child from pregnancy or sexually transmitted infection, protecting the physical safety of a child, or promoting a child's emotional well-being by the giving of advice. In all cases, the person must not be causing or encouraging the commission of an offence or a child's participation in it. Neither must the person be acting for the purpose of obtaining sexual gratification. In effect, these last two stipulations differentiate sexual advice made in good faith, from sexual talk carried out for the purposes of 'grooming' a child for sexual exploitation.

PRACTICAL GUIDELINES 11.2

Health professionals may supply contraceptive advice and treatment to those under 16 years providing that certain criteria under the Fraser Guidelines are met:

1 that the young person understands the advice and has sufficient maturity to understand what is involved
2 that the doctor could not persuade the young person to inform their parents or to allow the doctor to inform them

3 that the young person would be very likely to begin or continue having sexual intercourse with or without contraceptive treatment
4 that, without contraceptive advice or treatment, the young person's physical or mental health would suffer
5 that it would be in the young person's best interest to give such advice or treatment without parental consent (DoH 2004).

CASE STUDY REVIEW 11.2 Acting in Helen's best interests

In Helen's case, you might wish to advise her appropriately on how to avoid a second unwanted pregnancy. In doing so, you would have to discuss methods of contraception and advise her on how to obtain contraceptive treatment. In doing this, you would be acting entirely within the law, even though

Helen is under the legal age of consent, because you are providing this advice in order to prevent her suffering the mental and physical harm of another unwanted pregnancy and are, therefore, acting in her best interests.

This means that, providing the person is acting in the young person's best interests, it is not unlawful to advise a young person on sexual matters. This exception, in statute, covers not only health professionals, but anyone who acts to protect a child, for example teachers, Connexions personal advisers, youth workers, social care practitioners and parents (Sexual Offences Act 2003, Section 73). This 'exception' clause enables health professionals working with young people to provide sexual health advice or treatment for young people under the age of legal consent, without falling foul of the law. Provided it is judged to be in the child's best interest (and you must be prepared to defend this judgment), it is lawful to advise a young person in aspects of contraception and sexual health, even if they are under 16 years of age.

ACTIVITY 11.2 Markers of transition to adulthood

Think about possible markers of the transition between childhood and adulthood within various frameworks.

How might the biological framework be used to define adulthood?

What kind of social markers given by society signal that a person is an adult?

How do religious and moral frameworks understand and mark adulthood?

OUTCOMES OF SEXUAL ACTIVITY

Most people have sex for pleasure or to strengthen or express a loving relationship. These are desirable outcomes of sexual activity. However, sex can sometimes have undesirable outcomes that cause distress for young people. The next section deals with two outcomes of sexual activity that cause concern for young people and for society. These are unintended and unwanted pregnancy and sexually transmitted infections. Those who care for and advise young people who are sexually active are acting in the best interests of the young people in their care, when they help them to avoid these two undesired consequences of sex. In order to do this, it is helpful to have a basic understanding of contraception and of the common sexually transmitted infections.

Contraceptive Methods and Young People

Although not all sexual acts will lead to pregnancy, it is important to help young people avoid an unplanned or unwanted pregnancy, while they are beginning to explore their sexuality. In England in 2009 approximately 38 out of every 1000 girls between 15 and 17 years became pregnant. Of these 38,000 pregnancies 49 per cent ended in abortion, indicating that many girls become pregnant each year, when they do not wish to do so (ONS 2011):

- Half of all conceptions under 18 in England occur in the 20 per cent most deprived wards.
- Teenage pregnancy rates among the most deprived 10 per cent of wards are four times higher than in the 10 per cent least deprived wards.
- Teenage pregnancy 'hotspots', where more than 6 per cent of girls aged 15 to 17 become pregnant, are found in virtually every local authority in England.

If a contraceptive method is used consistently and correctly the vast majority of unwanted pregnancies could be avoided. There are many reasons why young people do not use contraception, some of which will be explored in this section. There is evidence that the younger a person is when she first has sexual intercourse, the less likely she is to use contraception and the more likely she is to regret having sex (Wellings et al. 2001). There are good reasons to encourage young people to delay having sex until they feel ready. Nonetheless, it is likely that some young people, for whom you will care as a child branch nurse, will be sexually active. Clear, consistent, factual advice on contraceptive methods from a trusted health professional can help young people prepare for sexual activity by taking steps to prevent unwanted pregnancy.

ACTIVITY 11.3 Advising Helen about contraception

Consider Helen's needs for contraceptive advice.

What kind of things might you discuss with Helen?

How might you try to assess whether she is Fraser competent?

Will you inform her parents about your discussion?

What is important when you give her advice about contraception?

The next section provides the background knowledge to discuss with Helen her contraceptive options, including the effectiveness and the side effects of the various methods.

How to Prevent a Pregnancy

For pregnancy to occur a sperm must be able to meet and fertilise an egg. Next that fertilised egg must be able to implant in the lining of a womb, in order to develop and eventually become a foetus. Contraceptive methods work by stopping one or more of these processes.

Methods that Prevent Ovulation (Egg Production)

Many contraceptive methods act by preventing a woman from ovulating. If no egg is produced then sperm have nothing to fertilise and pregnancy does not occur:

NO EGGS = NO PREGNANCY

Methods that prevent ovulation are highly effective. These include the combined pill, the contraceptive implant, the contraceptive injection, the contraceptive patch and the contraceptive ring.

Methods that Kill Sperm

Other methods kill sperm before it can get to the egg to fertilise it. The most important is the copper intrauterine device or IUD (sometimes called the 'coil'). The copper IUD also stops a fertilised egg from implanting in the womb and so is a highly effective method. Spermicidal gels, creams or pessaries kill sperm but, on their own, are not a very effective contraceptive method.

Methods that Block Sperm from Meeting the Egg

Stopping sperm from meeting an egg can be achieved by thickening the mucus plug in the cervical canal. This is the method by which most progesterone-only pills work. It is also the method of action of the intrauterine system (IUS), which is a progesterone-containing device that sits in the womb. The

one used in the UK is the Mirena.™ (The IUS also acts to prevent implantation of a fertilised egg and so is a highly effective method of contraception.)

Sperm can also be prevented from reaching the womb by blocking the path with a mechanical barrier, usually a piece of latex. Methods that do this are male and female condoms, diaphragms and caps. These are known as barrier methods because they act as a barrier to the sperm.

Methods that Block Implantation

The copper coil (IUD) and the Mirena™ coil (IUS) can also prevent a fertilised egg from implanting in the lining of the womb.

All these contraceptive methods can be used by young people. Some are much more effective than others and so are preferable when it is important to prevent a pregnancy. All have advantages and some disadvantages and these must be considered by the young person before she (or sometimes he) chooses a method. Although it is unlikely that you will be supplying contraceptive methods in your role as a child branch nurse, it is very helpful to be able to provide young people with the facts about contraception and to dispel any myths. You can also discuss any fears or anxieties they might have about particular methods.

The next section deals in more detail with individual contraceptive methods.

How Effective are Contraceptive Methods?

In Helen's case, a discussion with her should ensue about which methods are most effective with lowest failure rates. This is so that she does not become pregnant again until she really wants to. Not all contraceptive methods are equally effective. Some work better than others and some are easier to use properly. In general, methods that you have to remember to take or use (like pills, condoms and diaphragms) work less well in real life than methods that stay in place for a long time (like IUDs, IUS, implants and injections). Table 11.1 shows the effectiveness of each method when it is used perfectly and the effectiveness of each method when it is used 'in

Table 11.1 Efficacy rates of common reversible contraceptive methods

	Expected pregnancies when used perfectly (per 100 women per year)	Expected pregnancies when used typically (per 100 women per year)
Combined pill and progesterone-only pill	Less than one	Nine pregnancies
Male condoms	Two pregnancies	18 pregnancies
Implant	Less than one	Less than one
Injection	Less than one	Six pregnancies
IUD	Less than one	Less than one
IUS	Less than one	Less than one
Diaphragm	Six pregnancies	12 pregnancies
No contraception	N/A	85 pregnancies

Source: Trussell (2011)

real life'. This 'real-life' effectiveness is known as typical use. The figures refer to how many women would become pregnant if 100 women used the method for a year. If the number is less than one it means that it is possible that no women may accidentally fall pregnant in any one year, indicating a very effective method. The last line shows how many women would get pregnant per year if no contraception is used.

The methods most commonly used by young people (pills and condoms) are the ones that have quite high failure rates in typical use. Methods that are fitted and then can be forgotten about such as the implant, the copper IUD and the IUS are much more effective in typical use. For this reason, the Department of Health has been encouraging the use of these long-acting methods in young people. Together these long-acting methods are sometimes referred to as LARCs or long-acting reversible contraceptives. These are the implant, the injection, the IUD and the IUS. They are highly effective in everyday use and result in very few pregnancies. Everyone considering a new method of contraception should be told about the LARCS.

A summary of contraceptive methods runs thus:

- Long-acting reversible contraceptive methods:
  - implant
  - IUD
  - IUS
  - injection.
- Oral contraceptive pills:
  - combined oral contraceptive pill
  - progesterone-only pill.
- Combined hormonal patch.
- Vaginal contraceptive ring.
- Barrier methods:
  - male condom
  - female condom
  - diaphragms
  - caps.

Long-Acting Reversible Contraceptive Methods

The first four methods listed here last for more than 1 month before needing to be renewed. In fact, some IUDs can last for as long as 10 years. This group of long-acting reversible contraceptive methods are much less likely to be forgotten by the user.

Contraceptive Implants

This is a matchstick-sized rod that is inserted, under local anaesthetic, into the inner side of the upper arm. It slowly releases progesterone over a 3-year period. It stops pregnancy by stopping ovulation. It has very few health risks and is an extremely effective method. It is thought that only one in 2000 women using the method will get pregnant at the end of a year. This makes it more effective than female sterilisation.

Disadvantages

Many women experience irregular or intermittent bleeding with implants. Some women have no periods. Some women dislike the insertion procedure, which involves a needle-like device.

Advantages

The method is extremely effective and lasts for 3 years. Fertility returns immediately on removal. It can be used by women for whom the contraceptive pill might pose health risks, e.g. women or girls who suffer migraine headaches with aura.

Copper-Containing Intrauterine Device (IUD)

This is a small T-shaped device, which is inserted through the cervix and sits in the womb. It is inserted without the need for anaesthetic in a procedure similar to having a cervical smear. It prevents pregnancy primarily by killing sperm. It will also prevent a fertilised egg from implanting in the lining of the womb. The best IUDs last for up to 10 years. It has very few health risks and is a very effective method. It is thought that eight out of every 1000 women using a copper IUD will be pregnant by the end of the first year.

Disadvantages

Copper IUDs can make periods heavy and more painful in some women. Insertion can be uncomfortable in young women who have not yet given birth. If the cervix is infected with a sexually transmitted infection at the time of insertion of any intrauterine device, this can lead to a serious infection of the upper reproductive tract, known as pelvic inflammatory disease (PID). For this reason, swabs for chlamydia and gonorrhoea are taken before insertion. Young women should use condoms as well as a copper IUD to reduce the risk of acquiring a sexually transmitted infection.

Advantages

Copper IUDs are very effective and very long lasting. They are immediately reversible on removal. They can be used by young women for whom hormone use may be risky.

Intrauterine System (IUS)

This is a T-shaped plastic device that contains slow-release progesterone. It is inserted into the womb through the cervix. It prevents pregnancy by thickening the mucus at the cervix and preventing sperm from entering the womb. It also thins the lining of the womb, preventing implantation of a fertilised egg. It is an extremely effective contraceptive method and lasts for 5 years. It has very few health risks.

Disadvantages

Some women experience irregular, intermittent or absent periods with an IUS. Insertion can be uncomfortable in young women who have not given birth. If the cervix is infected with a sexually transmitted infection at the time of insertion of any intrauterine device, this can lead to a serious infection of the upper reproductive tract, known as pelvic inflammatory disease (PID). For this reason, swabs for chlamydia and gonorrhoea are taken before insertion of an IUS, just as before insertion of an IUD (see earlier).

Advantages

It is extremely effective and long lasting and fertility returns immediately when it is removed. It can help with heavy periods by making them lighter and less frequent. It is safe for women who cannot use a contraceptive pill because of fears about blood clots.

Contraceptive Injection

There is only one long-term contraceptive injection licensed in the UK. This is known by the trade name Depo-Provera™ and is often referred to as the 'depot injection'. The injection is given every 12 weeks into the buttock and is an extremely effective method. It works by turning ovulation off and also by thickening the mucus at the cervix. It is a progesterone-containing preparation and has very few health risks. There has been some concern that long-term use in teenagers may cause some thinning of the bones. For this reason, it is not the first recommended choice in women under 19 years but can be used if no other method is suitable.

Disadvantages

The depot injection can cause heavy intermittent bleeding in the first weeks of use. Eventually most users become amenorrhoeic (i.e. have no periods). The injection causes weight gain in some users. The injection can take some time to wear off and fertility can take up to a year to return to normal after stopping the method.

Advantages

It is an extremely effective method. Amenorrhea can be an advantage in women who have painful or heavy periods. Like all progesterone methods, the injection can be used by women for whom oestrogen containing methods are contraindicated, e.g. those who have had a clot in the leg (DVT).

Short-Acting Reversible Contraceptive Methods

The remainder of contraceptive methods act for less than one month before they need to be renewed. In some cases, like the oral contraceptive pills, they must be taken every day. This makes them easier to forget. The most commonly used method of contraception in the UK is the oral contraceptive pill (OCP). There are two types of OCP – the combined oral contraceptive pill (COCP) and the progesterone-only pill (POP). These are both short acting reversible methods.

Combined Oral Contraceptive Pill (COCP)

As the name suggests, this pill is a combination of oestrogen and progesterone. Common trade names in the UK are Microgynon,™ Mercilon,™ Marvelon™ and Cilest.™ There are, in fact, over 30 brand names of COCP in the UK, which vary slightly in their combination of oestrogen and progesterone. The COCP works by switching off ovulation. It is very effective if taken consistently. Unfortunately, its effectiveness is very much reduced if taken inconsistently. The COCP is designed to be taken for 21 days in a row, after which the user takes a 7-day pill-free week. During this time the pill user will have a 'period', which is in fact a bleed brought about by the withdrawal of hormones. Then the next pill packet is started after 7 days and a further 21 days of pills arc taken. This pattern of pill requires the user to remember to take her pill every day of the 21-day packet and to remember to restart the next packet after no more than a 7-day break. The COCP is also affected by enzyme-inducing drugs (e.g. some antiepileptic medication), which reduce its

effectiveness, and by vomiting, if the user is unable to absorb the hormones. The COCP is immediately reversible and fertility returns within days of stopping the method.

Disadvantages

The COCP is a short-acting method that requires the pill taker to be meticulous about remembering to take it. The oestrogen in the COCP makes blood more likely to clot. This means it can be unsuitable for women who have a predisposition to clotting or a medical history of already experiencing clotting problems. It is also unsuitable for migraine sufferers who experience an aura before their headache occurs.

Advantages

The pill is an extremely effective method if used consistently. It can be stopped without the aid of medical assistance. It may also help with painful or heavy periods. COCP users can usually predict exactly when a period is about to occur.

Progesterone-Only Pill (POP)

These pills do not contain oestrogen (unlike the COCP) but, as the name suggests, contain only progesterone. This greatly reduces any health risks associated with taking them. They work by creating a mucus plug at the cervix, which prevents sperm from swimming up the cervical canal and into the womb. A new version of the POP based on the progesterone desogestrel (Cerazette™) also acts by preventing ovulation. POPs are effective contraceptives but most cause a degree of irregular vaginal bleeding, which can limit their acceptability. Cerazette™ is as effective as the COCP in young women, with a failure rate of less than 1 per cent. Older POPs were slightly less effective in young women than the COCP and for that reason were used only as a second-line method. POPs are taken every day of the month, with no 7-day gap.

Disadvantages

POPs can cause irregular bleeding.

Advantages

POPs can be used by women for whom the COCP may be contraindicated, e.g. heavy smokers, those who suffer migraine with aura and those who are wheelchair bound or who have suffered a previous clot in the leg (DVT). They are taken every day, which reduces the possibility of the young user forgetting to restart her pill.

Combined Hormonal Patch

The combined hormonal contraceptive patch can be thought of as the ingredients of a combined pill that is absorbed through the skin. The patch available in the UK at present is known as Evra.™ The contraceptive patch contains both oestrogen and progesterone. It works by stopping ovulation. Three Evra™ patches are applied to the skin consecutively for 1 week each. During week four no patch is used, during which time the user will usually experience a vaginal bleed. Three new patches are then applied for a further 3 weeks. The contraceptive patch is as effective as the combined oral contraceptive pill in perfect use (more than 99 per cent) and has an identical effectiveness during typical use (91 per cent).

Disadvantages

The oestrogen in the combined patch makes blood more likely to clot. This means it can be unsuitable for women who have a predisposition to clotting or a medical history of already experiencing clotting problems. It is also unsuitable for migraine sufferers who experience an aura before their headache occurs. The patch is visible on the skin of the user and is only available in a beige colour. The user must remember to replace the patch after the 7-day break.

Advantages

The patch provides a highly effective method of contraception, which is rapidly reversible and under the woman's control. The woman does not have to remember to take a pill each day.

Vaginal Contraceptive Ring

The vaginal contraceptive ring contains both oestrogen and progesterone and can be viewed as the ingredients of a COCP absorbed through the vaginal mucosa. This has the effect of stopping ovulation. The woman inserts the ring high into the vagina where it is retained and slowly releases its hormones. The woman removes the ring after 3 weeks and allows a 7-day break, during which she will usually experience a vaginal bleed. On the eighth day she places a new ring in the vagina for a further 3 weeks. The vaginal ring is a highly effective method which, with perfect use, is 99 per cent effective. In typical use, it is 91 per cent effective. Fertility returns almost immediately once the ring is removed for more than 7 days.

Disadvantages

As with the COCP and contraceptive patch, the oestrogen in the contraceptive ring makes blood more likely to clot. This means it can be unsuitable for women who have a predisposition to clotting or a medical history of already experiencing clotting problems. It is also unsuitable for migraine sufferers who experience an aura before their headache occurs. The vaginal ring may not be suitable for those young women who dislike touching their vaginas.

Advantages

The ring provides a highly effective, readily reversible method of contraception that is under the woman's control. The ring, once inserted, stays in place for 3 weeks so the user does not have to remember to take a pill every day.

Barrier Methods

Barrier methods act by presenting a physical barrier to sperm, thus preventing fertilisation. The most commonly used barrier method is the male condom. Female condoms, diaphragms and caps are also barrier methods. The male condom is the second most frequently used method of contraception in the UK. However female condoms, diaphragms and caps are much less used by young people.

Male Condoms

These are most commonly made of latex rubber. It is possible to buy non-latex condoms, which are useful if either partner has a latex allergy. Male condoms are effective methods of contraception if used correctly and consistently. The effectiveness of this method varies between 82 per cent in typical use and 98 per cent in perfect use. Condoms also protect against most sexually transmitted infections, including HIV. Male condoms must be used before any genital contact is made. It is important to check that a condom is in date and that the packet is not damaged. Fingernails and sharp objects will tear the very thin latex of a condom, making it ineffective. Oil-based substances such as baby oil, massage oil, sun cream, Vaseline™ and some ointment and creams used for thrush treatment such as Canestan™ can also cause condoms to weaken and fail. Water based lubricants designed for use with condoms such as K-Y Jelly™ are safe. When the male partner has ejaculated the condom must be grasped firmly by the base to prevent it slipping off in the vagina as the penis becomes less rigid. Condoms must be used at every episode of sexual intercourse and cannot be re-used.

Disadvantages

Condoms are less effective than LARC methods or contraceptive pills. A degree of familiarity and practice is required to use condoms correctly. Condoms can split, tear and slip off. Condoms must be used every time intercourse takes place.

Advantages

Condoms can be bought without prescription or obtained free from sexual health clinics. Condoms do not pose any health risks and provide some protection from sexually transmitted infections.

Female Condoms

Female condoms are non-latex sheaths that are worn by the female partner. They work by collecting semen and thus preventing sperm from entering the womb. The one available in the UK is known as the Femidom.™ They are baggier than male condoms and have two rings at either end, which help with insertion. The woman places the smaller ring high in the vagina before intercourse and the larger ring sits outside the vagina, covering the labia. Femidoms are slightly less effective than male condoms in typical use (i.e. about 79 per cent) but work better if used correctly and consistently. They have the advantage of placing responsibility for condom use with the female. Because they are not made of latex, they are not damaged by oil based substances. However, care must be taken not to allow the man's penis to go around rather than inside the Femidom™ when entering the vagina. Like male condoms, they must be used before any penetration takes place and must be used every time intercourse occurs.

Disadvantages

They may interfere with foreplay. They can sometimes be noisy in use. They are more expensive than male condoms.

Advantages

They can be bought without prescription. They provide protection from sexually transmitted infections. They do not cause any health risks or systemic side-effects.

Diaphragms

Diaphragms are latex rubber rings with a compressible spring around the outside of the ring. They are designed to be inserted in the vagina, covering the cervix. They are used with spermicidal cream or pessaries. They act by preventing sperm from reaching the womb and any fertilisable eggs. They must be inserted before intercourse and retained in the vagina for at least 6 hours after intercourse. In practice, if sex takes place in the evening, this usually means they are removed the following morning. They are about 88 per cent effective in typical use and 94 per cent effective in perfect use. They have been shown to be more effective in an established relationship and in older women. Diaphragms are not frequently used by young women. They must be used correctly and inserted before every act of intercourse, to achieve maximum effectiveness. When inserted correctly the diaphragm should be comfortable and virtually unnoticed by either partner. A diaphragm once prescribed can be re-used and usually lasts for 2 to 3 years.

Disadvantages

They have a failure rate of 6 per cent even with perfect use. It takes practice and commitment to use one effectively and reliably. They require the user to be comfortable with touching her own genital area. They need to be fitted initially by a health professional to ensure they are the correct size for the woman.

Advantages

They are discreet and can be fitted before intercourse, thus not interrupting the flow of sex. They are within the woman's control. They do not pose any health risks or systemic side-effects.

Caps

Caps are similar in nature and action to diaphragms but are smaller and fit over the cervix itself. They have the same effectiveness as diaphragms. They require a little more dexterity to fit correctly since they must be placed exactly over the cervix. The method of use, advantages and disadvantages are the same as those for the diaphragm.

ACTIVITY 11.4 Choosing a suitable method

What are the most effective methods that Helen could use?

What methods might be less suitable in terms of effectiveness?

What side-effects might Helen need to think about?

ACTIVITY 11.5 Young people and the pill

Why might a young woman like Helen become pregnant even though she is being prescribed an oral contraceptive pill?

What kind of things might make the pill less effective for her?

Helen might also have been told a lot about using condoms for protection during sex. Although condoms do prevent most sexually transmitted infections they are not very effective at preventing pregnancy in typical use. The failure rate for condoms in typical use is 18 to 21 per cent (18 to 21 out of 100 women becoming pregnant per year). For this reason, although Helen should be encouraged to use condoms to protect against sexually transmitted infections, she should be aware that they do not provide the most effective means of contraception available to her.

ACTIVITY 11.6 Young people and condoms

What kind of things might make condoms less effective for Helen?

How might you advise her about using condoms?

Emergency Contraception

Despite her best intentions, Helen might find herself at risk from pregnancy due to having had sex without contraception or having had a condom burst or come off. If this happens she needs to know about emergency contraception (EC). This is contraception that can be used after intercourse, to stop a pregnancy occurring. It is important that Helen is aware that she can use emergency contraception. She also needs to know where to get it and how soon she needs to use it. If you can advise her about these things she will be better equipped to deal with an accidental unprotected act of intercourse. At the present time in the UK there are three forms of emergency contraception. Two involve taking a pill and one involves having a copper IUD or coil fitted.

Emergency Contraceptive Pills

The pills available are marketed as Levonelle,™ which has been available for a number of years and ellaOne,™ which has been available only since November 2009.

The most frequently used emergency contraceptive in pill form is Levonelle.™ This is a single tablet of Levonorgestrel, which is a progesterone hormone. Levonelle™ is available free of charge from contraception and sexual health clinics, GPs, some A&E units and some pharmacies. It can also be purchased for around £25 to £30 from pharmacies, without prescription.

Levonelle™ should be taken as soon as possible after an act of unprotected intercourse. However, it can be used up to 72 hours after unprotected sex. Levonelle's main mechanism of action is to delay ovulation by a few days. This gives time for any live sperm in the female reproductive tract to die before an egg becomes available. Overall Levonelle™ is thought to prevent around 80 per cent of conceptions that would otherwise have occurred.

Ulipristal is a new method of emergency contraception available in the UK. It was launched in November 2009. It is a pill and is marketed under the trade name of ellaOne.™ It is at least as effective as Levonelle™ at preventing pregnancies and research suggests it will prevent around 80 to 85 per cent of pregnancies that might otherwise have occurred. ellaOne™ is only available on prescription and so must be accessed through contraception and sexual health clinics, GUM clinics or GPs. It cannot be bought over the counter. The main advantage of ellaOne™ is that it is effective up to 120 hours after intercourse.

Emergency Copper Intrauterine Device (IUD)

Recent surveys have consistently shown that the majority of men and women have heard of the emergency contraceptive pill. However, only four out of 10 are aware of the possibility of using a copper coil as an emergency contraceptive method. This is regrettable because the emergency coil can be very useful in certain circumstances. The copper-bearing coil as an emergency contraceptive method prevents 99 per cent of pregnancies that might otherwise have occurred. This is an improvement on the 80 per cent of pregnancies prevented by Levonelle.™ If a young woman is adamant that she does not want to become pregnant, a copper-bearing coil may be a good option for her.

The copper coil also has the advantage of being effective up to 120 hours after the act of unprotected intercourse. This means that if, for example, a condom splits on a Friday night, before a bank holiday Monday, the coil can be fitted on the Tuesday or Wednesday following. Some people think that a coil cannot be fitted in a woman who has not delivered a baby. This is no longer the case. Even if a woman has not had a baby, a small copper-bearing coil can still be fitted either as an emergency method or as a permanent method of contraception.

When advising a young person who is sexually active and using a method of contraception that may fail (e.g. condoms), it may be helpful to remind him of the emergency contraceptive options that are available and how to access them. It is important to stress the time limits within which emergency contraception must be started. It is also worth pointing out that emergency contraception should only be used in 'emergencies' and that it is always better to have a regular method of contraception in place.

STIs and Young People

Pregnancy is only one of the unwelcome effects of sexual activity. Sexually transmitted infections are also a problem that may come to your attention when looking after young people. Young people under the age of 25 years are disproportionately affected by sexually transmitted infections (STIs). Young women aged 16 to 19 years have the highest rates of STIs of all women. Most STIs can be prevented by using a condom during sexual intercourse. Knowledge of the need to use a condom to prevent STIs is not enough to ensure that young people actually practise 'safe sex' on all occasions. Human behaviour is complex and many factors may mean that condom use is intermittent. Alcohol and drug use, young age, lack of experience and lack of negotiating skills can all mean that a condom is not used for every act of intercourse (McMunn and Caan 2007). There is some evidence to suggest that young people in established relationships stop using condoms as a mark of fidelity and trust (Bolton et al. 2010). This can be a problem if one of the couple has a previously acquired STI. Condoms may also be abandoned when the female partner becomes established on a more effective method of contraception such as an implant or the contraceptive pill.

The concept of 'double Dutch' is useful to stress in conversations with young people regarding contraception and STIs. This refers to using a highly effective method such as an implant, IUD, IUS pill or injection for contraception, while also using condoms to prevent infection.

ACTIVITY 11.7   Advising Joel about STIs

What is likely to be the cause of these lesions?

How might you advise Joel?

It is likely that Joel has genital warts which are the result of a sexually transmitted infection. Joel is 16 years old and so he is able to give consent to sexual intercourse. As long as Joel is not being coerced or abused by an adult in a position of trust (e.g. a teacher or social worker), there will be no legal concerns regarding his sexual activity. However, because he is a young person you may still have concerns about his welfare and wish to advise him on how to explore his sexuality safely.

If concerned that he lacked the mental capacity to consent despite being 16 years of age (e.g. because of a learning

---

CASE STUDY 11.2   Young person with an STI

Joel is admitted to your ward for rehabilitation following an operation to correct a contracture caused by his cerebral palsy. He is 16 years old. He attends mainstream school and is about to take his GSCEs. While you are helping him attend to his personal hygiene needs he mentions to you that he is worried about some 'cauliflower-like things' that have appeared on his penis.

CASE STUDY REVIEW 11.3 Attending a GUM clinic

Joel can attend a GUM clinic to have his warts treated. He will also be able to have a screening test for a number of other STIs. He can be assured of confidentiality when attending a GUM clinic. Even his GP will not be informed of his visit unless he gives permission for this.

Accessing a clinic may prove difficult for Joel, especially if he does not want his parents to know about this diagnosis. You may want to discuss with him how he might get to a clinic. You might also want to discuss with him whether he wants his parents to be involved.

disability), seek advice from more experienced colleagues on how to proceed to protect him from exploitation or harm. However, the Mental Capacity Act 2005 makes it clear that no assumption can be made that a person lacks capacity, simply on the basis of a learning disability. It would be necessary to explore his understanding of the situation and his ability to make an informed decision.

The next section will discuss some of the more common STIs in the UK in the 21st century.

Chlamydia

Chlamydia is by far the most commonly diagnosed sexually transmitted infection in the UK. In 2010 there were over 215,000 diagnosed cases in the UK (Health Protection Agency (HPA) 2011a). It affects young people under 24 years more than any other age group. More than half the cases in men and almost 90 per cent of the cases in women affect those under the age of 24 years (HPA 2011a).

Symptoms

Chlamydia may cause symptoms or it may be asymptomatic (i.e. the person is carrying the infection without experiencing any noticeable effects) (see Table 11.2). It is estimated that about 70 per cent of infections in women and 50 per cent of infections in men are asymptomatic. This means that the person does not realise that she is infectious or infected.

The complications of chlamydia include infertility in women (and less often in men). Because even asymptomatic infection can cause infertility in some people, it is important to screen for and to treat chlamydia in young people.

Testing

The test for chlamydia in a person who does not have symptoms is straightforward and painless. It involves a self-taken vaginal swab or a urine sample for women and a urine sample for men.

Treating

The treatment is a single dose of antibiotics. Sexual intercourse should be avoided until 7 days after treatment.

Follow-up

If someone is diagnosed with chlamydia, it is important to trace, test and treat her recent sexual partners as well. This is called partner notification or contact tracing. The person who has been diagnosed can contact her sexual partners personally or a sexual health clinic can do it on her behalf. Those affected should be given advice on using condoms to prevent or reduce re-infection.

Genital Warts

Genital warts are the second most commonly diagnosed sexually transmitted infection in the UK. In 2010 there were nearly 76,000 newly diagnosed cases in England (HPA 2011b). The rates of genital wart infection have increased in the last 10 years. Young people under 24 years are most affected. Genital warts are caused by human papilloma virus infection (HPV).

Table 11.2 Chlamydia symptoms in men and women

Symptoms of chlamydia in men	Symptoms of chlamydia in women
• Dysuria • Urethral discharge	• Dysuria • Vaginal discharge • Intermenstrual bleeding • Abdominal pain • Pelvic inflammatory disease (PID)
More rarely • Prostatitis • Proctitis • Conjunctivitis • Epididymo-orchitis • Reactive arthritis (Reiter's syndrome)	More rarely • Peri-hepatitis • Conjunctivitis • Reactive arthritis (Reiter's syndrome)

Symptoms

The symptoms are small warty growths on the genitals like those noticed by Joel. These are usually softer than warts on other parts of the body. Sometimes these warts affect only the cervix in women and so are not visible. If the person's immune system is weakened, as can occur in pregnancy, or in cases of HIV (human immunodeficiency virus), the warts can become very large.

Testing

Diagnoses are made by visual identification of the warty lesions.

Treating

Treatment involves removing the warts. The human papilloma virus that causes the warts is not treated. Warts can be removed chemically by applying caustic or immune moderating solutions. Alternatively, they can be frozen off using liquid nitrogen, burned off by electrocautery or removed surgically.

Follow-up

No follow-up is needed. Women with genital warts are reminded to attend for regular cervical smears since some strains of human papilloma virus (HPV) are also associated with cervical cancer. Wearing a condom that covers the lesions can partially protect a sexual partner from acquiring the virus. Current sexual partners may benefit from examination, diagnosis, treatment or advice but previous sexual partners are not usually contacted.

Genital Herpes

Genital herpes is the third most common sexually transmitted disease in England. In 2010 there were nearly 30,000 newly diagnosed cases in GUM clinics in England (HPA 2011b). The rates of genital herpes, like those of genital warts and chlamydia, have risen over the last 10 years and continue to rise. It is caused by infection with the herpes simplex virus, which also causes cold sores around the mouth. Herpes viruses infect an individual and then can lie dormant for many months or years, only to return periodically to produce symptoms.

Symptoms

Genital herpes can be asymptomatic in up to 50 per cent of people when they first contract the virus. Asymptomatic virus shedding (i.e. being infectious without symptoms) is also common. When symptoms do occur they differ slightly between the first exposure to the virus (the primary infection) and subsequent returns of symptoms (recurrences). On first exposure to the virus people can experience a flu-like illness with fever, muscle pains and headaches. Small, multiple, shallow, painful ulcers develop on the genitals. These can cause intense pain if urine passes over them during urination. Recurrent attacks of genital herpes can occur in the months and years after infection. These are usually milder than the original attack, and occur without the flu-like symptoms. However, the painful ulceration recurs. Recurrences usually become less frequent with time since infection.

Testing

If genital herpes is suspected swabs from the lesion are taken and sent for cell culture. Blood samples can show antibodies to the virus and can help differentiate between primary and recurrent infections.

Treating

The symptoms of primary genital herpes can be lessened and their duration shortened by using oral antiviral therapy (e.g. aciclovir tablets) usually for 5 days. The virus is not eliminated and recurrences are not prevented by taking these drugs. Advice on saline bathing of lesions and how to manage painful urination and analgesics are often helpful. Treatment may not be needed for recurrences but can be used if they are severe or troublesome.

Follow-up

Patients may need supportive advice and counselling after diagnosis and there are some self-help groups who can provide ongoing support (e.g. Herpes Alliance). Partner notification will help identify those with undiagnosed disease but it is not carried out in all areas or in all clinics. Advice on reducing transmission to partners is important. Condom use will lessen but not eliminate transmission of herpes between sexual partners.

Gonorrhea

Gonorrhoea is less common than the preceding three sexually transmitted infections. In the UK in 2010 there were just over 18,500 diagnosed cases (HPA 2011a).

Symptoms

It causes more acute and more noticeable symptoms than chlamydia (see Table 11.3). Despite this, 20 per cent of cases in men and 50 per cent of cases in women are thought to be asymptomatic and therefore the person does not know he or she is infected.

One of the complications of gonorrhoea is infertility in women due to ovarian tube damage.

Testing

The tests for gonorrhoea involve swabs of the affected areas. This means urethral (and sometimes rectal) swabs for men and women and a cervical swab for women. A urine sample in men or a self-taken vaginal swab in women may be used in some clinics.

Treating

Gonorrhoea has become increasingly resistant to many common antibiotics. For this reason, each region will treat it differently according to advice given by the laboratory that tests the samples. Treatment is usually with injectable antibiotics although in some circumstances oral antibiotics are used.

Follow-up

It is important to retest people diagnosed with gonorrhoea about 2 weeks after treatment to make sure that the treatment has been successful and the infection cured. Partner notification, testing and treating is also carried out. Condom use will reduce or prevent the transmission of gonorrhoea.

Table 11.3 Gonorrhea symptoms in men and women

Symptoms of gonorrhoea in men	Symptoms of gonorrhoea in women
• Dysuria • Urethral discharge • Tender inguinal nodes	• Dysuria • Vaginal discharge • Intermenstrual bleeding • Abdominal pain
More rarely • Epididymo-orchitis • Conjunctivitis • Pharyngitis • Rectal pain/discharge	More rarely • Conjunctivitis • Pharyngitis • Rectal pain/discharge

---

ACTIVITY 11.8 Advising Joel on safer sex

Joel tells you that he has a girlfriend who is also 16 years old. They started to have sex a few months ago. He has also had sex with one or two other friends at a party. He uses a condom with his casual partners but not with his girlfriend because she is on 'the pill'.

What might you like to explore with Joel?

What advice will you give him?

SUMMARY OF KEY LEARNING

About one in four young people becomes sexually active under the age of 16 years (Wellings et al. 2001). This means that when nursing young people discussion on personal matters to do with contraception and sexual health may occur. Although it is illegal to have sexual intercourse with a young person under the age of 16, this does not prevent your advising a young person on these matters, if it is in her best interest. Providing clear factual advice on contraception and sexually transmitted infections will allow young people to make informed decisions and may help them protect themselves from the unintended pregnancy and sexually transmitted infections.

- One-quarter of young people in the UK have their first experience of sexual intercourse under the age of 16.
- It is legal and good professional practice to provide young people with clear, accurate factual advice on sexual health and contraception even if they are under the age of consent (i.e. under 16 years).
- The oral contraceptive pill and condoms have higher failure rates than the LARCs methods of contraception. For this reason, LARCs should be discussed with young people who need contraception.
- Young people under the age of 24 years suffer from disproportionately high rates of sexually transmitted infection compared to the rest of the population.
- While condoms are not very effective methods of contraception, for young people they are important for reducing the risk of acquiring a sexually transmitted infection. Double Dutch methods, where condoms are used for protection against infection and another more reliable method is used to prevent contraception, should be encouraged.

FURTHER RESOURCES

BASHH guidelines: **http://www.bashh.org/guidelines**. This is the website of the British Association for Sexual Health and HIV. It contains guidelines for the diagnosis and treatment of STIs.

BASHH guide to treatment of genital warts: **http://www.bashh.org/documents/86/86.pdf**

BASHH guidelines for management of genital herpes: **http://www.bashh.org/documents/115/115.pdf**

BASHH guideline for management of chlamydia: **http://www.bashh.org/documents/61/61.pdf**

Faculty of sexual and reproductive health guidelines: **http://www.fsrh.org/pages/clinical_guidance.asp**. This site contains guidelines for all the contraceptive methods presently available. It is designed for health professionals and has freely downloadable summaries and guidelines.

RCN forum: sexual health for non-experts (RCN membership required): **http://www.rcn.org.uk/development/learning/learningzone/clinical_skills/sexual_health_for_non-experts**

Nursing and Midwifery Council (NMC): **http://www.nmc-uk. org**. This site contains advice on confidentiality, consent, safeguarding and other legal, ethical and professional issues that will affect your nursing practice.

NMC guidance on confidentiality: **http://www.nmc-uk.org/ Nurses-and-midwives/Advice-by-topic/A/Advice/ Confidentiality/**

NMC advice for nurses working with children and young people: **http://www.nmc-uk.org/Nurses-and-midwives/Advice-by-topic/A/Advice/Advice-on-working-with-children-and-young-people/**

Sexual Offences Act 2003: **http://www.legislation.gov.uk/ ukpga/2003/42/contents**. This site allows you to read the law that covers sexual offences, including the laws governing the age of consent. It makes it clear that health professionals can advise young people on sexual matters if they are acting in the best interests of the young people.

Mental Capacity Act 2005: **http://www.legislation.gov.uk/ ukpga/2005/9/contents**. This site allows you to read the law that covers decision making and consent in adults with learning difficulties or dementia.

ANSWERS TO ACTIVITIES

ACTIVITY 11.1 Acting in Helen's best interests

Consider the health and well being issues that arise as a result of Helen's diagnosis.

What might you wish to do to ensure the best outcome for Helen?

What anxieties might you have?

What difficult legal or ethical situations might you find yourself in?

Helen has clearly had sexual intercourse despite being under the age of sexual consent. It is in her best interests that this is discussed with her and that she does not become pregnant again unless she wishes to do so. She will therefore need advice on how to prevent a pregnancy and how to keep herself safe from sexually transmitted infections.

You may be concerned about whether Helen is being exploited or abused in her sexual relationship. Some young people are groomed by much older adults and coerced into having sex. You will want to find out who Helen has been having sex with and under what circumstances. You want to know the age of her sexual partner or partners.

This information has to be sought sensitively and without distressing or humiliating Helen.

You might be concerned about the balance between your duty of confidentiality and your duty to disclose information if a young person is at risk of harm. You might also be concerned about whether Helen's parents are aware that she has been sexually active and whether you should tell them.

You may not break your duty of confidentiality toward Helen, regardless of her age, unless you are concerned that she is being exposed to harm. Given that she nearly died as a result of her ectopic pregnancy, you might decide that in this case, disclosure is necessary. However, this does not mean you can tell anyone who might ask. You must always be able to defend your breach of confidentiality as being in the patient's interest and, in this case, social services are the appropriate agency to which to disclose the information.

In every case, you would seek the advice of your line manager and more senior colleagues.

You may not tell Helen's parents about her sexual activity but you should encourage Helen to do so, since the support of a responsible and caring adult is important for a young sexually active person.

You might also be concerned about whether it is legal for you to give sexual advice to a young person under the age of consent. Fortunately, the Sexual Offences Act makes it clear that you may do so provided it is in the young person's best interest.

ACTIVITY 11.2 Markers of transition to adulthood

Think about possible markers of the transition between childhood and adulthood within various frameworks.

How might the biological framework be used to define adulthood?

- Beginning or end of puberty
- First menstrual period
- Voice breaking
- Ability to grow a beard

What kind of social markers given by society signal that a person is an adult?

- Driving licence
- Voting rights
- Joining the army
- Consent to medical treatment
- Consent to marriage
- Consent to sexual intercourse

How do religious and moral frameworks understand and mark adulthood?

Maturity to accept full strictures or responsibilities of faith e.g. confirmation (Christian), bar/bat mitzvah (Jewish).

ACTIVITY 11.3 Advising Helen about contraception

You might like to discuss with Helen whether she wants to or thinks she might continue having sex.

If Helen is going to continue having sex, it is important that she does not become pregnant again without wanting to do so. She will therefore need advice on contraceptive methods. Before giving advice, you must assess whether she is Fraser competent.

You might like to start by finding out how much she knows about how pregnancy occurs.

You might also want to discus with her what methods of contraception she knows about and what methods she has used.

If you feel she has sufficient maturity to understand what is involved and that it is in her best interest to receive some advice on contraception, you might want to discuss with her the options that she has.

You are not obliged to inform Helen's parents or guardians about the fact that you are discussing contraception with her. If she is Fraser competent and does not wish you to break her confidentiality on this matter then you *must not* do so, unless you suspect she is at serious risk of harm. However, it is good practice, and probably in Helen's best interest, that her parents are aware that she is sexually active and considering using contraception. You should encourage her to involve her parents or guardians in this decision.

In Helen's case, you will probably want to discuss with her methods that are highly effective with low failure rates.

You will also want to discuss the benefits, risks and possible side-effects of the methods so that Helen is enabled to make a fully informed choice about her method of contraception.

ACTIVITY 11.4 Choosing a suitable method

What are the most effective methods that Helen could use?

What methods might be less suitable in terms of effectiveness?

What side-effects might Helen need to think about?

Helen will want to use a very safe but very effective method of contraception if she wishes to continue having sex. The most effective method available at present is the contraceptive implant. This has a pregnancy rate of less than one in 1000 women per year and carries virtually no health risks. However, it often causes irregular bleeding. It also has to be inserted in her arm under local anaesthetic and she will have to have another minor surgical procedure if she wants it removed.

Copper coils (IUDs) and Mirena coils (IUS) are both highly effective and very safe alternatives for teenagers. Each has a failure rate of less than one pregnancy per 100 users

per year and once inserted will last between 5 and 10 years depending on the device. However, IUDs and IUSs must be fitted through the cervix in a procedure similar to having a smear taken. Helen may not want to undergo this insertion procedure.

The depot injection is not a first-line choice for Helen because of the concerns around loss of bone minerals in young teenagers using the injection. However, if no other method is suitable Helen could use the injection which she will receive every 12 weeks.

Helen might have expected to use an oral contraceptive pill. This provides a good effective means of contraception provided it is taken properly. However, in typical use up to nine in 100 women using the pill get pregnant every year. This figure is often higher in younger women. This means that an oral pill might not be the best choice for Helen.

ACTIVITY 11.5 Young people and the pill

The oral contraceptive pill has a higher failure rate when used by young people than when used 'perfectly'. Because it is a short-acting method it is necessary for the young person to take it correctly and consistently, remembering the rules about how to take it.

Reasons for pill failure in young women include:

1 forgetting to take the pill every day

2 forgetting to restart the packet after a 7-day break
3 vomiting pills
4 going away for the weekend and forgetting to take the pills with her
5 taking other medication (such as St John's Wort or some drugs for epilepsy) that interferes with the pill and make it less effective.

ACTIVITY 11.6 Young people and condoms

Condoms fail quite often in typical, everyday use. If 100 women use only condoms for a year, about 18 of them will become pregnant.

Things which make condoms less effective:

1 not using one every time
2 tearing it before it goes on

3 using a condom that is out of date
4 putting a condom on after genital contact has already happened
5 condoms bursting or splitting
6 having oily substances (massage oil, lipstick, Vaseline) on your hands when handling a condom.

ACTIVITY 11.7 Advising Joel about STIs

It is likely that Joel has developed genital warts. Genital warts are a very common infection that develops as a result of becoming infected by the human papilloma virus (HPV). It is infectious and Joel is likely to have caught it from a sexual partner and will be at risk of passing it on to subsequent sexual partners.

You will want to advise Joel on what he should do about the warts that he has noticed.

You might also want to give him some general advice about sexually transmitted infections and how to avoid them.

You will probably want to advise Helen that she should use 'double Dutch' contraception. That means always using a condom to reduce the risk of catching an STI in addition to using a more effective method to prevent her becoming pregnant.

You might want to enquire tactfully about whether his sexual partners are male or female. You should not assume that all your young patients are heterosexual. The age of consent is the same whether his partners are male or female.

Joel will want advice on how to have his warts treated, where to go to get screened for other STIs and how to protect himself from other infections.

ACTIVITY 11.8 Advising Joel on safer sex

Joel tells you that he has a girlfriend who is also 16 years old. They started to have sex a few months ago. He has also had sex with one or two other friends at a party. He uses a condom with his casual partners but not with his girlfriend because she is on 'the pill'.

What might you like to explore with Joel?

What advice will you give him?

You might want to talk to Joel about the failure rate and the chances of pregnancy when using a condom. Is this the only method of contraception he is using with his 'casual' partners?

You will want to stress to Joel the importance of using a condom every time he has sex. 'Double Dutch', i.e. using the

pill and a condom, would be a good option with his regular partner.

You might also like to discuss how he can obtain condoms easily and where he can get them for free. You might want to discuss with Joel how to use a condom properly and the steps he can take to ensure it does not break or fail.

You might want to discuss with Joel whether it is a good idea to have more than one sexual partner at a time. This is a difficult judgement to make because you do not wish to appear judgemental or disapproving. However, having several sexual partners at once greatly increases the rate of transmission of sexually transmitted infections.

SELECTED REFERENCES

Bolton, M., McKay, A. and Schneider, M. (2010) Relational influences on condom use discontinuation: a qualitative study of young adult women in dating relationships. *Canadian Journal of Human Sexuality*, 19(3), 91–104.

Department of Health (DoH) (2004) Best practice guidance for doctors and other health professionals on the provision of advice and treatment to young people under 16 on contraception, sexual and reproductive health: **http://www.dh.gov.uk/en/Publicationsandstatistics/Publications/PublicationsPolicyAndGuidance/DH_4086960**

Health Protection Agency (HPA) (2011a) Number and rates of selected STI diagnoses in genitourinary medicine clinics and community settings in the UK 2008–10: **http://www.hpa.org.uk/webc/HPAwebFile/HPAweb_C/1317132033760**

Health Protection Agency (HPA) (2011b) Numbers of selected STI diagnoses made at genito-urinary clinics in England

2001–2010: **http://www.hpa.org.uk/webc/HPAwebFile/HPAweb_C/1215589013442**

McMunn, V. and Caan, W. (2007) Chlamydia infection, alcohol and sexual behaviour in women. *British Journal of Midwifery*, 15(4), 221–224.

Nursing and Midwifery Council (NMC) (2012) NMC guidance on confidentiality: **http://www.nmc-uk.org/nurses-and-midwires/advice-by-topic/A/advice/confidentiality.**

Okasha, A., Ragheb, K., Attia, A.H., Seif el Dawla, A., Okasha, T. and Ismail, R. (2001) Prevalence of Obsessive Compulsive Symptoms (OCS) in a sample of Egyptian adolescents. *Encephale*, 27(1), 8–14.

ONS (2011) Conception statistics in England and Wales 2009: **http://www.ons.gov.uk/ons/rel/vsob1/conception-statistics--england-and-wales/2009/index.html**

Trussell, J. (2011) Contraceptive failure in the United States. *Contraception*, 83, 397–404.

Wellings, et al. (2001) Sexual behaviour in Britain: early heterosexual experience. *The Lancet*, 1(12), 1843–1850.

CHAPTER 12
Mental Health and the Challenges of Mental Ill Health

Steven Walker and Dave Hawkes

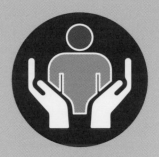

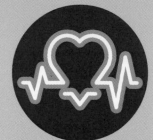

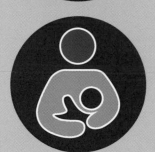

LEARNING OUTCOMES

On completion of this chapter, the reader will be able to:

- Explore the impact and implications of policy and legislation on the services for mental health delivered to children and adolescents.
- Evaluate the collaboration at the personal, organisational and societal level in providing child and adolescent mental health services.
- Analyse the evidence base for health promotion in child and adolescent mental health services.
- Reflect on the appropriate approaches when communicating with a child in distress.
- Review the evidence base for care or service delivery to children and adolescents for those with mental health problems and/or disorders.
- Understand and explore the therapeutic interventions used with children who have mental health issues.
- Explore the overview of family and system therapies for children and young people.

TALKING POINT

'Grown-ups never understand anything for themselves, and it is tiresome for children to be always and forever explaining things to them' (Saint-Exupery 1943).

'Parents and their children should be central to the process of decision-making about their care, and receive appropriate information to exercise choice. They need to be fully informed and provided with information about the nature of the illness, different interventions and treatment options available to them and relevant support groups and voluntary organisations that might help them.'

NSFC YPS (2004) Standard 6

INTRODUCTION

The chapter aspires to provide a foundation of theoretical ideas and practical guidance that will offer support and create the basis for informed, reflective, confident practice. For a minority of young people, the issues for mental health become more challenging and they will require further support to resolve the problems that arise and this will also be explored. While there is a real need for mental health nurses specialising in children and young people's mental health, it is not the role of this chapter to explore this specialist training, rather it is important in any setting where children and young people are to offer guidance on how to assess, offer simple interventions that cause no harm to the child or young person and refer to the appropriate services, including child and family consultation (CAFC) or Child and Adolescent Mental Health Services (CAMHS). Early intervention to build mental well-being and resilience in infancy and childhood can prevent mental health problems in adult life and lead to better outcomes in health, education, employment and relationships (Teatheredge 2012).

Protective factors that may reduce the incidence of mental health challenges may include:

- low distress
- sociability
- good self-help skills
- impulse control
- strong motivation
- keen interests or hobbies
- supportive peer group
- positive self-image
- self-confidence
- independence
- good communication skills
- good problem-solving skills
- reflective learning style
- assertion
- positive set of values.

'Mental health' is usually a measure of how well a person is able to cope with daily challenges and difficulties. For example, children and young people are considered mentally 'healthy' if they are able to:

- develop physically, emotionally, intellectually and socially
- enjoy personal relationships and have an awareness of others
- develop a sense of right and wrong
- play and learn.

However, there is a problem with this definition, in that even if a child may not be able to do some of these things listed, it does not mean that they are mentally 'unhealthy' or mentally ill. In addition, there are also times when children feel stressed, anxious, worried, upset or angry as these are all part of development and indeed show a healthy range of emotions. But when these experiences continue and negatively impact on everyday life, they can become signs of problems with emotional well-being and may lead to mental health difficulties.

The need to support children and young people's mental health has attracted more attention in recent years due to increased demands on specialist resources by parents, nurses and primary healthcare staff. Adolescents are generally perceived as a healthy age group and yet 20 per cent of them, in any given year, experience a mental health problem, most commonly depression or anxiety. In many settings, suicide is among the leading causes of death among young people (WHO 2012, page 1). Attempting to meet the needs of children such as Nina who have emotional and behavioural problems as well as their carers/families has proved onerous. The evidence suggests the need for policy and practice changes to ensure a sufficient range of provision and skills to improve the effectiveness and efficiency of Child and Adolescent Mental Health Services (CAMHS). This chapter aims to provide a resource for a variety of contexts in which health and social care professionals may encounter situations where concerns are expressed about the behaviour, emotional state, or mental health of a child or young person.

CASE STUDY 12.1

Nina who has a history of self-harm

A multi-agency meeting on the children's ward is considering the case of Nina, a young South Asian female, 15 years of age with a history of self-harm and school refusal. She is described by her parents as 'moody' and 'uncommunicative' (see Figure 12.1). The nurse noticed old parallel cut marks on her arm when Nina was admitted following alcohol intoxication. Nina did not respond to questions about the marks and voices her concern that the nurses on the ward are trying to poison her. The police have been involved in the past due to incidents of shoplifting and gang-related alcohol abuse. The teacher reports that Nina is hard working but low on ability when she does attend lessons. As far as social services are concerned there has been sporadic contact with the family over the past few years with one younger brother sustaining one incident of non-accidental injury. There are four other children in the household and the father has a history of domestic violence.

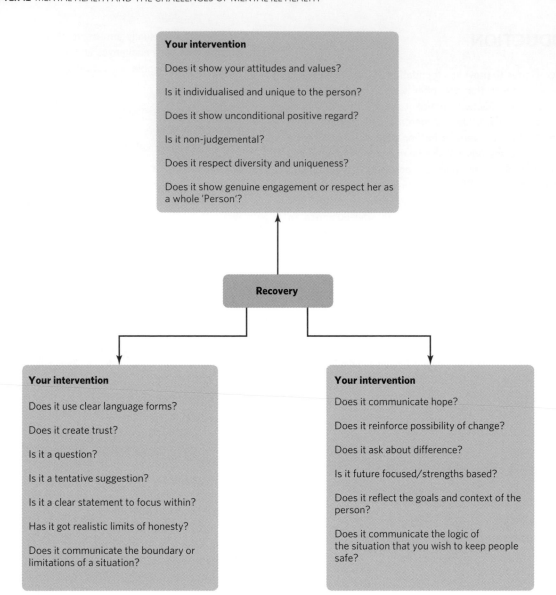

Figure 12.1 Recovery generator

HISTORY, BACKGROUND AND CONTEXT OF DEVELOPMENT OF MENTAL HEALTH SERVICES

Evidence of the rising numbers and specific characteristics of child and adolescent mental health problems has been thoroughly documented prompting widespread professional, public and private concern. Nearly 10 per cent of children aged 5 to 16 have a clinically recognisable mental disorder (ONS 2005). Data from several economically developed countries agree fairly closely that the prevalence of mental health problems in children up to the age of 18 years is 10 per cent, with higher rates among groups that suffer a number of risk factors such as those who live in many poor, inner city environments (WHO 2012). Nurses are at the heart of this phenomenon working in the frontline where children, families, parent/carers, schools and communities are experiencing the destructive consequences in self-harm, suicide, drug and alcohol abuse, crime and antisocial behaviour.

The traditional model of service delivery in community child and adolescent mental health care in Britain began to emerge after the child guidance council was set up in 1928 to 'encourage the provision of skilled treatment of children showing behaviour disturbances and early symptoms of disorder'. This was the result of pressure from education and health officials, who were concerned about the abilities and behavioural problems of children brought into the new state compulsory education system at the beginning of the 20th century. These developments were also influenced by innovations in the USA, where the first child guidance clinic was established in a deprived neighbourhood in 1909 in Chicago.

The interplay between social deprivation and children's emotional problems had begun to be correlated, highlighting the need for a social dimension to assessment and intervention in this area that has endured to this day (Crutcher 1943, cited by Walker 2001a). The service was comprised of a multidisciplinary team of various professionals with health, education, and social work backgrounds who all brought their separate training, theoretical models and working practices under one clinical umbrella. Over the next 50 years child guidance clinics grew in number and became accessible to more and more children and families. Their aims were to intervene with children and families referred for help in a variety of ways where there were concerns about a child's mental health, behaviour or emotional development. Each team member had distinctive skills and worked with the child, parents or whole family. Traditionally, the psychiatrist would lead the team and be responsible for clinical diagnosis. Social workers would support parents. Psychotherapists or specialist nurses

worked with children individually, while education staff focused on learning ability and liaison with teachers. However, their success in offering support to young people, parents and other professionals resulted in increasing demand, the creation of long waiting lists, delays in treatment and pressure to prioritise the most urgent and worrying cases. These would invariably include children with severe and longstanding mental health problems, aggressive or disturbed behaviour, school learning problems, physical, sexual or emotional abuse, depression, acute anxiety and suicidal behaviour.

The need to develop Child and Adolescent Mental Health Services (CAMHS) has attracted more attention in recent years due to increased demands on specialist resources by parents, teachers, social workers, and primary healthcare staff. The evidence has suggested the need for policy and practice changes to ensure a sufficient range of provision and skills to improve the effectiveness and efficiency of CAMHS (Walker 2001a).

RESEARCH NOTE 12.1 Mental Health Foundation (1999)

The Mental Health Foundation estimates that in Britain, one in five children and young people manifests mild emotional or behavioural difficulties or the early stage of significant problems that do not require long-term specialist intervention. However, only a small proportion of these children actually present to services for help, manifesting difficulties in a variety of contexts in which the cause of the problem is not adequately addressed. Many staff lack confidence in assessing and intervening even when they suspect a mental health component to the difficulties being presented.

LEGAL AND POLICY FRAMEWORK

The legal framework for child and adolescent mental health encompasses a wide spectrum of health and social policy including juvenile justice, mental health, education and children and family legislation. An important point is that the term 'mental illness' is not defined in law relating to children and young people. The variety of legal frameworks affecting them provide the context for work undertaken by a number of health and social care staff concerned about children and young people whose behaviour is described as disturbed or disturbing. The relevant legal and ethical issues for nurses are linked to practice principles and values best embedded in a psychosocial approach. Of particular interest to staff in the context of empowering practice are the issues of consent and confidentiality: this is especially true for young people such as Nina. The Coram Children's Legal Centre (2008) draws attention to a number of issues regarding the rights of children and young people who might have contact with agencies on the basis of their mental health problems (Table 12.1).

Challenges for Children and Young People with Mental Health Issues

Children and young people such as Nina with mental health problems may move between four overlapping systems: the health service, criminal justice, social services and education.

They are not always helped by the appropriate service since this often depends on the resources available in the area at the time. It also depends on how different professional staff may perceive the behaviour of a particular child or young person and the vocabulary used by the service in which they work. A children's nurse could identify concerns about depression, a youth offending team member may talk about a young person engaged in antisocial activity, a teacher about poor concentration and aggressive behaviour and a social worker may perceive a needy, anxious, abused child. All are describing the same child. The pathway of a child into these systems is crucial because the consequences for subsequent intervention can either exacerbate the behaviour or help to reduce it. The Mental Health Act 1983, the Children Act 1989 (2004) and the Human Rights Act 1998 are currently the three significant pieces of legislation providing the context for practice in child and adolescent mental health.

ACTIVITY 12.1 Challenges for Nina

What challenges do you think a children's nurse would see as the greatest priority for Nina?

What challenges do you think other professionals would see as the greatest priority for Nina?

Table 12.1 Rights issues for children and young people and mental health problems

Lack of knowledge	Lack of knowledge and implementation of legal rights for children and young people to control their own medical treatment A general lack of rights to self-determination
Discrimination	Discrimination against children and young people on grounds of disability, race, culture, colour, language, religion, gender, and sexuality, which can lead to categorisation as mentally ill and subsequent intervention and detention
Unlawful restriction of liberty	Unnecessary and, in some cases, unlawful restriction of liberty and inadequate safeguards in mental health and other legislation for children and young people
Inadequate assessment	Inadequate assessment and corresponding lack of care, treatment and education in the criminal justice system
Use of drugs for containment	Use of drugs rather than any other forms of treatment purposes in the community, hospitals, schools, and in other institutions, combined with a lack of knowledge of consent procedures
Placement of children	Placement of children on adult wards in psychiatric hospitals or inappropriate general paediatric wards
Lack of clear ethical guidelines	Lack of clear ethical guidelines for extreme situations such as force feedings in cases of anorexia, care of suicide risk in young people and care of HIV positive or AIDS patients

Mental Health Act 1983

The Mental Health Act Commission has repeatedly expressed concern about the safety of children in adult psychiatric wards. The Mental Health Act 1983 is a piece of legislation designed mainly for adults with mental health problems and, among other things, sets the framework for the assessment and potential compulsory admission of patients to hospital. The majority of children in psychiatric hospitals or units are informal patients. They do not have the same access to safeguards available to adult patients detained under the Mental Health Act 1983. Children under 16 such as Nina are frequently admitted by their parents even though they may not have wanted to be admitted. This is de facto detention. The number of children admitted to NHS psychiatric units has risen in recent years (see Table 12.2).

In 2009–2010, official statistics reveal that 175,941 inpatient bed days were recorded for young people suffering mental health problems. It has been estimated that each young person spends an average of 20 days in inpatient settings; this translates to 8797 young people. According to the 2000 National In-patient Child and Adolescent Psychiatry Study (O'Herlihy et al. 2007) there were 758 children admitted inappropriately to general paediatric or adult psychiatric wards (177 and 581, respectively).

In 2003 more than 270 children were detained under the Mental Health Act and placed in unsuitable adult psychiatric establishments according to the Mental Health Act Commission (2004). Despite several years of campaigning against this inhuman and inappropriate treatment, 91 children were still admitted onto adult psychiatric wards in England and Wales in 2009. This is a worrying trend, which is also reflected in the adult statistics for compulsory admissions. Health and social care policy is meant to be shifting resources away from institution-based provision to community care, but in the context of troubled young people the reverse appears to be the case.

Parts 2 and 3 of the Mental Health Act 1983 provides for compulsory admission and continued detention where a child or young person is deemed to have, or suspected of having, a mental disorder. The mental disorder must be specified as mental illness, psychopathic disorder, learning disability, or severe mental impairment. Learning disability is not stated as such in the Act, and as with psychopathic disorder, it must be associated with abnormally aggressive or seriously irresponsible conduct. Full assessment and treatment orders under Sections 2 and 3 require an application to be made by the nearest relative or an approved worker under the Mental Health Act, together with medical recommendation by two doctors. Nurses could have a role whether as approved mental health professional (AMHP) or not in safeguarding the rights of children and young people at these rare and acute episodes

Table 12.2 Number of children and young people under 19 who were admitted to psychiatric hospitals or units in England and Wales

Year	Number
1995	4891
2000	5788 (increase of 18%)
2004	7977
2010	8797

Source: ONS (2005)

Table 12.3 Mental Health Act 1983

Section 2	For assessment for possible admission for up to 28 days
Section 4	For an emergency assessment for up to 72 hours' admission
Section 5 (2)	For emergency detention by one doctor for up to 72 hours
Section 5 (4)	For emergency 6-hour detention when no doctor or AMHP available
Section 3	For inpatient treatment for a treatable disorder for up to 6 months

in their lives. The sections of the Mental Health Act 1983 most likely to be used with children and young people are shown in Table 12.3.

Consent

Defining the capacity of a child to make her own decisions and consent to intervention is not easy especially in the area of child and adolescent mental health. The concept of 'Gillick competence' arose following a landmark ruling in 1985 in the House of Lords (3 All ER 402, 1985). That ruling held that competent children under 16 years of age may consent to and refuse advice and treatment from a doctor. Since then further court cases have modified the Gillick principle so that if either the child or any person with parental responsibility gives consent to treatment, doctors can proceed, even if one or more of these people, including the child, disagrees.

The concept of competence refers to a child having the capacity to understand the nature, terms and consequences of proposed treatment or the consequences of refusing such treatment, free from pressure to comply (Walker 2010). In practice, children are considered to be lacking in capacity to consent although this could be as a result of underestimating children's intelligence or, more likely, reflect an inability to communicate effectively with them. Courts have consistently held that children do not have sufficient understanding of death, therefore the force feeding of children and young people with anorexia and giving blood transfusions to children who are Jehovah's Witnesses.

Court of Appeal decisions have since overturned the principle that Gillick-competent children can refuse treatment. Such cases involved extreme and life-threatening situations involving anorexia, blood transfusion and severely disturbed behaviour. Importantly, the courts have indicated that any person with parental responsibility (PR) may, in certain circumstances, override the refusal of the competent child. This means that children under a care order or accommodated by the local authority, even if considered not to have the capacity to consent, still retain the right to be consulted about proposed treatment. If a child is accommodated, the nurse should always obtain the parents' consent since they retain full parental responsibility (Brammer 2003). If the child is under a care order, the parents share parental responsibility with the local authority. Good practice requires the nurse in these situations to negotiate with parents about who should give consent and ensure that all views are recorded in the care plan.

> **ACTIVITY 12.2** Consent to treatment
>
> Nina is refusing to drink as she is vomiting frequently; she is refusing treatment.
>
> How are you going to encourage her to have intravenous fluids and an antiemetic?

Confidentiality

Children and young people require the help and advice of a wide variety of sources at times of stress and unhappiness in their lives. There are voluntary, statutory and private agencies as well as relatives or friends who they find easier to approach than parents. They may want to talk in confidence about worrying feelings or behaviour. The legal position in these circumstances is confused, with agencies and professional groups relying on voluntary codes of practice guidance. A difficult dilemma frequently arises when children are considering whether a helping service is acceptable while the nursing staff are required to disclose information to others in certain situations, for example where child protection concerns are raised.

The agency policies should be accessible to children and clearly state the limits to confidentiality. But in doing so many practitioners know they could be discouraging the sharing of important feelings and information. Nurses know only too well the importance of establishing trust and confidence in vulnerable young people and constantly have to tread the line between facilitating sensitive communication and selecting what needs to be passed on to parents, colleagues or to third parties. Ideally, where disclosure needs to be made against a young person's wishes it is good practice to inform the young person in advance and give her or him the chance to disclose the information first.

The Data Protection Act 1984 and the Access to Personal Files Act 1987 give individuals the right to see information about themselves, with some limitations. Children 'of sufficient understanding' have the right of access except in certain circumstances. These are particularly relevant to child and adolescent mental health:

- where disclosure would be likely to cause serious harm to the child's physical or mental health
- where the information would disclose the identity of another person

- where the information is contained within a court report
- where the information is restricted or prohibited from disclosure in adoption cases
- where the information is a statement of special education needs made under the Education Act 1981.

Updates to the Mental Health Act 1983 came into force in 2008 with the Mental Health Act 2007. These included a single definition of mental disorder; changing the criteria for detention by abolishing the treatability test and introducing a new appropriate treatment test. Importantly, changes also included a directive to ensure that age-appropriate services are available for any young person admitted to hospital who are aged under 18. Broadening the professional groups that can take particular roles has concerned many social workers who fear their vital independent role separate from the health service has been weakened. Conversely, nurses may feel uncomfortable in new roles that create ethical and professional dilemmas. Young people now have the ability to apply to court to change their nearest relative, and ensuring the right to an advocacy service when under compulsion.

Importantly, the UK at long last signed up in full to the United Nations Convention on the Rights of the Child. The United Kingdom government had maintained an opt-out since 1991, which meant it did not fully accept responsibilities to asylum-seeking children to appropriate protection and assistance. Now asylum-seeking children have the same protection and access to services as other children although such children are still subject to inhuman detention and financial constraints that adversely affect their mental health.

Children Act 1989 (2004)

Professional practice was, prior to the Children Act 1989, perceived as intrusive, legalistic and biased towards child protection investigation. The new Act tried to redress the balance towards identifying needs and providing support to parents to prevent harm or neglect of children and young people. Contemporary debate about the Children Act is still concerned with how to translate the widely endorsed principles of the legislation into practical help for child welfare service users and providers (Walker and Thurston 2006). In the context of child and adolescent mental health, this requires nurses to optimise professional knowledge, skills and values in a very complex area of practice.

A child who is suffering with mental health problems may behave in ways that stretch their parents'/carers' capacity to cope, which can result in the potential for significant harm. On the other hand, a child who is being abused or neglected may come to the attention of professionals concerned initially about his mental health. The interactive nature of mental health and child abuse presents a considerable challenge for nurses tasked with conducting assessment work in child and family contexts. In terms of the Children Act, staff operate within deceptively clear guidelines. In practice, however, the provisions within the Act and subsequent practice guidelines have sought to bring simplicity to what are inevitably highly complex situations. The duties under the terms of the Children Act are straightforward and underpinned by the following principles:

- The welfare of the child is paramount. Nina's health and social care needs have to come first.
- Children should be brought up and cared for within their own families wherever possible. Professionals need to work with the family as long as the risk to Nina's health is not compromised.
- Children should be safe and protected by effective interventions if at risk. Nina requires support for challenging behaviours not punitive measures.
- Courts should avoid delay and only make an order if this is better than not making an order. Professionals should endeavour to undertake work with Nina and her family rather than using legal chastisement wherever possible.
- Children should be kept informed about what happens to them and be involved in decisions made about them. Nina should be involved with all the discussions about her present and future needs and interventions.
- Parents continue to have parental responsibility for their children even when their children are no longer living with them. Nina should benefit from a continuing relationship with her family, even if she is not residing with them.

The shift in emphasis heralded by the Children Act from investigative child protection to needs-led assessment for family support services is particularly significant for nurses engaged in work involving children's mental health. In harmony with a broad range of fiscal and social policy measures and neighbourhood renewal projects, it means family support is enjoying something of a renaissance and enabling staff to practice creative interventions. There is a specific legal requirement under the Act that different authorities and agencies work together to provide family support services with better liaison and a corporate approach (Brammer 2003).

Together with the four-tier integrated child and adolescent mental health services structure, the framework is there to achieve better coordination and effectiveness of services to help any family with a child who has a mental health problem:

- **Tier 1 services:** all professionals working within the community, e.g. teachers, GPs or youth workers.
- **Tier 2 services:** counsellors, therapists and mental health specialists work individually (in the community) in the Tier 2 level of the mental health system.
- **Tier 3 services:** specialist clinics comprising multidisciplinary teams of counsellors, therapists, social workers, nurses, psychologists and psychiatrists work within the Tier 3 level of the mental health system. These clinics often provide a service for those who may be causing harm or risk to themselves or others; they may have substance misuse difficulties, offending behaviour, phobias or emotional and behavioural disorders.
- **Tier 4 services:** community psychiatric nurses, social workers, psychiatrists, psychologists and therapists all work within specialist teams or clinics within Tier 4 services. These services are often hospital based and involve seeing people as outpatients or admitting them for treatment. These specialist

teams work with people who have mental disorders that affect them in such a way as to risk putting themselves or others at serious risk of harm (Teatheredge 2012).

This is made clear under the terms of Section 17 of the Children Act that lays a duty on local authorities to provide services for children in need. The definition of 'in need' has three elements:

- The child is unlikely to achieve or maintain, or to have the opportunity of achieving or maintaining, a reasonable standard of health or development without the provision for the child of services by a local authority.
- The child's health or development is likely to be significantly impaired, or further impaired, without provision for the child of such services.
- The child is disabled.

The Act further defines disability to include children suffering from mental disorder of any kind. In relation to the first two parts of the definition, health or development is defined to cover physical, intellectual, emotional, social or behavioural development and physical or mental health. These concepts are open to interpretation of what is meant by a 'reasonable standard of health and development', as well as the predictive implications for children having the 'opportunity' of achieving or maintaining it. However, it is reasonable to include the following groups of children within this part of the definition of, 'in need' and to argue the case for preventive support where there is a risk of children developing mental health problems (Ryan 1999):

- children living in poverty
- homeless children
- children suffering the effects of racism
- young carers
- children who are described as delinquent
- children separated from parent/s.

Some children from these groups may be truanting from school, getting involved in criminal activities or have behaviour problems at school and/or home. Agency responses will tend to address the presenting problem and try an intervention to apparently address it. Assessment of the needs of individual children and families is often cursory, deficit-oriented and static. The Common Assessment Framework (DoH 2005) offers the opportunity for nurses, in collaboration with other professionals, to conduct more positive, comprehensive assessments that permit the mental health needs of children and adolescents to be illuminated.

Section 47 of the Children Act gives the local authority a duty to investigate where they suspect a child is suffering or is likely to suffer significant harm. Guidance suggests the purpose of such an investigation is to establish facts, decide if there are grounds for concern, identify risk and decide protective action. The problem with child and adolescent mental health problems is that this guidance assumes certainty within a time-limited assessment period. The nature of emotional and behavioural difficulties is their often hidden quality combined with the child's own reluctance to acknowledge them.

The interpretation of a child or young person's emotional or behavioural state is usually decided by a child and adolescent psychiatrist who may be brought into a Section 43 child assessment order that has been sought following parental lack of cooperation. The nurse in situations like this, and in full care proceedings, has a crucial role in balancing the need to protect the child with the future consequences for them and their family of oppressive investigations and interventions.

In cases where the child's competence to consent to treatment, or capacity to express her wishes and feelings, is impaired, it is likely that the Children Act 1989 should be used in preference to the Mental Health Act 1983. The Children Act does not carry the same stigma and consequences of the Mental Health Act and it provides for a children's guardian to consider all the factors and act as an independent advocate in legal proceedings. The Children Act aimed to consolidate a number of childcare reforms and provide a response to the evidence of failure in children's services that had been mounting in the 1980s (DHSS 1985).

ACTIVITY 12.3

In negotiating Nina's long-term interventions, what elements of the Children Act (1989; 2004) should be given priority?

Which professional should lead on the interventions?

PRACTICAL GUIDELINES 12.1 Role of the nurse as an advocate

One of the distinctive roles for nurses in this context is that of advocate in supporting a complaint as a member of staff involved in CAMHS. Section 26 of the Children Act provides for a complaints procedure through which children and young people can appeal against decisions reached by members of the interprofessional team. There are informal and formal stages to the procedure with an expectation that an independent person is included at the formal stages. When these procedures have been exhausted, a judicial review can be applied for within 3 months of the decision being appealed against.

The three grounds for succeeding with judicial review are:

- ultra vires – the social services department did not have the power to make the decision
- unfair – the decision was reached in a procedurally unfair manner or by abuse of power
- unreasonable – all relevant matters were not considered, the law was not properly applied or there was insufficient consultation.

Human Rights Act 1998

The Human Rights Act (UN 1998) came into force in 2000 and incorporates into English law most of the provisions of the European Convention on Human Rights. The Act applies to all authorities undertaking functions of a public nature, including all care providers in the public sector. The Human Rights Act supports the protection and improvement of the health and welfare of children and young people throughout the United Kingdom.

Article 3 concerns freedom from torture and inhuman or degrading treatment. Children and young people who have been subjected to nursing staff using restraint, seclusion or detention as a result of alarming behaviour could use this part of the Act to raise complaints.

Article 5 concerns the right to liberty and, together with **Article 6** concerning the right to a fair hearing, is important to children and young people detained under a section of the Mental Health Act, the Children Act or within the youth justice system. Nurses involved in such work must ensure that detention is based on sound opinion, in accordance with clearly laid out legal procedures accessible to the individual and only lasts for as long as the mental health problem persists. In the context of youth justice work, particular attention needs to be paid to the quality and tone of pre-sentence reports which can be stigmatising. The formulaic structure of pre-sentence reports might not enable an assessing social worker, working under deadline pressure, to provide an accurate picture of a young person.

Article 8 guarantees the right to privacy and family life. Refugees and asylum-seeking families can become entangled in complex legal procedures relating to citizenship and entitlement. This provision can be invoked when UK authorities are considering whether a person should be deported or remain in this country. Compassionate grounds can be used for children affected by the proposed deportation of a parent or in cases where a parent is not admitted. Staff attuned to the attachment relationships of often small children can use this knowledge to support Article 8 proceedings. In such circumstances, the maintenance of the family unit is paramount. The Convention emphasises that care orders should be a temporary measure and that children should be reunited with their family as soon as possible, where appropriate. In the case of a parent with a mental health problem detained in a psychiatric hospital, the Convention could be employed by their children to facilitate regular visits if these have been denied.

Article 10 concerns basic rights to freedom of expression and in the context of children's mental health, is a crucial safeguard to ensuring that practitioners work actively to enable children and young people to express their opinions about service provision. Nurses have an opportunity within this specific provision to articulate and put into practice their value principles of partnership and children's rights.

Article 14 states that all children have an equal claim to the rights set out in the Convention 'irrespective of the child's or his or her parent's or legal guardian's race, colour, sex, language, religion, political or other opinion, national, ethnic or social origin, property, disability, birth or other status'. This provision could be used to argue for equality of service provision and non-prejudicial diagnosis or treatment.

Staff need to ensure they are employing antiracist and non-discriminatory practice as well as facilitating children and young people to:

- access information about their rights
- contact mental health services
- access advocates and children's rights organisations
- create children's service user groups.

ACTIVITY 12.4

How would you approach your care to Nina to ensure her rights as a young person are maintained but that she also is kept safe?

Resource Implications

Mind gained information on budgets, service cuts and reductions in CAMHS posts. Of the 55 who responded, more than half (29) said they had cut their budgets for children and young people's mental health services for 2011/2012. The biggest reductions are in councils, with some reporting cuts of up to 30%, leaving essential early intervention services at risk.

Draining money from early intervention services is short-sighted, and just stores up problems for the future as young people are left without access to early help, meaning mental health problems become more serious and entrenched. It is therefore vital that councils and NHS commissioners prioritise funding comprehensive CAMHS services as they begin to set their budgets for next year, to avoid deepening the potential damage that further cuts could cause to children and young people's mental health. (Sarah Brennan, Chief Executive, YoungMinds) (**http://www.youngminds.org.uk/ about/our_campaigns/cuts_to_camhs_services**)

ASSESSMENT OF MENTAL HEALTH IN A NON-MENTAL HEALTH SETTING

Children and young people may face mental health challenges in a number of settings; it is not the role of the children's nurse to rectify the problem. Rather, the nurse needs to be able to initially assess the child's distress and refer the child to the appropriate services. The use of an RCN toolkit for nurses who are not mental health specialists (2009) (see Table 12.4) highlights this and explores mental health in children and young people:

Most children with mental health problems are managed outside specialised mental health services. Consequently, all staff should have an understanding of how to assess and address the emotional wellbeing of children and young people. They should be able to recognise if a child or young person may be suffering from a mental health problem and

Table 12.4 Mental health problems and disorders

Mental health problems	Mental health disorders
Sleeping difficulties	Affective (mood) disorders, such as depression
Feeding difficulties	Chronic fatigue syndrome
Unhappiness	Conduct disorders
Bed wetting without a physical cause	Temper tantrums beyond the usual age
Faecal soiling without a physical cause	Disorders of thought, such as delusions and hallucinations
Over-activity	Eating disorders, such as anorexia and bulimia
Tantrums, oppositional and deviant behaviour	Hyperkinetic disorders, such as attention deficit disorder
	Posttraumatic syndromes
	Self-harm and suicide

Source: Adapted from RCN (2009)

liaise with the appropriate services. Mental health promotion should be an underpinning principle for all who come in contact with children and young people, whether they are well or unwell (RCN 2009; page 2).

While mental health problems are often seen as less of a concern to professionals than mental health disorders, for the young person and the family it is still very distressful. It is therefore important to listen to Nina and give her the opportunity to voice her concerns. As Nina appears to have symptoms of both problems and disorders, it is important to undertake a general assessment. Children and young people such as Nina can be difficult to assess accurately. Assessing Nina and giving her a label is a very dangerous procedure as errors are easily made, and once the label has been assigned it may stick (Teatheredge 2012). Errors can occur due to professionals making assumptions about the child's and family religion, culture or even the child's stage of development. Nina needs to be taken seriously by professionals, including her in the whole process of assessment, and allowing her to make discoveries to determine her own self-worth within the context of her growing and being.

PRINCIPLES OF THE COMMON ASSESSMENT FRAMEWORK FOR CHILDREN AND YOUNG PEOPLE (CAF)

The Common Assessment Framework for children and young people (CAF) is a shared assessment tool used across agencies in England. It can help various agencies to develop a shared understanding of children in order for the needs including mental health to be addressed more effectively. It has been designed for practitioners/agencies to assess need at an early stage, not, however, for children at harm or risk (see Table 12.5). It has been designed because all children need to have better

lives and the best way of doing this is for all involved with children to keep an eye on their well-being (Teatheredge 2012).

Main themes are:

- information handling
- clear communication
- engagement
- knowledge
- importance of information sharing
- role and responsibilities
- awareness of complexities
- awareness of laws and legislation
- child-centred
- rooted in child development
- ecological in approach
- ensure equality of opportunity
- involve working with children and families
- build on strengths as well as identify weaknesses.

When exploring the issues for Nina and how the challenges relate to the Common Assessment Framework (DoH 2005), it is clear that there are many risk factors for Nina. This may mean that while the framework can be used as a starting point it may not be able to assess all her issues. When interviewing Nina professionals should talk to her first on their own, making her aware of confidentiality. This way Nina may feel the professionals view her needs as important. The professionals should show respect, interest and acceptance avoiding judgement, surprise or disapproval. This may help Nina feel more secure and less fearful or apprehensive. There are professionals that advocate innovative ways to work with these situations.

R.D. Laing (1927–1989) was a psychiatrist noted for his views on the causes and treatment of mental illness, which went against the psychiatric orthodoxy of the time by taking the expressions or communications of the individual patient or client as representing valid descriptions of lived experience

Table 12.5 Potential Common Assessment Framework initiated for Nina

Missing developmental milestones	Nina is making slower progress than expected at school
Challenging or aggressive behaviours	Nina has been abusing/misusing substances and committing offences
Physical or mental ill health or disability, either their own or their parents	Nina has been self-harming for some time
Exposure to substance abuse/misuse, violence or crime within the family	Nina's younger brother sustaining one incident of non-accidental injury
Bereavement or family breakdown	No specific knowledge known for Nina
Bullied or bullying	Nina is part of a gang
Disadvantaged for race, gender, sexuality, religious belief or disability	Nina is a young South Asian female
Homeless, threatened with eviction, or living in temporary accommodation	No specific knowledge known for Nina
Teenage mother/father or being the child of teenage parent	No specific knowledge known for Nina
Persistent truancy	Nina does not often attend school

Source: adapted from RCN (2009)

or reality rather than as symptoms of some separate or underlying disorder (**http://www.psychologistanywhereanytime .com/famous_psychologist_and_psychologists/psychologist_ famous_r_d_lang.htm**).

Milton Erickson (1902–1980) had an approach that departed from traditional hypnosis in a variety of ways. While the process of hypnosis has customarily been conceptualised as a matter of the therapist issuing standardised instructions to a passive patient, Ericksonian hypnosis stresses the importance of the interactive therapeutic relationship and purposeful engagement of the inner resources and experiential life of the subject. Erickson revolutionised the practice of hypnotherapy by coalescing numerous original concepts and patterns of communication into the field (**http://erickson-foundation.org/**).

A specific intervention tool that uses an innovative approach to communication is VERA:

- **V**alidation
- **E**ngagement
- **R**eassurance
- **A**ctivity

VERA is a cycle of intervention based on validation approach (Feil 2002). It addresses the fact that nurses often do not know how to respond to confused communication, whether that be linked to memory loss or anxiety states, panic or psychosis, where attempts to communicate may be unusual to us or a metaphor for the person's experience. This approach developed in the earlier part of this century has been used very successfully with the older person who is confused, but will work well with any age group or any individual who is anxious or confused including children and young people.

Nina saying 'You're trying to poison me' can be seen as an attempt to communicate fear and anxiety rather than just 'mad' or 'paranoid'. By working on the fear with Nina as she refuses treatment and particularly 'What would make you feel safe at the moment?' represents two people talking about 'What is safety for you?', 'When were you last feeling you were safe? And could live as freely as you liked and go out' etc. 'Are there times when you feel safe and more relaxed? When do you feel safe from harm?' The nurse is not colluding with the particular idea but working with the implications and emotional content of the communication (Hawkes et al. 2011).

This allows a conversation and engagement to take place without the nurse having to agree with the cause or focusing on the delusion or a particular inferred diagnosis. 'You're trying to poison me' from Nina can be seen as genuine attempts to engage with another human being and is a clue about her emotional state and priorities. They provide opportunities for sharing communication as, traditionally, these types of communication are seen as evidence that communication is not possible or that therapeutic communication or intervention should not take place (the person is 'too confused' or 'don't talk to them at all it will make it worse').

Reality orientation (RO) is often misunderstood by nurses and students and its wholesale and blunt application (An answer to an exam question recently was 'I would say no. Your father is not visiting because he is dead' and 'I would do this because the NMC code says we must tell the truth') shows a rather naive reading of the NMC, a lack of awareness of how to respectfully apply RO and could be said to retraumatise the client. A practical stepped approach to engagement with confusion or different reality experiences in clients would seem to be very useful and the mnemonic VERA is used to structure a cycle of engagement and communication in response to confusing communications.

COMMUNICATION TAKES PLACE BETWEEN PEOPLE WITHIN A CONTEXT

Communication takes place between people and within a context and this needs to be recognised. It is not the client who is confused but it is this unique exchange in this setting in this context between these two people that is confusing, e.g. the client knows that this brightly lit place with the cars speeding past and all the echoing noises should be a station and so he approaches a uniformed person to ask for a train to get him home. He also hears someone crying or a noise like it, and also thinks it is important to get to his children who must be home alone as he can't see them here, so the train is vitally important. This is understandable. But to the nurse who is dressed in a nurse's uniform so often they have forgotten it is not everyday wear and is so used to the cavernous and brightly lit surroundings (and the noise of passing food trolleys so they no longer sound like underground trains), the client's question 'when is the 5:15 porter? The kids need me to snuggle them down' is almost unfathomable.

Communication can become confused the individual's and experiences may not be easy to link to the current situations, most situations are of course more complex than the one presented as the example above. However, remembering that communication is between people, it is the professionals' responsibility to learn from the individual child or young person what they are trying to say and try and connect this with them, that redresses the usual balance of the nurse as the listener and the client with the responsibility to make themselves understood. Here the nurse and Nina are in this together. Systems theorists and linguistic philosophers have known that it is a process in communication. Communication is to humans what water is to fish. Nina is not confused; it may be the nurse who cannot understand or has not allowed them to share an emotional contact, desire or need with her.

VERA is a communication cycle that stands alone as an intervention but may also allow further techniques or models to be used as part of its action phase. At the very least, instruction advice or support could be seen to be achievable after the VERA stages have been explored. Reality orientation or prescriptive interventions can becomes the stage of action and may fit there with less of a clash with the child's own world experience than as a simple statement as suggested earlier. It may form a practical way of implementing rather complex ideas such as validation and also showing respect and a commitment to the recovery model and holistic care.

So Nina says: 'I feel really sick; the drinks you are giving me must be poisoned.'

V is Validate the Experience

'Sometimes it is hard to trust that the people caring for you have your interests at heart isn't it?'

'We all worry occasionally about what happens around us?'

'It must be especially hard when you cannot stop being sick?'

E is Engage with the Emotional Content and Show Empathy

'Are you feeling like you aren't in control of your own actions at the moment, that you are a bit frightened about what the staff team are like?'

R is Reassurance and Respect

'Because you are ok, you are safe here and we are doing all we can to look after you and give you any help you require.'

Talking about the aim of the intervention, nutritional supplement, etc. and linking this to a goal Nina might have such as going home, or being able to develop friendships that last etc. may come into play here. But the main aim is to invite further communication and engagement, reduce anxiety by reassurance and respectful engagement linked to the emotional content that may be being displayed.

A is Activity, Some Meaningful Joint Action

You can undertake communication with the person:

'Shall we prepare the next drink together?'

'Do you want to decide what flavour you would like to drink?'

Action can also be more communication, for example:

'Tell me the best ways you have found to deal with these drinks so that you can feel they are "no big thing".'

Action could also be engaging in another therapeutic activity or model, e.g. distraction techniques (relaxation tapes, videos) or perhaps reality orientation.

When the nurse has hopefully given a positive initial response, shown interest and empathy, accepted Nina, de-escalated the initial anxiety and fear of asking for help or approaching a 'stranger', the anxiety of the initial approach will decrease. The nurse may be able to talk to Nina about how she is actually feeling and who she is gently. It is cruel to argue with Nina before the nurse has used other steps to engage.

Overarching Rules for Communicating With Nina

Respect for Nina:

- Accept each new communication from Nina as a genuine attempt.
- Match the sensory level of the initial approach as far as possible. Even a 'mmm?' can be a comforting and appropriate communication.

- Show empathy and respect for Nina and be willing to learn from her.
- Be open to the new opportunity to communicate as unique.
- Be creative and see Nina as an expert: the nurse needs to learn from her what the communication means to her and how to engage.

Nina should not be seen as faulty or damaged in **VERA** but as a person teaching the nurse how to communicate with them. It is an ongoing process and so this view takes **blame** out of the equation. The nurse need not blame herself for a lack of technical skills or patience and need not blame Nina for confusing the issue or repeating what has just been said. It should be seen as a new attempt for both to communicate for a while in a way that shows care and respect. This introduces the idea of an ongoing creative process of engagement rather than seeing Nina as simply not listening. The focus is on what does change in this cycle; what is different about this approach is the nurse and Nina.

Further communication skills and language patterns may develop that may fit with Nina and show a commitment to diversity, individuality and recovery.

Examples of questions that achieve this would be:

- Questions that ask about the future rather than the past.
- Questions that ask about strengths.
- Questions that ask about smaller goals.
- Scaling questions or questions that partition off part of the problem or solution to concentrate on a priority or on a small step forward.
- Questions that ask about difference.
- Questions that ask about exceptions, times when people do cope or have a better experience.

A list of questions could be:

- What do you think needs to change in your life? (future focused question).
- Have you ever been confronted with a problem similar to this in the past? What skills did you use to get to grips with it then? (partitioning and looking for strengths).
- What's different about this time to other times in your life? (difference focused).
- What bits of your life are still how you want them to be? Just tiny glimmers of hope that, yes, that bit of my life is better than it was or is still ok? (exception).
- When things change what would they notice you will be doing differently? (future focus and relationship).
- What would they say works for you at the moment? (relationship and existing strengths).
- How did you get yourself to do that? (existing strengths).
- How did you know this was the right thing to do? (existing strengths).
- Thinking back over the last month what was the best day you have had, just a single day? What happened? What did you do on that day that helped? What did others do that made it better than other times? (exceptions).

- Is there anything you want us to leave well alone? Anything that might look like a problem but you feel is part of a solution? (partitioning).
- Is there any bit of your current behaviour/thinking/feelings/relationships that keeps you safe and that you need to keep in place for the time being? (partitioning – focus on risk).
- What else has worked for you this time? (existing strengths).
- How come the situation is not worse? Is there anything that you are doing instinctively or something you have thought about and learned that stops this situation getting worse? (existing strengths – focus on resilience).
- If you can't have a miracle at this time, what is the least you will settle for? (partitioning).
- What would you like to start on first? What is the most manageable bit of this situation? (partitioning).
- On a scale of 0–10 where 10 was where you want your life to be and 0 was the worst it has been, where are you now? What does one step up the scale look like? What would get you just 1 point up the scale? What would you be doing (at 5) that would tell you 'this is better'? (future focus/partitioning).
- Can you think about a time when you had a difficult problem to solve in the past and how you went about solving it? (existing strengths).
- What does this tell us about how you prefer to solve problems? About where your skills might lay? (goal setting and future focus on possible change).
- Any times when you surprised yourself and were able to . . . ? (exception).
- How did you manage to keep going? (exception with focus on resilience).
- What is it about you as a unique person that might help you in these circumstances? (future focus and existing strengths).
- How would you advise someone else in this situation to cope ? (relationship question).
- What would you say they should do if you were asked to help them come up with a plan of action? (goal-setting relationship question).
- What are you going to do differently now to make this the shortest/most useful stay you have ever had with us? (future focus, goal setting and relationship question).
- How would you like things here to be different this time? What should we do differently from any other service you have received in the past? (future focused, emphasis on difference as possible relationship based on service).
- How will we know that we have become part of a real healing process for you? What would be different, what would we see different about you and about these conversations? How would we know ? (future-focused goal setting).
- What would the staff here do that would allow you to tell yourself 'this is a really good idea', 'being involved with this team at this time is really helping me'? (relationship focus on possibility of change).
- How do we make this the best/shortest/most valuable meeting yet?

Note that it is not advisable to use these questions unless the individual professional has the knowledge, training and experience to use them.

These questions could also be connected to Heron's model of six-category intervention in that they are facilitative interventions; they facilitate thought change and are involving the young person collaboratively. Heron's framework provides a model for analysing how you deliver help. His model identifies six primary categories or styles of helping intervention. Based on studies in counselling, his categories became widely used to study and train health and education professionals (**http://www.mindtools.com/ CommSkll/HeronsCategories.htm accessed 24/7/12**).

There are two main approaches: **authoritative**, where you directly help the person and often used in supervision, and **facilitative**, where helping the person requires support to enable the individual to develop themselves.

Authoritative

- **Prescriptive:** this would not work with Nina as it tells her what to do rather than working with her and she may well reactive negatively.
- **Informative:** this approach gives Nina information and guidance, but may not encourage her to make her own decisions.

- **Confronting:** while this could be seen as positive for some young people, it does mean challenging Nina and may have a detrimental effect and should only be attempted in a safe environment with an appropriately qualified professional, not on an acute children's ward.

Facilitative

- **Cathartic:** as Nina may again be adversely affected by this approach, this should only be attempted in a safe environment with an appropriately qualified professional.
- **Catalytic:** this approach encourages reflection and Nina may start to be able to problem solve and make changes in her life, however, this should be with an appropriately qualified professional.
- **Supportive:** this approach will enable Nina to build up her confidence and helps her to acknowledge her strengths.

As Nina appears to have multiple issues with multifactual factors involved, it would seem good practice to refer her onwards to mental health services. Treatments offered for mental health challenges will vary according to the needs of the child and the state of her mental health (see Table 12.6). All interventions offered need to be undertaken in a safe environment and with the appropriate professional. This may mean that Nina is discharged

Table 12.6 Potential treatment for Nina

Therapy	Effect	Appropriates for Nina
Psychopharmacology	Use of drugs that affect mood, behaviour and cognition. It includes treatments for psychiatric disorders as well as substances that can be abused	May help Nina with her mood and behaviour, however, should only be offered once other avenues have been explored
Talking treatments	Involves talking to someone who is trained to help deal with negative feelings or experiencing distress	May help Nina with her mood and behaviour, needs to be undertaken by appropriately qualified professional
Psychotherapy	Is a talking therapy, sometimes other methods may be used. This could be art, music, drama, play or movement rather than talking	This could be supportive, especially if art, music and drama are activities that Nina enjoys. Also enable other forms of non-verbal communication
Counselling	Provides a regular time and space for people to talk about their troubles and explore difficult feelings in an environment that is dependable, free from intrusion and confidential	This could be supportive if Nina is in an environment in which she feels safe to talk
Cognitive behavioural therapy (CBT)	Is a psychotherapeutic approach that addresses dysfunctional emotions, behaviours, and cognitions through a goal-oriented, systematic process. The name refers to behaviour therapy, cognitive therapy	May help Nina with her mood and behaviour, however, should only be offered once other avenues have been explored
Psychosocial treatments	Including certain forms of talk therapy and social and vocational training, helpful in providing support, education, and guidance to people with mental illnesses and their families. As with medication, it is important to follow the treatment plan for psychosocial treatments to gain the greatest benefit	This has positive elements for Nina as the approach is holistic, dealing with her mood and behaviour through talking. Also giving her support and guidance for future plans

Source: adapted from Teatheredge (2012)

home and continues to have care from community teams such as CAMHS. If, following the initial assessment on the ward by the mental health team, she is seen to be at risk of harm by returning home, she could be transferred to a young person (adolescent) mental health unit.

When engaging children to assess their needs or work with them therapeutically, the professional needs to use other strategies than just verbal communication. These may include play or what Geldard (2008) terms 'media', such as art, sand, clay and the use of miniatures with or without the above. He also suggests encouraging the child to use their imagination or encourage them to tell stories. These strategies can help to engage the child therapeutically and this can help therapeutic change to occur.

CASE STUDY REVIEW 12.1

Children's nurses on the ward were able to have supportive and non-judgemental conversations with Nina, using VERA. Her observations settled very quickly once the alcohol was excreted from her body.

Following a mental health assessment, the next day Nina was successfully discharged from hospital back home after 48 hours. The CAMHS was informed and provided a key worker.

Once at home, the mental health key worker role included managing the organisation of care, liaising with the interprofessional team including her school and GP, also providing ongoing emotional, psychological and developmental support for Nina and her family, finally coordinating therapy appointments.

SUMMARY OF KEY LEARNING

This chapter has identified, through the care of Nina, just a few of the aspects of caring for children who have mental health issues on a children's ward. It is important to offer information and advice on discharge so that Nina and her parents can support her safely at home. It is of paramount importance to promote the mental health of all children and young people such as Nina by providing universal and targeted support for families and at-risk groups. Early intervention builds mental well-being and resilience in infancy and childhood, and can prevent mental health problems in adult life and lead to better outcomes in health, education, employment and relationships. However, once the challenges arise it is the appropriate use of resources that will help to ensure that young people such as Nina receive safe, timely and appropriate interventions to reduce the risk of escalation and long-term challenges to mental health.

FURTHER RESOURCES

Childhood Anxiety

Hadwin, J. et al. (2006) The development of information processing biases in childhood anxiety: a review and exploration of its origins in parenting. *Clinical Psychology Review*, 26, 876–894. **https://pathwayshrc.com.au/images/assets/info%20 processing%20biases.PDF**

Craske, M. et al. (2009) What is anxiety disorder? *Depression and Anxiety*, 26, 1066–1085. **http://www.dsm5.org/Documents/ Anxiety,%20OC%20Spectrum,%20PTSD,%20and%20 DD%20Group/Anxiety%20Disorders/Craske_What%20 is%20an%20Anxiety%20DO.pdf**

Childhood Depression

Bhatia, S. and Bhatia, S. (2007) Childhood and adolescent depression. *American Family Physician*, 75 73–80; **http://www.sepeap. org/archivos/pdf/10456.pdf**

Costello, E. et al. (2006) Is there an epidemic of child or adolescent depression? *Journal of Child Psychology and Psychiatry*, 47(12), 1263–1271. **http://devepi.duhs.duke.edu/library/ pdf/20208.pdf**

Young mind YouTube clip: **http://www.youtube.com/user/ youngmindscharity#p/u/18/NYPTI4-gwNE**

NICE (2005) Clinical guideline 28. Depression in children and young people: identification and management in primary, community and secondary care. NICE: London. **http://www.nice .org.uk/nicemedia/pdf/CG028NICEguideline.pdf**

Childhood Trauma

Stickley, T. and Bassett, T. (2008) Learning about mental health practice. Wiley. London.

Larkin, W. and Read, J. Childhood trauma and psychosis: evidence, pathways, and implications. *J Postgrad Med*, 54, 287–293; **http:// www.jpgmonline.com/text.asp?2008/54/4/287/41437**

Psychosis

Morgan, C. and Fisher, H. (2007) Environment and schizophrenia: environmental factors in schizophrenia: childhood trauma – a critical review. *Schizophrenia Bulletin*, 33(1), 3–10. **http://schizophreniabulletin.oxfordjournals.org/content/33/1/3.full**

Freeman, D. and Fowler, D. (2009) Routes to psychotic symptoms: trauma, anxiety and psychosis-like experiences. *Psychiatry Research*, 30, 169(2), 107–112. **http://www.ncbi.nlm.nih.gov/pmc/articles/PMC2748122/**

YouTube clip: **http://www.youtube.com/watch?v=D4GNL8jz3jA**

Eating Disorders

Nicholls, D. (2011) Childhood eating disorders: British national surveillance study. *British Journal of Psychiatry*, 198, 295–301. **http://www.rcpch.ac.uk/sites/default/files/BJPsych%20April%202011%20-%20childhood%20eating%20disorders%20Paper.pdf**

Herpertz-Dahlmann, B. (2008) Adolescent eating disorders: definitions, symptomatology, epidemiology and comorbidity. *Child Adolesc Psychiatric Clin N Arn*, 18, 31–47. **http://hka.stein-dev.de/doc/HDCHC409.pdf**

YouTube clip: **http://www.youtube.com/user/youngmindscharity#p/u/19/E4jBMre1aok**

Self-Harm

Nock, M. et al. (2006) Non-suicidal self-injury among adolescents: diagnostic correlates and relation to suicide attempts. *Psychiatry Research*, 144, 65–72. **http://www.wjh.harvard.edu/~nock/nocklab/Nock%20et%20al_Psychiatry%20Research_2006.pdf**

Skegg, K. (2005) Seminar paper. *The Lancet*, 366(10), **http://dnmeds.otago.ac.nz/departments/psychological/pdf/skegg_lancet%20seminar.pdf**

YouTube clip: **http://www.youtube.com/user/youngmindscharity#p/u/17/-IZviOSzOGU**

OCD

Lewin, A. and Piacentini, J. (2010) Evidence-based assessment of child obsessive compulsive disorder: recommendations for clinical practice and treatment research. *Child Youth Care Forum*, 39(2), 73–89. **http://www.ncbi.nlm.nih.gov/pmc/articles/PMC2847172/**

NICE (2005) *Obsessive-compulsive disorder: core interventions in the treatment of obsessive-compulsive disorder and body dysmorphic disorder.* NICE: London. **http://www.nice.org.uk/nicemedia/live/10976/29947/29947.pdf**

Copy of the children's Y-BOCS (CY-BOCS) assessment tool: **http://www.jfponline.com/pdf/5503JFP_AppliedEvidence3-upt3.pdf**

YouTube Clip: **http://www.youtube.com/user/youngmindscharity#p/u/16/5s3BFD9qPNg**

Conduct Disorder

NACRO (2011) New responses to vulnerable children in trouble: improving youth justice. NACRO: London. **http://www.nacro.org.uk/data/files/nacro-new-responses-to-vulnerable-children-jan11-878.pdf**

Sainsbury Centre for Mental Health (2010) The chance of a lifetime: preventing early conduct problems and reducing crime. SCMH: London. **http://www.centreformentalhealth.org.uk/pdfs/chance_of_a_lifetime.pdf**

ANSWERS TO ACTIVITIES

ACTIVITY 12.1 Challenges for Nina

What challenges do you think a children's nurse would see as the greatest priority for Nina?

What challenges do you think other professionals would see as the greatest priority for Nina?

A children's nurse could identify concerns about depression and physical safety, by undertaking regular observations on LOC. Monitor fluid input and number of times she is vomiting, and intervene to ensure hydration including infusions is achieved.

It also depends on how different professional staff may perceive the behaviour of Nina and the vocabulary used by the service in which they work.

Youth offending team members may talk about Nina being engaged in antisocial activity.

Teachers may focus on Nina's poor concentration and aggressive behaviour.

Social workers may perceive Nina as a needy, anxious, abused child.

Mental health support workers would see communication challenges.

ACTIVITY 12.2 Consent to treatment

Nina is refusing to drink as she is vomiting frequently; she is refusing treatment.

How are you going to encourage her to have intravenous fluids and an antiemetic?

Nurses know only too well the importance of establishing trust and confidence in vulnerable young people and constantly have to tread the line between facilitating sensitive communication and selecting what needs to be passed on to parents, colleagues or to third parties. Respect for Nina should accept each new communication as a genuine attempt and show empathy and respect for Nina and be willing to learn from her. Also see Nina as an expert – the nurse needs to learn from her what the communication means to her and how to engage. This could then lead to negotiation with Nina and a plan to move forward to ensure her safety that she is happy to comply with.

ACTIVITY 12.3

In negotiating Nina's long-term interventions, what elements of the Children Act (1989; 2004) should be given priority?

Which professional should lead on the interventions? The welfare of the child is paramount:

- Nina's health and social care needs have to come first.
- While in hospital the children's nurse will lead on this.

Children should be brought up and cared for within their own families wherever possible:

- Professionals need to work with the family as long as the risk to Nina's mental health and well-being is not compromised, a social worker needs to be allocated to support Nina and her family.

Children should be safe and protected by effective interventions if at risk:

- Nina requires support for challenging behaviours not punitive measures, and the mental health key worker can offer a range of solutions (see 'therapies' in this chapter).

Courts should avoid delay and only make an order if this is better than not making an order:

- Professionals such as probation officers from the youth offending team should endeavour to undertake work with Nina and her family rather than using legal chastisement wherever possible.

Children should be kept informed about what happens to them and involved in decisions made about them:

- Nina should be involved with all the discussions about her present and future needs and interventions; this may mean that Nina has a social worker to work as her advocate, rather than a social worker for the whole family.

Parents continue to have parental responsibility for their children even when their children are no longer living with them:

- Nina should benefit from a continuing relationship with her family, even if she is not residing with them; it is the role of the professional to ensure that communication lines remain open.

Once at home, the mental health key worker role includes managing the organisation of care, liaising with the interprofessional team including her school and GP and providing ongoing emotional, psychological and developmental support for Nina and her family; lastly, coordinating therapy appointments.

ACTIVITY 12.4

How would you approach your care to Nina to ensure her rights as a young person are maintained but that she also is kept safe?

The Human Rights Act (UN 1998) came into force in 2000 and incorporates into English law most of the provisions of the European Convention on Human Rights. The Act applies to all authorities undertaking functions of a public nature, including all care providers in the public sector. The Human Rights Act supports the protection and improvement of the health and welfare of children and young people throughout the United Kingdom (see articles highlighted in the chapter). Nina should be involved in all decisions about her care. Where there is a conflict of opinion, it is the children's nurse's role while Nina is in hospital to ensure as her advocate that Nina's voice is heard and her wishes taken into consideration, even if the interventions are not what she requests.

SELECTED REFERENCES

Brammer, A. (2003) *Social work law.* Pearson Education: Harlow.

Coram Children's Legal Centre (2008) Coram Children's Legal Centre: Promoting Children's rights in the UK and worldwide: **http://www.childrenslegalcentre.com.**

Department for Education and Skills (DfES) (2003) Every child matters: change for children. DfES: Nottingham.

Department for Education and Skills (DfES) (2005) Common core of skills and knowledge for the children's workforce. DfES: Nottingham.

Department for Education and Skills and Department of Health (DfES/DoH) (2004) National Service Framework for children, young people and maternity services. DfES/DoH: London.

Department of Health (DoH) (1998) Modernising mental health services: safe, supportive and sensible. HMSO: London.

Department of Health (2005) Mental health of children and young people in Great Britain, 2004. HMSO: London.

Department of Health and Department for Children, Schools and Families (DoH/DCSF) (2004) Children act. HMSO: London.

Department of Health and Department for Children, Schools and Families (DoH/DCSF) (2005) Common assessment framework. HMSO: London.

Department of Health and Social Security (1985) Social work decisions in child care. HMSO: London.

Feil, N. (2002) The validation breakthrough: simple techniques for communicating with people with Alzheimer's-type dementia, 2nd ed. Vicki deKlerk-Rubin Health Professions Press.: Baltimore Maryland.

Geldard, K. and Geldard, D. (2008) *Counselling children: a practical introduction*, 3rd ed. Sage: London.

Green, H. et al. (2005) *Mental health of children and young people in Great Britain*. Palgrave Macmillan: Basingstoke.

Hawkes, D. Blackhall, A. Hingley, D. and Wood, S. (2011) VERA framework: communicating with people who have dementia. *Nursing Standard*, 26 (10) 35–39.

House of Commons (1997) Health Committee Report into Child and Adolescent Mental Health Services. HMSO: London.

Mental Health Foundation (1993) Mental illness: the fundamental facts. Mental Health Foundation: London.

Mental Health Foundation (1999) The big picture: a national survey of child mental health in Britain. Mental Health Foundation: London.

Mental Health Foundation (2001) Turned upside down. Mental Health Foundation: London.

Mental Health Foundation (2006) Truth hurts: report of the national inquiry into self-harm among young people. Mental Health Foundation: London.

National Institute for Clinical Excellence (NICE) (2002) Schizophrenia – core interventions in the treatment and management of schizophrenia in primary and secondary care. HMSO: London.

National Institute for Clinical Excellence (NICE) (2004) Eating disorders, core interventions in the treatment and management of anorexia nervosa, bulimia nervosa and related eating disorders. HMSO: London.

National Institute for Clinical Excellence (NICE) (2005) Depression in children and young people: identification and management in primary, community and secondary care. HMSO: London.

National Institute for Clinical Excellence (NICE) (2008) Attention deficit hyperactivity disorder: diagnosis and management. HMSO: London.

O'Herlihy, A., Lelliott, P., Bannister, D. et al. (2007) Provision of child and adolescent mental health in-patient services in England between 1999 and 2006. *Psychiatric Bulletin*, 31, 454–456.

Royal College of Nursing (RCN) (2009) Toolkit for nurses who are not mental health specialists. RCN: London.

Ryan, M. (1999) *The Children Act 1989: putting it into practice.* Ashgate: Aldershot.

Saint-Exupery, A. de (1943) *The Little Prince.* Reynal & Hitchcock: New York.

Teatheredge, J. (2012) Lecture notes, Anglia Ruskin University.

TNS UK (2009) Attitudes to mental illness, research report. *JN*, 189997.

Walker, S. (2001a) Developing child and adolescent mental health services. *Journal of Child Health Care* 5(2), 71–76.

Walker, S. (2001b) Consulting with children and young people. *International Journal of Children's Rights*, 9, 45–56.

Walker, S. (2001c) Tracing the contours of postmodern social work. *British Journal of Social Work*, 31, 29–39.

Walker, S. (2002) Family support and social work practice: renaissance or retrenchment? *European Journal of Social Work* 5(1), 43–54.

Walker, S. (2003a) *Social work and child and adolescent mental health.* Russell House Publishers: Lyme Regis.

Walker, S. (2003b) Social work and child mental health – psycho-social principles in community practice. *British Journal of Social Work*, 33, 673–687.

Walker, S. (2003c) *Working together for healthy young minds.* Russell House Publishers: Lyme Regis.

Walker, S. (2003d) Interprofessional work in child and adolescent mental health services. *Emotional and Behavioural Difficulties*, 8(3), 189–204.

Walker, S. (2004) Community work and psychosocial practice – chalk and cheese or birds of a feather? *Journal of Social Work Practice* 18(2), 161–175.

Walker, S. (2005) *Culturally competent therapy: working with children and young people*. Palgrave: Basingstoke.

Walker, S. (2010) *The social worker's guide to child and adolescent mental health: a multidisciplinary handbook of child and adolescent mental health for front-line professionals*, 2nd edn. Jessica Kingsley Publishers: London.

Walker, S. and Akister, J. (2004) *Applying family therapy – a guide for caring professionals in the community*. Russell House Publishers: Lyme Regis.

Walker, S. and Beckett, C. (2004) *Social work assessment and intervention*. Russell House Publishers: Lyme Regis.

Walker, S. and Thurston, C. (2006) *Safeguarding children and young people – A guide to integrated practice*. Russell House Publishers: Lyme Regis.

World Health Organisation (2005) *Mental health policy and service guidelines: child and adolescent mental health policy and plans*. World Health Organisation: Geneva.

World Health Organisation (2012) *Adolescent mental health: mapping actions of nongovernmental organisations and other international development organisations*. World Health Organisation: Geneva.

CHAPTER 13

The Challenges for Children and Young People with Learning Disability from Black Asian Minority Ethnic (BAME) Background

Rena Williams

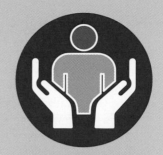
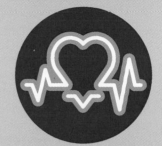
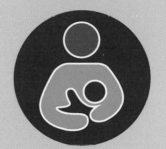

LEARNING OUTCOMES

On completion of this chapter, the reader will be able to:

- Explore the term learning disabilities and have an understanding of the categories of learning disabilities.
- Have an awareness of the impact that a child with severe learning disabilities has on the family unit.
- Analyse some of the dynamics faced with providing support to families from a BAME background.
- Plan a package of health and social care based on holistic and multicultural needs.
- Analyse and evaluate your skills in providing family-friendly care and support within diverse communities.

TALKING POINT

Valuing People Now: The Delivery Plan 2010–2011

'Some joint strategic needs assessments have failed to include the needs of people with learning disabilities and, in others, there are insufficient data on which to plan and commission services effectively.

People with profound and multiple disabilities and their families still struggle to receive appropriate services that focus on total communication, holistic health and social care assessment, support and care.

There is still insufficient awareness of the particular needs of people with learning disabilities and their families from black and minority ethnic and newly arrived communities – across all agencies.'

Department of Health (2012)

INTRODUCTION

Remember the UK poll tax riots of 1990 where several people were arrested and injured during protests against the new community charge? It was a time when Labour had a 12-point lead over the Conservatives, the fatwa placed on the author Salman Rushdie was renewed, fears over a recession were rife due to the lowest highstreet sales recorded since 1980, the IRA bombed the Stock Exchange in London, a heatwave was recorded at 37.1°C (99°F), pavements and roads were melting and a major piece of legislation was published called the National Health Service and Community Care Act.

Some of the key things that happened in 1990 have come full circle: the riots in 2011 triggered by a police shooting, the recession, Labour having a lead in the opinion polls over the coalition of Conservatives and Liberal Democrats and a greater community presence of people with learning disabilities, leading more fulfilling lives compared to previous years of being housed in institutions such as large campus hospitals.

The term learning disabilities (LD) has several connotations attached to it in today's society, one of which is the misunderstanding of what a learning disability is and the impact it may have on the individual and her family. The term LD has been used in England since 1996 (BILD 2012) and has replaced previous terms such as mental handicap and learning difficulty, however, it is often confused with the current meaning of learning difficulty, which refers to educational difficulties such as dyslexia. Nursing practitioners need to have a baseline understanding of the difference between learning disability and learning difficulty in order to be effective in delivering and evaluating a plan of care, which will be discussed later.

The images used throughout this chapter are drawn from Picture Bank devised by CHANGE. This is an organisation committed to international human rights, social inclusion and equality, co-led by people with disabilities for over 15 years. One of their many initiatives is to translate information into easy-read format by using illustrations that matches the theme of the written content. Easy read text is highly promoted within the LD field but also recommended for people with a range of needs, from English as second-language speakers to people with dementia.

One key factor to effective LD care is interprofessional and interagency team work with an approach that focuses on the 'team around the child' process. This process will have a lead agent coordinating the care, which may often be the parents/main carers (DoE 2012). A person-centred approach to the young person and family will endeavour to diminish the expert power that can often act as a barrier towards families as well as encourage engagement, mutual learning, peer support and partnership working. Such working practice will have more therapeutic effect for the family and young person as opposed to a prescriptive model of care. The health practitioner should be working alongside a theme of family focus and well-being, which is also paramount to the delivery of effective care for people with LD as the family more often takes on the full time caring role, which can lead to family burn out, resentment and breakdown, all of which have physiological and psychological pitfalls.

Over the last 15 to 20 years extensive work has been done by specialists in the fields of learning disability nursing and social care to change and amend various policies at national and local level, to highlight the health needs of this population and to raise awareness of the disparities in healthcare access that many face, in turn causing the LD population to fall into a marginalised community. However, common social factors can cause the LD population to encounter double or triple discrimination in health and social care environments: some of these factors include the ageing population, sexual choice and expression, parenting, ethnicity and culture.

This chapter will be exploring a number of issues that affect a family with a child with a LD from a BAME background who have a long journey ahead in navigation around the health and social care systems in place, while maintaining their cultural dignity and belief systems. This will allow the reader to fine-tune their practical skills in supporting/advocating and implementing effective health and social care, to heighten the reader's awareness to cultural issues and possible professional bias that may create a barrier in partnership working, as well as to focus on the complex health needs of the child that could impede their quality of life, especially if the LD remains the sole focus of the practitioner rather than healthcare needs which can often be overshadowed.

The case study acts as the anchor throughout this chapter, in order to link theory to practice and provoke thoughts around the care package required for Myah and her family, at this stage looking at Myah as a person first and not a condition or label; this will help keep the plan of the care person-centred with a holistic focus. Person-centred focus or planning is a concept widely used in caring for people with LD and this will be explored in greater depth within the chapter.

DEFINING LEARNING DISABILITIES (LD)

The definition of what a LD is has been blurred over the years as it is often confused or referred to as learning difficulties (Table 13.1). For the purpose of this chapter, the definitions offered by the World Health Organisation (WHO 2011) and the Department of Health (2001b) are used as baseline definitions.

WHO (2011) defines learning disabilities as 'a state of arrested or incomplete development of mind' as well as having 'significant impairment of intellectual functioning' and 'significant impairment of adaptive/social functioning'.

From the DOH (2001b) perspective, a learning disability includes the components of:

A significantly reduced ability to understand new or complex information, to learn new skills (impaired intelligence), with a reduced ability to cope independently (impaired social functioning); which started before adulthood, with a lasting effect on development.

LD is a label that includes several issues where a person has difficulty learning in a typical manner, usually caused by an unknown factor or factors. The unknown factor is the disorder

CASE STUDY 13.1

Myah is 12 and has a diagnosis of unknown etiology/severe global developmental delay (learning disabilities) and is wheelchair dependent. Myah commenced her menstrual cycle at 11, which she does not understand and reacts to the pain and discomfort through crying, mood change and non-engagement. Myah was born in the UK of Caribbean ethnic heritage, she attends a special educational needs school, has two brothers who do not have learning disabilities aged 14 and 16 years and lives at home with both parents who work part-time in order to provide shared care for their three children as well as to provide an income.

Myah is incontinent, requires full-time 24-hour care and her parents take it in turn to sleep in her room due to her muscular spasms, which can occur at any time for varying durations. During these muscular spams, Myah's parents will often massage and sing to her to try to relax and pacify her. This often results in her parents having very little sleep on alternate nights; Myah's parents have not used respite services and are not keen on strangers who may not understand their culture to care for Myah in their absence.

Working alongside the school nurse based in the special needs school, the following must be addressed:

- Myah's menstrual cycle and the pain she is going through.
- Muscular spasms that do not seem to have been investigated further.
- Myah is not responding to the current treatment of Baclofen 50 mg twice a day.
- Myah's mobility needs as she is wheelchair dependent.
- Myah's parents report exhaustion due to lack of sleep, but are resistant to home respite despite their and her siblings' needs within the family unit.

that affects the brain's ability to receive and process information. One of the most important issues to be aware of is that a learning disability must have been present in a person before their 16th birthday, as 16 is the accepted age for when the majority of formative learning should have taken place in the UK. For example, Myah in the scenario is 12 and her learning disability, although unknown, was diagnosed before she was 16. If she had progressed through the normal developmental milestones and reached the age of 16 any complication that occurs afterwards would be classified as a disability rather than a learning disability.

Table 13.1 Categories of disability with indicators

Category of disability	of the learning disability in the general population	Previous indicators	Current indicators 2000 – 2011
		Intelligence quotient (IQ). Average IQ ranges between 80 – 120	
Mild	Mild and moderate learning disability suggests a prevalence rate of around 25 per 1000	IQ 50 – 70	Several self-help skills, can live independently with minimal support, often vulnerable within the community
Moderate	Mild and moderate learning disability suggests a prevalence rate of around 25 per 1000	IQ 35 – 50	Some self-help skills, communication/level of understanding can be limited, may be vulnerable and require some health and social support
Severe	Estimation of around 210,000 people with profound and severe learning disabilities in England, of which 65,000 are children	IQ 20 – 35	Two or more health or physical issues, poor communication and understanding, 18 – 24 hour care
Profound	Estimation of around 210,000 people with profound and severe learning disabilities in England, of which 65,000 are children	IQ 20 and below	Complex health/physical care needs, subtle communication gestures, 24-hour care

(Not definitive and overlaps exist between categories.)

ACTIVITY 13.1   Can you name causes of LD:

- before birth (prenatal)?
- after birth (postnatal)?

ACTIVITY 13.3

Myah has a number of factors that make up her overall diagnosis. Where would you place her using the table of terms for LD?

Why did you place her in that category?

OVER A MILLION AND COUNTING

The population of the UK is estimated at 62 million, (Office for National Statistics (ONS)) (2010) and the number of people with a learning disability in the UK is estimated to be over 1.2 million, however, this is an estimation based on client contact or visibility to education, health and social care services. The true number is unknown due to several factors:

- hidden population: people who do not access any statutory services
- non-engagement with services: borderline mild learning disabilities/autistic traits and Asperger's
- missed or unconfirmed diagnosis: unable to come to a conclusion around the diagnosis.

Although medical intervention, health promotion or health education and social environments have advanced greatly over the last 20 years, there is also a recorded increase of illness within the learning disabled population.

Ethical Consideration

At this point, it is important to add that there should not be an ethos of eradication of LD due to medical and social advances. Ethically, it would be wrong to see medical intervention as a cure to LD. However, as a proactive health practitioner there is a need to have an awareness of the demographics of the population, as well as of the options that may be given to a family if the expectant mother is carrying a child with a known disability. Parents have often found the choices offered to them once a disability is confirmed as stark and hard to cope with, especially if the decision needs to be made within a short period of time.

Consent

Before considering any interaction between the family, Myah and the nurse, consent needs to be obtained and reconfirmed throughout the working partnership. Without consent, it could be questioned that any intervention with Myah and her family that they did not agree to or with could be seen as professional abuse of trust (GMC 2008). There is a mistaken belief that because a person has a disability, she will automatically require healthcare to be administered, especially with children who are seen as delicate or fragile and in need of specialised support. One explanation is that in the past the medical model of care, which is a prescriptive model, was thought to be the best model to use with people with learning disabilities, rather than looking at the person as a whole, so only the medical issue was addressed. The medical model is sometimes referred to as the 'individual model': it is a model of care used within healthcare settings and its primary focus is to identify the healthcare issue, treat the healthcare issue and then discharge once the issue has been treated (DoH 2009b). Therefore assumptions are made that if the health issue is removed the person would be better and no longer in need of healthcare.

In light of having a learning disability that cannot be cured or removed, the medical model would not be best placed in addressing the various needs of Myah as a disabled child: some needs may be of a social nature, unless, of course, there is a medical need in the first place. Although Myah has a medical need, it is not of the severity that she requires emergency treatment; in such cases, consent becomes secondary to the preservation of life.

ACTIVITY 13.4

Reflect on and list as many of Myah's needs as possible; make a decision as to whether a medical model intervention is required and, if so, explain why.

ACTIVITY 13.2

What could the reasons be for people not declaring that they have learning disabilities or that their child has?

Think of the psychological factors that could influence such a decision.

1. hidden population?
2. non-engagement?
3. missed or unconfirmed diagnosis?

Obtaining consent can be seen as a task, tickbox exercise or, in worst cases, not even required because it is assumed by the nature of the nurse and client interaction that the client gives automatic consent.

CLOTHES SHOP SCENARIO PART 1

What would you do if every time you walked into a clothes shop, the shop assistant assumed that you had definitely come to buy something, ushered you to the till and gave you a list of prices to choose from, without allowing you to browse or indeed leave the shop without a purchase? You could possibly avoid going into a clothes shop again until you really had to and at that point you could be left with very little option as to what you want to buy and accept the first thing that was given to you.

CLOTHES SHOP SCENARIO PART 2

Let's go back to the clothes shop example. Once you have entered and the shop assistant says 'Can I help you?', you reply 'Not at the moment, thank you' and the shop assistant then ignores you for the entire time you are in the store. It might make you feel that you only have one opportunity to gain their assistance. However, if the assistant comes back to you after observing you for some time, again asking if they can help you, she gives you another option to accept their help. The shop assistant does not assume that because you have remained in the shop, you automatically now need to make a purchase.

Therefore, the nurse should never assume that because a client is in professional care, no matter how informal, that consent is automatically given. The client may well be browsing for information, comparing present information with the internet or other people in the same position. So just like the good shop assistant asking if any help is needed today, nurses must ask the client whether it is acceptable to intervene. Gaining consent does not have to be an exercise; it can be something that is part of daily healthcare vocabulary, by obtaining consent by using friendly language such as 'is it ok if I' and 'let me know if this is what you want me to do' or even 'would you like me to'. Gaining consent does not stop at the first agreement from the client, it is something that needs to be offered at each intervention or offer of care. So there is a need to find several ways of changing the consent request so that it does not feel or seem like a tickbox exercise.

Another important factor is that choice is given to the person, so the control is not held with the nurse; this is another criticism of the medical model of care as the power is often assumed to be with the professional and very little choice or option is given to the client. This leads to who can and who cannot give consent. Not everyone who has the ability to breathe has the ability to give consent. The General Medical Council (GMC 2008) published easy-to-use guidance on consent issues and partnership working between patients and medical practitioners. The guidance sums up the ability for the doctor to assess the ability of the client to make a decision, or have the capacity to make decisions in practice. Capacity is an important starting point or baseline for nurses to be aware of, as without capacity, the client may not be best placed to make a decision or give consent.

PRACTICAL GUIDELINES 13.1

The client needs to be able to	What the nurse needs to be able to summarise	People with a learning disability	Action plan: an interprofessional approach
Understand the information being given	Can the client understand the spoken language? Is it their first or second language? Can the client repeat what you have told them? Can the client put the information given into their own words?	The client may not understand all the vocabulary or may only understand a limited number of words	Seek advice and assessment from the speech and language therapist Does the client have a communication passport? Does the client have a carer that knows them well and has up to date information on the client's communication ability? Has the client's hearing been assessed? If not audiology may need to be involved for a baseline assessment Does the information need to be placed into easy-read format with symbols and pictures?

(continued)

The client needs to be able to	What the nurse needs to be able to summarise	People with a learning disability	Action plan: an interprofessional approach
Repeat the information so that they can gain clarity of the information	Can the client ask relevant questions in relation to the information that has been given?	Are the questions being asked relevant? If not, is the client nervous or scared causing misunderstanding of information? Is there a need to rephrase the information? If so to what degree? Is there an underlying confusion or mental health issue?	Depending on the client's ability to understand information, relevant questions may or may not be asked A person with LD may need time to digest the information and may need to be asked the same questions over a period of days to make sure that each answer is consistent
Question the information	Can the client ask about the alternatives?	Does the client understand the alternatives being given? May be a need to repeat the processes in the action plan Can the client explain why they have chosen an alternative?	See action point above An advocate may also be enlisted to help the client discuss the options further
Weigh up the pros and cons of the information	Can the client tell you the benefits and disadvantages of the procedure?	As action point above	As action points above
Understand what the implications are to themselves if they choose not to do anything	If the client is refusing, are they giving a logical reason that has not been explored in any of the action points above?	If all the reasons above have been explored and there are a great number of concerns, if the client chooses not to have the procedure there will be a need to seek further advice and support	There will be a need to make contact with the children's/adult learning disability team The issue may need to go through the local safeguarding policy

ACTIVITY 13.5

Read through the case study again and then answer the questions. Why would Myah's parents be fearful of professionals or others that do not understand their culture?

Although Myah is in the care of her parents this does not mean that she should be left out of decision-making processes. A major criticism of professionals is that decisions are made without including the person with LD thus minimising the real choice they have over their lives (DoH 2009b). By the same token, Myah's parents know their daughter's needs and should be seen as equal partners in the care and advice that you wish to share with them. Families caring for people with LD may see accepting help from professionals as a threat to their ability to care (Mencap 2012). They may already be at breaking point with first contact and this will also reveal a lot of emotions

that may have been bottled up and just like a fizzy drink, once shaken enough, the eruption may go far and wide. Therefore, as a sensitive practitioner, seeking consent is more of a preparation to forging a therapeutic bond between the nurse and the client and family and should never be taken for granted. Simply asking the family 'how can I be of help?' will go much further than prescribing a plan of action.

Another factor would be the parents' or main carer's view point on capacity and consent; they may see it as their right to consent on behalf of their child with LD as they have been responsible for the majority of care that the child requires. They may see the option of giving consent as theirs alone and this could be due to several factors:

- having to make several major decisions on the discovery that their child has a learning disability
- no one knows their child as well as they do thus their decision should be the only decision listened to
- parents' or main carer's cultural and social viewpoint on the role and responsibility of the parent
- distrust of professionals through past experience
- feeling left out of the decision-making process causing greater need to stay 'in control'

- seeing the child as a more vulnerable person than he actually is, leading to overprotection
- feeling that the options and decisions required are not within the child's capacity to understand.

Bearing these points in mind, the reaction received from parents and main carers when discussing the need for the child to be given as much choice and opportunity to give consent will need to be handled with sensitivity. Offence may be taken from their point of view, where none was intended and the nurse needs to be as inclusive as he can. Therefore, for Myah, it is important to include her in the conversation, address questions to her and look for positive or negative body cues or vocalisations that may indicate that she is aware of being included. Each practice area will have capacity testing tools/questionnaires; however, it is advisable to work in partnership with members of the local learning disability team, who will be experts in assessing capacity and ability to give consent for people with LD and lack of clear communication ability.

BASELINE ASSESSMENTS

As a health practitioner, there is a need to have an understanding of Myah's current health situation in order to discuss and introduce a plan of care, based on her health needs. Gathering Myah's current health concerns as well as her abilities in one document will be a 'baseline assessment'. This document will act as an anchor during the working relationship with Myah and her carers as well as a way to measure a plan of care, so that continual assessment and evaluation of the effectiveness of the care plan can be made. Without such a baseline, the evidence of the plan of care as a success is not quantifiable, or whether it needs adjusting or indeed has failed. The baseline assessment acts as an agreement between the client, carers and the nurse, therefore the client should have just as much ownership, if not more, over the assessment than professionals – there should be nothing written on the assessment that the client is not aware of. Once summarised the information gathered should always be proofread to allow the client and carers to view the information to make sure an accurate account of what was said has been recorded.

PRACTICAL GUIDELINES 13.2

If there are safeguarding issues highlighted in the initial assessment or referral, a baseline assessment may not always be appropriate. You will need to seek direction from the safeguarding lead and follow the healthcare trust procedure on documentation and safeguarding assessments (see Chapter 5).

The baseline assessment usually has headings that come from the activity of daily living model (Roper et al. 2000). (Note that other models of health assessment are often used in conjunction with or instead of Roper et al., when there is more specific information to be gathered.) The Roper et al. model is one that is very well accepted and researched as being effective in the UK thus gives a firm base to launch a baseline assessment from.

ACTIVITY 13.6

Look at Roper, Logan and Tierney's activity of daily living model.

List and number the headings from this model down one side of paper leaving enough space under each heading to write a short statement.

After each heading, decide a user-friendly term that you could use to the client and carer that they would understand. For example, elimination = going to the toilet.

ACTIVITY 13.7

Using the sections of information from Activity 13.6, under the heading that you think is relevant, write down other terms that you could use for explanations. For example, under the heading elimination/going to the toilet, you could add 'Myah is incontinent, requires full-time 24-hour care.'

Note that you may find that some information in the scenario can go under more than one heading and some headings will not have any information as you have yet to do a full baseline assessment.

A baseline assessment is usually done at the first meeting or very soon after meeting the client; it would be good practice to make an appointment with the client and carers without having to launch into the assessment straightaway, as this would allow the client and carers a chance to get to know the nurse before disclosing their personal details; however, it is often expected in a busy healthcare service that the first meeting for practitioners will be the meeting at which the baseline assessment is attempted. For a successful assessment, adequate time must be set aside so that the process does not feel like the sole focus of the meeting. The client may wish to ask questions or give some insight into their lives; this is an important part of the pre-assessment phase as empathy, gaining subtle information and allowing a professional personality to shine through can emerge without being too clinical in the first instance.

At this stage, it is hard to say whether the nurse should be taking notes of the information being given, trying not to come across as too clinical but also not wishing to miss vital clues that will help plan the care package. Develop nursing practice to establish when it is alright to take notes at the pre-assessment stage or not. Some clients and carers may feel intimidated by the practitioner taking notes of everything that is said. Myah's parents do not seem to have much faith in the healthcare service and may feel threatened by the practitioner as they may presume that they are being judged by the professional rather than being listened too. Reflecting on the scenario 'Myah's parents have not used respite services and are not keen on strangers who may not understand their culture to care for Myah in their absence', there is a fear of professionals or others who do not understand their cultural background and norms.

ACTIVITY 13.8

Why would Myah's parents be fearful of professionals or others who do not understand their culture?

- Make a list of all the things that come to mind.
- Reflect on your list when reading the practical guidance that follows.

PRACTICAL GUIDELINES 13.3

During a pre-assessment phase, always ask the client and carers if it is alright to make notes as you go along, just in case they mention something that you might forget later on or may not be triggered by the assessment. This acts as another way of gaining informal consent and also takes away the clinical feel of assessment. There is no harm asking the client and carers to highlight the areas that you should be taking note of as this allows them to have more control of the clinical feature of note taking.

It is always good practice to offer the baseline assessment in two sessions; this allows for the client and carer to have a break if the assessment is too taxing for them and allows them to have control as to when the baseline assessment should finish. Although this may prolong your information gathering, the client will not forget that you had the time to offer a split session. Carers of people with learning disabilities have often complained that they are not given enough time to convey and discuss the presenting health issues (DoH 2001a/b, 2009a/b).

NB Some specialist assessments may not be able to be done in two parts due to the information they are trying to capture.

There are some specific health and social plans that are well known and used with the LD population. You will need to be aware of these plans as it can save you valuable time when doing a baseline assessment to be able to compare and discuss the information in these plans when compiling your information. It will also act as a trigger, if the client does not have such a plan, to discuss working with members of the learning disability team in the area to create one. The most common plans used are the health action plan, the hospital passport and the person-centered plan.

HEALTH ACTION PLANS

The health action plan is an initiative that was highlighted in the 2001 White Paper (DoH) 'Valuing people' and acts as a way of collating the service users' current health needs, and should be completed in collaboration with the person with LD and his family and support workers. It is a live working document that should be reviewed on a regular basis and updated whenever there is a new development. It follows the theme of the health assessment, but is usually in a portable hand-held format that the client and carers have ownership over. It is often illustrated using easy read pictures and writing. Such plans are unique and tell the health story of the client but most important how the client will be best treated within the health services.

A major driver for the use of a health action plan is that people with LD are often more prone to secondary health problems than the general population and these health needs were often misdiagnosed, overshadowed or ignored by healthcare professionals (Mencap 2009) (see Table 13.2). People with LD are 2.5 times more likely to have health problems than other people (Disability Rights Commission 2005/2006).

HOSPITAL PASSPORTS

A hospital passport is a useful way of documenting essential information about the health of a person with LD, so that they can take it with them if they need to go to hospital. It is often one sheet of paper with the most up-to-date information on treatment and healthcare plans. The purpose of the hospital passport is to let medical staff know as much about the client as they need to know to reduce the time necessary to give the client the treatment she may need and to communicate with her. This is particularly important if, like Myah, the client has communication problems. The passport may also be linked to a fast track admission system set up via the GP.

PERSON-CENTRED PLANS

An initiative that came out of the DoH (2001b) 'Valuing people' was a recommendation that people with LD should be offered a person-centred plan (PCP). PCP is a collection of tools that help a family, individual or collection of people who share the same goals to make purposeful and meaningful changes to their life. The plan can be pictorial, written or a mixture of both. It

Table 13.2 Common health concerns in the LD population

Health issue	Fact
Obesity	One in three people with LD is obese compared to one in four for general population
Mortality	People with LD are four times more likely to die of a preventable cause than people in general population People with LD are 58 times more likely to die before the age of 50 than general population
Mental health	Children and young people with LD are six times more likely to have mental health problems than other young people One in three adults with LD has problems with his mental health
Dementia	21.6% of people with LD, compared to 5.7% of the general population, have dementia People with Down's syndrome are also at a high risk of developing dementia younger
Sight problems	People with LD are more likely to have sight problems
Hearing problems	40% of people with LD have hearing problems
Dental health	36.5% of adults and 80% of adults with Down's syndrome have unhealthy teeth and gums
Epilepsy	22% of people with LD, compared to 1% in the general population, have epilepsy
Thyroid problems	People with LD have a greater risk of having thyroid problems, particularly those with Down's syndrome
Gastroesophageal reflux disease (GERD)	This is a more serious form of gastroesophageal reflux and is common in people with profound physical and cognition disabilities
Weight	People with LD are more likely than the general population to be either underweight or overweight
Osteoporosis	People with LD tend to have osteoporosis younger than the general population and have more fractures

Source: DoH (2001a/b), DRC (2005/2006) and Mencap (2009)

can take many formats from small pocket-held documents to large murals. PCP either follows a theme or is a mix of the following themes:

- **personal futures planning:** used to highlight and unearth people's future goals and aspirations
- **essential lifestyle planning:** used to highlight and imbed the essential factors that need to happen in someone's life. Good to use with people with profound and severe LD such as Myah
- **maps:** used to record a history of events leading up to the present. Good to use with any level of LD for making a permanent meaningful record of the clients' history that allows their story to be told their way
- **paths:** used to highlight things that should happen in the client's life or identify areas of change and plan towards making the change happen. Good to use with people with a mild to moderate LD; however, it can be used with any level of LD.

Anyone can have a PCP. It is not exclusive, but is based on liberating the person or group by making dreams turn into reality no matter how big or small the ambition may be. It enables the person or group to plan for themselves, as well as the person or group having more control over their life. It allows for the person or group to have real choice over

who they want to help them with achieving their dreams and goals. It uses practical ways of making things happen with the minimum amount of resources possible so that the plan has a greater chance of sustaining itself without the dependence on statutory funding or support, unless this is a major requirement; for example someone with profound LD will require a 24-hour support system that may have to be funded through the health or social care budget. The best type of PCP for someone who requires 24-hour care would be an essential lifestyle plan.

There is no jargon in PCP, it is straightforward and is based on simple processes. A PCP is not held by everyone with a LD but awareness during the baseline assessment is useful to know what the client wants to achieve in their life, as this would be a holistic lead into healthy lifestyle choices surrounding the health interventions that will be discussed with the client and carers. At the Helen Sanderson Associates website there is further information on person-centred planning:

In the UK the government policy 'Putting People First' stated that person-centred planning must become mainstream. In 2010 guidance was issued to help councils use person-centred thinking and planning to deliver the personalisation agenda. **http://www.helensandersonassociates.co.uk/reading-room/how/person-centred-planning.aspx**

PRIORITISATION

Following the health assessment, the practitioner needs to assess and prioritise the aspects of care that need immediate, short-term and long-term or ongoing actions. Making an order of priority will give the practitioner a sense of urgency and logical order when planning interventions within an interprofessional setting. It is important for the practitioner not to act alone in relation to interventions and also to check with the family and person with LD that the order of prioritisation is agreed and simultaneous. The key theme here is also empowerment as the family should be encouraged to do as much for themselves as possible so that they feel the greatest sense of control over the care package being offered. With ever decreasing budgets, care packages (health or social care or a mixture of both) need to be cost effective, sustainable and fit for purpose. Personalised budgets is one way that sustainability and empowerment has been factored into care packages for people with LD. (For more information around personalised budgets see the DoH website: **http://www.dh.gov.uk/health/category/policy-areas/ nhs/personal-budgets/**.)

Have a look at Table 13.3 to see how the order of priority can become disjointed if there is no interprofessional approach.

Although each agency, including Myah and her parents, has its own order of priority, working as an interagency team will allow for several priorities to be worked on simultaneously, hence the importance for the interagency to agree on what the immediate, short-term and long-term actions are.

ACTIVITY 13.9

Looking back on the assessment carried out in Activity 13.6 and Myah's scenario, prioritise the actions that need to be addressed. They should fall into three categories:

- immediate actions
- short-term actions
- long-term or ongoing actions.

Each action should be followed by the name of an interagency professional or a parent as the person who would be responsible for this action.

VULNERABILITY AND SAFEGUARDING

Children and young adults with LD are vulnerable members of society by nature of their disability and are more likely to be in a vulnerable situation than the average member of society. This is mainly due to the dependency that individuals with LD may have on others from making healthy lifestyle choices to 24-hour care (Cooke and Sinason 1998). A practitioner needs to be aware that signs of vulnerability may be extremely hard to detect if the client does not have the words or means to express what has caused their vulnerability to be compromised further; although this can be said of young children on the whole, children without disabilities may be able to give noticeable signs and clues that their safety has been compromised. Therefore, there exists

Table 13.3 Disjoints in the order of priority of care

Interagency team around the child	Priority	Possible rationale
Parents	Myah to remain in the family unit with as minimal intervention from professionals as possible	Lack trust in professional services Cultural differences in the understanding of the role of the professionals Feeling of failure by allowing professionals to assist
GP/health	Myah's muscular cramps	An immediate health issue that can be minimised or curtailed with a suitable intervention
Care manager/social services	Needs of the family unit	Maintaining an ethos of family bonding and togetherness Implementation of packages that will prevent family unit breakdown
Physiotherapist	Assessment of the wheelchair Assessment of the spine	Postural issues and growth spurts could be a factor to the muscular spasms
Teacher	Myah's lack of engagement and comfort during her menstrual cycle	Myah's well-being is affected by her monthly cycle and impeding her ability to enjoy education

a double risk of compromised vulnerability for children with LD and the practitioner should be aware that a child with LD may have very subtle and nondescript ways of showing vulnerability. It is important for the practitioner to have an understanding of what the normal behaviour patterns for the child are, as discussed in baseline assessment. If there is behaviour to compare the changed behaviour with, it may be clear that there is an issue to investigate, however, you will also need to rule out underlying health concerns that may not be visible or reportable by the child, while looking into the cause of the change in behaviour. Such concerns need to be investigated following strict guidelines that have been drawn from policy and relate to the trust or place of work in which the practitioner operates.

> ## ACTIVITY 13.10
>
> List Myah's areas of vulnerability.
>
> List the subtle and non-descript ways in which Myah may manifest her compromised vulnerability.
>
> Think about how your answers would alert you to concerns in a non-disabled child.

It cannot be stressed enough that a practitioner needs to be aware of the duty of care that they have towards the disabled child and overarching policies should be referred to such as the Children Act 1989 and 2004, as well as the United Nations Convention on the Rights of the Child.

CULTURAL REFERENCES

From a cultural frame of reference, there may be customs and rituals that are widely accepted or supported by the culture that are illegal outside that culture or country. There may be plausible excuses given for circumstances that raise a cause for concern or trigger a safeguarding investigation. It is important for the practitioner to have an understanding of the cultural background of the family or main carers but this should not blur investigations as the safety of the child is paramount within the UK and will nullify any customary norms that may be supported within the cultural circle.

In Myah's situation, her behaviour has changed; however, this change of behaviour seems linked to her menstrual cycle and muscular spasms, as in all other times in her life she seems content. Such information should be consistent at home as it is in school, thus parents and school staff should report similar concerns. From a cultural viewpoint, Myah's parents may see any discomfort that Myah displays as a failure on their part to keep her free from pain with minimal use of medication and they may be resistant to using medication especially if the side-effects cause further discomfort. It may be the case that Myah's parents report that there is nothing wrong at home, as

they are totally devoted to making Myah comfortable, whereas in the school setting staff may not have the capacity to give dedicated one-to-one attention to Myah and medical intervention may seem the logical choice in alleviating her pain. This can leave the practitioner in the middle ground trying to do the best for Myah as the main concern but also trying to mediate between the staff and parental viewpoint. It may also trigger a safeguarding concern where staff feel that Myah is suffering during her menstrual cycle. Forceful intervention may alienate Myah's parents, therefore a reasonable solution would be to discuss a trial period of the mildest analgesic with the least side-effects that both parents and school staff could monitor in order to get feedback from both parties, but also to give a time limit so that the parents do not see the intervention as a permanent fixture. This is where the negotiation skills of the practitioner are paramount when addressing issues that could offend or ostracise a particular culture based on its cultural value. The end result should always promote the safety and well-being of Myah in relation to the Every Disabled Child Matters Campaign (2006).

EVERY FATHER MATTERS

Recognition given to fathers has, on the whole, increased within the UK with campaigns spearheaded by groups such as Fathers for Justice (**http://www.fathers-4-justice.org/**), 100 Black men (**http://www.100bmol.org.uk/**), Contact a Family (**http://www.cafamily.org.uk/**) and Gingerbread, a support group for lone parents (**http://www.gingerbread.org.uk**). These groups have been campaigning tirelessly to have the same positive media and rights given to fathers as there are to mothers.

The role of the mother often supersedes that of the father, as mothers are often seen as the primary care giver who takes on the major role of family care and coordination. It is perceived that it is often mothers who take the child with the disability to hospital appointments, do the school run, activities and social gatherings, often because the mother has given up her employment or further education to be a full-time carer. Therefore, main contact with service provision often takes place with the mother and not the father. The Contact a Family support group comments that fathers may see themselves as the main wage provider and feel further burden through the increasing costs of looking after a child with disabilities. Fathers who hold a strong cultural viewpoint that parentage, offspring and continuation of the family line should be without any impairment of mind or body may see having a disabled child as a slight to their family line or a reflection that something has gone wrong in the family line, thus they may struggle with their cultural expectations and natural feelings of love towards their child. All fathers will need the same support service as offered to mothers and the practitioner needs to be sensitive to cultural viewpoints that may be held thus, in turn, being able to source culturally sensitive support groups for fathers. However, a safeguarding issue may become apparent if the cultural viewpoints of the family go completely against the nurturing aspects of being parents to the disabled child. There is also a fine line between cultural superstition and cultural myth, which may influence the family rather than the evidenced-based rationale. An example of this is where people with epilepsy were thought to be witches and were killed in the UK during the Middle Ages. However, with advances in research and medicine, epilepsy is no longer seen as an indicator for witchcraft, although these myths may still be meaningful within the UK through families or groups who continue to maintain this belief.

A practitioner needs to include and engage with both parents unless there is a valid reason not to, for example, a court order, foster or adoptive care and safeguarding issues. Such reasons must be valid and supported with legal documentation and not because there is a dispute between the parents, which may lead to one parent being excluded from the life of the client. Keeping both parents in the loop is vital for giving equal respect but also aiding family decision making and maintaining healthy bonds. Simple salutations for example addressing formal letters to 'Mr and Mrs' or 'to the parents of' to requesting a time to see both parents rather than just the mother will allow fathers greater involvement in the care of their child. Every Disabled Child Matters (2006) highlights the need for family support to be given to both partners in order to promote the family staying together as a unit.

RESEARCH NOTE 13.1 Afro-Caribbean fathers and their presence in the UK

The Fatherhood Institute (2010) conducted research into Afro-Caribbean fathers and their presence in the UK. It looked at the negative stereotypes that can be placed on this group due to several factors. It also looked at the similarities between young Afro-Caribbean fathers and white fathers of the same age. Awareness is required from the practitioner as to how fathers from BAME backgrounds are viewed in society as this may be a hidden burden on the father who has a disabled child.

A summary of this study can be found at **http://www .fatherhoodinstitute.org/2010/fatherhood-institute- research-summary-african-caribbean-fathers/**.

RESEARCH NOTE 13.2 Growing together or drifting apart? (Devenney 2008)

In 2008 Devenney, head of policy and dissemination at One Plus One, looked at parents of disabled children and published a literature review entitled 'Growing together or drifting apart? Children with disabilities and their parents' relationship' (Glenn 2008). He found that couples caring for a child with a disability were at increased risk of relationship issues and divorce. (More information can be found at **http://www.careforthefamily.org.uk/article/?article=634**.)

Myah's father takes an active role in her care, providing an income for the family as well as giving support to his wife by sharing the night-time routine. The practitioner needs to be subtle and sensitive to the father's needs as a care giver, as he may feel a duty to provide even more so than a father who does not have a disabled child. There may be hidden emotions linked to common themes of being a parent to a child with LD. The themes range from negative to positive such as:

- guilt or shame: cultural comparatives with friends and families, personal aspirations
- bereavement or loss: of the child that was hoped for – 9 months of waiting and planning for a non-disabled child
- over-compensating: siblings may be neglected as more attention is given to the disabled child
- campaigner: becomes an activist for the disabled and may stigmatise people who do not have a disabled child.

As mentioned earlier, some of the hidden feelings may also be linked to the cultural perspective held by the family in relation to having a child with LD. Some cultures may see a child with LD as a blessing or a gift from God, whereas other cultures may see a child with LD as being a sign that forefathers have done something wrong, a curse or indeed an indication that either the mother or father is not of good reproductive stock (O'Hara 2003); wherever possible, promotion of positive attributes of having a child with LD should the practitioners focus in their conversations with the family and dismissive or negative comments made by families should be explored and if there are triggers for safeguarding, as mentioned earlier, this will promote the safety of the child. However, the father must be supported in his role of caregiver and provider as well as given support to come to terms with new roles that he has taken on in light of his child's LD.

CULTURAL DIVERSITY AND AN APPRECIATION OF CARING FOR INDIVIDUALS

Interpretation of culture to each individual is a unique set of thoughts, rules and norms that underpin how that person sees himself within the society in which he lives. All individuals belong to something that shares the same culture; this may be a close family unit, a wider family circle or a group that share a set of common features. Some of the common features that a group of the same culture may share may include faith, music, food, sexual orientation, dress sense and ritual behaviours.

Other than a person's own cultural features, it can be hard to think of the many differences that an individual may come across in everyday life and nursing practice. However, recognising cultural differences is not about how much detail that you know about each culture, as it would be impossible to know every detail about every culture; it is about recognising, valuing and respecting the many differences that exist and taking the time to make reasonable adjustments to ensure equal access to healthcare is achieved. This may not be an easy task as we can often take it for granted that one service will fit all recipients; this can be an unconscious quality to our working practice and it is only when someone points out that the service offered does not meet their cultural needs that the unconscious working practice is brought into the conscious.

Minority ethnic communities will have various subcultures within them, however, it is important for the practitioner to remember that just as with your own cultural themes, minority ethnic communities will also have common themes that make up their cultural norms (Royal College of Psychiatrists (RCP) 2011). One of the issues facing minority ethnic communities is the double discrimination faced by having a LD as well as coming from a minority group. This is echoed by the DoH (2012), which found such barriers: lack of cultural sensitivity, wrong assumptions, language barriers and discrimination.

Thinking about the morning routine from wake-up to leaving for school, there are often things that may seem trivial but are actually unique to the person and that is repeated day in day out. These trivial things are often the very aspects of life that make people who they are and the fact that they are automatically undertaken mean that they are firmly a part of nature. Someone with LD and families caring for that person will also have similar trivial things that they may do, which may not be interpreted as being part of their routine; if misinterpreted these trivial factors may lead to further distress to the person or family. These trivial routines may look very different from what is expected or considered conventional and this is why actions may be misinterpreted. The more profound the LD the more we may see non-conventional routines being part of the family culture.

> Myah requires full time 24-hour care and her parents take it in turn to sleep in her room due to her muscular spasms, which can occur at any time for varying durations. During these muscular spasms, Myah's parents will often massage and sing to her to try and relax and pacify her – often resulting in her parents having very little sleep on alternate nights.

Looking at this part of the scenario there are some assumptions. These assumptions may be natural when interviewing the parents to get a family history, however, it must be remembered that the parents' routine is logical to them and part of their family culture, which allows them to cope and keep the family unit together. Some assumptions may occur about the way a family functions with a child with LD when comparing them with what is expected of a family without a child with LD. This list is just a snapshot of some of the assumptions that may arise and are to act as thought provokers rather than hard and fast rules.

PRACTICAL GUIDELINES 13.4

Assumptions of Myah's family situation	Average family unit	Assisting the family while respecting cultural norms
Myah will never be able to sleep independently	A 12-year-old may be sleeping independently or sharing a room with a sibling	Discuss the use of a visual or auditory monitor that could alert the parents to any distress Myah may be in Discuss the use of a mattress epilepsy alarm; this will alert the family of spasms Discuss with external family members the use of direct payments that could be paid to provide night-time support, if parents do not feel comfortable with strangers
Parents have not detached from sleeping in the same room as their child	It is encouraged for an infant to be sleeping independently as soon as possible	Discuss with the parents if they are happy with the current sleeping arrangement. If so, ask them is there anything that could possibly enhance what they are doing? It may be too early to introduce the concept of respite or strangers sleeping in the house. Using external family members may increase the bond between external and immediate family members. It will also keep the cultural norms

(continued)

Assumptions of Myah's family situation	Average family unit	Assisting the family while respecting cultural norms
Parents will never have private time together at bed time due to the shared night time care	Parents will need to find times to be intimate and private away from their children; this often gets easier as the child becomes more independent	This is a tricky subject to broach, however, tackling the issues above may automatically free up quality time for the parents to be together. If not tactful ask the question of how the parents have quality time with each other. They may or may not disclose their feelings and they may perceive their parental role as much more important than their role as partners to one another. However, if trust is built up over time the parents may become more trusting of having a form of respite that works for them and allows them to have more personal time together Research other families of the same cultural background to act as buddies to Myah's family, as they may feel more comfortable discussing personal issues with people that share the same cultural norms and stories
Myah does not have friends over to visit	A 12-year-old will be inviting friends over possibly leading to sleep-overs	Are there after-school clubs that Myah could attend? Could the school facilitate a service to bring friends from school together using their transport? Could a person-centred plan be created to address Myah's circle of support?
Siblings may feel neglected or resentful of Myah: siblings may take on the role as young carers	You need to be aware of the average developmental stages of young boys and be able to plot where they should be aiming towards educationally and emotionally You also need to be aware of the needs of young black males as research by the Office of National Statistics in 2009 has shown that young black males may be at risk of lower achievement if they do not have the right motivation and role models Myah's parents may expect the boys to share the role of caring for Myah as part of their cultural development and rite of passage into adulthood	Myah's brothers may need concentrated attention not only from their parents but from their own friends as well as support groups if they wish to engage Their aspirations and development need to be encouraged and nurtured They will need to make sense of their own role within the family unit as they may be torn between the role of carer, sibling and advocate for their sister. Barnardo's estimate that the average age of a young carer is 12 If there is too much responsibility placed on the siblings, resentment may creep into their feelings towards Myah and their parents
Other cultural factors that will need to be taken into consideration: faith food language gender	These issues are not highlighted within the scenario but need to be at the back of the practitioner's mind when working with all families and service users	Always try and research the cultural needs of the family that you are working with Always ask the family and service user's questions about their culture even as an ice breaker in order to show that you are interested in them as a whole rather than starting with the presenting problems

RESEARCH NOTE 13.3 Unemployment

The Office of National Statistics reports that unemployment for young black male jobseekers has risen from 28.8% in 2008 to 55.9% in the last three months of 2011, which is double the rate for young white people. (More information can be read at **http://www.guardian.co.uk/society/2012/mar/09/half-uk-young-black-men-unemployed**.)

Cultural interpretation of statutory services will differ due to the exposure that the culture has had to such services, for example, if Myah's parents were born outside the UK, their understanding of the health service and its provision may be different from what they have been used to previously, depending on how much contact they have had with the service thus far. There may be some suspicion as to how they will be judged as carers and parents due to their cultural norms. This may be more apparent if the health service workforce that they engage with does not have staff representation from the same or similar background. However, if Myah's parents have been living in western society for some time, they may be more comfortable with engaging with the service irrespective of the staff cultural mix and be willing to accept help and support.

Never make assumptions that a difference in culture will create a barrier to acceptance of healthcare, but be aware of the need to tailor the services on offer so as not to offend or encroach on the cultural norms of the clients. There is also a need to be sensitive that the care package that suits one culture may not suit another, therefore reasonable adjustments can be made in order to tailor the service provided. Cultural understanding of the service on offer may lead to refusal or only part-uptake and this can be seen by the professional as a difficulty – take care not to label families as difficult as it is often the care package that does not fit the client's needs rather than the family being difficult. Myah's parents have had to devise a package of care that works for them and their other two children and their package may seem strange to us as professionals but very logical to them. There is a fine line between enhancing the family's quality of life and completely restructuring their life when trying to introduce what you think is best, based on British cultural norms.

RESPITE SUPPORT

Mencap 2003 published a report titled 'Breaking point' highlighting the massive strains that families who care for someone with a profound learning disability are under.

The report highlighted the following:

- eight out of 10 families have reached breaking point
- six out of 10 families are getting no short-break service or a minimal service that does not meet their needs

- three out of 10 families received fewer short breaks than in the previous year
- two out of three families who are on a waiting list for short-break services have been waiting for at least 6 months
- eight out of 10 families have never been offered a choice of service
- three out of 10 families do not trust the service offered to them
- five out of 10 families have found services unsuitable.

Within the average family, parents or main carers expect and sometimes look forward to natural periods of respite as their child becomes independent. Starting from play group, to nursery, school, sixth form or college, then on to higher education and work. Entwined within the child's journey of independence is the ability to self-care, make decisions, spend longer time in the company of friends, find a partner or soulmate and then make a home independent from their parents. This journey may have several pauses along the way dependent on the developmental path of the child as well as the financial constraints of the society that they are in; however, there is an aspiration to be seen as an individual providing for himself and making choices based on his own needs and desires.

Young people with LD often have greater limitations in relation to the average child and are often thought of as 'eternal children'; despite the actual age of the person with learning disabilities, they are often spoken to, treated and thought of as their developmental age. You may often see or hear professionals and lay people justify the learning disabled person's behaviour or actions to that of a 2-year-old or indeed an age that their learning or development is thought to have ceased.

A summary of Erikson's (1968) child developmental stages, Table 13.4 shows a concept that children have to reach each stage successfully in order to progress to the next. If the child becomes stuck in a stage, due to disability, or lack of positive social role models for example, there may be a consensus that this is the stage at which the child will function throughout their life with slight variances either side of the developmental stage, this in turn will determine their 'ego', and their level of developmental maturity in adulthood. Therefore respite for carers who wish to care for their child is vital to alleviate the caring role that can be a 24-hour, 365-day activity. (Further information on Erikson's developmental stages can be found in Chapter 2.)

Table 13.4 Erikson's developmental stages

Actual age of child	Stage of ego (concept)	Developmental milestones	Learning disability comparison
Infancy Oral stage Birth–18 months	**Trust vs. mistrust** Visual contact with the mother or main carer creates a loving bond Fascination with objects that are often placed in the mouth If basic needs are met trust is built and the child has confidence that the future will be ok	**Drive and hope** Respond to sound and notice bright lights, be able to focus and stare at faces, make gurgling sounds, follow close objects, know familiar voices, smile, laugh and hold head steady Reach for toys and roll over, recognise familiar faces, kick legs and discover both hands, stand steady when being held, reach out for and hold toys/roll over Respond to their name Imitate sounds and gestures Sit without support Make more babbling and chatter sounds Hold simple food and feed themselves	Profound
Early childhood 18 months–3 years	**Autonomy vs. shame** Self-esteem and achievement is being driven by the things the child can do for themselves Using the word 'no' allows the child's will to develop If encouragement is not given by the main carer the child may feel shame in completing tasks	**Self-control, courage and will** Walking, talking, self-feeding, toilet training Fine motor skills developing	Profound/severe
Play age 3–5 years	**Initiative vs. guilt** Children take the opportunity to copy or mimic adults around them Storytelling and play acting becomes a main feature of play activity Exploration of the world around by continually asking 'why' if the child feels let down with their own achievements	**Purpose** Milestones begin to be defined and modified for problem solving	Severe/moderate
School age Latency 6–12 years	**Industry vs. inferiority** Learning and creativity is a main feature of development especially acquiring new skills The child begins to form stronger attachments to school and peers and parents become less important However, problems can occur when unresolved feelings transfer into this stage of development	**Method and competence** Milestones should have formed a strong basis for continual learning to take place for the rest of the child's life	Moderate/mild

(continued)

Actual age of child	Stage of ego (concept)	Developmental milestones	Learning disability comparison
Adolescence Moratorium 12–18 years	**Identity vs. role confusion** In between child and adult, the young person will have several experiences that will play a major role in their life choices Establishing one's identity is a key focus and can be very confusing as the distance from parents or main carers expands Role confusion is common as the young person withdraws from responsibility Peer group bonding is at its strongest and ideals are based on notations that do not have conflict, however, this is often far from real life Without resolve this period of development can leave the young person searching for answers without conclusions	**Devotion and fidelity** Major life events, such as puberty, can be seen as milestones but are more aligned to transition to adulthood	Mild

MEDICAL INTERVENTIONS AND ACCESS TO ACUTE SERVICES

The person-centred plan may also indicate the level of respite required in the form of independent activity that the person with LD has. If there is little activity away from the main carers there will be a greater respite need as the parents get older. Respite does not need to be an expensive care package; a person-centred plan could highlight the client's circle of support, which can either be paid through direct payments or personal budgets or employ one-to-one workers to offer meaningful activities that relieve the carers of the 24-hour caring role.

Myah has ways of communicating her discomfort and her parents are tuned into her method of communication, however, without her parents' translation of Myah's communication channels the outside world may not readily tell when or if Myah is trying to convey pain or discomfort until it becomes so severe that Myah becomes distressed. Although this chapter has highlighted the use of health action plans and hospital passports, there are times when acute services do not respond to the subtle signs or the verbal reports of parents and carers.

Living with a LD does not mean that life is less fulfilling than that of the average person, however life will be different from what was expected and reasonable adjustments will need to be made throughout the journey so that the child with LD has the potential to stay safe, be healthy, enjoy/achieve, be supported economically and make a positive contribution to life (DoH 2004).

RESEARCH NOTE 13.4 'Death by indifference: 74 deaths and counting' (Mencap 2007, 2012)

These reports highlight the untimely demise of people with LD in hospital settings due to several factors, which included lack of confidence in staff to deal with LD, diagnostic overshadowing where the behaviour was thought to be the presiding issue, non-cooperation and lack of engagement with parents and carers who were trying to highlight that something was wrong and lack of awareness in the needs of the LD population.

CASE STUDY REVIEW 13.1

This chapter has given an insight into the information a practitioner needs in order to have a greater awareness; however, there will still be major healthcare concerns for people with LD when it comes to accessing medical healthcare. In Myah's case, this could lead her to face double discrimination based both on her LD and the cultural viewpoints of her family. The document 'Valuing People Now' (DoH 2009b) looks at the double discrimination faced by marginalised groups with LD, such as BAME, gays and lesbians and the travelling population.

As a practitioner, the first question to ask is when did Myah have her last medical, either in school or with her GP? This would act as a trigger for the parents who should have the latest information to hand, if not it may be a turning point for greater interaction with medical staff. Every child, irrespective of disability, should have a school medical and Myah's parents will be able to relate to this from Myah's brothers. Especially if Myah's parents are trying to promote equity across the three children, then Myah should not be left out of having a periodical medical in order to address any presenting issues. A medical can be phrased as a 'review of health status', which may seem less clinical and threatening to Myah and her parents and this is where her current medication regime as well as any presenting problems should be looked into (see Table 13.5).

Table 13.5 Overview of Myah's presenting needs and possible medical/allied health intervention

Presenting health status to be reviewed	What could be the cause?	What investigations and referrals could be made?
Myah's menstrual cycle and the pain that the client seems to be going through	Dysmenorrhea: period pain may be within average levels	Date and record Myah's cycle so there is a baseline over 3–4 months
	A pelvic disorder that is overshadowed by assumption that it is 'regular menstrual pain'	Pelvic scan
		Analgesic to be given during menstrual cycle
	Lack of understanding of what is going on causing further distress to Myah	Speach And Language Theraphy (SALT) – discuss using a symbol card that shows Myah is in pain and use this card during her facial and body expressions
Muscular spams that do not seem to have been investigated further and are not responding to the current treatment of Baclofen 50 mg twice a day	Connection to Myah's unknown diagnosis of severe LD	Review of medication
	Undiagnosed epilepsy	Sensory assessment
	Undiagnosed nervous reaction	Occupational therapy
	Undiagnosed sensory reaction – hyper/hypo-sensitivities	Neurological assessment
Myah's mobility needs as she is wheelchair dependent	Growth spurts	Physiotherapy assessment
	Inappropriate wheelchair	Wheelchair clinic
	Wear and tear of seating	Motorised wheelchair that can follow tracking in the school setting
	Lack of independence if Myah relies on others to propel	

SUMMARY OF KEY LEARNING

This chapter has followed Myah and her family through a number of issues that may seem challenging to the professional at face value, but offer a number of rewards in relation to perso-centered care, breaking down barriers and boundaries and adjusting the pitch and tone of care delivery. Being sensitive to cultural aspects is a fundamental part of nursing/care provision in today's ever increasing multicultural society and Myah and her parents need to feel a sense of identity while preserving their cultural values and navigating their way through healthcare systems. A valuable service that will aid the practitioner to provide a personalised plan of care is the local learning disability team who will have the remit to work

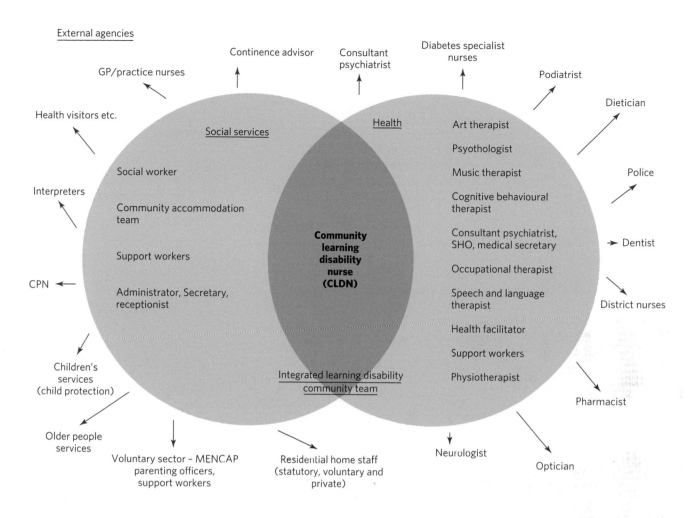

Figure 13.1 Integrated learning disability community team
Source: (taken from the Barking and Dagenham community LD term presentation)

across all disciplines within the health and social care service (see Figure 13.1). Myah should not be excluded from decisions about her healthcare, nor should she be denied healthcare due to her limitations or disability. Every endeavour should be made to investigate and resolve presenting health and social care issues in order to give Myah and her family the confidence to access services that are culturally sensitive and promote inclusiveness. Inclusivity crosses many agencies and this chapter ends with a community learning disability team's pictorial overview of interprofessional working.

FURTHER RESOURCES

National Advisory Group on Learning Disability and Ethnicity (NAGLDE): **www.learningdisabilities.org.uk**

National Learning Disability and Ethnicity Network: **www.lden .org.uk**

Ethnicity Training Network: **www.etn.leeds.ac.uk**

Office for Disability Issues (ODI): **http://odi.dwp.gov.uk/disa-bility-statistics-and-research/index.php**

Helen Sanderson Associates: **http://www.helensanderson-associates.co.uk/reading-room/how/person-centred-planning. aspx**

Janet Cobb Network: **http://www.jan-net.co.uk/**

Access to Acute Network: **http://a2anetwork.co.uk/**

Picture Bank at Change People: **http://www.changepeople .co.uk/**

Personal budgets: **http://www.dh.gov.uk/health/category/ policy-areas/nhs/personal-budgets/**

ANSWERS TO ACTIVITIES

ACTIVITY 13.1

Before birth: lack of oxygen/micro or hydrocephalic/fetal alcohol syndrome/chromosomal disorders/congenital disorders.

   After birth: poor developmental delay due to unknown aetiology/slow or late onset of condition, such as Rett syndrome/ childhood accidents leading to brain damage/viral infections/ extreme or poor social environments.

ACTIVITY 13.2

1. ● Travelling communities – people who are on the move and do not register for services due to their nomadic lifestyle.
   ● Cultural beliefs that people with learning difficulties are taken care of at home, therefore do not have access to services.
   ● People may not understand what they are entitled to therefore they cope without engaging with services.
   ● People who speak English as a second language may not know how to access help.

2. ● Fear of stigma of being labelled, which is common among people with mild LD, may often have social circles who are unemployed or at risk from poor life/health choices.
   ● Families who have had poor relationships with statutory services and choose not to engage due to previous experiences.

   ● Fear of the child being taken into care – or their coping skills being scrutinised.
   ● On rare occasions people with learning difficulties who are parents themselves may distance themselves from services due to fear of criticism.

3. ● Behavioural issues may lead to blurring of diagnosis.
   ● The presenting issue does not fit criteria for either a learning disability service or a mental health service. (This can leave a client without a service or a poor service.)
   ● Diagnostic overshadowing – the main issue being treated masks the underlying LD, common in children who have major physical disabilities, which distorts a true gauge of developmental milestones.

ACTIVITY 13.3

Reflect and discuss your answer and focus on why Myah did not fit into any other category.

ACTIVITY 13.4

The list is exhaustive and will change during your development and ability to see beyond the obvious needs of the written scenario

ACTIVITY 13.5

Some of the ideas that may have come to mind:
● Fear of being judged or blamed for having a child with LD.
● Fear of being seen as parents unable to cope.
● Fear of being seen as abnormal – taking it in turns to sleep in Myah's room.
● Fear of being blamed for not using more pharmacology to suppress the spasms – there may be a resistance to the overuse of medication as this may be seen as a more restrictive form of dealing with the problem.
● Being compared to other families who are not of the same cultural/ethnic background.
● Previous bad experiences with accessing the health service.

● Previous negativity from people within the health service.
● Previous or current negativity from their cultural community.
● Previous or current negativity from neighbours and strangers within the community.
● Poor or no representation of health professional of the same ethnic background.
● Fear of losing their child to services that may misinterpret their method of care – 'her parents take it in turn to sleep in her room due to her muscular spasms, which can occur at any time for varying durations. During these muscular spasms, Myah's parents will often massage and sing to her to try and relax and pacify her'.

ACTIVITY 13.6 AND ACTIVITY 13.7: ROPER, LOGAN AND TIERNEY'S ACTIVITIES OF DAILY LIVING

These questions will be answered by the whole family.

	Appropriate terms	Plan
Maintaining a safe environment	What things make Myah and her family feel safe	Support Myah and her family to feel physically and emotionally safe in the short and longer term
Communicating	How would Myah and her family like to be called and what help does the family need to make decisions	Take time to explain to Myah and her family what is going to happen Answer questions
Breathing	I am going to count how many times a minute you are breathing in and out	N/A
Eating and drinking	What does Myah like to eat and drink?	Support Myah and her family if required
Eliminating	How does Myah let people know she needs to go to the toilet or has been to the toilet?	Support Myah's family in taking care of elimination needs, including resources required Ensure that pain relief is given as required
Personal cleansing and dressing	How does Myah like to have a wash, bath, or shower? What clothes would you like to wear?	Maintain normal routines as far as possible
Controlling body temperature	What is the best way for Myah to cool down? How does Myah like to keep warm?	
Mobilisation	Do you have any difficulties in moving about?	Encourage rest to aid pain relief Encourage movement and play activities as able Support her family and enable Myah to receive specialist medical care for her menstrual pain
Working and playing	What games does Myah enjoy playing?	Provide toys around, which enable quieter activities to promote rest
Expressing sexuality	How does Myah let her family know she is in pain due to her menstrual bleed?	Support her family to seek and receive specialist medical care for her menstrual pain
Sleeping	What time do you like to go to bed or get up?	To maintain routines as far as practicable
Dying	As with any other child, this needs to be discussed sensitively.	

ACTIVITY 13.8

Why would Myah's parents be fearful of professionals or others who do not understand their culture?

Some ideas that may have come to mind:

- fear of being judged or blamed for having a child with LD
- fear of being seen as parents unable to cope
- fear of being seen as abnormal – taking it in turns to sleep in Myah's room
- fear of being blamed for not using more pharmacology to suppress the spasms – there may be a resistance to the overuse of medication as this may be seen as a more restrictive form of dealing with the problem
- being compared to other families who are not of the same cultural/ethnic background

- previous bad experiences with accessing the health service
- previous negativity from people within the health service
- previous or current negativity from their cultural community
- previous or current negativity from neighbours, and strangers within the community
- poor or no representation of health professional of the same ethnic background
- fear of losing their child to services that may misinterpret their method of care

ACTIVITY 13.9

Priority of actions.

This is a snapshot of Myah's presenting issues and are not in any order of importance.

Immediate	Short term	Long term/ongoing
Review medication and annual medical health check up (school doctor or GP)	Is there a PCP/circle of support?	Independence and transition
Investigate mentrual pain (school doctor or GP)	Is there a Health Action Plan (HAP)?	Personal budget for further education and day-time activity post-school
Request wheelchair assessment (wheelchair clinic via physio department)	Review respite provision and alternatives	
Request physio and occupational therapy assessment to address muscular spasms (physiotherapist/OT and school doctor)	Support for siblings	Motorised wheelchair
Request a carer's assessment/review benefits/direct payments (social worker or case manager)	Support for parents	
Request speech and language report	Is there a communication passport?	
Continence assessment (continence nurse or advisor)		Long-term aim of keeping Myah dry through baseline toileting

ACTIVITY 13.10

List Myah's areas of vulnerability.

Myah is vulnerable for a number of reasons:

- limited communication
- reliant on others for 24-hour care
- no independent mobility.

Myah has very subtle and non-descript ways of communication:

- facial expression – may show happiness or fear

- may be able to make vocal sounds which indicate pain or joy
- body tremors and spasms – may show fear and be a reaction to something she does not like as well as being involuntary
- non-engaging – Myah may opt out of engaging through lack of eye contact, vocal sounds, lack of appetite and general low mood.

Some of these signals are very similar to ones displayed by non-disabled children (see Chapter 5).

SELECTED REFERENCES

Ball, J., Milmo, D. and Ferguson, B. (2012) Half of UK's young black males are unemployed. *Guardian*, March. http://www.Guardian.Co.Uk/Society/2012/Mar/09/Half-Uk-Young-Black-Men-Unemployed

Barnardo's (2012) Young carers: http://www.Barnardos.Org.Uk/What_We_Do/Our_Projects/Young_Carers.Htm

BILD (2012) Definitions of learning disability factsheet. BILD. http://www.Bild.Org.Uk/; www.Bild.Org.Uk/Easysiteweb/Gatewaylink.Aspx?Alid=3961

Children's Act (2004) Children's Act: http://www.Legislation.Gov.Uk/Ukpga/2004/31/Pdfs/Ukpga_20040031_En.Pdf

Cooke, L. and Sinason, V. (1998) Advances in Psychiatric treatment (APT). Journal of continuing Professional Development, 4, 119–125.

Department of Education (DoE) (2004) Every child matters: https://www.Education.Gov.Uk/Publications/Standard/Publicationdetail/Page1/Dfes/1081/2004

Department of Education (DoE) (2012) Team around the child: http://www.Education.Gov.Uk/Childrenandyoungpeople/Strategy/Integratedworking/A0068944/Team-Around-The-Child-Tac

Department of Health (DoH) (2001a) Seeking consent: working with children: http://www.Dh.Gov.Uk/En/Publicationsandstatistics/Publications/Publicationspolicyandguidance/DH_4007005

Department of Health (DoH) (2001b) Valuing people: http://www.Archive.Official-Documents.Co.Uk/Document/Cm50/5086/5086.Pdf

Department of Health (DoH) (2009a) NHS continuing healthcare checklist: http://www.London.Nhs.Uk/webfiles/continuing%20healthcare/checklist.pdf

Department of Health (DoH) (2009b) Valuing people now: a new three-year strategy for people with learning disabilities: http://www.Dh.Gov.uk/En/Publicationsandstatistics/Publications/Publicationspolicyandguidance/DH_093377

Department of Health (DoH) (2012) Valuing people now: the delivery plan 2010-11: http://www.dh.gov.uk/en/publicationsandstatisctics/publication/publicationspolicyandguidance/DH_115173

Disability Rights Commission (2005/2006) Equal treatment: closing the gap interim report, parts one and two: http://www.Leeds.Ac.Uk/Disability-Studies/Archiveuk/DRC/Health%20FI%20main.Pdf

Emerson, E. and Hatton, C. (2008) People with learning disabilities in England. CeDR research report. CeDR, Lancaster University: Lancaster.

Equality and Human Rights Commission (2012) The duty to make reasonable adjustments for disabled people: http://www.Equalityhumanrights.Com/Advice-And-Guidance/Guidance-For-Employers/The-Duty-To-Make-Reasonable-Adjustments-For-Disabled-People/

Every Disabled Child Matters Campaign (2006) Every disabled child matters campaign: http://www.Edcm.Org.Uk/

Fatherhood Institute (2010) Fatherhood Institute research summary: African Caribbean fathers: http://www.Fatherhood institute.Org/2010/Fatherhood-Institute-Research-Summary-African-Caribbean-Fathers/

Fertleman, C., Gallagher, A. and Rossiter, M. (1997) Evaluation of fast track admission policy for children with sickle cell crises: questionnaire survey of parents' preferences. *British Medical Journal*: http://www.Bmj.Com/Content/ 315/7109/650

Gask, L. (1999) Acquisition of clinical skills. *Advances in Psychiatric Treatment*, 5, 311–316.

General Medical Council (2008) Consent guidance: patients and doctors making decisions together: http://www.Gmc-Uk.Org/Guidance/Ethical_Guidance/Consent_Guidance_Index.Asp

Glenn, F. (2008) http://www.Oneplusone.Org.Uk/Wp-content/Uploads/2012/03/Thecoupleconnection.Net-Evaluation.pdf

Mencap (2003) Breaking point: http://www.Longtermventilation.Nhs.Uk/_Rainbow/Documents/Breaking%20point%20report%20on%20short%20breaks.%20

Mencap (2007/2012) Death by indifference and follow up report 74 deaths and counting: http://www.Mencap.Org.Uk/Sites/Default/Files/Documents/Death%20by%20Indifference%20-%2074%20Deaths%20and%20counting.Pdf

Mencap (2009) Death by indifference: http://www.Mencap.Org.Uk/Campaigns/Take-Action/Death-Indifference

Mencap (2012) Help and support: http://www.Mencap.Org.Uk/All-About-Learning-Disability/Information-Parents-Carers-And-Family/Hearing-News-Getting-Diagnosis/Help-And-Support

Mir, G. et al. (2001) Learning difficulties and ethnicity report to the Department of Health: http://www.Dh.Gov.Uk/En/Publicationsandstatistics/Publications/Publicationspolicyandguidance/DH 4002991

NHS Choices (2012) Consent to treatment: http://www.Nhs.Uk/Conditions/Consent-To-Treatment/Pages/How-Does-It-Work.Aspx

Office for Disability Studies (2012) Easy read and Makaton: http://Odi.Dwp.Gov.Uk/Inclusive-Communications/Alternative-Formats/Easy-Read-And-Makaton.Php

Office for National Statistics (ONS) (2009) Children and young people around UK: http://www.ons.gov.uk/ons/index.html/

Office for National Statistics (ONS) (2010) Population UK: http://www.Statistics.Gov.uk/Hub/Population/Index.Html

O'Hara, J. (2003) Learning disabilities and ethnicity: achieving cultural competence. *Advances in Psychiatric Treatment*, 9, 166–174.

Parley, F. (2011) What does vulnerability mean? *British Journal of Learning Disabilities*, 39(4), 266–276.

Roper, N., Logan, W.W. and Tierney, A.J. (2000) The Roper-Logan-Tierney model of nursing: based on activities of living. Elsevier Health Science: Edinburgh.

Royal College of Psychiatrists (RCP) (2011) Minority ethnic communities and specialist learning disability services: http://www.rcpsych.ac.uk/pdf/fr_ld_2%20for%20web.pdf

Scope (2012) The social model of disability: http://www.Scope.Org.Uk/About-Us/Our-Brand/Talking-About-Disability/Social-Model-Disability

World Health Organization (WHO) (2011) World report on learning disabilities. WHO Press: Geneva.

CHAPTER 14
Children and Young People with Life-Limiting Conditions

Sharon Clarke

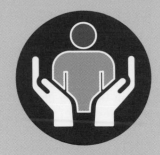
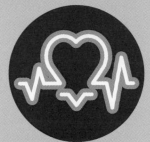
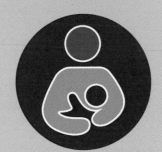

LEARNING OUTCOMES

On completion of this chapter, the reader will be able to:

- Analyse the needs of children, young people and their families requiring respite and palliative care.
- Review the evidence base for care or service delivery to children and young people and their families with respite and palliative care needs.
- Critically appraise the effectiveness of personal, organisational and societal collaboration in providing respite and palliative care for children and young people and their families.
- Critically reflect on the impact that cultural, psychological, social and spiritual perceptions of death and dying can have on the delivery of palliative care to children, young people and their families.

TALKING POINT

'On this journey, we're the "invited guest", we will join them for part of the journey as a guest and, accordingly, we should behave like a guest. Sometimes we just want to fix things but we may need to acknowledge that we can't, though we may be able to help. The beginning of wisdom is being able to say, "I don't know".'

Brother Francis (2006)

INTRODUCTION

'Death leaves a heartache no one can heal, love leaves a memory no one can steal.' (author unknown)

The ultimate aim of palliative care is to achieve quality of life and a dignified death, preferably in a place of the child or young person's and family's choosing. It incorporates the provision of short-break care and the management of distressing symptoms, not just in the dying stages, but in the weeks, months and years before a child's death (WHO 1998; ACT/RCPCH 2003; DoH 2004, 2007). Palliative care forms a thread through the lives of many children and young people with life-limiting conditions. Palliative care should support family and community, ideally extending to siblings, school friends and involved teachers (DoH 2004, 2008b, 2009; DfES DoH 2005; ACT/Children's Hospices UK 2009a).

Evidence suggests there is an enormous overlap between children with disabilities and complex health needs and those requiring palliative care. Children and young people typically move into and out of different services depending on the progress of their condition (ACT/RCPCH 2003). Services for children and young people with palliative care needs have developed over the last 25 years in a largely unplanned way. Although progress has been made in joint working in children's services as a whole, evidence suggests that there is little evidence of this in the planning, commissioning and delivery of care for children and young people requiring palliative care. The health service must adapt the way it works to provide safe, effective services for this group throughout their childhood and into young adulthood.

This chapter is intended for professionals working with children and young people and/or their families who require palliative care. The purpose of this chapter is to develop knowledge and understanding of the needs of children and young people who require palliative care and the evidence-based interventions and strategies that might be used to better enable the care of such individuals. Consideration will also be given to the needs of the child and young person's family, carers and society and how these might be most effectively met. Finally, this chapter will identify good practices in how children's needs require health, education and social services to work together.

CASE STUDY 14.1

Owen's story

Owen is a 7-year-old boy who had been diagnosed with a brain tumour, a medulloblastoma, at the age of 6. His parents, John and Sue, had noticed that there had been changes in Owen's behaviour, with tiredness and clumsiness. Owen's teacher was concerned that there had been a gradual decline in his school work and noted that Owen was finding tasks such as drawing and writing difficult.

Owen has two sisters, Victoria, aged 11 and Grace, aged 5 years.

Over the course of his illness, Owen had undergone two surgeries, one course of chemotherapy and one of radiation therapy.

Throughout the course of his treatment Owen has had a 6-month duration of remission. Then just after his 7th birthday it was decided that there were no further curative treatment options and the parents wanted palliative care provided at home.

DEFINING CHILDREN AND YOUNG PEOPLE'S PALLIATIVE CARE

Owen's palliative care, as with all children and young people with a life-limiting condition, embraces a philosophy that emphasises an active and total approach to care that attends to the physical, emotional, social and spiritual needs of the child or young person and their family (WHO 1998; ACT/RCPCH 2003). There is a shift in emphasis from conventional care that focuses on quantity of life towards a commitment to care that enhances a quality of life (Craft and Killen 2007).

Advances in technology and breakthroughs in medical science mean that more children than ever before with serious illness or disabilities are surviving. As a result, the number of children with long-term complex health needs is growing. While the entire trajectory of some diseases occurs within childhood, others may persist into adulthood and the need for palliative care may range from days to years or even decades (ACT/RCPCH 2003; DoH 2004, 2005, 2008b, Craft and Killen 2007).

ACT has described the conditions that result in life-limiting conditions within four broad groups (2009). These four medical diagnostic categories form the basis for identifying children with palliative care needs. However, categorisation is not easy and the examples used are not exclusive. The range of life-limiting conditions in children is wide and although cancer is the single most common diagnosis, more children have non-malignant conditions. They outline which conditions might be included and which therefore excluded from palliative care services. Those that are not encompassed by the categories may be better met through provision via other pathways.

In terms of services provision, these categories have also become a criterion for acceptance for some hospice and short-break services. Many authors consider it has been vital in the development and provision of services, making the children's palliative care definition more clear and palliative care needs more

Table 14.1 Four categories of children and young people's palliative care

Group	Conditions	
Group 1		Life-threatening conditions for which curative treatment may be feasible but can fail Palliative care may be necessary during periods of prognostic uncertainty and when treatment fails (e.g. cancer and cardiac anomalies)
Group 2		Conditions in which there may be long periods of intensive treatment aimed at prolonging life and allowing participation in normal childhood activities, but premature death is still possible (e.g. cystic fibrosis and muscular dystrophy)
Group 3		Progressive conditions without curative treatment options, in which treatment is exclusively palliative and may commonly extend over many years (e.g. Batten's disease and mucopolysaccharidosis)
Group 4		Conditions involving severe neurological disability that may cause weakness and susceptibility to health complications and may deteriorate unpredictably, but are not considered to be progressive (e.g. severe cerebral palsy)

Source: ACT (2009b)

recognised. A word of caution is needed as to the broad diagnostic mix, as prevalence can still be inaccurate and inconsistent. In addition, categorisation in this way creates a 'label' for children and their families (see Table 14.1). For some children and young people who do not have a definitive diagnosis or 'label', this can make accessing services very difficult and poses the argument that services should not be based on a 'label' but on individual need. Diagnosis is only part of the process – the spectrum of disease, severity of disease and subsequent complications and the impact on the child and family also need to be taken into account.

Defining children and young people's palliative care enables epidemiological studies to be carried out; consequently, our knowledge of the epidemiology of children with life-limiting conditions is improving. The number of children dying is small compared with that of adults (McCulloch et al. 2008). Familial disorders often affect more than one family member.

Earlier reports published by the charity ACT (2009a) and the Department of Health (2007) estimated the numbers of children and young people in the population with life-limiting conditions. A more recent report by Fraser et al. (2011) is the first to provide empirical data on the numbers of children and young people with life-limiting conditions using national data on children who are currently alive. Their findings demonstrated that the prevalence of life-limiting conditions in children and young people was more than double previous prevalence estimates in England with figures for Scotland, Wales and Northern Ireland also confirming higher prevalence (Table 14.2).

An important note for services development is that as a result of these data there may be a need for further specialist palliative care services, should this increase in prevalence continue. If the previous prevalence estimates of 16 per 10,000 are being used to plan services then there may be underprovision

of services. Also the largest proportional rise in prevalence in this study was in the 16- to 19-year-olds who may require services for young adults which are currently lacking.

Children and young people's palliative care has developed as a small but distinct specialty in recent years in the UK, alongside the emergence of the children's hospice movement, the further development of paediatric oncology outreach services and the expansion of community children's nursing teams with a specialist remit for this area of practice (Price et al. 2005; Brown 2007; Craft and Killen 2007; Pfund 2007). A number of recent policy documents have reflected the UK government's increasing commitment to children requiring palliative care and their families.

ACTIVITY 14.1

What are the main principles for children's and young people's palliative care practice?

THE POLICY CONTEXT FOR CHILDREN WITH LIFE-LIMITING CONDITIONS

Palliative care is a current priority for the UK government and a recent independent review has published findings relating to funding of palliative care for adults and children in England. Indeed, a number of recent policy documents have reflected the UK government's increasing commitment to children requiring palliative care and their families (Table 14.3). Other related policies include the public service agreement targets for long-term

Table 14.2 Summary of prevalence of life-limiting conditions

Double previous prevalence estimates in England with figures for Scotland, Wales and Northern Ireland also confirming higher prevalence
The highest prevalence in the under-1 age group and decreased with age
Higher prevalence in the male population compared to the female population
Highest prevalence in areas of high deprivation
Highest prevalence in numbers of neonates (babies under 28 days old)
Highest prevalence observed in children with life-limiting congenital anomalies
Significantly higher prevalence in the South Asian, black and other ethnic minority groups compared with the white population

Source: Fraser et al. (2011)

conditions, access to services, and patient and user experience, building on the five key outcomes that are set out in 'Every child matters: change for children' (DfES, 2003) and the Children Act 2004. Standard 8 of the Children's NSF expects high-quality palliative care to be available to all children and young people who need it (DoH 2004). It is to be coordinated by a network of agencies including the NHS, children's hospices, the voluntary sector, social care and education. Primary care trusts (PCTs), NHS trusts and local authorities are required to ensure provision takes account of the child or young person's and their family's physical, emotional, cultural and practical needs in a way that promotes choice, independence, creativity and quality of life. The government is now encouraging organisations to invite children and their parents to play an active role in the development of local services and to design their own packages of care using individual budgets. At the same time, local authorities and PCTs are being tasked to gather more and better data on the needs of this group.

Table 14.3 Policy drivers

ACT/RCPCH 2003. *A Guide to the Development of Children's Palliative Care Services*
ACT and Children's Hospices UK 2009. *Right People, Right Place, Right Time*
ACT and Children's Hospices UK 2009. *Making the Case for Children's Palliative Care*
Children Act 1989
Commission for Service Improvement (CSIP) 2007. Developing Multi-agency Planning and Commissioning for Services for Disabled Children and Young People, those with Long-term Health Conditions and/or Requiring Palliative Care. A Ten-Step Guide
Craft and Killen 2007. *Palliative Care Services for Children and Young People in England: an independent review*
DfES 2003. *Every Child Matters: Change for Children*
DoH 2004. *National Service Framework for Children, Young People and Maternity Services*
DoH 2005. *Commissioning Children and Young People's Palliative Care Services*
DoH 2007. *Palliative Care Statistics for Children and Young Adults*
DoH 2008. *Aiming High for Disabled Children*
DoH 2008. *Better Care, Better Lives. Improving outcomes and experiences for children, young people and their families living with life-limiting and life-threatening conditions*
DoH 2009. *Better Care, Better Lives. Achieving the vision for the palliative care of children and young people in the East of England*
Marie Curie 2008. *Supporting the Choice to Die at Home*
National Institute for Clinical Excellence 2004. *Supportive and Palliative Care for Adults*
National Institute for Clinical Excellence 2005. *Improving Outcomes in Children and Young People with Cancer*

BREAKING BAD NEWS/ COMMUNICATING WITH CARE AND COMPASSION

'I think that conveying difficult news to parents is just as much of an art form as doing an operation and it's just as important to be self-critical.' (Professor Sir David Hall, President of the Royal College of Paediatrics and Child Health 2000–2003)

Owen's journey started, as it does for many children, with attendance at or admission to hospital following a professional concern, a parental concern or a critical event, although this may not always be the case. The National Service Framework for children, young people and maternity services (DoH 2004) encourages healthcare professionals to consider the child's journey through our healthcare system.

VOICES 14.1 Breaking bad news

Consider the scenario.

Owen's parents' recall:

'Following Owen's second surgery we noticed his recovery was more difficult and the radiation therapy made him so tired.

We were due to return to the oncologist to get the results of Owen's last MRI. We always dreaded these appointments. It felt like we were on a rollercoaster ride; would it be good news or bad?'

Straightaway, I noticed that the nurse was looking concerned and went to inform the consultant of our arrival. When they came back I noticed how anxious they both looked. We were taken to a room with some chairs and a box of tissues! We knew something was dreadfully wrong and all John and I could do was wait for the bombshell.'

Think about the sorts of decision that the parent will have to make on behalf of their child.

Breaking bad news is one of the most challenging and difficult tasks faced by health professionals causing considerable anxiety (ACT 2004). A US study by Contro et al. (2004) reported the distress caused by uncaring delivery of bad news. Furthermore, it is suggested that recipients of bad news can often remember where, when and how bad news was communicated. In addition, ineffective or insensitive news disclosure can have a long-term adverse impact on recipients (Fallowfield and Jenkins 2004), remaining a potential bitter focus of distress. To break bad news effectively requires careful planning and sensitivity; however, health professionals seldom receive specific training in undertaking this difficult task (Buckman 2005; Walter 1996).

VOICES 14.2

'I was told over the telephone that my daughter was life limited. I was on my own in the house'

(Square Table Local Learning and Evaluation Report 2011)

The principles of breaking bad news are the same in any situation, whether with children or adults. Psychological defence mechanisms have a profound impact on our ability to handle and communicate distressing information. It is an unnatural subject to discuss with children and young people; however, it is an important one to ensure that their dreams, hopes and wishes are respected.

ACTIVITY 14.2 Breaking bad news

Your mentor has invited you to attend the meeting in which the oncologist will give the results of investigations to Owen's parents, John and Sue. These indicate that, despite radical treatment, there is no further curative treatment options available. During the meeting John and Sue are adamant that they do not want Owen to receive this information.

What are the key goals in breaking bad news?

Read the information in Figure 14.1 and consider what the nurse's role is in breaking bad news

What ethical dilemmas may occur?

According to Baile et al. (2000) the interprofessional team has four goals in breaking the news:

1. learn what is already known about the situation and determine readiness to hear the news
2. provide clear information tailored to needs and desire to know
3. provide empathy and emotional support
4. develop a treatment plan that takes wishes into account.

Every family should receive the disclosure of their child's prognosis in a face-to-face discussion in privacy and should be treated with respect, honesty and sensitivity. Information should be provided both for the child and the family in language that they can understand (Scope 1993). As can be seen in Figure 14.1, Price et al. (2006) explore the role of the nurse in breaking bad news in relation to the family and the interprofessional team. The health professional should prepare in advance by making sure they have obtained and been informed about the patient's condition and management to date (Buckman 2005). The health professional will need to plan the location of where to break the news. Make sure it gives the family complete privacy, and ensure the right people are present (Scope 1993; DHSSPS 2003). If some family members have different levels of knowledge or are approaching the situation very differently,

Manager/leader
Before

- Prepare self
- Prepare venue – consider privacy
- Liaise with doctors
- Ensure X-rays, results, information leaflets available
- Organise the necessary people to be present
- Allocate another member of team to care for child

After

- Ensure follow-up as required
- Document clearly in nursing notes

Facilitator/supporter
During

- Support family during interview
- Show empathy/be attentive during interview
  – take notes for parents if desired/appropriate
- Ensure parents have time to express their emotions
- Supportive presence for doctor during interview

Immediately following meeting

- Give choices – do they want to be left alone?
- Answer any questions they may have, clarify any points, use simple language

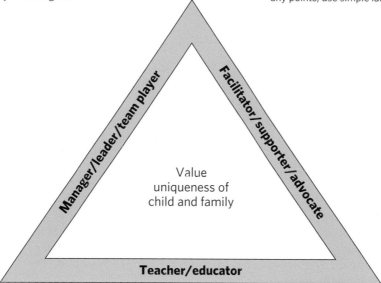

Teacher/educator
Following meeting

- Provide family with any further information they require
- Practical help and written information to back up verbal if appropriate

Advocate/team player
Following meeting

- Communicate with other members of MDT
- Document and record in nursing notes
- Promote needs of child/support parents regarding how and why to tell their child

Figure 14.1 Breaking bad news
Source: Price et al. (2006)

it might be useful to speak to them separately. However, it is important to get all the key decision makers in the same time-frame or risk causing tensions and conflict. It may or may not be appropriate for the child to be there (Scope 1993; DHSSPS 2003). Often, and particularly with smaller children, parents tend to prefer having the news broken to them first and then take part in breaking significant news with the child herself.

When a child and family are confronting a life-limiting diagnosis, it is possible for them to be in one of four different 'awareness contexts' as listed by ACT (2011). As can be seen in Figure 14.2, open awareness is the ideal as it allows for fears and concerns to be voiced and addressed, for better care plans to be negotiated and agreed and for the child and family to feel more in control. Often child, family and professionals are each in different awareness contexts or stuck in 'mutual pretence', usually because the truth is too distressing or difficult to handle. Generally, it is fine to allow everyone to reach open awareness in her own time, but where blocked

RESEARCH NOTE 14.1

The goal of the Schmid Mast et al. (2005) study was to show that physician communication style of breaking bad news affects how the physician is perceived, how satisfied recipients of bad news are with the consultation and how they feel after the consultation.

The study concluded that a patient-centred communication style has the most positive outcome for recipients of bad news on a cognitive, evaluative and emotional level.

The results of this study provide guidelines to physicians on how to convey bad news.

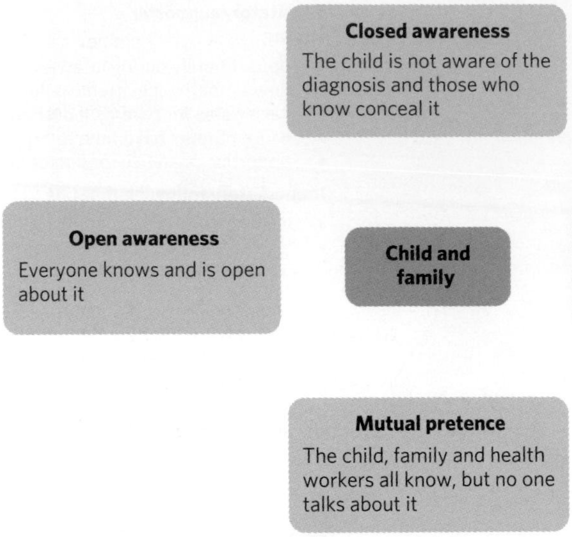

Figure 14.2 Awareness contexts
Source: ACT (2011)

communication risks increasing a child's suffering (e.g. where a child is isolated and anxious), or where events are proceeding so fast that communication is crucial to plan, prepare and adapt, then intervention may be needed. This is a continuum along which parents have to make decisions about what to divulge and when. This situation may be more problematic for children and young people with cognitive impairment and judgements have to be made on how much they understand and how fully they can contribute to decision making about their care. The literature clearly indicates that an open awareness context is the best way to prepare a child or young person for death and that this can also act as a preparation for bereavement for the family.

Warn, Pause, Check (WPC) Chunk Method

Although there is a plethora of frameworks or models for breaking bad news in the literature (Buckman 1992; Rabow and McPhee 2000; Bloom 2001; DHSSPS 2003), few focus specifically on children's nursing and the role of the children's nurse. Amery (2009) as can be seen in Figure 14.3, provides a useful strategy for accomplishing the goals in breaking bad news, employing a four-step protocol, known as 'WPC chunk' method. This method is a simple approach for presenting distressing information in an organised manner to patients and families.

Following the breaking of bad news, the next stage is to wait for a reaction and respond to the child's and family's feelings.

PRACTICAL GUIDELINES 14.1

Establishing awareness

How much each person knows:

- Ask each one individually and try to prevent others blocking or interrupting; but this takes time and the healthcare professional will need to allow silence and space.
- When they speak, reflect what they have said and make sure you have understood exactly what they know before moving on.

Levels of denial

Find out the level of denial the child or family members have, either consciously or subconsciously:

- If they signal they are not ready to be open, stop and review this later. Don't push for information if they don't want to give it.

- Managing denial and collusion is an art, not a science, so there are no clear, 'one-size-fits-all' answers.
- You need to try and balance the risks and the benefits of allowing the denial to continue.
- Where the motivation is love (rather than control), collusion and denial tend to melt away as events progress and as people adapt to the situation. In this case, all you need to do is support and wait until this happens naturally.
- Where things are deteriorating fast and time is not a luxury you have, or where the child is clearly being isolated and upset by the collusion or denial, you need to explain to the whole family that you recognise that everyone is acting as they are purely to prevent others being hurt; but that, by not allowing open communication, they may be inadvertently hurting their child (ACT 2011).

PREPARE	**1** Start by mentally breaking the significant news into chunks **2** Don't overwhelm with large pieces of information as people stop hearing **3** There may be several bits of news: • That he or she will die • That they will die soon, or may have a long-term condition with slow degeneration and complex care needs • That he or she might suffer with unpleasant symptoms unless carefully managed • That the family will need to learn what to do if any of these eventualities arise **4** Decide which chunk you are going to share
WARN	This gives the person a chance to prepare and helps them to absorb the difficult information
PAUSE AND PRESENT	This gives the person a chance to decide whether or not they still want to go ahead and also to react. If they assent (either verbally or non-verbally), go ahead and share the first chunk of news
CHECK BACK	• Ask what they have understood and correct or reinforce. This allows you to ensure they have understood you and also acts to embed the news properly in the person's memory. This is important because, after traumatic events, people often forget what happened and what was said • Decide whether they are ready to move on and, if they are, then share the next chunk of news using the same method

Figure 14.3 Warn, pause, check (WPC) chunk method
Source: Amery (2009)

Most importantly, whatever the response is, validate it. Once the response settles, you should repeat the process until one of four things happens:

1. There is no more news to share.
2. They signal that they have had enough.
3. You get the feeling that they have stopped hearing or absorbing.
4. You feel you personally cannot do anymore (which is fine, as long as you make sure you arrange to come back).

Once all the news has been given the health professional needs to take on a more active role. Begin to identify options, suggest sources of support and start negotiating care management plans for the various problems and issues that you have identified. Lastly, make sure the family is able to make contact with a health professional over the next few days (DHSSPS 2003; Amery 2009).

REFLECTION Difficult Questions

• Reflect on your own practice and list the main barriers to communication with children that affect you.
• List those things you will do to make your communication and practice more child friendly.
• Here are some common 'difficult' questions in children's palliative care:

  • Will it hurt when I die?
  • Where will I go when I die?
  • What will happen to my brother when I die?
  • Will mummy be sad when I die?

CHILDREN'S AND YOUNG PEOPLE'S CONCEPTS OF DEATH AND DYING

'Death in childhood is uncommon, but for those families who have to confront the problems of caring for a terminally ill child, the burden is great.' (Goldman et al. 2006)

In today's society, people do not generally have direct experience of being with, talking about or observing death and dying, therefore discussion of death and dying does not generally take place openly. Concepts of death and dying can often be 'medicalised'. Parents and carers may feel overwhelmed. Klassen et al. (2008) reported that parents of children with cancer report poorer quality of life with many parents experiencing distress from having to make difficult end-of-life care decisions, withholding or withdrawing life-sustaining treatments, foregoing cancer chemotherapy, talking to their children about death or deciding on the location of their last days (Dunlop 2008; Dussel et al. 2009).

There has been increased recognition of children's participation in making treatment decisions. Over recent years attention has been given to children's experience of their illness; this is essential not only to enhance their quality of life, but also as a guide to clinical decisions and goals of care. The complexities of involving children and young people can become more challenging as an illness progresses, especially if the family and healthcare professionals are reticent to discuss death with children. A landmark study by Kreicbergs et al. (2004) discovered that among the Swedish parents surveyed, those who had talked to their dying child about death reported no regrets about having had that discussion. Conversely, the parents who had not talked to their child about the impending death did regret having omitted this conversation.

CORE THEME Ethics

A useful guide to the duties of health professionals is that of the Royal College of Paediatrics and Child Health (UK). It describes four aspects of child involvement in decision making that health professionals should ensure are addressed wherever possible. These include the child:

- being informed
- being consulted
- views taken into account in decision making
- being respected as the main decision maker.

INVOLVING CHILDREN AND YOUNG PEOPLE

CORE THEME Children's Rights

Dying children or young people are afforded the same rights enshrined in law, both nationally in the 1989 Children Act and internationally in the UN Convention on the Rights of the Child 1991.

The current emphasis on the rights of children to have access to information and participate in decisions is far from universal.

A cautionary note: in the urgency to include children, this may inadvertently create a burden on the child that he does not feel equipped to manage.

Many researchers have sought to define the child's complex concept of death and dying. Children's concept of death has been shown to be influenced by:

- age/cognitive development
- life-limiting illness
- religion
- nationality
- personal experience of death
- family attitudes to death.

A child's understanding of death generally follows her cognitive development and matures with age. As can be seen in Table 14.x, one of the challenges of palliative care is the child's ever changing physical, emotional and cognitive development and its impact on the understanding of disease and death. A child's response may be limited by her verbal ability but she may understand more than she can articulate.

Much of the literature on children's views of death and dying is dominated by a developmental perspective. Table 14.4 provides a developmental perspective on the child and young person understanding of death and grief. While younger children (as can be seen in Table 14.4) may not be able to take an abstract or time-based perspective, her expressed fears and concerns can provide the basis for her decisions. Older children and adolescents who have more capacity to plan over time can engage in complex end-of-life decisions

---

RESEARCH NOTE 14.2

The observational study of Kreicbergs et al. (2004) discovered that, among the Swedish parents surveyed, those who had talked to their dying child about death reported no regrets about having had that discussion. Conversely, 27% of the parents who had not talked to their child about the impending death did regret having omitted this conversation.

This study provides valuable guidance for optimal family-centred care.

The study had little to say about the implications of the findings as such unjustifiable implications could harm some parents and children.

that may be driven by relationships, culture and spirituality. Health professionals are often left to rely on their own judgement to assess children's understanding of the contingencies they face. The difficulty with this perspective is that it is seen as a linear process, which makes assumptions that, at points in the child's and young person's developmental maturation, they cast aside immature notions. Indeed, scholars have differed about the particular age or stage at which a particular view emerges.

Freyer et al. (2006) address the issues of adolescence and end-of-life care, pointing out that the comprehension of death and grief is complex and is complicated by their cognitive abilities, personal experiences, cultural background and emotional responses. Their views require consideration of these factors as well as the context of the conversation, the environment and how the issues are presented.

Children often express their understanding, awareness, and thoughts about treatment options and living or dying to individuals other than their parents. Owen had asked the nurse on the children's ward: 'Why has the medicine stopped? Will they give me some new medicine?' Children are often quite perceptive about the changes to treatment or life-prolonging options available and members of the interprofessional team are essential at this point. Nurses can play an important role in assisting parents to understand specific cognitive concepts of death and reactions to death.

Developmental Considerations

Cognitive development and age form the foundation for a child's understanding of the concept of death. Understanding emerges over time in a sequential pattern, but the process is diverse and varies with each child. There are general considerations in caring for children of different ages at the end of life.

Infancy to 2 Years

Normal developmental tasks for infants include developing trust in parents, while achieving a sense of differentiation. Separation from parents is a primary fear. Infants have no concept of death and are most affected by the family's emotional and physical state. Reactions occur in relation to separation from caregivers and alterations in routines or surroundings. To support a child this age, encourage parents to stay with the child as much as possible, and provide physical relief and comfort (Corr and Balk 2010).

Toddlers' developmental tasks include establishing small amounts of independence from parents, wanting a sense of control over their environment, and learning basic self-care skills. Children under 2 years of age have limited understanding of the dying process. Because differentiation from others is not complete, children at this early age are influenced by the emotions of others, often reacting as they see their parents react. Hospitalisation is extremely stressful (Corr and Balk 2010).

PRACTICAL GUIDELINES 14.2

The nurse's support may include:

- minimising the child's separation from parents as much as possible
- if a parent cannot be available, encouraging the parents to find a consistent, reliable adult to stay with the child
- encouraging the family to maintain familiar routines or explain reasons why the routine must be changed.

- providing opportunities for the child to continue to achieve her developmental skills
- providing the necessary materials and resources to help the child succeed at the tasks
- encouraging regular play activities
- providing maximum physical relief and comfort.

Early Childhood (2–6 Years)

Development of autonomy begins during this age and children enjoy making decisions and expressing themselves. Children of this age are becoming increasingly independent from their parents and enjoy self-sufficiency. The world is viewed in terms of good or bad, and magical thinking leads children to believe they have a direct impact on the events in their lives.

For the preschooler, the concept of death is limited, and death may be seen as reversible or temporary. Illness and separation from parents may be perceived as punishment for bad thoughts or actions; feelings of guilt and responsibility for causing illness/death may develop. Children may regress behaviourally in an attempt to feel secure (Corr and Balk 2010).

PRACTICAL GUIDELINES 14.3

The nurse's support may include:

- assuring the children that he is not being punished
- providing clear, honest explanations of the illness and treatments
- minimising separation from parents and significant others where possible
- providing outlets for normal childhood emotions
- providing an environment that encourages curiosity
- providing maximum physical relief and comfort.

Middle Childhood (6–9 Years)

Peers are important at this age, yet children return to the security of home and family for comfort. Children have the ability to master and learn; constant activity is normal. Feelings of independence, self-confidence and individuality are emerging.

Rules and order are internalised and every act is thought to have a punishment or reward (Corr and Balk 2010).

Hospitalisation or illness may be seen as a punishment for any wrongs. A child's evolving sense of self may be impacted by the illness, creating feelings of anger and confusion. Parents may be held responsible for the illness.

PRACTICAL GUIDELINES 14.4

The nurse's support may include:

- providing children with concrete details and truthful, open communication about the illness
- providing opportunities for children to exercise their skills and abilities so they can feel a sense of achievement and control
- maintaining interaction with friends
- minimising separation from parents
- allowing children to be involved in planning or carrying out treatment procedures, if possible
- providing maximum physical relief and comfort.

Late Childhood (10–12 Years)

Through socialisation with friends and the onset of puberty, children begin to develop a body image, self-esteem and identity. Peers are critical, and privacy is extremely important. Young adolescents begin to incorporate information to solve problems and want more independence from parents. Children of this age have a realistic view of death as inevitable, irreversible and universal. They understand that biological life ends in death (Corr and Balk 2010).

When terminally ill, young adolescents may struggle between the developmental need to begin separating from parents and the natural tendency to regress due to the illness. Peer groups may feel their own independence threatened and may withdraw, leaving adolescents feeling alienated from parents and rejected by peers. There is a marked concern among adolescents for how the illness will affect their physical appearance.

PRACTICAL GUIDELINES 14.5

The nurse's support may include:

- allowing children as much control and independence as possible
- providing opportunities for them to interact with the medical staff
- providing opportunities for involvement in the decision-making process
- providing opportunities to share feelings and ask questions
- treating adolescents with respect and dignity
- providing clear, honest and direct communication
- encouraging association with friends
- providing privacy and maximum physical relief and comfort.

Young Adult (13–18 Years)

The development of identity, body image and self-esteem continue; additionally, a sexual identity is being formed. Young people of this age seek to establish emotional and economic independence from parents. An adult view of death exists, yet they often believe they are infallible and immortal.

The young adult with a terminal illness may worry that they may not be able to attract a partner and that peers may reject them. The young adult may be more concerned about the physical side-effects of treatment than about dying. They are concerned that their independence from parents will be impeded. As the illness has its effect on the body, they feel a loss of control (Corr and Balk 2010) (see also Table 14.4.).

PRACTICAL GUIDELINES 14.6

The nurse's support may include:

- treating the young person with respect
- providing clear, honest and direct communication
- providing for privacy
- finding ways to recognise and support the individual's unique identity
- offering opportunities to express emotions
- encouraging association with friends
- allowing as much control and independence as possible
- recognising and addressing issues of sexuality
- providing maximum physical relief and comfort.

VOICES 14.3

This is an extract from a poem written by a group of young people from Y-Plan, Young People Looked After Network, Gloucestershire, as part of a film project with Catcher Media about their experiences of loss and grief.

A thousand daggers twist in my guts,
the hurt like spiders crawling up my throat,
worry wriggles under my skin.
My legs are stiff as steel, My arms are stiff as trees.

My eyes puff up like bags of crisps ready to be popped
Stomach an erupting volcano
Numb body full of ice,
Mouth is clamped shut
My head holds an electric storm
Body frozen, everything stops
and my eyes just stare.
(Catcher Media 2007)

Table 14.4 Children and young people's understanding of death and expressions of grief

Age (Piaget)	Understanding of death	Expressions of grief
Sensorimotor stage Infancy to 2 years	Not yet able to understand death and its finality	Quietness, irritability, decreased activity, poor sleep, and weight loss
		Clings to others
		Reaction to non verbal cues
	Separation from mother causes changes (Bowlby 1959)	
Preoperational stage 2–6 years	Death is like sleeping	Concerned about own well-being
		Feels confused and guilty
		May use imaginative play
		Withdraws
		Irritable
		Regresses
		Asks many questions (How does she go to the bathroom? How does she eat?)
		Language may be taken very literally
		Denial is a common defence mechanism
		Problems in eating, sleeping and bladder and bowel control
		Fear of being abandoned
		Feelings of guilt, especially siblings
		Tantrums
	Dead person continues to live and function in some ways	'Magical thinking' (Did I think or do something that caused the death? Like when I said I hate you and I wish you would die?)
		May see death as a punishment

(Continued)

Age (Piaget)	Understanding of death	Expressions of grief
	Death is not final	
	Dead people can come back to life	
Concrete operational stage 6–11 years	Begins to understand concept of death	May seem outwardly uncaring, inwardly upset
	Death is thought of as a person or spirit (skeleton, ghost)	May attempt to 'parent'
		May play death games
	May be superstitious about death	Curious about death
	May be uncomfortable in expressing feelings	Asks specific questions
	Worries that other important people will die	May have fears about school
	Death is final and scary	May have aggressive behaviour (especially boys)
		May act out in school or home
		Worries about imaginary illnesses
	Death happens to others, it won't happen to me	May use denial to cope
		May feel abandoned
Formal operational stage 11 and older	Mature understanding of death Everyone will die	May respond better to peers than adults/parents
		Strong emotions, guilt, anger, shame
		Increased anxiety over own death
		May be interested in theological theories
		Moodiness and irritability
	Death is final	Fear of rejection; not wanting to be different from peers
	Even I will die	Try to retain independence and autonomy
		Changes in lifestyle habits, i.e. eating
		Sleeping problems
		Regressive behaviour (loss of interest in outside activities)
		Impulsive behaviour
		Feels guilty about being alive (especially related to death of a brother, sister or peer)

Source: adapted from Himelstein et al. (2004)

From even a very young age children will be able to give information about their abilities and, provided with an atmosphere in which their views are respected and given validity, they will be able to describe feelings and needs (Sourkes, cited in Goldman et al. 2006). The health professional should therefore consider how to involve children in the assessment process taking into account their age, development, disability and culture. It will be necessary to build a rapport that will help the child to feel understood, establishing the most appropriate method of communication (West Midland Paediatric Macmillan Team 2005). Non-verbal communication using signs, body language or even eye movement have been used to great effect with children who have severe disability. Play using props can also be effective in gaining insight into children's feelings. These themes are discussed in other chapters.

Childhood is socially constructed, therefore it is essential to consider the ethnic and spiritual culture of the family as a significant factor in how the child's voice is heard and how it is incorporated into the decision-making process. In ensuring that the child and siblings are given opportunities for participation, it will be necessary to take care to respect the family's culture. Some children and young people may not have previously been involved in decision making or expression of views and it may challenge the parents' approach to care. It may also be a painful experience for the parents and the worker to witness emotions in children that have not been expressed before (West Midland Paediatric Macmillan Team 2005).

DEFINING NEED

VOICES 14.4

'It's also about giving permission for a parent to be a parent as well so that they can enjoy being a parent. This time is their special time with their child and that time may be short. We should not expect them to do all the caring and nursing things.' (Square Table Local Learning and Evaluation Report 2011a)

Palliative care affects the whole family, with the burden of care falling on parents and siblings or grandparents. Some illnesses are 'familiar' and more than one child may be affected. In most cases, the direct family are the primary carers for the child/children. It is recognised that family members and carers provide 24-hour care and support for a child, many of whom have very complex health care needs and disabilities. An estimated 63 per cent of children and young people requiring palliative care have a need for social care services (DoH 2007, 2008a, 2008b).

Health professionals are experienced in caring for children and young people as individuals within a context of family-centred care (Brown and Mercer 2011). These concepts are explored in other chapters. Indeed the philosophy of holistic family-centred care has become a core principle of children and young people's nursing and recognises that there are many different factors that come together to influence quality of life (West Midland Paediatric Macmillan Team 2005). There are particular challenges in caring for children and young people with palliative care needs. Children and young people have ongoing developmental, educational, identity and dependency needs that have to be identified and managed.

The needs of children and young people with a life-limiting illness and their families are summarised in the report by ACT and the Royal College of Paediatrics and Child Health (2003).

Families need support from the time of diagnosis and throughout treatment as well as when the disease is far advanced. Professionals must be flexible in their efforts to help. Each family and individual within a family is unique, with different strengths and coping skills. The needs of siblings and grandparents should be included. The family of a child or young person with an inherited condition have additional difficulties. They may have feelings of guilt and blame, and they will need genetic counselling and information about prenatal diagnosis in the future. When an illness does not present until some years after birth several children in the same family may be affected (West Midland Paediatric Macmillan Team 2005).

Assessing and Planning Care

A central tenet of Owen and his family's care and advocated by ACT documents is that good children's palliative care planning means 'hoping for the best and planning for the worst' (ACT 2011).

Many texts refer to two different levels of needs assessment:

- first, the assessments of the needs of an individual child within the context of family and environment
- second, the needs of a population to inform service planning.

CASE STUDY REVIEW 14.1 ASSESSING OWEN'S NEEDS

Owen's brain tumour is causing escalating intracranial pressure and seizures. These symptoms have resulted in Owen and his family being very anxious about being at home.

Owen and his family live in a flat in a rural setting.

Owen's mother, Sue, gave up work to care for Owen and his sisters, while Owen's father, John, is a self-employed contractor. Owen has two sisters, Victoria, aged 11 and Grace, aged 5 years, who have missed having Owen at home. The family has relied on Sue's parents to help with the day-to-day care of Victoria and Grace.

- Consider how you would assess and plan Owen's care.
- What anxieties might Owen and his family be experiencing?
- What anxieties might you have?

These activities are interlinked, as data is collected from individual assessments and used to inform the planning of local and national services.

Over the last decade there have been a number of national paediatric palliative care needs assessments which have helped determine service planning (Contro et al. 2004; DfES and DoH 2005). These studies have identified the specific needs of children, young people and their families, as well as providing data on mortality and location of death. The central themes from these studies are that children and their families want to be at home but that community resources are inadequate in enabling the families to achieve this goal. Essential services such as short-break care are still inadequate. The services available to children, young people and their families often depends on where they live and their diagnosis, as services for children and young people with cancer are often better developed (ACT 2003, 2004; West Midland Paediatric Macmillan Team 2005). As the result of these nationally identified needs, ACT has developed a number of care pathways as an approach to delivering care and support to children and families throughout their journey; from diagnosis to end of life and into bereavement (as can be seen in Figure 14.4).

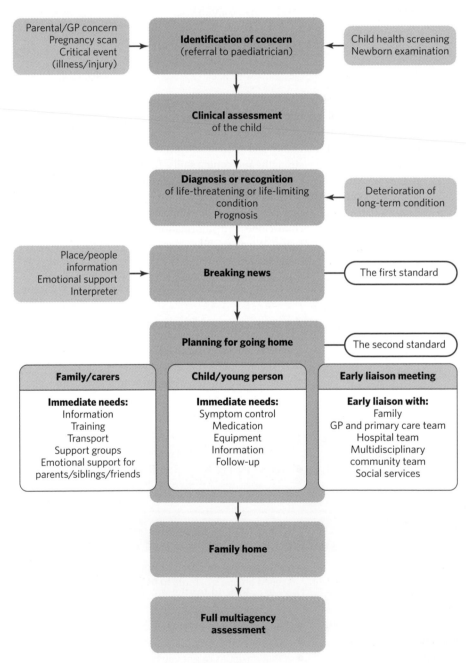

Figure 14.4 The ACT (2004) integrated multi-agency care pathway for children with life-threatening and life-limiting conditions, stage 1

Care Pathway Approach

Care pathways are a systematic approach in utilising knowledge to improve acute and community services. They are a means of achieving coordinated care reflecting individual and local need by seeking user involvement. Care pathways complement guidance from NSF children, young people and maternity services (DoH 2004) by following the patient's journey with the use of interprofessional assessment, protocol and standards.

> ### ACTIVITY 14.3 Care pathways
>
> Consider and list why care pathways are needed
>
> What are the stages and standards of ACT Care Pathways?

The care pathway approach, now widely adopted across the UK, has helped to improve the family's journey throughout their child's life. In 2004 ACT published the first multiagency, integrated care pathway for children and young people with palliative care needs: the ACT integrated multiagency care pathway for children with life-threatening and life-limiting conditions, commonly referred to as the ACT Care Pathway. This was followed by a transition care pathway in 2007 designed to encourage better planning and support for those young people who receive palliative care and need to make the transition to adult palliative care services.

More recently, ACT has published a dedicated neonatal care pathway for babies with palliative care needs and a care pathway to support extubation within a children's palliative care framework. ACT's Care Pathways for professionals have been complemented by a family companion to the ACT Care Pathway, which has been designed to guide families through the complex and often bewildering journey that takes place following diagnosis (ACT 2004, 2007a and b, 2009c). The Department of Health is developing a continuing healthcare pathway, and ACT is contributing to this. The Liverpool care pathway for the dying child is being developed. Work on gold standard framework for children's palliative is under way. The preferred place of care tool can be adapted for use in children's services.

ASSESSMENT OF THE CHILD OR YOUNG PERSON WITH PALLIATIVE CARE NEEDS

Assessment is central to health professional activity as a process for understanding what is happening to Owen and his family and to inform decisions about action to be taken or services to be provided. Assessment is also an intervention in itself. The process of assessment may create change and lead to help from the extended family and/or the provision of services. Assessments of children in need should be undertaken in partnership with children and families. Although the feasibility of

full partnership can be questioned when professionals hold disproportionate power and resources, research shows that practitioners can engage in effective working with families that builds on strengths, enables their participation and promotes their involvement in decision making and planning (ACT 2003, 2004, 2009a, 2009b; DoH 2004).

Without a full assessment and an agreed, achievable and realistic care plan it is very difficult to provide good children's palliative care. Many studies have shown how professionals sometimes delay difficult discussions and care planning until it is too late, leaving the child and family to suffer unnecessarily or spend their last days in hospital, rather than at home. Having been assessed, one family may require little in the way of direct services, while another whose child has the same condition may require considerable input. A detailed assessment of need in partnership with the family ensures, first, that the family's concerns are heard and, second, that finite resources are directed to those most in need (ACT 2003, 2009a; DoH 2004, 2008b; West Midland Paediatric Macmillan Team 2005).

Care planning offers the health professional a process of discourse with the child (where possible), family and other relevant people. Good care planning involves clarification and agreement on specific and realistic management objectives, contingency planning, and arrangements for appropriate review and 'handover' to the family as endorsed by the NSF for children, young people and maternity services (DoH 2004).

Assessment Skills for Children's Nurses

The International Council of Nurses' position statement reflects on the responsibility of nurses to alleviate suffering, as well as their essential role in the provision of palliative care (ICN 2006; IMPaCTT 2007). All children and young people with palliative care needs will require variable components of both generic and specialist palliative care provided in a planned, coordinated, timely and flexible manner (Brown 2007; Pfund 2007; ACT/Children's Hospices UK 2009; Wolfe et al. 2011).

Within the delivery of children's palliative nursing care, there is diverse range of professional roles (DoH 2008, 2009; Wolfe et al. 2011). These include community children's nurses, school nurses, children's hospice nurses and health visitors. Those undertaking needs assessments should have appropriate skills and knowledge. As can be seen in Figure 14.5, circle 1 indicates the skills a nurse is expected to understand and demonstrate: these include the basic concepts of holistic assessment in recognising and meeting the needs of caring for children and young people in a family unit thus providing family centred care, while circles 2 to 4 indicate the developing competencies of the qualified nurse to the expert practitioner. Consequently, there is a demand for the provision of training and education for this expanding group of nurses (Pfund 2007).

Palliative Care Education

The European Association for Palliative Care (EAPC) and the World Health Organization considers training in palliative

1 Basic concepts of holistic assessment to meet needs, recognising caring for children and young people in a family unit

4 Expert practitioner in advanced holistic assessment. Leader of interagency/professional sharing of assessment and care pathway developer

Assessment skills

2 Recognition of dying and last offices. Holistic needs of the child, young person and family Interagency working Application of end-of-life care tools

3 Evaluation of holistic needs assessment and use of management plans, including end-of-life plans, ways of coping, interagency/professional sharing of assessments

Figure 14.5 Nurses' assessment skills
Source: ACT (2009a)

care for healthcare professionals a priority (IMPaCCT 2007). ACT (2003) believes that every life-limited child and her family should have access to the best possible care and support delivered by a skilled, experienced and confident workforce. The Department of Health in their first children's palliative care strategy 'Better care: better lives' (DoH 2008b, page 43) proposes that the importance, contribution and value of a fit-for-purpose workforce are critical to achieving the improvements.

As previously discussed, it is essential for staff delivering children's palliative care to be competent and have had appropriate education, experience and support in the healthcare of children (ACT/Children's Hospices UK 2009). At its most basic level, palliative care training must be a core part of the curriculum for all paediatric healthcare professionals, as well as related subspecialties (Craft and Killen 2007; ACT/Children's Hospices UK 2009). To accommodate the educational needs of senior specialist nurses in palliative care, there must be designated

centres of excellence that can provide formal teaching and postgraduate training in all aspects of paediatric palliative care (Craft and Killen 2007; ACT/Children's Hospices UK 2009a).

As well as ensuring that the necessary skills are developed within the existing workforce, it is important to consider succession planning to ensure sustainability. The strategy reinforces many of the views expressed in the Independent Review of Children's Palliative Care, which acknowledges the need for developing a career pathway for nurses specialising in palliative care for children and young people (Craft and Killen 2007; ACT/Children's Hospices UK 2009a).

ACT and Children's Hospices UK (2009a) suggest that formal palliative care training is on the increase, although, there is a dearth of published evidence on children and young people's palliative care education with few higher education institutions (HEIs) offering distinct programmes or modular components within programmes.

RESEARCH NOTE 14.3

This UK study from Neilson et al. (2010) aimed to explore the experiences of community children's nurses (CCNs) and children's palliative care nurses (CPCNs) who provide end-stage palliative care to children with cancer in the family home.

A qualitative approach was adopted with one-to-one interviews and facilitated case discussions were undertaken with 30 community nurses who had provided palliative care to a child or young person with cancer. A grounded theory approach was used for data analysis.

Because of the relative rarity of childhood cancer many CCNs and CPCNs engage infrequently in the palliative care of children or young people. This makes it difficult for them to develop and maintain knowledge and skills. There is a variation in the out-of-hours service provision available to families.

Further funding is needed to develop teams of trained, experienced CCNs and CPCNs who can provide palliative care for children and young people 24 hours a day, 365 days a year.

A Key Worker

VOICES 14.5

'The most valuable thing in the whole package of care was a key worker doing all the liaison. They had a dedicated budget to spend on anything the family needed. They could buy in anything within days. They brought the agencies together to meet the family' (Square Table Local Learning and Evaluation Report 2011).

Key workers are seen by many families and professionals as critical in promoting a better quality of life for children and young people with palliative care needs (Greco and Sloper 2004). A key worker or lead professional is responsible for co-ordinating the child's comprehensive care package, coordinating and liaising with all the professionals and services involved with the child and being a main point of contact for the family. The key worker is often a community children's nurse or a professional within the interprofessional community team. Key workers have ongoing and long-term relationships with families, have assessment and care management planning skills, and are used to networking and coordinating care for patients. Keyworkers help the family to build and maintain appropriate professional support systems ensuring access to practical support, education and social services (Greco and Sloper 2004). In addition, keyworkers provide continuity ensuring that the care provided is consistent with the needs of the family. Despite the benefits of having a keyworker, children, young people and families should only have a key worker if they want one. Yet despite these obvious benefits, the majority of parents report that they did not have access to a key worker (Care Co-ordination Network UK 2006; ACT/Children's Hospices UK 2011).

The coordination of services can pose significant challenges for overstretched and under-resourced health services, working across different agencies (statutory and voluntary) and settings (hospital, hospice, school, short-break centre, home). What should be a smooth, integrated and reassuring process for the family can become a disjointed, fragmented and distressing one. This is why it is essential that a key worker or lead professional is identified as soon as possible (Greco and Sloper 2004).

Nursing Models of Care

Nursing models of care provide 'a descriptive picture of practice which adequately represents the real thing' (Pearson and Aylott 2007). There are a number of nursing models available with Casey's model being widely utilised within children's nursing. The Mercer model provides a framework for continuity of care and informs the whole nursing process, aiming to meet the holistic needs of families, including spiritual, emotional and social elements (see Figure 14.6).

Mercer's model of nursing care is reminiscent of Bronfenbrenner's ecological systems theory. Bronfenbrenner's theory defines complex 'layers' of environment, each having an effect on a child's development. The central core of the Mercer model is that the child or young person is at the centre of the concentric rings. Each child is depicted as being at the centre of his or her own family. Detailed preadmission and admission assessment takes into account the physical systems and daily activities of living, such as eating and digestion, breathing and the respiratory system, posture and so on. The second layer represents the child's family and how their relationships and needs affect the child. The third dimension describes local influences that affect the care of the child, for example, education, voluntary agencies, statutory welfare benefits and the services of the local hospital and the local authority. The fourth layer represents national and international factors, including legislation and political influences (Brown and Mercer 2005).

Children and families should have their needs assessed as soon as possible after diagnosis or recognition. A comprehensive and multiagency approach should be used to avoid the need for multiple assessments. Assessment of needs should be in

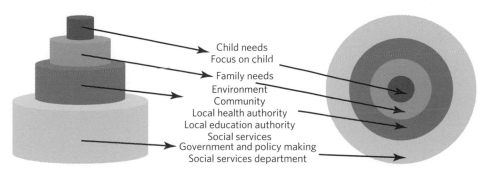

Figure 14.6 Mercer's Model of nursing care
Source: Brown and Mercer (2005)

partnership with the child, the immediate family, any other family members or statutory services who have a decision-making function regarding the child and other community or voluntary individuals or agencies involved with the child's care. In the assessment process, it is easy to focus on the views of the parents or main carers and the difficulties they face in caring for a child with a life-limiting condition. The child or young person should be kept in focus and involved in the process. The health professional should respect the child and family's individuality and ethnicity with issues of confidentiality and consent addressed. It is essential that straightforward, non-jargon language is used and information should be recorded systematically to ensure consistency (ACT 2003, 2004, 2009a, 2009b; DoH 2004).

Assessment should be seen as an ongoing process rather than a single event and, depending on the individual family's needs, may take days or even weeks. Assessment information gathered should be made available to the family. The following text and Table 14.5 provides clarity to some of the aspects to consider when assessing the needs of children, young people and families.

Once the assessment process has been completed, it is important to put meaning to the information collected. This can be provided through a continuing care approach, which includes reviewable personalised care plans, helping to improve the flexibility of care and coordination of services to these children, for whom the application of time limits on care is quite inappropriate. As set out in the NSF, children requiring NHS continuing care should receive coordinated multiagency packages of care according to their individual need (DoH 2004, 2010a; DfE 2009).

The term 'care plan' has been found to have different interpretations. It is often used to describe the child's personal detailed nursing and care record held in the home. Health professionals involved in direct care of the child will use this record to deliver medical and personal care. There should be a distinction between the hands-on care plan and the programme of care designed for delivering a range of services. We have adopted the term 'care package' used by some services to refer to the holistic care plan. It may also be called a 'care agreement' (DfE 2009; DoH 2010a).

THE INTERPROFESSIONAL TEAM

VOICES 14.6

'My life would be easier if…"There were nurses who could look after me at home rather than going into hospital."' (DoH 2008b).

Table 14.5 Aspects to consider when performing a needs assessment

Family	Child or young person	Environment
Information – care choices	Symptom and pain management	Place of care
Financial/benefit advice	Personal care needs	Adaptations
Emotional support	Therapies	Risk assessment
Siblings' well-being	Emotional needs	Home assessment
Family functioning	Information needs	Equipment needs
Short breaks	Short breaks	Transport needs
Quality of life	Education	School/college/university
Interpreter	Leisure/play	
Spiritual, cultural and religious needs	Quality of life	
Transition to adult services	Nursing support	
Genetic counselling	Spiritual, cultural and religious needs	
Contact details for professionals	Transition to adult services	
	Independent living needs	
	Follow-up (routine/emergency)	

Source: ACT (2004)

ACTIVITY 14.4 The interprofessional team

'It's a minefield and you get frightened going through it. Services don't join up and people don't explain things to you ... they don't tell you what all the services actually do ... by the time I had made it all fit together my child had passed away. That makes me sad that he could have had so much more out of life' (Parent, Square Table 2011).

Consider these comments:
- What factors need considering when collaborating with the interprofessional team?
- How does the disparity of services impact on the child, young person and family?

Partnership working is seen as essential to ensuring the best outcomes for children and young people with a life-limiting condition. The interprofessional team should recognise the individuality of each child, young person and her family, upholding her values, wishes and beliefs unless this exposes the child or young person to avoidable harm.

As with Owen and his family, many children and young people with palliative care needs will already be known, through the universal services of health and education, to a range of professionals, and collaboration between agencies and professionals is therefore essential. Often these services are provided through child development centres, local clinics and special schools. Input from a physiotherapist, dietician or speech therapist can make a significant difference to the child's quality of life, particularly one with severe multiple disabilities. Figure 14.7 illustrates the interprofessional team with the child and family at its core.

A series of national collaborative events were conducted in 2011 by ACT and Children's Hospices UK. These events were designed to explore children's palliative care and brought together children, young people and families alongside a range of statutory and non-statutory services. One of the themes that emerged was the awareness of services. Many parents were surprised about the breadth of services available, at least in theory, to them. Similarly, some hospital-based professionals (particularly those working in an acute hospital setting) and GPs were unaware of the range of support available through children's hospice services and other community-based palliative care providers (ACT/Children's Hospices UK 2011b).

It is essential that the interprofessional team ensures continuity of care at home, in the hospital and in the hospice through careful assessment and planning. The review of children's palliative care services in England (Craft and Killen 2007) noted that a range of accessible services were important elements of good practice. The Palliative Care Funding review in 2011 utilises the Craft/Killen triangle (as can be seen in Figure 14.8) to define three levels of dedicated palliative care for both children and adults as containing all the following elements (DoH 2007):

- **universal palliative care services** – this level should be appropriately applied by all health professionals, as care is delivered by generalist (non-palliative care specialists) health and social care providers such as GPs and social workers
- **core palliative care services** – at an intermediate level care is delivered by people whose primary focus is palliative care, e.g. community children's nursing teams. Community children's nurses, although not engaged full time in palliative care have had some training and experience of palliative care
- **specialist palliative care services** – specialist care delivered by expert providers whose core activity is the provision of palliative care, e.g. children's hospices, children symptom management teams, e.g. True Colours.

Community-Based Support

The UK model of home care is based around an identified key worker who supports local professionals and coordinates palliative care in the community: in children with cancer, the paediatric outreach oncology nurse (POON), community children's nursing (CCN) teams and, in some areas, hospice outreach services. (The role of the community children's nurse is discussed in Chapter 6.)

Access to 24/7 children's community nursing services forms the bedrock of children's community palliative care service provision, providing families with choice to be able to receive their care at home where appropriate. It is also important that local medical support (usually a paediatrician) is identified to support palliative care provision to an individual child and also to the local population of children and families with palliative care needs.

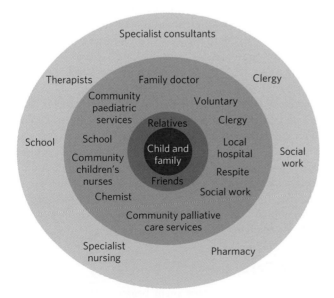

Figure 14.7 The interprofessional team

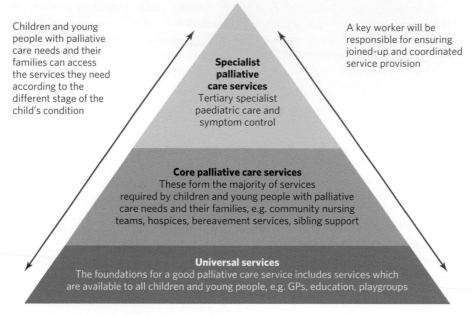

Palliative care for children is about providing a continuum of care–from the provision of universal services for children (e.g. education, social care, transport, home help, short breaks etc.) through acute care and the management of the individual child and family, to very specialist support such as that provided by tertiary centres and specialist bereavement services (*BCBL, page* 15).

Children and young people with palliative care needs and their families can access the services they need according to the different stage of the child's condition

A key worker will be responsible for ensuring joined-up and coordinated service provision

Specialist palliative care services
Tertiary specialist paediatric care and symptom control

Core palliative care services
These form the majority of services required by children and young people with palliative care needs and their families, e.g. community nursing teams, hospices, bereavement services, sibling support

Universal services
The foundations for a good palliative care service includes services which are available to all children and young people, e.g. GPs, education, playgroups

Figure 14.8 Different service levels in a children's palliative care service
Source: Department of Health (2007)

As identified by Craft and Killen (2007) and 'Better care; better lives' (DoH 2008b), community-based medical support should be provided by a paediatrician who has been identified to take the lead for palliative care in each locality, whether that be in a geographical locality or a hospice-based locality. They will work alongside the child's specialist and local paediatricians, children's nursing teams, GP, interprofessional teams and family to support safe and effective delivery of palliative care in an anticipatory manner.

PLACE OF DEATH

> **REFLECTION** The Right Place in which to Die?
>
> Owen's parents wanted to care for him at home but as his symptoms had escalated, the family were frightened that they would not be able to manage the symptoms and care at home.

There is much discussion in the literature about the 'right place in which to die'. Many parents would elect for their child to die at home, although it is likely that they are choosing 'place of care' rather than 'place of death'. Care is often intense, requiring frequent assessment of needs and frequent input from

professionals as symptoms develop, yet with around-the-clock access to appropriate advice and support, parents are able and confident to care for their child at home. Vickers et al. (2007) reported that, in the UK, families of children with incurable cancer stated a preference for home death in the last month of the child's life. Over a 7-month period 77 per cent of children/ young people enrolled in this study died at home.

Several studies have highlighted the relationship between the type of malignancy and place of care at the end of life. Bradshaw et al. (2005) found that patients with a solid tumour or brain tumour who are dying of progressive disease are more likely to have time for end-of-life decision making and more likely to die at home than those dying of leukaemia or treatment-related toxicity.

The role of the children's hospice in end-of-life care for children with cancer is also developing. Historically, relatively few paediatric oncology children have accessed children's hospices for end-of-life care. However, as experience in symptom control increases and with new networks of care evolving, the numbers of children with cancer using these services is increasing. Often, once the families have been introduced to the hospice and become familiar with the facilities provided, the hospice provides a reassuring alternative to home care if the need arises.

Hospice Care

The Children's Hospice Movement began in the early 1980s. Children's hospice services provide palliative care for children

Table 14.6 Range of children's hospices and provision of care

Services offered	Children's Hospice Provision 2009/2010
Management of common symptoms, primarily physical but also psychosocial and spiritual	• 97% in hospice environment • 62% in the hospital environment • 78% in the home environment
End-of-life care, helping children and young people with advanced illness to live as comfortably as possible until the end of their lives	End-of-life care was the most commonly provided service: • 100% in hospice environment • 38% in the hospital environment • 69% in the home environment
24-hour access to emergency care as and when needed	• 94% in hospice environment • 15% in the hospital environment • 66% in the home environment
Short breaks to support the family in the care of their child in a dedicated children's hospice building or at home	• 85% reported provision of care in hospice settings • 32% provided support in hospital settings • 78% described home-based provision
Support for the entire family, including siblings and grandparents	Sibling support services: • 94% in hospice environment • 23% in the hospital environment • 91% in the home environment Family support services: • 97% in hospice environment • 62% in the hospital environment • 94% in the home environment
Bereavement support for all family members for as long as it is needed	• 88% of hospice services reported the provision of bereavement support • Remainder of hospices were new or developing services and had not yet developed this type of service
Specialist therapies, including physiotherapy, play and music therapy	• 80% in hospice environment • 15% in the hospital environment • 50% in the home environment
Information, support, education and training to carers, where needed	• All hospices provided information on their services and 85% published the eligibility criteria on access to them

and young people with life-limiting conditions and their families from the moment of diagnosis for as long as it is needed. Care is delivered by a multidisciplinary team and in partnership with other agencies, children's hospice services take a holistic and flexible approach to care and are shaped by the physical, emotional, social and spiritual needs of both child and family. There are currently 44 hospices in the UK providing a range of services within purpose-built centres, as well as providing hospice at home. As can be seen in Table 14.6, the services offered by hospices are extensive and are delivered in a variety of environments which includes the home and hospices (Children's Hospices UK 2010).

SYMPTOM MANAGEMENT
Assessing Symptoms

'It focuses on enhancement of quality of life for the child and support for the family and **includes the management of physical symptoms**, provision of respite, and care following death and bereavement. It is provided for children for whom curative treatment is no longer an option and may extend over many years.' (ACT/RCPCH 2003)

Assessing symptoms is an essential step in developing a plan of management. Often a picture must be built up through

RESEARCH NOTE 14.4

Previous research suggests a preference for home as the location of death, but these studies have primarily focused on adults, children with cancer or settings without paediatric hospice facilities available as an option.

This retrospective study (Siden et al. 2008) analysed data for 703 children who died from 2000 to 2006 to examine where children with a broad range of progressive, life-limiting illnesses actually die when families are able to access hospital, paediatric hospice facility and care at home. There was an overall even distribution for location of death in which 35.1% of children died at home, 32.1% died in a paediatric hospice facility, 31.9% in hospital and 0.9% at another location.

Our results suggest that the choice of families for end-of-life care is equally divided among all available options. Given the increasing numbers of children's hospices worldwide, these findings are important for clinicians, care managers and researchers who plan, provide and evaluate the care of children with life-limiting illness.

discussion with the child or young person, if possible, combined with careful observations by parents and staff. There are formal assessment tools for assessing pain in children that are appropriate for different ages and developmental levels, but assessment is more difficult for other symptoms and for preverbal and developmentally delayed children. It is also important to consider the contribution of psychological and social factors for a child and family and to enquire about their coping strategies, relevant past experiences and their levels of anxiety and emotional distress. A key reminder is for health professionals to assess symptoms on individual merit (Wolfe et al. 2008; Goldman et al. 2006; Brown 2007).

REFLECTION Prevalence of Symptoms

- Reflect on the types of symptom you have experienced in practice.
- What were the main symptoms?
- Which were more prevalent?
- Which were more pervasive?
- Consider which symptoms cause you the greatest anxieties

Much of the evidence in symptom assessing and managing is heavily biased towards cancer and the adult sector. Consequently, further research is urgently required regarding prevalence of symptoms and effectiveness of interventions for children with progressive degenerative disorders and profound disability related conditions during the 'living with' stage of the care pathway.

Most studies published are on bereaved parents of children with cancer. In one such study, 96 bereaved Australian parents of children with cancer reported that, in the last month of life, 84 per cent of children suffered from at least one physical symptom (pain, fatigue, poor appetite, constipation, dyspnoea, nausea/vomiting, diarrhoea or seizures), with pain, fatigue and poor appetite the most frequent (Heath et al. 2010). Nearly half (43 per cent) of children suffered from three or more physical symptoms. Parents also reported that 42 per cent of children had been 'more than a little sad,' 38 per cent experienced 'little or no fun' and 21 per cent were 'often afraid'. In a Swedish study of 449 bereaved parents of children with cancer, physical fatigue was the most frequently reported symptom (86 per cent) to have a higher or moderate impact on the child's well-being, with reduced mobility (76 per cent), pain (73 per cent) and decreased appetite (71 per cent) also major concerns (Jalmsell et al. 2006). In this study, parents were more likely to report anxiety in children older than 9 years of age than in younger children. Children also suffered from difficulties in swallowing, depression, reduced mobility, impaired speech, swelling, disturbed sleep due to anxiety and urinary problems.

The most commonly reported symptoms for children with cancer in the last month of life are:

- pain
- fatigue/weakness
- anorexia
- weight loss
- mobility
- nausea
- constipation
- vomiting.

Managing Symptoms

ACTIVITY 14.5 Symptom management

List the core principles of symptom management.

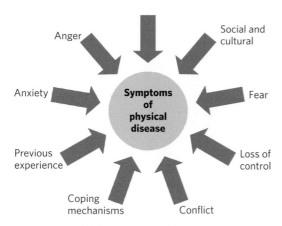

Figure 14.9 Child's experience of pain
Source: Goldman et al. (2006)

Managing symptoms requires assessment of psychological, social, spiritual and physical symptoms assessed on a regular basis, as illustrated in Figure 14.9. The use of an interprofessional team in the assessment and management of symptoms is paramount and information on symptoms must be sought from all relevant sources. The health professional should utilise practical, cognitive, behavioural and supportive therapies combined with appropriate drug treatment (Pfund 2000; Goldman et al.

2006; Sourkes 2006; Jassal and Hain 2011). The identification of persistent physical symptoms should be treated with medication given at regular intervals and severe uncontrolled symptoms should be regarded as medical emergencies where active intervention may be appropriate (Goldman et al. 2006; Jassal and Hain 2011).

Some hospitals provide outreach nurses who deal with only one type of disease. Local expertise can also be provided by those professionals who see many children with a range of different life-limiting conditions. They will liaise closely with the paediatrician to ensure that each child is receiving optimum care. For all families, 24-hour access to a health professional is required.

The degree to which the child or parent believes symptoms are well managed can influence other outcomes, such as where a family might choose to care for their child for the end-of-life phase. An example of poorly controlled pain can militate against a family caring for a child at home. Good pain control, by way of contrast, can mean the difference between memories of distress and angst or memories that soften the inevitable transition from life to death. As can be seen in Figure 14.9, symptoms that are not managed can have a psychological, social, spiritual and physical effect on the child, young person and family (Pfund 2000; Goldman et al. 2006; Sourkes 2006; Jassal and Hain 2011).

RESEARCH NOTE 14.5

This study from McCluggage and Elborn (2006) aimed to identify the symptoms that cause anxiety to staff working in children's hospices. More than 70% of all staff groups felt that identifying the symptom correctly caused more anxiety than treating identified symptoms.

A postal questionnaire was sent to children's hospice staff who were asked to identify symptoms experienced by life-limited children that caused them anxiety. Staff in 23 hospices were sent questionnaires. Twenty eight questionnaires were returned from 10 doctors and 18 nurses. Just under half of the hospices contacted were represented. The staff were very experienced but had significant anxieties about treating.

For doctors, the top five symptom problems were, seizure control, spasms, pain assessment, unidentified distress and vomiting.

For nurses, the main concerns were the non-verbal child in distress, psychiatric or psychological problems, assessing pain, seizures, pain management and vomiting.

Doctors and nurses perceive seizures, pain management and vomiting as the most troublesome symptoms for children with life-limiting conditions. Further research is needed into symptom management in genetic syndromes.

Specific Symptoms

Pain

Pain is a major symptom in children and young people's palliative care both for children with cancer and those with non-malignant life-limiting disease (Breau et al. 2003). Pain is a subjective experience, not an objective fact and it can vary from person to person and situation to situation. In the context of living with a life-limiting illness, the experience of pain is potentially the result of a complex interplay among physical, psychological, social, spiritual and other factors. The severity of a child's pain, for example, may be exacerbated by anxiety,

depression or suffering (Pfund 2000; Sourkes 2006). All these factors must be considered, assessed and treated in order to effectively alleviate suffering related to the experience of pain, as can be seen in Figure 14.10. Quality of life is often related to a child's experience of pain and it is therefore vital that the child receive excellent pain assessment and management. Successful pain management often needs the combined efforts of the interprofessional team (Pfund 2000; Goldman et al. 2006; Sourkes 2006; Hendricks-Ferguson 2008; Jassal and Hain 2011).

Pain is therefore hard to quantify and without a good pain assessment, it is difficult to treat pain effectively and promptly. Therefore, it is important to think about the possibility of pain

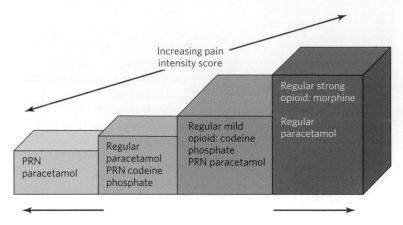

Figure 14.10 Analgesic pain relief plan
Source: World Health Organisation (2010)

being present in any palliative situation and look for symptoms that are known to be painful or that can cause anxiety and pain. It is also important to remember to always consider the most obvious causes of pain prior to starting treatment. Chronic pain is potentially hard to assess and sometimes the only way to find out is to try analgesia and see if the child appears brighter, eats better, is less miserable or more interactive. Remember that there may well be more than one pain and each one needs to be identified, quantified and treated. Communication about pain can be difficult: it is essential to try and support any information with as much evidence and common sense as possible (Hendricks-Ferguson 2008; Jassal and Hain 2011). Acute pain and pain assessment tools are discussed in other chapters.

The World Health Organization (2010) states that a certain standard of pain management must be available to every child receiving palliative care irrespective of location, and the pain relief ladder forms the basis of the analgesic pain relief plan (Figure 14.10). It recommends that if pain occurs there should be prompt oral administration of drugs then as necessary, mild opioids followed by strong opioids, until the patient is pain free. Medication should be given 'by the clock', that is every 3 to 6 hours, rather than on demand.

Many of the drug doses and routes used in palliative care are not licensed for children and responsibility lies with the clinician prescribing them. In all situations the management plan should consider both pharmacological and psychological approaches along with practical help (Hendricks-Ferguson 2008; Jassal and Hain 2011). The health professional must anticipate the side-effects of medication and actively treat. Children often find it difficult to take large amounts of drugs and complex regimens may not be possible. Doses should be calculated according to a child's weight. Oral drugs should be used if possible and children should be offered the choice between tablets, whole or crushed and liquids. Long-acting preparations are helpful, reducing the number of tablets needed and simplifying care at home. If an alternative route is needed some children find rectal drugs acceptable; they can be particularly useful in the last few days of life. Otherwise, a subcutaneous infusion can be established or, if one is in situ, a central intravenous line can

be used. Parents are usually willing and able to learn to refill and load syringes and even to resite needles.

Figure 14.11, which provides an example of a child with a rare genetic disorder requiring palliative care, is used to illustrate how one aspect of the support needs of parents can be met through the use of therapeutic flow charts. The case study shows how a symptom management flowchart was developed to help one family feel more confident in caring for their dying child. It enabled them to focus less on the illness and more on spending quality time as a family. The development of symptom care flowcharts enabled the professional team and parents to think through problems before they arose and to make joint decisions. They boosted the confidence of family and carers by providing them with clear information and advice. Flowcharts of this kind can help support parents and carers in ongoing situations where multiple carers are involved and the child's care needs change over time (Willis 2007).

ACTIVITY 14.6 Owen's symptom management

Owen has developed raised intracranial pressure, therefore a comprehensive symptom management plan encompassed pain relief for the pain associated with raised intracranial pressure, anti-convulsant medication to control increasing seizure activity as well as medication to reduce anxiety and nausea.

Consider the care that Owen requires in relation to the symptoms he may be experiencing.

Spiritual Care

Holistic care encompasses the care for the 'whole' person in terms of spiritual as well as psychological, physical and social needs (DoH 2010b). Yet there has been little evaluation of the impact of spiritual care on patients. Palliative care philosophy

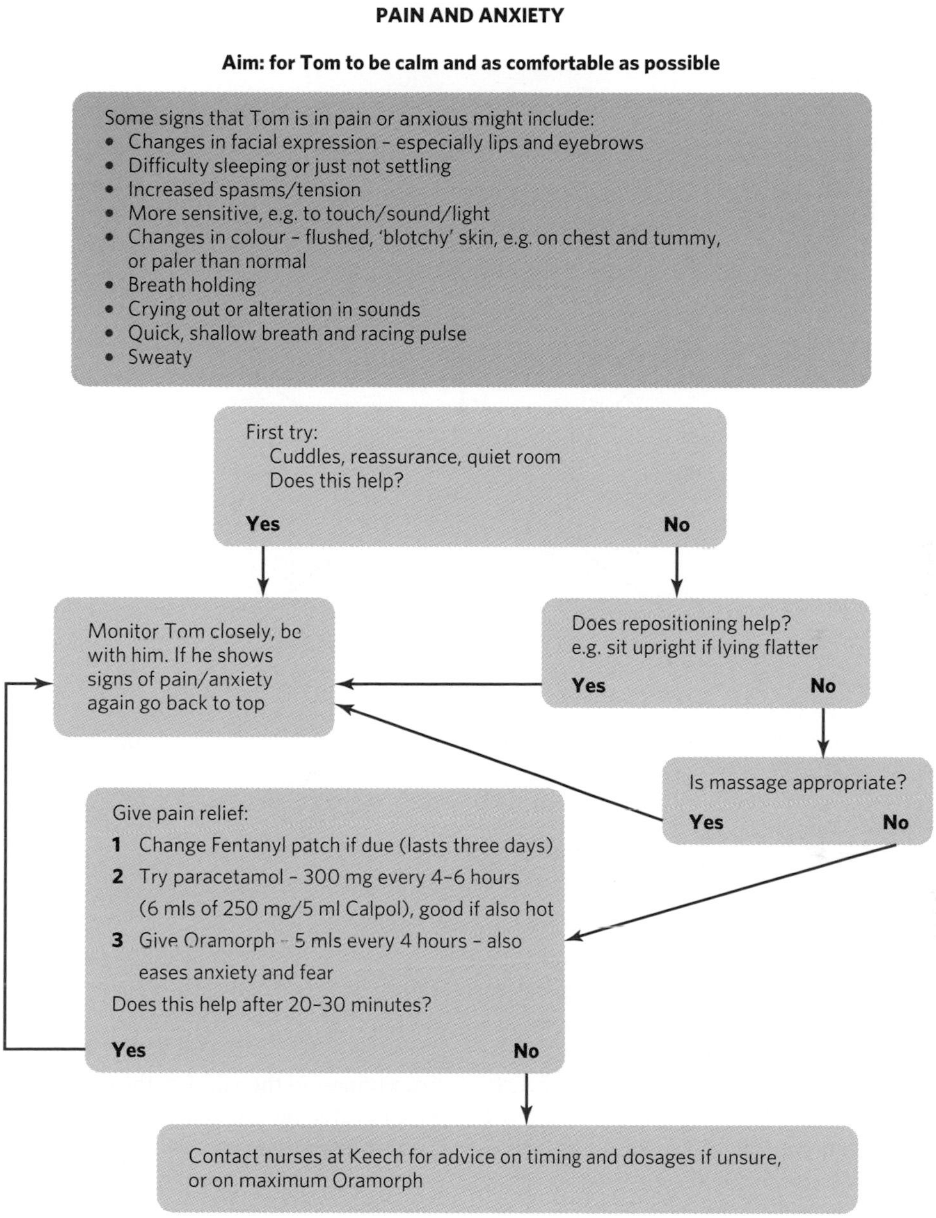

PAIN AND ANXIETY

Aim: for Tom to be calm and as comfortable as possible

Some signs that Tom is in pain or anxious might include:
- Changes in facial expression – especially lips and eyebrows
- Difficulty sleeping or just not settling
- Increased spasms/tension
- More sensitive, e.g. to touch/sound/light
- Changes in colour – flushed, 'blotchy' skin, e.g. on chest and tummy, or paler than normal
- Breath holding
- Crying out or alteration in sounds
- Quick, shallow breath and racing pulse
- Sweaty

First try:
Cuddles, reassurance, quiet room
Does this help?

Yes   **No**

Monitor Tom closely, be with him. If he shows signs of pain/anxiety again go back to top

Does repositioning help? e.g. sit upright if lying flatter

Yes   **No**

Is massage appropriate?

Yes   **No**

Give pain relief:
1. Change Fentanyl patch if due (lasts three days)
2. Try paracetamol – 300 mg every 4–6 hours (6 mls of 250 mg/5 ml Calpol), good if also hot
3. Give Oramorph – 5 mls every 4 hours – also eases anxiety and fear

Does this help after 20–30 minutes?

Yes   **No**

Contact nurses at Keech for advice on timing and dosages if unsure, or on maximum Oramorph

Figure 14.11 Example of an individual symptom care flow chart
Source: Willis (2007)

acknowledges the importance of spiritual values and beliefs in contributing to making us who we are (Bull and Gillies 2007). Beliefs provide a dependable framework of meaning, within which people are able to make sense of their lives. Children and adults need to receive, and share with others, the gifts of faith, hope and love that are the heart of spirituality. Faith describes the need for safety, protection and trust. Hope brings the ability to dream, to wish and to make meaning out of one's life story. Love encompasses the relationships we cultivate, the value that we feel as unique individuals and the legacy we leave with those whose lives we touch. For parents finding out that the life that they had planned for their child will not be fulfilled and that they may die before reaching adulthood is devastating. It can leave parents questioning their beliefs and wondering 'why me?'.

Despite much of the literature focusing on definitions there is a general lack of clarity with regard to the meanings of the terms 'spirituality' and 'religion' (Bull and Gillies 2007; DoH 2010). The meaning of spirituality has shifted and changed as cultural assumptions have altered. Spirituality relates to the way in which people understand and live their lives in view of their beliefs and values and their perception of ultimate meaning. Spirituality includes the need to find satisfactory answers to ultimate questions about the meaning of life, illness and death. Therefore, spirituality refers to what it is to be human: it is deeply personal and subjective and it gives meaning to the value of life. Spirituality is an integral part of any religion but it can also be a meaningful part of the life of someone who does not have a religion or a faith in a god (Bull and Gillies 2007).

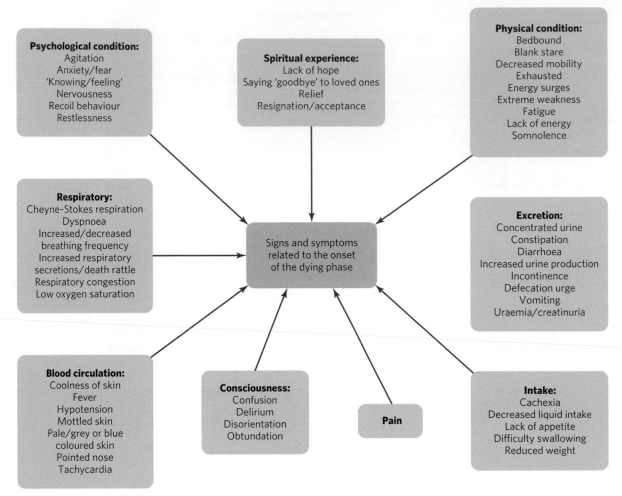

Figure 14.12 Conceptual model of changing signs and symptoms related to the onset of the dying phase
Source: van der Werff et al. (2012)

Religion is defined as participation in the particular beliefs, rituals and activities of traditional religion. Guidelines are offered to deal with religious patients and to ensure that their specific traditions are understood and their particular needs met. Religion is respected as a mode of spirituality but is not considered to be synonymous with it. The importance of both religion and spirituality is that they provide a context in which people can make sense of their lives, explain and cope with their experiences and find and maintain a sense of hope and peacefulness in the midst of the challenges of life. While not all writers agree on the benefits of religion within an end-of-life context, there remains evidence that religious spirituality can have clear benefits in terms of coping with illness and the threat of death.

In their qualitative study van der Werff et al. (2012) provide a model (as illustrated in Figure 14.12) which brings together many of the concepts discussed in this section and highlights the changing signs and symptoms related to the onset of dying.

RESEARCH NOTE 14.6

Klepping's (2012) article is a reflective case study of the symptom control strategies implemented by a hospice team caring for Jack, a teenage male with metastatic nasopharyngeal cancer who was experiencing severe pain. The concept of a 'total' approach to pain assessment and management is introduced and Jack's pain is analysed in the context of total pain, including the psychological, social, spiritual and physical dimensions that contributed to his overall pain experience during his final months.

This paper examines the elements of Jack's life that caused him anxiety and triggered pain episodes, including familial and cultural issues, and discusses the pharmacological and non-pharmacological interventions used by the hospice to address these. The article demonstrates how the care delivered by local services was informed by UK strategies for palliative and oncological care of young people.

Palliative Care or 'Just-In-Case' Boxes

Following the assessment and compilation of a written plan, it will become apparent that certain drugs and supplies need to remain with the child so that they can be easily accessed in an emergency or out of hours. It is therefore very useful to provide a 'palliative care box'. This is a locked medicine box containing medication, a prescription form, infusion equipment and supplies that can be used by medical and children's community nursing or children's hospice nursing staff. The medication placed in the box is chosen to address specific and commonly occurring anticipated symptoms. The route prescribed is mainly subcutaneous and/or intravenous, reflecting the box's purpose to provide rapid symptom relief at the end of life. Alder Hey Hospital has done some research suggesting that the following six drugs can be considered essential (Anderson et al. 2010):

- Diamorphine
- Cyclizine
- Haloperidol
- Levomepromazine
- Midazolam
- Hyoscine hydrobromide.

END-OF-LIFE CARE – ENCOUNTERING DEATH FOR THE FIRST TIME

The last moments spent with a dying child are *'often filled with awe and with emotional pain'*. (Rosenblatt 2000)

The Sick Child touches on the fragility of life (see Figure 14.13). It draws on Munch's personal memories, including the trauma of his sister's death.

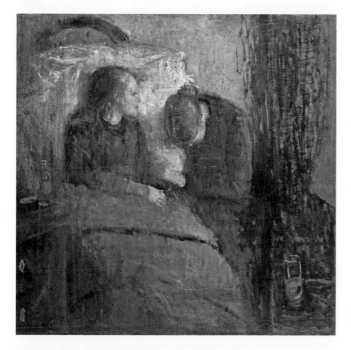

Figure 14.13 *The Sick Child,* by Edvard Munch

ACTIVITY 14.7 End-of-life care

John and Sue want Owen to die at home but they are concerned about the symptoms he may experience at the end of life.

What are the core principles for end-of-life care?

The principles of end-of-life care services for children are broadly the same as those for adults. Communication with family and professionals (both verbal and written) is crucial to effective end-of-life care (ACT 2004; DoH 2008). Good end-of-life care requires equally good teamwork and planning. The 'gold standards framework' for end-of-life care in adults in the UK details three steps (identify, assess, plan) and its emphasis is on the importance of communication, coordination and control of symptoms (Becker 2010). These principles work just as well in children's palliative care.

Carefully considered and managed care of the child and family at the time surrounding and after death can have a positive impact on their memories (Brown 2007; Davies 2009). Well-managed and well-supported end-of-life care is a key component of palliative care services. It is impossible to overestimate the extent to which the level and type of care provided can affect the family's experience of the loss of a child (Pfund 2007; Grinyer 2012).

End-of-life care focuses on preparing for an anticipated death and managing the end stage of a terminal condition from the point of recognition that the end of life is approaching. This includes care during and around the time of death and for the family immediately afterwards. It enables the supportive and palliative care needs of both child and family to be identified and met throughout the last phase of life and into bereavement (ACT 2004; Pfund 2007).

Recognition of End of Life

An essential step in end-of-life care is recognising that the child has probably reached the end of her life and then 'naming' that for the child, family, carers, colleagues and yourself. Some discussions should take place, while the child is in relatively good health, in preparing practically for acute, distressing symptoms and making realistic but flexible end of life and advance care plans. A decision needs to be made about emergency treatment options and resuscitation and if necessary a personalised resuscitation plan set out and documented for use by ambulance crews, A&E departments and primary Care Services (DoH 2005). The end-of-life care plan may include an advanced care Plan (ACP) which may include decisions regarding withdrawal of treatment and DNACPR decisions (ACT 2003, 2004, 2009a, 2009b; DoH, 2004).

Unfortunately, determining the end-of-life stage for a child with a life-limiting condition can be difficult for a number of reasons: children can be remarkably resilient and survive what

Table 14.7 End-of-life assessment

Family	Child or young person	Environment
Practical support	Pain and symptom control	Place of death
Sibling involvement	Quality of life	Ambience
Grandparents	Friends	Place of body after death
Emotional support	Emotional support	
Spiritual/religious issues	Spiritual/religious issues	
Cultural issues	Cultural issues	
Funeral planning	Funeral planning	
Organ donation	Organ donation	
	Resuscitation/withdrawal of treatment (ACP/DNACPR)	
	Special wishes or activities	
	Life goals	
	Children's 'will'	
	Memory box	

Source: ACT (2011)

we may think is the 'last event'. By the same token, children can also decline very rapidly and unexpectedly. This is why it is ideal to have made some of the difficult end-of-life decisions beforehand, but also important to have parallel planning in place, where the carer prepares for the worst, but hopes for the best. This is especially important as there is considerable unpredictability of disease trajectory for many of these children. The difficulty in accurately predicting death means families often face many acute life-threatening events thinking each one is a terminal event. This is unsurprisingly emotionally and physically exhausting for them (see Table 14.7). There could also be reluctance on the part of both parents and professionals to use certain drugs which often become necessary at the end of life for fear of 'causing death' (ACT 2003, 2004; ACT/Children's Hospices UK, 2009).

An Advanced Care Plan (ACP)

VOICES 14.7

'One family in our area had an advanced care plan but did not know that they had to show it. At a very difficult time for the family they ended up with the police and the coroner involved because the ambulance crew did not know that the child was not to be resuscitated' (Square Table Local Learning and Evaluation Report 2011).

It is often difficult to anticipate the course of an illness, but as a death may occur suddenly and unexpectedly such discussions need to take place. An advanced care plan is an important part of an end-of-life plan, and is designed to communicate the child's and family's wishes for the child's care, as part of the broader end-of-life care plan. The extent to which a child or young person is included in this discussion is usually a matter of judgement and agreement between parents and professionals. Often the child or young person's inclusion will depend on his chronological age but also his capacity, competence and cognitive abilities. An advanced care plan is usually initiated by a senior clinician who knows the family well and sets out an agreed plan of care to be followed when critical events occur and/or when a child's condition deteriorates. It provides a framework for discussing and documenting specific care choices. This includes decisions regarding the withdrawal of life-sustaining treatment which may include a do not attempt cardiopulmonary resuscitation (DNACPR) order and remains valid when parent(s) or next of kin cannot be contacted. It is designed to be used in all environments that the child or young person encounters: home, hospital, school, hospice, short-break care and for use by the ambulance service (ACT 2003, 2004; ACT/Children's Hospices UK 2009b).

According to the Royal College of Paediatrics and Child Health (RCPCH) guidance on 'Withholding or withdrawing of life-sustaining treatment in children' (2004), clinical staff who are involved in completing an ACP are advised to read the RCPCH document. The document describes five circumstances in which it may be ethical and legal to consider withholding or withdrawing of life-sustaining medical treatment, as can be seen in Table 14.8.

During or Following a Death

During and following Owen's death, care was taken to ensure that the family's spiritual, religious and cultural beliefs and rituals were fully respected (Komaromy 2004). It is important that professionals have awareness that different cultures and religions have varying customs and rituals when a person dies e.g. touching of the body, position or placing of the body and different funeral arrangements, as can be seen in Table 14.9 (Brown 2007). Parents/carers should be consulted as to whether they wish to be involved in caring for their child after death and to the level of handling appropriate to their needs and beliefs. For many faiths it is customary to wash and dress the child following death, once death has been confirmed (ACT 2003, 2004; ACT/Children's Hospices UK 2009b).

PRACTICAL GUIDELINES 14.7

If the death takes place at home:

- Practical advice about reducing the room temperature and quantity of bedding should be given.
- If the family wish the body to stay at home for more than 24 hours, consideration may need to be given to the use of a mobile cooling unit to slow the natural deterioration of the body.
- Parents appreciate advice from the care team or funeral director about care of the body at home.

Legal Issues

- The doctor who is treating the child or the general practitioner should have seen the child within the previous 14 days.

- If this is not the case, the doctor is required to contact the coroner to discuss whether there is a need for a post-mortem.
- The medical certificate of cause of death will be issued by the doctor and collected by the family at a time convenient to them both.
- The need for a post-mortem may be also considered and the family should be prepared for this. Particularly if the death is accidental, suspicious or unexpected and therefore handling of the body or removal of tubes may be restricted in these circumstances.
- The child's body may not be moved to a different venue until a doctor has verified the death.

Table 14.8 Five circumstances for withholding or withdrawing life-sustaining treatment in children

No-chance situation	The child has such severe disease that life-sustaining treatment simply delays death without significant alleviation of suffering Treatment to sustain life is inappropriate
No-purpose situation	Although the patient may be able to survive with treatment, the degree of physical or mental impairment will be so great that it is unreasonable to expect them to bear it
Unbearable situation	The child and/or family feel that in the face of progressive and irreversible illness further treatment is more than can be borne They wish to have a particular treatment withdrawn or to refuse further treatment irrespective of the medical opinion that it may be of some benefit
Permanent vegetative state	
Brain stem death	

Source: RCPCH (2004)

Table 14.9 Religious beliefs and rituals at the end of life

Religion Considerations	Buddhist	Christianity	Hinduism	Judaism	Muslim	Sikhism
Beliefs and rites	• Believe in rebirth • Suffering is universal and is eased by not being selfish • Call a faith representative to facilitate peace and quiet for meditation	• Belief in life after death in heaven or hell • Infants assured of heaven • Roman Catholic and some Church of England require a priest for last rites, blessing or baptism	• Believe in rebirth • Children enter heaven first • A priest may be required • Reading from holy books	• Belief in life after death in heaven or hell • Infants assured of heaven in most traditions • A rabbi may visit • Readings are normally lead by the family	• Belief in life after death and in heaven and hell • Infants are assured a place in heaven • Imam may visit • Prayers are normally led by the family • Death is seen as the will of god • Life span is allocated to individual at the beginning of time	• Believe in rebirth • A priest or chaplain may visit but the reading can be led by the family
End-of-life care	• May not wish sedatives • Family may wish to wash the body • Provide a place of peace and quiet • Families may not want the body to be touched for a period of time to allow the mind to leave the body	• Offer baptism or a blessing for the child if this has not happened	• Any jewellery or sacred threads should not be removed • Close eyes and straighten body • May wish to be placed on the floor • Family may wish to wash the body and wrap it in a white cloth • Holy water may be applied to the lips	• The body should be handled as little as possible • After death close eyes, clothing remains and cover with a sheet • Family may wish to wash the body • Some tradition may wish for same gender contact only • Most tradition wish for the child not to be left alone • Separate undertakers	• May wish for a reading before death • Eyes and mouth closed and body straightened, turn head to the right and cover with a clean sheet • May wish to face Mecca • Privacy for the family to grieve • Any sacred jewellery should not be removed • Washing has to be in accordance with Islamic faith	• The 5 Ks should not be removed • Family will read from holy books, there are no priests • Music or prayer may be played • Close eyes and straighten body • Family may wish to wash and dress the body • If the boy is over 5 or puberty, he will wear a turban • Eldest son represents the family

(continued)

Religion Considerations	Buddhist	Christianity	Hinduism	Judaism	Muslim	Sikhism
					• Families may wish to have the child at home • Separate undertakers	
Funeral	• Cremation is preferred	• No general preference of burial or cremation	• Funeral takes place ASAP • Children may be buried • A gift of a toy in the coffin for the child to play with while they are waiting in heaven for rebirth • Photo / candle / religious symbol displayed at home for 12 days after the funeral • Adults cremated • Close female relatives only at the crematorium	• Funeral takes place ASAP after death • A 'watcher' sits with body in some traditions • May prefer burial in separate cemetery • Mourners do not leave the house • Mourning for a child is 30 days	• Funeral takes place ASAP after death, 24 hours • Always buried • Funeral prayer will he led by imam • Young children are assured a place in paradise • Segregation at the funeral	• Always cremated, although babies without teeth may be buried • Mourners sometimes wear white • Ashes poured into flowing water • Will sit separately at the funeral

Source: adapted from RCN (2005)

CARING FOR THE BEREAVED

'Every child and family should receive emotional, psychological and spiritual support to meet his or her needs. This shall begin at diagnosis and continue the child's lifetime, death and in bereavement.' (ACT 2004)

The death of a child before that of her parents is regarded as unnatural, as it undermines the natural order (Davies 2004). Parents lose not only their child but also all their child represents, such as a future together and grandchildren. Life, as they assumed it would be, ends with the child's death and the role of parent changes to that of bereaved parent (Talbot 2002).

VOICES 14.8

'It's hard when nobody talks about her and anything to do with my   sister's death is avoided' (a sibling, The Child Bereavement Trust).

It is important to distinguish between grief and bereavement as people are often confused and see them as the same (Davies 2004). **Bereavement** is a state of having lost someone or something dear to you. **Mourning** is our external expression of loss. It is a style of expressing loss. Families, communities and cultures may mourn differently. Rituals help to bring healing and closure. **Grief** is the emotional and social reaction to loss. In children, grief can come from the loss of parents, siblings, failure of exams, death of pets, etc. Grief after the death of a child is described as the most painful and enduring:

- Parents suffer multiple losses.
- Siblings suffer too and may have difficulty adjusting; they often feel isolated and neglected.
- Families, communities and cultures may grieve and mourn differently.
- Rituals can help to bring healing and closure.
- While there are parallels, children do not grieve in the same way as adults.
- Health professionals can play a huge part in helping people grieve, simply by being a point of stability and a

professional, experienced listener, as well as a gatekeeper to important practical support such as benefits, sickness certification and mental health support.

Bereavement and grief can be shaped by the interaction the family experiences prior to the death and by the services available to family in their loss. According to Contro and Scofield (2006) most parents say they would have benefited from more preparatory information prior to the death of child. In some cases, this involves not only the parents' preparation but that of the young person and siblings, what to tell them, how much and when.

The traditional models of grief centre on the belief that the resolution of grief lay in detachment from the deceased. However, as Walter (1996) points out, while the models may be useful in working with grieving spouses or relatives, they are not appropriate for bereaved parents, for whom it is impossible to detach and reinvest. Table 14.10 demonstrates how theories of grief have evolved over the last 30 years.

Over the last 30 years there has been an enormous shift in attitude from Worden's assertion that keeping the deceased's possessions or room intact was a denial of reality and a sign of being stuck in pathological grief (1982), to the new model of

Table 14.10 Traditional and modern theories of grief

Traditional models of grief		
Theorist	**Main points**	**Advantages and disadvantages**
Sigmund Freud (1961)	- Grieving involved a process of detaching from the deceased person - Recovery took place when the detachment was complete and the bereaved person could then move on to form new attachments	- Oversimplifies complex experiences - Implies an end to grieving - Misinterpret normal grieving as pathological - Grievers are alike and predictable - Imposing inappropriate expectations on grievers - Reinforces helplessness. - Provides little guidance for caregivers. - Implies that caregiving means waiting, comforting and listening to grievers or treating symptoms. (Davies, Attig and Towne, 2006)
John Bowlby (1961)	Freud's theory was further developed by Bowlby, who classified grief into **three stages:** - searching - despair - reorganisation	
Colin Murray Parkes and John Bowlby (1970)	Bowlby added another stage: - numbness	

(continued)

Traditional models of grief		
Theorist	**Main points**	**Advantages and disadvantages**
Elizabeth Kubler-Ross (1969)	Identification of **five stages of grieving:** <ul><li>denial</li><li>anger</li><li>bargaining</li><li>depression</li><li>acceptance</li></ul>	
Colin Murray Parkes (1972)	Medical model emphasising ways in which grieving is a matter of recovering from symptoms Sometimes seen as 'complicated' or 'pathological' grief	
Modern models of grief		
William Worden (1982)	Grief work theory Developed a **four-task model:** <ul><li>accepting the reality of the loss</li><li>working through the pain of grief</li><li>adjusting to life without the deceased and withdrawing emotional energy</li><li>re-investing in another relationship</li></ul>	<ul><li>Emphasises that grieving takes time and effort</li><li>Recognises that grieving is an active response to emotional, psychological, behavioural, social, intellectual and spiritual challenges in loss</li><li>Respects individuality</li><li>Appreciates how grievers address their helplessness as they actively engage with the challenge of loss</li><li>Provides guidance for caregiver's roles beyond passively waiting and supports the efforts of addressing the tasks of grieving</li></ul>
Dennis Klass, Phyllis Silverman and Steven Nickman (1996)	<ul><li>Sustaining the relationship by developing a set of memories, feelings and actions that keep them connected to the deceased child or parent</li><li>Reiterating that when children die the bond does not break</li></ul>	
Thomas Attig (2000)	<ul><li>Sustaining the relationship</li><li>Understanding grieving through biographies, the sharing of stories of journeys in grief</li><li>Grief is an active coping process of relearning relationships with others, the deceased, God and ourselves, including our daily life patterns</li></ul>	

Source: Davies et al. (2006)

parental bereavement based on studies of bereaved parents and the ways in which they maintain bonds with their dead children, through keeping possessions, sharing stories, establishing rituals and memorials and talking about and to the deceased (Klass 1993, 1996; Rosenblatt 2000; Talbot 2002; Davies 2004). The parents in these studies showed that it was only through continuing bonds that they were able to go on with their lives without their children as a physical presence. Rosof (1994, page 48) describes this process as 'simultaneously building a life in which the child does not live and keeping the child alive in your heart'.

The language of grief in western society is often clichéd, incorporating phrases such as 'passed away', 'gone to heaven' and 'laid to rest'. Schiff (1977, page 7) urges avoidance of such expressions and suggests that a move to a less death-denying culture might begin with something as simple as changing this language and using instead the unambiguous 'death', 'died' and 'dead'.

The poem by Moran (1999) describes her frustration with language and expressions of death and offers nurse's insights that are useful in practice.

VOICES 14.9   The Language of Grief

Please don't ask me if I'm over it yet,
I'll never be over it.
Please don't tell me she's in a better place.
She's not with me.
Please don't say at least she isn't suffering,
I haven't come to terms with why she had to suffer at all.
Please don't tell me you know how I feel,
unless you have lost a child.
Please don't ask me if I feel better.
Bereavement isn't a condition that clears up.

Please don't tell me at least you had her for so many years.
What year would you choose for your child to die?
Please don't tell me God never gives us more than we can bear.
Please just tell me you are sorry.
Please just say you remember my child, if you do.
Please just let me talk about my child.
Please mention my child's name.
Please just let me cry. (Moran 1999)

REFLECTION   Care in Bereavement

1 What are some of the most important things to consider when a child has died?
2 Can you reflect on caring for a child who is dying and write some key learning points?
3 Where can you find further information for supporting families in bereavement?

Parents

While the finality of death may be better acknowledged by using unambiguous language, the enormity of experiencing the death of one's child cannot adequately be conveyed within the limitations of spoken language (Davies 2005). Grinyer's study (2012), based on the written narratives of parents of young adult children with cancer, identifies the difficulty parents have in finding words to speak of their experiences. Indeed, Ann-Marie Dickason told me how the written words to her poem

---

VOICES 14.10   Dear Connie

A week has passed since you have gone
A week where we've had to carry on
We never thought that we'd get through
A week that seemed so long without you

The care you needed all day through
Has left us wondering what to do
We've had to plan so much for this day
When all we hoped was that you'd stay

But you decided your time was near
We saw you struggle and felt our fear
The time we've had still feels so small
Your life so full of love from all

And so dear Connie, we want to say
Thank you for the time you stayed
We've learnt so much and loved you so
We just don't want to let you go

But let you go we now must do
When all we want is to hold and kiss you
So with all our hearts and souls we pray
That we will be with you again some day
With all our love from Mummy and Daddy.

(Ann-Marie Dickason, mother of Connie; reproduced with kind permission).

'Dear Connie' seemed to flow easily at a particularly difficult time for the family.

The death of a child is an overwhelming emotional experience for parents and associated family members. Bereavement starts long before the time of death and bereavement support may be needed from the time of diagnosis, particularly for families who have no treatment hopes or options or for families with multiple bereavements and a family is still coming to terms with the previous death of a child. Those who have been involved with the family throughout are often the best placed to offer support and the key worker will play an important role at this time. Parents should be enabled to take control of events after death, and make their choices at their own pace. Grief and how each individual deals with loss are unique to that person. They should feel able to ask for help if they need it. Often someone to listen and provide emotional support is all some families need.

Siblings

Siblings of life-limited children have particular needs. Bluebond Langner (1995) describes brothers and sisters as 'living in houses of chronic sorrow' and Smith and Pennells (1995) refer to siblings as becoming 'forgotten mourners'. Care and consideration should be given to the needs of siblings as they are affected not only by the loss of their brother or sister, but also by the impact this has on the family and the relationships within it. Siblings should be included and not shielded from grief felt by others so that they do not feel they have to hide their feelings (ACT 2004). Siblings' reactions and feelings are influenced by their developmental stage and maturity level. However, more often than not, children of any age feel a sense of isolation and may withdraw or act out. Honest communication and

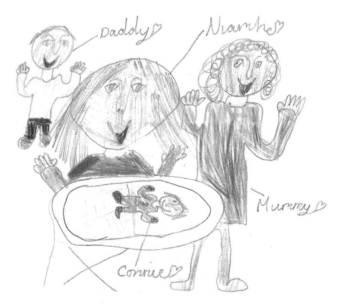

Figure 14.14 Death of Niamh's little sister

participation in the care of their dying sibling and after death, often helps to provide a sense of connectedness and importance. It can also provide a clearer understanding of the situation. In a similar way to their parents, siblings may not have the language to fully express their grief and therefore alternative forms of expression need to be utilised, as can be seen in the picture drawn by Niamh (Figure 14.14). It is interesting to note that Niamh's picture was drawn 4 months after the death of her little sister and yet the picture depicts Connie as being very much a part of her family and with all the individuals in it smiling.

Many children's hospice services have a sibling support worker who is able to facilitate groups and individual sessions for bereaved siblings to share experiences and feelings in a safe environment. There are other agencies that provide bereavement support for siblings, for example CRUSE for young people (rd4u), and Winston's Wish. Table 14.11 provides some practice guidance, taken from the child bereavement charter, produced by Winston's Wish.

Children do not react to loss in the same ways as adults. These are some of the ways children's grief is different:

- Children may seem to show grief only once in a while and for short times.
- A grieving child may be sad one minute and playful the next.
- Often families think the child does not really understand the loss or has got over it quickly. Usually, neither is true.
- Children's minds protect them from what is too much for them to handle emotionally.
- Mourning is a process that continues over years in children.
- Feelings of loss may occur again and again as the child gets older. This is common at important times, such as going to school, getting married or having children.
- Grieving children may not show their feelings as openly as adults. Grieving children may throw themselves into activities instead of withdrawing or showing grief.
- Children cannot think through their thoughts and feelings like adults. Children have trouble putting their feelings about grief into words. Strong feelings of anger and fears of death or being left alone may show up in the behaviour of grieving children. Children often play death games as a way of working out their feelings and worries. These games give children a safe way to express their feelings.
- Grieving adults may withdraw and not talk to other people about the loss. Children, however, often talk to the people around them (even strangers) to see how they react and to get clues for how they should respond to the loss.
- Children may ask confusing questions. For example, a child may ask, 'I know grandpa died, but when will he come home?' This is a way of testing reality and making sure the story of the death has not changed.

Table 14.11 Practice guidelines: charter for bereaved children (Winston's Wish)

B	**Bereavement support**
	Bereaved children need to receive support from their family, from their school and from important people around them
E	**Express feelings and thoughts**
	Bereaved children should be helped to find appropriate ways to express all their feelings and thoughts associated with grief, such as sadness, anxiety, confusion, anger and guilt
R	**Remember the person who has died**
	Bereaved children have the right to remember the person who has died for the rest of their lives; sharing special as well as difficult memories
E	**Education and information**
	Bereaved children need and are entitled to receive answers to their questions and information that clearly explains what has happened, why it has happened and what will be happening
A	**Appropriate response from schools and colleges**
	Bereaved children need understanding and support from their teachers and fellow students without having to ask for it
V	**Voice in important decisions**
	Bereaved children should be given the choice about their involvement in important decisions that have an impact on their lives such as planning the funeral and remembering anniversaries
E	**Enjoyment**
	Bereaved children have the right to enjoy their lives even though someone important has died
M	**Meet others**
	Bereaved children benefit from the opportunity to meet other children who have had similar experiences
E	**Established routines**
	Bereaved children should, whenever possible, be able to continue activities and interests so that parts of their lives can still feel 'normal'
N	**Not to blame**
	Bereaved children should be helped to understand that they are not responsible, and not to blame, for the death
T	**Tell the story**
	Bereaved children are helped by being encouraged to tell an accurate and coherent story of what has happened. These stories need to be heard by those important people in their lives

CASE STUDY REVIEW 14.2

Owen had spent considerable periods of time in hospital while undergoing treatment with some community children's nursing support when at home. Despite repeated active interventions of chemotherapy, radiotherapy and surgery these proved unsuccessful. Following lengthy conversations with Owen's parents and the interprofessional team, a decision was made to cease all active intervention.

However, Owen had signs of raised intracranial pressure which needed to be managed. Owen's parents considered the possibility of caring for Owen at home but also agreed to consider hospice care.

Owen and his family visited their local children's hospice and quickly settled into hospice life. This allowed the family time to consider the implications of the withdrawal of active treatment and to start to decide what their wishes for

end-of-life care might be, especially as the timescale of deterioration was unclear. Owen was assessed and a symptom management plan was developed.

While at the hospice, Owen and his family enjoyed some brief time using the facilities. Owen particularly enjoyed being in the garden with his sisters and in the hydrotherapy pool before his symptoms prevented these activities.

While at the hospice, Owen started to experience pain related to his raised intracranial pressure and had increasing seizure activity, both needing medication. In addition, medication was given to reduce anxiety and nausea.

As Owen deteriorated, he could no longer swallow and a nasogastric tube was required to maintain nutrition and hydration. At this point, medication was administered via the nasogastric tube and eventually a syringe driver. Although

Owen's saturations were satisfactory, he was more settled with continuous low-flow oxygen via nasal cannulae.

Owen was very settled on this regimen and, as his intracranial pressure increased, his medication was altered. Owen had minimal monitoring as his parents and the hospice staff were confident in monitoring him visually and behaviourally. As Owen's symptoms had escalated, his parents and his sisters decided to stay at the hospice. Owen was discharged from the community children's nursing and continuing care package, but with the parents' consent they were kept informed of Owen's progress and visited the family in the hospice should the family decide to go home.

Owen's family felt that to stay at the hospice as a family meant that they could focus all their time enjoying being with Owen and together as a family. The family were fully involved with Owen's care and found the sibling support crucial for Owen's sisters. Owen's extended family and friends were frequent and regular visitors to the hospice throughout Owen's stay.

Owen died peacefully 6 weeks later, with the hospice supporting the family through the formalities of after-death and funeral care. The music teacher was on hand to play some of Owen's favourite music at the funeral. The family received ongoing bereavement and sibling support. They attend the annual family remembrance days.

SUMMARY OF KEY LEARNING

Palliative care for children and young people with life-limiting conditions is an active and total approach to care, embracing physical, emotional, social and spiritual elements. It focuses on enhancement of quality of life for the child and support for the family and includes the management of distressing symptoms, provision of respite and care through death and bereavement (Association for Children's Palliative Care (ACT)/Royal College of Paediatrics and Child Health (RCPCH) 2003).

Children and young people with palliative care needs, as well as their parents, siblings and extended families need a range of support from health, social services and education, to enable them to continue to be cared for at home and to have access to suitable care outside the family home, when required. The need for palliative care begins as soon as it is clear that a child or young person has a life-limiting illness. Active palliative care approaches to support children, young people and families to lead as normal lives as possible include:

- symptom management
- partnership between the child, young person and family
- listening to and responding to children, young people and their families
- services that are integrated and reflect longer term continuing care
- delivering care where the child, young person and family want it, such as in the home, hospital or hospice, school or nursery

- psychological and social support including formal counselling and therapy
- attention to cultural, spiritual and practical needs
- interprofessional and multiagency teamwork and partnership
- supporting children, their families and education professionals to enable children to continue to access education.

A wide range of professionals from both the statutory and voluntary sectors provide care to children who have life-limiting conditions and their families. These children, young people and their families need access to high-quality palliative care throughout their care journey: this means they receive care from universal services such as education and health services as well as access to specialist paediatric palliative care including hospices, community children's palliative care teams and hospital symptom management services. Recent UK government documents set out the general direction for service development for children's palliative care services and there is considerable guidance available to support best practice in the care of children and young people: this includes care pathways and best practice charters. The combination of this information, the interest and skills, knowledge and expertise of the workforce provide opportunities for nurses and other practitioners to continue to develop family-focused, child-centred palliative care.

FURTHER RESOURCES

Assessment frameworks

Department of Health (2010) National framework for Children and Young People's Continuing Care: **www.dh.gov.uk/en/Publicationsandstatistics/Publications/PublicationsPolicyAndGuidance/DH_114784**

Department for Education (2009) Early identification, assessment of needs and intervention – The Common Assessment Framework (CAF) for children and young people: A guide for

practitioners. **www.education.gov.uk/publications/standard/publicationDetail/Page1/IW91/0709**

ACT (2011) Basic symptom control in paediatric palliative care – the children's rainbows Hospice guidelines, 8th edn: **www.act.org.uk/symptomcontrol**

Children's BNF: **bnfc.org/bnfc/index.htm**

Cancerpage.com (2007) Pain relief for children: **www.cancerpage.com/centers/pain/pediatrics_p.asp**

Paediatric Pain Profile (2011): **www.ppprofile.org.uk**

Decisions relating to cardiopulmonary resuscitation. A statement from the BMA and RCN in association with the Resuscitation Council (UK) (2007): **www.bma.org.uk/ethics/cardiopulmonary_resuscitation/CPRDecisions07.jsp**

Royal College of Paediatrics and Child Health (1997, 2004) Withholding or withdrawing life-sustaining treatment in children: a framework for practice: **www.rcpch.ac.uk/Publications/Publications-list-by-title#W**

BMA (2006) Parental responsibility: guidance from the British Medical Association: **www.bma.org.uk/ethics/consent_and_capacity/Parental.jsp**

General Medical Council (2007) 0–18 years: guidance for all doctors: **www.gmc-uk.org/guidance/archive/GMC_0-18.pdf**

Association of Anaesthetists of Great Britain and Ireland May (2009) DNAR decisions in the perioperative period: **www.aagbi.org/publications/guidelines/docs/dnar_09.pdf**

BMA (2007) Withholding and withdrawing life-prolonging medical treatment, 3rd edn: **http://www.bma.org.uk/ethics/end_life_issues/Withholdingwithdrawing.jsp**

Department of Health, Social Services and Public Safety (DHSSPS) (2003) Breaking bad news. Regional guidelines developed from partnerships in caring. DHSSPS: Belfast.

Scope (1993) Right from the start – template document. A guide to good practice in diagnosis and disclosure. Scope Publications: London.

You may also like to view an article written by Francis called 'Bereavement starts at diagnosis', which describes the journey that parents of children with life-limiting conditions take and the challenges in the work of those who support them: **http://www.thinkingfaith.org/articles/20090323_1.htm**

ANSWERS TO ACTIVITIES

ACTIVITY 14.1

Main principles of children and young people's palliative care are:

- Care should be child and family focused.
- Care should take account of children's rights.
- Care should encompass symptom management, emotional support, practical support, spiritual needs and bereavement for the whole family and should respect cultural and religious differences.

- Service delivery should be based on assessment of needs starting as soon as possible after diagnosis or recognition.
- The delivery of care should be well coordinated, with an emphasis on continuity of services.
- Care plans should be flexible to accommodate changing needs and choices.
- Regular review of needs should be undertaken and care plans adjusted to take account of changes in circumstances. (ACT 2004)

ACTIVITY 14.2 Breaking bad news

- Parents should be treated with openness and honesty.
- Parents should be acknowledged as experts in the care of their child.
- Significant news should be shared in a place of privacy.
- Professionals should allow plenty of time for sharing news and discussing what this means with families.
- Parents should be given the opportunity to hear news together.
- Advocates and interpreters should be readily available to support families.

- News should be shared using clear, jargon-free and readily understandable language.
- There should be open communication between professionals and the family.
- Parents should be given time to explore care options and ask questions.
- Breaking significant news should be backed up by helpful written material.

ACTIVITY 14.3 Care pathways

Consider and list why care pathways are needed.

- Wide range of palliative conditions, therefore meeting needs can be difficult.
- Disparity in services.

- Wide range of services – statutory and voluntary.
- Seamless provision of care is still problematic.
- Varying range of knowledge in hospital and community.
- Disparity in the development of the keyworker role.
- Disparity in shared documentation.

The ACT Care Pathways detail the essential steps of the patient's journey. Each care pathway is divided into three stages with 5 or 6 evidence-based standards. These include:

Stage 1, diagnosis or recognition of the condition:

- Standard 1 – breaking bad news
- Standard 2 – planning for going home

Stage 2, living with the condition:

- Standard 3 – multiagency assessment of the family
- Standard 4 – multiagency care plan

Stage 3, the end-of-life care phase:

- Standard 5 – end-of-life plan.

ACTIVITY 14.4 The interprofessional team

What factors need considering when collaborating with the interprofessional team?
How does the disparity of services impact on the child, young person and family?

For Owen and his family, collaborative interprofessional working is crucial but trying to establish collaborative working systems with families and co-workers can be frustrating, and time consuming in the initial stages. Nevertheless, to be effective, it is fundamentally important to work within this collaborative, comprehensive framework.

There are critical issues for these professionals in working together, for example, sharing the same understanding of what a child needs and having ways to exchange information to form a holistic view of what is happening to that child. Professionals need a clear understanding of the roles and responsibilities of others so they know what information they can seek from others and what that information might contribute to an assessment. The failure to achieve holistic assessments undermines opportunities for children and young people to achieve a 'good death'.

ACTIVITY 14.5 Symptom management

- Treating the underlying cause of a symptom may be equally as appropriate as providing symptom control.
- Practical, cognitive, behavioural, physical and supportive therapies should be combined with appropriate drug treatment.
- Persistent symptoms should be treated with medication given at regular intervals.

- Severe and uncontrolled symptoms should be regarded as a medical emergency and active interventions may be appropriate.
- Inappropriately invasive and painful routes of drug administration should be avoided whenever possible.
- Side-effects of medication must be anticipated and actively treated.

ACTIVITY 14.6 Owen's symptom management

Owen has developed raised intracranial pressure, therefore a comprehensive symptom management plan encompassed pain relief for the pain associated with raised intracranial pressure, anticonvulsant medication to control increasing seizure activity as well as medication to reduce anxiety and nausea.

Consider the care that Owen requires in relation to the symptoms he may be experiencing.

Feeding

Children with neurodegenerative disorders or brain tumours are particularly affected. Being unable to nourish their child causes parents great distress and often makes them feel that they are failing as parents. Sucking and eating are part of children's development and provide comfort, pleasure and stimulation. These aspects should be considered alongside a child's medical and practical problems with eating. In general, nutritional goals aimed at restoring health are secondary to comfort and enjoyment, although assisted feeding, via a nasogastric tube or gastrostomy, may be appropriate for those with slowly progressive disease.

Nausea and Vomiting

These are common problems. Antiemetics can be selected according to their site of action and the presumed cause of the nausea. In resistant cases, combining a number of drugs that act in different ways or adding an antagonist can be helpful. Vomiting from raised intracranial pressure should be managed.

Neurological Problems

Observing a child having a seizure is extremely frightening for parents and they should always be warned if it is a possibility and advised about management. A supply of anticonvulsants at home is valuable for managing seizures. Subcutaneous midazolam can enable parents to keep at home a child with severe repeated seizures. Children with neurodegenerative disease will often already be taking maintenance antiepileptic drugs and the dose and drugs may need adjusting as the disease progresses. Agitation and anxiety may reflect a child's need to express his or her fears and distress. Drugs such as benzodiazepines and haloperidol may help to provide relief, especially in the final stages of life.

Sources: Goldman et al. 2006, Hendricks-Ferguson 2008 and Jassal and Hain 2011

ACTIVITY 14.7 End-of-life care

- Professionals should be open and honest with families when the approach to end of life is recognised.
- Joint planning with families and relevant professionals should take place as soon as possible.
- A written plan of care should be agreed, which includes decisions about resuscitation.
- Emergency services should be informed of these decisions.
- Care plans should be reviewed and altered to take account of changes.

- There should be 24-hour access to pain and symptom control, including access to medication.
- Those managing the control of symptoms should be suitably qualified and experienced.
- Emotional and spiritual support should be available to the child and family.
- Children and families should be supported in their choices and goals for quality of life to the end.

SELECTED REFERENCES

Amery, J. (ed.) (2009) *Children's palliative care in Africa.* Oxford University Press: Oxford.

Amery, J. (2011) *Children's palliative care handbook for GPs*, 1st edn. Association for Children's Palliative Care: Bristol.

Anderson, A., Breen, M., Sebastian, N. and Mycroft, J. (2010) The use of emergency boxes for children with advanced cancer. *European Journal of Palliative Care*, 17(2), 80–83.

Association for Children with Life-threatening or Terminal Conditions and their Families (ACT) (2004) *A framework for the development of integrated multi-agency care pathways for children with life-threatening and life-limiting conditions.* ACT: Bristol.

Association for Children with Life-threatening or Terminal Conditions (ACT) and Children's Hospices UK (2007a) *Transition care pathway.* ACT: Bristol.

Association for Children with Life-threatening or Terminal Conditions (ACT) and Children's Hospices UK (2007b) *TA Care pathway to support extubation within a children's palliative care framework.* ACT: Bristol.

Association for Children with Life-threatening or Terminal Conditions (ACT) and Children's Hospices UK (2009a) *Right people, right place, right time.* ACT: Bristol.

Association for Children with Life-threatening or Terminal Conditions (ACT) and Children's Hospices UK (2009b) *Making the case for children's palliative care.* ACT: Bristol.

Association for Children with Life-threatening or Terminal Conditions (ACT) and Children's Hospices UK (2009c) *The neonatal care pathway.* ACT: Bristol.

Association for Children with Life-threatening or Terminal Conditions (ACT) and Children's Hospices UK (2011a) *Square table local learning and evaluation report.* ACT: Bristol.

Association for Children with Life-threatening or Terminal Conditions (ACT) and Children's Hospices UK (2011b) *Children's palliative care handbook for GPs.* ACT: Bristol.

Association for Children with Life-threatening or Terminal Conditions (ACT) and the Royal College of Paediatrics and Child Health (RCPCH) (2003) *A guide to the development of children's paediatric services*, 2nd edn. ACT: Bristol.

Baile, W.F., Buckman, R., Lenzi, R., Glober, G., Beale, E.A. and Kudelka, A.P. (2000) SPIKES – a six-step protocol for delivering bad news: application to the patient with cancer. *Oncologist*, 5, 302–311.

Becker, R. (2010) *Fundamental aspects of palliative care nursing: an evidence-based handbook for student nurses*, 2nd ed. Quay Books: London.

Bloom M. (2001) Breaking bad news: parents' perspectives. *Pediatric Nursing*, 13, 16–20.

Bluebond Langner, M. (1995) Worlds of dying children and their well siblings, in K. Doka (ed.) *Children mourning, mourning children.* Hospice Association of America: Washington: DC.

Bradshaw, G., Hinds, P.S. and Lensing, S. (2005) Cancer-related deaths in children and adolescents. *Journal of Palliative Medicine*, 8(1) 86–95.

Breau, L.M., Camfield, C.S., McGrath, P. and Finley, A. (2003) The incidence of pain in children with severe cognitive impairments. *Archive of Pediatric Adolescent Medicine*, 157, 1219–1226.

Brother Francis (2006) The spiritual life, in A. Goldman *et al.* (eds) *Oxford textbook of palliative care for children.* Oxford University Press: Oxford.

Brown, E. (2007) *Supporting the child and the family in paediatric palliative care.* Jessica Kingsley Publishers: London.

Brown, E. and Mercer, A. (2005) The Mercer model of paediatric palliative care. *European Journal of Palliative Care*, 12(1), 22–25.

Buckman, R.A. (1992) *How to break bad news: a guide for health care professionals.* Johns Hopkins University Press: Baltimore, MA.

Buckman, R.A. (2005) Breaking bad news: the S-P-I-K-E-S strategy. *Community Oncology*, 2, 138–142.

Bull, A. and Gillies, M. (2007) Spiritual needs of children with complex healthcare needs in hospital. *Paediatric Nursing*, 19(9), 34–38

Care Co-ordination Network UK (2006) Care Co-ordination Network Cymru: the key working charity: **http://ccnukorguk.site.securepool.com/ccnuk/default.asp**

Children's Hospices UK (2010) *Children's hospice care from March 2009 to September 2010. A report based on visits to all children's hospice services in the UK.*

Children's Hospices UK and ACT (2011) *Square table: local learning and evaluation report.* Children's Hospices UK and ACT: Bristol.

Contro, N. and Scofield, S. (2006) *The power of their voices: child and family assessment in pediatric palliative care*, in A. Goldman, R. Haines and S. Liben (eds) *Oxford textbook of pediatric palliative care.* Oxford University Press: London.

Contro, N., Larson, J., Schofield, S., Sourkes, B. and Cohen, H. (2004). Hospital staff and family perspectives regarding quality of pediatric palliative care. *Pediatrics*, 114(5), 1248–1252.

Corr, C. and Balk, D. (2010) *Children's encounters with death, bereavement, and coping.* Springer Publishing Company: New York.

Costello, J. and Trinder-Brook, A. (2000) Children's nurses' experiences of caring for dying children in hospital. *Paediatric Nursing*, 12(6), 28–32.

Craft, A. and Killen, S. (2007) *Palliative care services for children and young people in England. An independent review for the secretary of state for health.* Department of Health: London.

Davies, B., Attig, T. and Towne, M. (2006) Bereavement, in A. Goldman, R. Hain and S. Liben (eds) *Oxford textbook of palliative care.* Oxford University Press: Oxford.

Davies, R. (2004) New understandings of parental grief: literature review. *Journal of Advanced Nursing*, 46(5), 506–513.

Davies, R. (2005) Mothers' stories of loss: their need to be with their dying child and their child's body after death. *Journal of Child Health Care*, 9(4), 288–300.

Davies, R. (2009) Caring for the child at the end of life, in J. Price and P. McNeilly (eds) *Palliative care for children and families: an interdisciplinary approach.* Palgrave Macmillan: Basingstoke.

Department for Education and Skills (DfES) (2003) *Every child matters.* Stationery Office: London.

Department for Education and Skills (DfES) (2009) Early identification, assessment of needs and intervention – the common assessment framework (CAF) for children and young people: A guide for practitioners: **http://www.education.gov.uk/publications/standard/publication Detail/Page1/IW91/0709**

Department for Education and Skills (DfES) and Department of Health (DoH) (2005) *Commissioning children's and young people's palliative care services: a practical guide for the NHS commissioners.* HMSO: London.

Department of Health (DoH) (2004) *National Service Framework for children, young people and maternity services.* HMSO: London.

Department of Health (DoH) (2005) *Commissioning children and young people's palliative care services.* HMSO: London.

Department of Health (DoH) (2006) *Palliative care statistics for children and young adults.* DoH: London.

Department of Health (DoH) (2007) *Palliative care statistics for children and young adults.* HMSO: London.

Department of Health (DoH) (2008a) *Aiming high for disabled children.* HMSO: London.

Department of Health (DoH) (2008b) *Better care: better lives (BCBL). Improving outcomes and experiences for children, young people and their families living with life-limiting and life-threatening conditions.* HMSO: London.

Department of Health (DoH) (2010a) National framework for children and young people's continuing care. DoH: London.

Department of Health (DoH) (2010b) *Spiritual care at the end of life: a systematic review of the literature.* HMSO: London.

Department of Health, Social Services and Public Safety (DHSSPS) (2003) *Breaking bad news . . . regional guidelines developed from partnerships in caring.* DHSSPS: Belfast.

Dunlop, S. (2008) The dying child: should we tell the truth? *Paediatric Nursing*, 20(6), 28–31.

Dussel, V., Kreicbergs, U. and Hilden, J.M. (2009) Looking beyond where children die: determinants and effects of planning a child's location of death. *J Pain Symptom Manage*, 37(1), 33–43.

Fallowfield, L. and Jenkins, V. (2004) Communicating sad, bad, and difficult news in medicine. *The Lancet*, 363(9405), 312–319.

Fraser, L., Miller, M., Aldridge, J., McKinney, P. and Parslow, R. (2011) *Life-limiting and life-threatening conditions in children and young people in the United Kingdom; national and regional prevalence in relation to socioeconomic status and ethnicity. Final Report For Together For Short Lives.* University of Leeds: Leeds.

Freyer, D.R., Kuperberg, A., Sterken, D.J., Pastyrnak, S.L., Hudson, D. and Richards, T. (2006) Multidisciplinary care of the dying adolescent. *Child Adolesc Psychiatr Clin North Am*; 15(3), 693–715.

Goldman, A., Hewitt, M., Collins, G.S., Childs, M. and Hain, R. (2006) Symptoms in children/young people with progressive malignant disease: United Kingdom children's cancer study group/paediatric oncology nurses forum survey. *Pediatrics*, 117(6), 1179–1186.

Greco, V. and Sloper, P. (2004) Care coordination and key worker schemes for disabled children: results of a UK wide survey. *Child Care, Health and Development*, 30, 13–20.

Grinyer, A. (2012) *Palliative and end of life care for children and young people: home, hospice, hospital.* Wiley-Blackwell: Chichester.

Heath, J.A., Clarke, N.E., Donath, S.M., McCarthy, M., Anderson, V.A. and Wolfe J. (2010) Symptoms and suffering at the end of life in children with cancer: an Australian perspective. *Med J Aust*, 192(2), 71–75.

Hendricks-Ferguson, V. (2008) Physical symptoms of children receiving pediatric hospice care at home during the last week of life. *Oncology Nursing Forum*, 35(6), 108–115.

Himelstein, P., Hilden, M., Boldt, M. and Weissman, D. (2004) Pediatric palliative care. *New England Journal of Medicine* 350, 1752–1762.

Hughes-Hallett, T., Craft, A. and Davies, C. (2011) *Independent palliative care funding review.* DoH: London.

IMPaCCT (2007) Standards for paediatric palliative care in Europe. *European Journal of Palliative Care*, 14(3), 109–114.

International Council of Nurses (ICN) (2006). *The ICN code of ethics for nurses.* Imprimerie Fornara: Geneva.

Jalmsell, L., Kreicbergs, U. and Onelov, E. (2006) Symptoms affecting children with malignancies during the last month of life: a nationwide follow-up. *Pediatrics*, 117, 1314–1320.

Jassal, S. and Hain, R. (2011) *Basic symptom control in paediatric palliative care. The Rainbows children's hospice guidelines*, 8th edn. ACT: Bristol.

Klass, D. (1993) Solace and immortality: bereaved parents' continuing bond with their children. *Death Studies*, 17, 343–368.

Klass, D. (1996) *Continuing bonds: new understandings of grief.* Taylor & Francis: London.

Klassen, A., Klassen, R., Dix, D., Pritchard, S., Yanofsky, R. and O'Donnel, Mr. et al. (2008) Impact of caring for a child with cancer on Parent's health-related life. *Journal of clinical Oncology* 26(36), 5884–5889.

Klepping, L. (2012) Total pain: a reflective case study addressing the experience of a terminally ill adolescent. *International Journal of Palliative Nursing*, 8(3), 115–123.

Komaromy, C. (2004) Nursing care at the time of death, in S. Payne, J. Seymour and C. Ingleton (eds) *Palliative care nursing principles and evidence for practice*. Open University Press: Buckingham.

Kreicbergs, U., Valdimarsdottir, U., Onelov, E., Henter, J.I. and Steineck, G. (2004) Talking about death with children who have severe malignant disease. *N Engl J Med*, 351(12), 1175–1186.

McCluggage, H. and Elborn, S. (2006) Symptoms suffered by life-limited children that cause anxiety to UK children's hospice staff. *International Journal of Palliative Nursing*, 12(6), 254–258.

McCulloch, R., Comac, M. and Craig, F. (2008) Paediatric palliative care: coming of age in oncology? *European Journal of Cancer*, 44(8), 1139–1145.

National Institute for Clinical Excellence (NICE) (2005) *Improving outcomes in children and young people with cancer*. HMSO: London.

Neilson, S., Kai, J., MacArthur, C. and Greenfield, S. (2010) Exploring the experiences of community-based children's nurses providing palliative care. *Paediatric Nursing*, 22(30), 31–36.

Pearson, H. and Aylott, M. (2007) Fundamental aspects of end-of-life care, in A. Glasper et al. (eds) *Fundamental aspects of children's and young people's nursing procedures*. Quay Books: London.

Pfund, R. (2000) Nurturing a child's spirituality. *Journal of Child Health Care*, 4(4), 143–148.

Pfund, R. (2007) *Palliative care nursing of children and young people*. Radcliffe Publishing: Oxford.

Price, J. McNeilly, P. and McFarlane, M. (2005) Paediatric palliative care in the UK: past, present and future. *International Journal of Palliative Nursing*, 11(3), 124–126.

Price, P., McNeilly, P. and Surgenor, M. (2006) Breaking bad news to parents: the children's nurse's role. *International Journal of Palliative Nursing*, 12(3), 115–120.

Rabow, M. and McPhee, S. (2000) Beyond breaking bad news: how to help patients who suffer. *BMJ* 8, 45–88.

Rosen, H. (1990) *Unspoken grief: coping with sibling loss*. Lexington Books: Lanham, MD.

Rosenblatt, C. (2000) *Parent grief: narratives of loss and relationship*. Brunner/Mazel: Philadelphia.

Rosof, B.D. (ed.) (1994) *The worst loss*. Henry Holt: New York.

Royal College of Nursing (RCN) (2005) A guide to cultural and spiritual awareness. *Nursing Standard*, 17(19), 1–19.

Royal College of Paediatrics and Child Health (RCPCH) (2004) *Withholding or withdrawing life-sustaining treatment in children: a framework for practice*, 2nd edn. RCPCH: London.

Schiff, S. (1977) *The bereaved parent*. Crown Publishers: New York.

Schmid Mast, M., Kindlimann, A. and Langewitz, W. (2005) Recipients' perspective on breaking bad news: how you put it really makes a difference. *Patient Education and Counseling*, 58, 244–251.

Scope (1993) *Right from the start – template document. A guide to good practice in diagnosis and disclosure*. Scope Publications: London.

Siden, H., Miller, M., Straatman, L., Omesi, L., Tucker T. and Collins, J. (2008) A report on location of death in paediatric palliative care between home, hospice and hospital. *Palliative Medicine*, 22, 831–834.

Smith, S.C. and Pennells, M. (eds) (1995) *Interventions with bereaved children*. Jessica Kingsley: London.

Sourkes, B. (2006) *The psychological impact of life-limiting illness*, in A. Goldman, R. Haines and S. Liben (eds) *Oxford textbook of pediatric palliative care*. Oxford University Press: London.

Talbot, K. (2002) *What forever means after the death of a child*. Brunner-Routledge: London.

van der Werff, G., Paans, W. and Nieweg, R. (2012) Hospital nurses' views of the signs and symptoms that herald the onset of the dying phase in oncology patients. *International Journal of Palliative Nursing*, 18(3), 143–149.

Vickers, J., Thompson, A., Collins, G.S., Childs, M. and Hain, R. (2007) Place and provision of palliative care for children with progressive cancer: a study by the Paediatric Oncology Nurses' Forum/United Kingdom Children's Cancer Study Group Palliative Care Working Group. *J Clin Oncol*, 25, 4472–4476.

Walter, T. (1996) A new model of grief: bereavement and biography. *Mortality*, 1, 7–25.

West Midland Paediatric Macmillan Team (2005) *Palliative care for the child with malignant disease*. Quay Books: London

Willis, E. (2007) Symptom care flowcharts: a case study. *Paediatric nursing*, 19(1), 14–17.

Wolfe, J., Hammel, J.F., Edwards, K.E., Duncan, J., Comeau, M. and Breyer, J. (2008) Easing of suffering in children with cancer at the end of life: is care changing? *J Clin Oncol*, 26(10), 1717–1723.

Wolfe, J., Hinds, P. and Sourkes, B. (2011) *Textbook of interdisciplinary pediatric palliative care*. Elsevier: Philadelphia.

Woodgate, R.L. (2006) Living in a world without closure: reality for parents who have experienced the death of a child. *J Palliat Care*, 22(2), 75–82.

Worden, W. (1982) *Grief counselling and grief therapy*. Springer Publishing: New York.

Worden, W. (1991) *Grief counselling and grief therapy: a handbook for the mental health practitioner*, 2nd edn. Routledge: London.

World Health Organization (WHO) (1998) *Guidelines for analgesic drug therapy in cancer relief and palliative care in children:* **http://whqlibdoc.who.int/publications/9241545127 .pdf**

World Health Organization (WHO) (2008) *Definition of palliative care*. WHO: Geneva.

World Health Organization (WHO) (2010) *Guidelines for analogies drug theraphy. Cancer pain relief and palliative care in children*. WHO: Geneva.

CHAPTER 15
Preparation for Professional Practice

Sue Collier

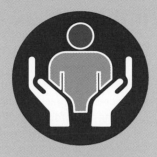
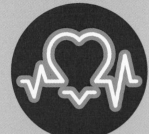
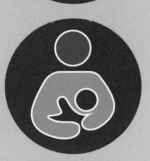

LEARNING OUTCOMES

On completion of this chapter, the reader will be able to:

- Critically explore political drivers to protect patients and promote health and well-being.
- Assess the mechanisms and processes that are utilised in monitoring, evaluating and improving standards of care delivered.
- Critically reflect on team working in terms of leadership qualities, management skills, communication skills and evidence-based practice.
- Critically evaluate the concepts of professional/interprofessional collaboration and issues around accountability and responsibility in managing the delivery of care.
- Explore how organisational systems facilitate the quality of care delivery and safeguard quality.
- Understand the key skills required to lead a team of nurses and to effectively manage the care of a group of patients.

TALKING POINT

'In 1996/7 the budget for the NHS in England was 33 billion, in 2008/9 it is 96 billion.'
Lord Darzi

High Quality Care for All: NHS Next Stage Review Final report (2008)

'Of all medication incidents reported...[from acute hospital settings] nearly 10% involve patients aged between 0 and four years.'

Review of patient safety for children and young people (2009)

'Safety is a very complicated business. It requires thinking about the clinical environment, how people behave, about the equipment and the technology.'

Prof Charles Vincent, DOME lead psychologist (2012)

http://www.bbc.co.uk/news/health-16812134

INTRODUCTION

Current policy statements emphasise the need for clinical governance and interprofessional collaboration to reflect the necessity for risk assessment, risk management, research and evidence-based practice, in the provision of healthcare. Leading, managing or coordinating care for a group of children and young people can be a rewarding experience yet it requires practice and a range of honed skills. Preparing to extend those experiences to include overseeing an entire ward requires a 'fluency' with the skills, knowledge and understanding of the key concepts on which the organisation operates and a contemporary knowledge of key professional issues. This chapter will enable the reader to consider aspects of organisation and management of care and to gain an understanding of the organisational processes that influence the delivery of care.

This chapter will seek to explore leadership, management conflict, clinical governance and the maintenance of professional standards in relation to Woodland Ward. The purpose of this chapter is not to recapitulate the extensive general and nursing works on leadership or management in great depth but rather to present well-known theories in context.

Children's and young people's nurses are in a pivotal role within the care and day-to-day management of children, young people and their families through their healthcare journeys. There is a range of different inpatient journeys and the impact they have on each family will differ. Whatever the context or setting the children and young people's nurse will always be required to follow the guiding political and professional principles, underpinning theories, assess, plan and implement care, to discern when care is not progressing appropriately and to build a therapeutic relationship with the child, young person, parents or carers and the interprofessional team. This requires effective leadership, management, communication, team work, appropriate decision making and trust (Bricher 1999). In order to understand why we do what we do in children's and young people's nursing, it is important to understand the interface between different disciplines. To that end, a working knowledge of the ethos of the organisation and other agencies in order to work collaboratively for seamless care between inpatient and community care is vital.

As healthcare practitioners, children's and young people's nurses are in a pivotal position to build a therapeutic relationship with the child, young person or their families and at the same time, network with a range of professionals. The children

---

CASE STUDY 15.1

Rebecca has worked on Woodland Ward for 6 years and is a loyal and valued member of staff. Rebecca is a caring and passionate person; she frequently takes on work with people that alleviates the stress of the rest of the team. Rebecca has been known to stay on after her shift in order to 'give the children and families a little extra care and attention'.

Louize is a newly qualified member of staff who has just completed her period of preceptorship. Louize is surprised by the speed with which she has been left managing the ward and is 'still finding her feet'. Louize has very good technical knowledge and often reads research articles and engages the rest of the team in interesting discussions on best practice guidelines. Although new in the team, Louize clearly 'shines', although her interpersonal communication is rather brusque and she comes across as rather authoritarian, even though she is actually quite shy.

On leaving her office, Erin, the matron, overhears a heated discussion between Rebecca and Louize. Voices are raised and

it is evident that children, young people and their families/carers can hear the exchange between them.

Rebecca: 'Look, I have been qualified longer than you and I do a really good job. Due to tiredness, I make one tiny, little mistake leaving the medicines on the nurse's station. It does not really matter, I have done it before and so have other staff nurses. I don't need a little upstart, just out of university, telling me what I can and cannot do.'

Louize: 'I appreciate it must be really hard for you to accept that you are in the wrong. I have worked hard to achieve my PIN number and I am just advocating for the safety of the children and young people. I mean, the trust will not want bad publicity if this gets into the local paper.'

Rebecca: 'Just what I mean, an arrogant little upstart.'

Erin: 'Ladies, shall we just take this conversation into my office?'

Source: adapted from Hawkes (2012)

---

and young people's nurse is required to integrate professional values and directives into the evidence-based care of children and young people to ensure that all appropriate care interventions are met. All registered nurses are accountable and responsible for their actions and omissions during the care process and have a duty of care to children and young people (NMC 2008; Cornock 2011a).

Medicines management is synonymous with the role of all children's nurses with clear direction from policies, reports and protocols. Medicine containers are clearly labelled, 'Keep out of

the reach of children' yet, in the melee of a busy children's ward, Rebecca had left unknown medication laying around, which had the potential to compromise the safety of the children on the ward. Children and young people have the right for care they receive to be in their 'best interest' yet, leaving unattended medications on a nurses' station has risk associated implications. Working as a children's and young people's nurse requires effective communication, effective team working and effective leadership and management of the nursing environment and consideration of every single task or activity. This case study follows on from an incident where Rebecca may feel under threat from Louize who is newly qualified and has highlighted a significant issue with an administration of medicines processes.

PUBLIC SOCIETY THROUGH PUBLIC LAWS, POLICY AND PRESSURES

In order to understand the situation involving Rebecca, Louize and Erin, it is important to place the children's nurse in the context of the contemporary children and young people's nursing and how it fits with the context of key structures and systems within the United Kingdom. Lewis and Bately (1982) identified clear spheres of nursing in relation to the notion of accountability. Dimond (2011) makes it clear that in order to have accountability, the children's nurse will have completed a nurse education programme to qualify and as such will have demonstrated appropriate knowledge gained throughout the study. Griffith and Tengnah (2008) point out that every nurse must uphold the law the same as any other member of the public. Cornock (2011a) clarifies that being responsible for an act and being accountable are not the same issue, and further adds that the focus is on being responsible for an act. The NMC 'Guidance on professional conduct for nursing and midwifery students' (2008) also identifies that students must 'act with integrity'. This means that students are required to uphold professional principles and values, work closely with staff that support them in acquiring clinical skills and adhere to the directions given professionally through the NMC, politically through policy and through law.

The children's and young people's nurse also needs to comply with the 'law of the land': the policies of the employer and students are required to follow and uphold the policies of the placement provider and university. Changing clinical environments may require familiarisation with new policies and guidelines. To this end, student nurses need to be nurtured in an environment that fosters accountability and responsibility at every level. New members of staff also require a period of time to become familiar with the policies and guidelines in order to be able to follow them appropriately. Louize had been afforded this opportunity as her period of preceptorship had been completed.

In order to be accountable children's nurses have some conditions that need to be met.

Knowledge and Expertise

Typically, those who are accountable in a professional context need to have the required expertise in order to be held to account. Erin, Rebecca and Louize are all professionally accountable to the NMC and have varying degrees of knowledge, experiences and expertise. Erin, Rebecca and Louize are accountable contractually to their employer and those delegated to have authority on their behalf. Erin will have authority over Rebecca and Louize due to her position in the organisation.

A Degree of Autonomy and Freedom

A person who has no alternative course of action cannot be held to account. The scenario does not give the background of events leading to Rebecca leaving unattended medication on the nurses' station. The NMC (2008) is clear on the area of responsibility as 'actions and omissions' are identified. Policies and guidelines are in place to guide actions and although these may be comprehensive there are some 'unsaid common sense' assumptions that apply. Administration of medications with children should mean that the medication is never left unattended.

A Person or Body to Whom One is Accountable

The concept of accountability makes no sense unless there is someone who can demand the explanation or justification. Erin, Rebecca and Louize are all accountable to the NMC and their employer (see Figure 15.1). Rebecca and Louize will also be accountable to Erin due to her position in the organisation (see 'power' later in chapter).

It is almost unthinkable that children's and young people's nurses need to think about the 'law of the land' in relation to the care of the young and vulnerable patients. While the majority of children's nurses will be law-abiding people and have the interests of their patients at heart, there have been reported incidents where serious untoward incidents have occurred. While the majority of these are managed within organisations, there are rare occasions on which an organisation is brought under the public microscope because a particular incident has gained notoriety. An example of this would be the actions of Beverley Allitt and the subsequent legal proceedings.

Unfortunately, the case of Beverley Allitt and her crimes are not an isolated incident. Innocent lives have been ended by murder or the quality of life has been irreversibly changed by other catastrophic events. Harold Shipman, a general practitioner, also committed heinous crimes in the community setting with older adult patients. Both these events demonstrate that younger and older patients are vulnerable and may have influenced the public to distrust healthcare professionals. Yet, it is not just the vulnerable patients at opposing ends of the age spectrum who are vulnerable. Laurance (2011) reports that Anne Grigg-Booth was charged in 2005 with the murder of three elderly patients in hospital; Benjamin Green was convicted in 2006 of murdering two patients and harming 15 others in hospital; Colin Norris was jailed for 30 years in 2008 for killing four elderly patients at two hospitals. The events at another hospital raised further alarm bells during 2011 where adult patients died (Tozer and Hull 2012). Naturally, the general public are alarmed that healthcare professionals could act in this manner. Media coverage plays an important role in reporting key information that raises 'alarms' with the general public, potentially causing fear and anxiety until the culprits have been found. Questions and concerns are raised about healthcare professions, but it is important that these events

Contemporary society
influenced by European and global political decisions

	RN (child)	

Society through public law, policies and pressures
Through public law (generally)
Law of Murder
Criminal Justice Act (2003)
Youth Justice Act (1999)
Medicines Act (1968)
 	
(Specifically)
Children Act (1989, 2004)
 	
Through political systems
Office of the Children's Commissioner
Department of Health
  National Institute of Clinical Excellence
  National Patient Safety Agency
  Health and Safety Executive
National Audit Office
Care Quality Commission (CQC)
 	
Through media
Television, documentaries and newspapers
 	
Changes through
trade union pressures
Public lobbying/outcry
Public inquiry
		Employers
		Through contract of employment
		
		Through adopting and adapting public policies and/or systems
		Clinical governance
		Benchmarking
		Pathways
		Care bundles
		
		Through government strategies
		CQC monitoring
		
		Through public perceptions
		Service-user feedback systems
		Media
		
		Through adverse events
		Actual or perceived negligence
		
		Media
		Positive reporting increases public trust
		
		Negative reporting decreases public trust

	RN (child) Adherence to Department of Health, NMC and employers' directives and policy Accountable and responsible practitioner Achieve evidence-based practice to high standard Contemporary evidenced-based knowledge Competent and proficient skills	
Professional *Through statute law* Nursing and Midwifery Council Order (2001) **NMC quasi-government** Public protection through standards Self-governing NMC code NMC standards of care NMC professional publications NMC hearings *Through unions* Royal College of Nursing *Through professional media* Nursing press		**Child/young person and family/carer** Through tort law Through right to safe, effective care (Article 3) Through the voices of children, young people as consumers of healthcare Through parents/carers as advocates

Service user and public perspectives of healthcare

Figure 15.1 The 'big picture': public/professional, employer, child and family
Source: Adapted from Lewis and Bately (1982), Griffith and Tengnah (2009) and Dimond (2011)

have not been silenced and that justice has been served. These healthcare professionals were appropriately dealt with by public law and statute law. In all these events, the patients were at the mercy of the healthcare professionals who had been educated to provide high-quality, effective care and with whom the patients had developed rapport and trust. Abuse of the administration of medication played a key part in the majority of these cases.

ACTIVITY 15.1 NMC hearings

Access the NMC website and consider how many hearings relate to medicine misuse in nursing and in particular children's nursing (**http://www.nmc-uk.org/Hearings/**).

An example of errors from a children's nurse case:

1 Prepared to administer 2.5 mls of xxxx to Patient A who was prescribed 2.5 mgs of xxxx, to be administered in two doses of 1.25 mls.

2 a Failed to check adequately the identity of Patient B before administering medication to him at around 6 am

   b intravenously administered approximately 350 mgs of an antibiotic to Patient B that should have been administered to Patient C

   c failed to record the administration of 350 mgs of an antibiotic to Patient B in Patient B's chart

   d failed to administer 350 mgs of an antibiotic to Patient C

   e recorded in Patient C's drugs chart that 350 mgs of an antibiotic had been administered to Patient C at around 6 am when it had not been.

As a result of the above, your fitness to practice is impaired by reason of your misconduct.

How much information is displayed about the registrant, the reasons for the hearing or the outcome?

Government strategies have ensured that the Department of Health has a comprehensive system of organisations that oversee a particular area related to care. Each organisation reports its findings and formulates strategies to improve the situation under scrutiny. The National Institute for Clinical Excellence (NICE) produces guidance for healthcare professionals, patients and carers. The work includes the management and care of specific conditions, the use of new and existing health technologies and new surgical procedures. The guidelines assist professionals to both provide evidence-based care and to protect patients. NHS healthcare professionals will be responsible for applying the NICE guidelines at local level. The range of evidence NICE produces includes recommendations for further research and give 'do-not-do' recommendations. Some of these relate to the administration of medications in children and young people.

A change occurred on 1 June 2012, when some of the work set up by the National Patient Safety Agency transferred to the NHS Commissioning Board Special Authority, which would facilitate the patient safety incident data to analyse risk, drive learning and improve patient care (Figure 15.2).

The Department of Health provided the national service frameworks, which give insight to key priorities and key interventions which lay the blueprint for care. A selection from the range of national service frameworks may be used in combination when applicable to children and young people. NSFCYPMS Standard 10, in particular relates to the issues related to the prescribing, dispensing and administration of medicines.

The National Service Framework for children, young people and maternity services (2004) outlines a vision and key standards for operation. There are also a series of national service exemplars that map a journey of a child and where the sources with supporting evidence from the national service framework can be found (DoH 2004) (see Table 15.1). This was a proactive step in the modernisation agenda of the NHS and it guides the planning and standard of service provision and development for all service users (DoH 2003) (see section on transformational leadership).

Table 15.1 Frameworks and exemplars

Range of national service frameworks	Some national service framework exemplars
• NSFCYPMS	• Asthma
• Cancer	• Acquired brain injury
• Diabetes	• Autistic spectrum disorders
• Mental health	• Complex disability
• Renal	• Maternity services
• Chronic obstructive pulmonary disease (COPD)	• Chronic fatigue syndrome (CFS)
• Coronary heart disease	• Myalgia encephalopathy (ME)
• Long-term conditions	• Continence
• Older people	

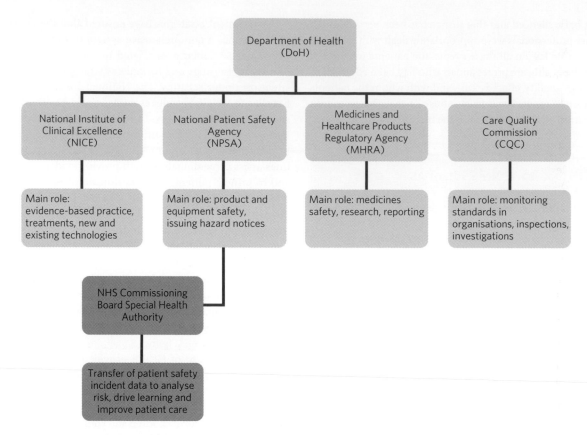

Figure 15.2 Organisational relationships between Department of Health and associated organisations

Over time, the NHS has strived to deliver quality healthcare, ensuring the service provided meets both the needs of the patient and provider (see Table 15.2 for a timeline). Currently, one of the strategies for delivering quality care is through clinical governance (DoH 1998; Scally and Donaldson 1998). Clinical governance sets out to ensure that there are systems in place to monitor the quality of clinical practice and that they are functioning properly and supporting the data collection required to demonstrate statistics or to lead to an 'intuitive' commissioning of services. The Audit Commission (2001) identifies that medicines administration should be linked to clinical governance. Clinical practice is reviewed and improved as a result of monitoring and achieving targets. This requires evidence-based practice, audit, training and proactive planning.

The major components of clinical governance relate to:

- professional self-regulation
- matching professional development with local plans to improve service quality
- forging links between theory and practice
- setting standards
- promoting evidence-based practice
- promoting clinical/cost effectiveness
- developing strong leadership.

It is essential to have robust and systematic monitoring of care interventions and processes. To this end, the Department of Health and NHS have also considered the quality of care being delivered and have responded by showing ways in which time for delivering good-quality, safe care to children and young people will include:

- releasing time to care: the productive leader
- quality and outcomes framework (QOF)
- safeguard quality.

ACTIVITY 15.2 Evidence-based practice: guiding the care and management of feverish illness in children

Review the NICE Guidance CG47 feverish illness in children (**http://guidance.nice.org.uk/CG47**) (see also Chapter 7).

What does NICE CG47 say about temperature taking in children 0 to 5 years old?

PROFESSIONAL SOCIETY

The Nursing and Midwifery Order 2001 exists through statute law, which enables them to protect the public through standards (Griffith and Tengnah 2008). The NMC acts as a quasi-government, providing all registrants with a clear set

Table 15.2 Timeline of political drivers

1968	Medicines Act
1996	Promoting Clinical Excellence (NHS Executive)
1998	New NHS, Modern and Dependable (DoH)
1998	First-Class Service (DoH)
1999	Making a Difference (DoH)
1999	Review of the Prescribing, Supply and Administration of medicines, Crown Report
2001	Organisations with a Memory (DoH)
2001	A Spoonful of Sugar (Audit Commission)
2002	NHS Plan (DoH)
2003	Medicines Management in NHS Trusts: hospitals' medicines management framework (DoH)
2004	National Service Frameworks (NSFs) (DoH)
2004	Patient and Public Involvement (DoH 2004)
2004	Building a Safer NHS for Patients – Improving Medication Safety
2005	Patient Choice When and Where (DoH 2005)
2005	Waiting, Booking and Choice (DoH 2005)
2008	High-quality Care for All: NHS Next Steps Review Final Report
2008	High-quality Care for All: our journey so far
2008	Health and Social Care Act
2010	Equity and Excellence: liberating the NHS
2012	NHS Reform Act

of professional values and standards for professional conduct (NMC 2008). All clinical registrants are required to meet standards such as those issued by the national regulatory bodies. To this end, the NMC provides detailed publications of key concepts in nursing which include confidentiality and the administration of medicines (2007, 2010). The media play a role in directing the NMC to take action by exposing poor practices by clinical practitioners/registrants that could bring the profession into disrepute if no sanctions were taken by the professional body. Children's nurses may have to decide whether to become a 'whistleblower' (Cornock 2011b). Being a self-regulatory body enables the NMC to take action against a registrant if poor, dangerous or catastrophic events have occurred. The NMC is open and transparent about its work and the website is open to both professionals and the general public. Information related to hearings of registrants can be found on a specific area of the website before they take place and the results are given following the hearing. The Audit Commission (2001, page 6) identified that 'hospital medication errors are unacceptably common'. Medicines management systems have changed since 2001 but the human factor means there will be room for potential errors to occur. Blair (2008) points out that medicines should be calculated according to the child's body weight and that children's nurses must ensure this is performed prior to the administration of the medicine because they are accountable for administering incorrect doses.

The NMC inform all registrants about forthcoming changes, listening events and publications that will impact on conduct in practice, patient care or political changes. The professional media also play a role in keeping practitioners updated with current research, consultations, policies and new innovations. There is an array of nursing journals from which clinical practitioners can be inspired by studies, reports and research. The unions also provide key information to their members. Union membership is also important for providing the clinical practitioner/registrant with indemnity insurance, support, legal and professional representation should there be questions.

Employers

The media play a key role in contemporary society in reporting positive and negative issues arising from patient care. Over time, the media has brought many high profile NHS issues related to patient care, systems failures and resources to the attention of the general public through television and newspaper reporting. The influences of the media and subsequent government responses have been influential in the management of key situations. The media reporting about events can cause public outcry and the Healthcare Commission (forerunner to the CQC) has acted on these reports and launched investigations into undesirable events. The government has debated the situation in the Houses of Parliament. It was evident that there had been a breakdown in leadership, resource allocation and opportunities for staff to report issues. There have been other reports of patients who appear to experience substandard care, cruelty and squalour and there has been a catalogue of rude nurses, dirty wards and cancelled operations.

The CQC has identified other issues including:

- a poor care environment in A&E
- a lack of privacy for patients
- inadequate arrangements to treat children
- few specialist paediatric staff
- breaches of infection control standards.

Naturally, these events and issues of poor care can impact on any organisation and cause the public to have a low opinion of their local hospital and the care they or their children may receive. For this reason, any trust will wish to provide excellent, evidence-based care and take active steps to ensure that policies and standards cover the care of all patients including children and young people.

RISK ASSESSMENT

Children and young people are taught risk assessment strategies from a young age in order to enable them to make decisions about their lives. A common example of this can be seen in the time parents and teachers invest to ensure that children are taught how to safely cross the road. In essence, children are taught to assess the risks of crossing the road at a particular time by looking and listening for traffic. There have been a number of strategies to reduce risks for children when crossing the road from the kerb drill, to the Tufty Club to the Green Cross Code (RoSPA 2012). These principles stay with children and young people through to adulthood and are passed on to the next generation. Parents may not always be aware of a conscious decision to teach risk assessment but consider that it is part of a child's experience in the social world of the day. Historically, health promotion messages have been given to children by communication methods appropriate to children. At the time of the Plague children were taught 'Ring o' ring of roses' as a rhyme to pass on a message of the risk of infection. During 1933 RoSPA analysed the causes of road traffic accidents. In 1942 during the Second World War, the kerb drill was devised (RoSPA 2012). The social culture of the day was about explicit routine to facilitate survival, which is reflected in the language of the time. As the social culture changed during times of peace, Tufty appeared as a cartoon animation to pass on the road safety message. As society changed, the approach to road safety needed to change and the Green Cross man reflected the symbol of the superheroes for children to identify with. There was also a strategy to use a celebrity to deliver the road safety message. Whether parents were implicitly or explicitly aware of the background to these road safety strategies, RoSPA have moved with the changing society to deliver the risk assessment message to children (see Voices 15.1).

VOICES 15.1

Cross the Road Safely, Children!
Tune: Nicola Every
Author: Nicola Every

Verse 1

When you're out with Mummy, hold her hand (repeat three times)
   [Hold adult's hand and swing arms as you sing]
   Cross the road safely, children.
   (ACTIONS)
   Stop – do action with hands
   Look – point to eyes
   Listen – hands to ears

Chorus

Stop, look, stop, look and listen
Stop, look, stop, look and listen
Stop, look, stop, look and listen –
Stop, look, stop, look and listen.
Cross the road safely, children.

Verse 2

When you're out with Daddy, hold his hand (repeat three times)
   Cross the road safely, children.

Verse 3

When you're out with Nanny, hold her hand (repeat three times)
   Cross the road safely, children.

Verse 4

When you're out with [can put in any name, e.g. school teacher's] hold her hand (repeat three times)
   Cross the road safely, children. [And so on …]

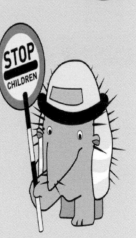

Risk Reduction Strategies

As healthcare professionals, children's nurses need to assess the risks that care interventions may pose to children and their families. It is important that practitioners learn from mistakes that occur within their own organisation and from lessons learned in other situations. The NHS Plan (1999) set out to modernise the NHS. Part of the process concerned the issue of risk. The policy document, 'An organisation with a memory' (DoH 2000) identified four key targets related to:

- maladministration of spinal injections following an incident in practice

- serious errors in the use of medicines
- harm to patients in obstetrics, gynaecology and midwifery care
- suicides of mental health patients as a result of hanging from non-collapsible bed or shower rails.

Building a safer NHS for patients (2004) sets out to plan the way forward with recording adverse events and near miss events at local level, undertaking an analysis of these and looking for the root cause. It was from these key documents that the structures within the NHS changed and the National Patient Safety Agency came into being. The seven steps to patient care are (NPSA 2004):

1 Build a safety culture.
2 Lead and support your staff.
3 Integrate your risk management activity.
4 Promote reporting.
5 Involve and communicate with patients and the public.
6 Learn and share safety lessons.

7 Implement solutions to prevent harm.

The National Patient Safety Agency (2008) produced guidance on risk assessment and identified a matrix format for identifying the likelihood and severity of a situation. This tool aids the prioritisation of risk in the clinical area.

RESEARCH NOTE 15.1

The elements in risk management include:

- The possibility of something harmful happening that involves exposure to danger or a hazard.
- Elements include a combination of the likelihood of something harmful happening and the seriousness of the potential injury. A hazard is less likely to cause harm if certain controls are in place.
- Controls are the steps taken to either eliminate the hazard or reduce the associated risk to an acceptably low level.
- Risk is managed by assessing it, avoiding it if it is unnecessary or reducing it to a level which is 'reasonably practicable'.

- When considering what is 'reasonably practicable,' the needs of both the child and staff should be taken into account.
- Reasonably practicable, as defined by the Health and Safety Executive (HSE), means 'an employee has satisfied his/her duty if he/she can show that any further preventative steps would be grossly disproportionate to the further benefit which would accrue from their introduction' (HSE 1992, page 8; Carlin 2005).

RESEARCH NOTE 15.2

Key: L = low , M = medium, H = high, E = extreme

Likelihood	Consequences				
	Insignificant	Minor	Moderate	Major	Severe
Almost certain	M	H	H	E	E
Likely	M	M	H	H	E
Possible	L	M	M	H	E
Unlikely	L	M	M	M	H
Rare	L	L	M	M	H

Management of Risk in the Clinical Area

In order to achieve a degree of excellence there is a set of standards to work towards. The Care Quality Commission reviews the performance of individual organisations and provides information for both the professionals and the general public (see Figure 15.1). The national service frameworks also provide a framework on which to make judgements about care. The National Surveys of Patient and User Experiences also enable stakeholders to judge their performance and provide an opportunity to review care (see Figure 15.3). Trust boards and MONITOR, the government's auditors, are other ways of assessing performance. It is evident that steps need to be taken in order to change poor and dangerous practice which may have been complicated and may have been caused by more than one event.

ROLE OF CHILDREN AND YOUNG PEOPLE'S NURSES

Children's nurses can be pivotal players in ensuring that evidence-based quality care is being delivered and awareness that the systems for monitoring them are robust. Ownership of the care interventions and processes are crucial when delivering care to children or young persons. The facilitating health trust will have professional development structures in place. It is essential that there is agreement of strategies for improvement. Quality standards, monitoring and performance is at every level of care from the government through to the organisation through to staff at all levels (Weir-Hughes 2011). To this end, a range of quality monitoring tools are provided by the Department of

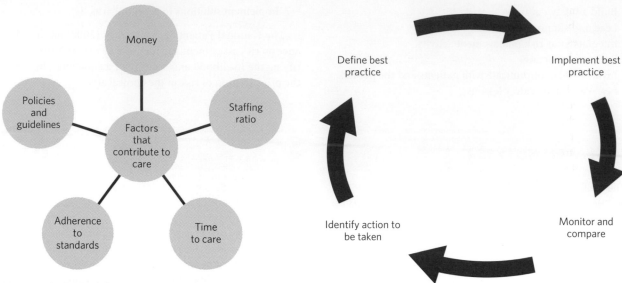

Figure 15.3 Factors that contribute to care

Figure 15.4 Audit cycle

Health, the NHS, the trust organisation and professional organisations such as the Royal College of Nursing (RCN), all of which aim to support children's nurses to deliver quality care and minimise risk. Quality improvement strategies can be implemented and/or generated at local level by children's nurses and other key stakeholders. Developing quality improvement strategies at local level can raise anxiety and stress levels. As making changes can be a stressful experience, it is important that there are support systems to combat the stress of change. There are also systems in place for supporting children's nurses at all levels with forums for clinical supervision.

The notion of audit is borrowed from the financial world and has been adapted to fit the clinical situations. The Department of Health (1989) identify that clinical audit is the systematic and critical analysis of the quality of clinical care, including the procedures used for diagnosis, treatment and care, associated use of resources and the resulting outcome and quality of life for the patient. Clinical audit should be professionally led and be a part of the educational processes (see Figure 15.4). Clinical audit should also be part of routine clinical practice and an action plan may be required to improve the issue under scrutiny. Clinical audit is based on standard settings and is able to generate results that can

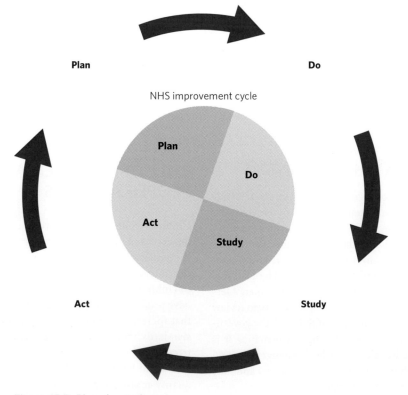

Figure 15.5 Plan, do, study, act

be used to improve patient care, but it is not the answer to every issue or a substitute for good practice (Saunders 2003). Clinical audit involves management of processes and outcomes. Clinical audit should be confidential at the patient level and informed by the views of the patient (Moules 2005, 2009; Gibbens 2010).

The NHS is always changing but issues would not necessarily need to be subjected to audit or highlighted as a result of it. Sometimes, children's nurses have an insight to an innovation or improvement that will lead to an enhanced care journey. A children's nurse may have an idea to enhance the care journey for children and young people, for example a sink or clock in the wrong place or the introduction of an interactive whiteboard to the clinical area (Davis 2011). The NHS improvement projects can be seen as ways forward. By implementing a 'plan, do, study, act' (see Figure 15.5) strategy you may direct the way forward when identifying an area for change.

There are a number of ways in which children's nurses can work to secure quality improvements for children and young people. The first steps are to ensure that the care being delivered is evidence based. By encouraging reflective practice, opportunities will arise for identifying areas for improvement or change. The thoughts and ideas can be followed up by sharing ideas with colleagues in appropriate forums for discussion, such as staff or unit meetings. At this point, an exploration of appropriate strategies for improvements to care interventions can be facilitated. From the discussions, a consensus of agreement could be reached to consider the way forward.

ACTIVITY 15.3 NHSi improvements

Risk taking is a part of everyday life. Risks are a part of children and young people's care journeys too. Look at an NHSi improvement that considers ways of identifying those factors which pose risks (**http://www.institute.nhs.uk/ safer_care/paediatric_safer_care/the_paediatric_trigger_tool.html**).

The paediatric trigger tool (PTT) measures harm caused by healthcare and can be adopted as part of routine monthly case note review. Through using the tool, it is possible to calculate the adverse event rate and identify areas of care in which most harms are occurring. It provides organisations with an unbiased measure of the incidence of iatrogenic harm experienced by their patients. It informs priorities for action and tracks improvements over time.

Second, by measuring care interventions against contemporary and projected national guidelines there is potential to identify possible discrepancies between best practice and the care interventions being received by the child or young person. The identification of a discrepancy means changing the current state of the care intervention in order to make changes to care. The children's nurse will need to identify appropriate education strategies and devise appropriate change strategies.

Third, the children's nurse needs to consider the skills and tools required to ensure that the child and young person receive appropriate care. Good effective communication skills are essential to facilitate appropriate care at the point of delivery and can reduce anxiety (Mooney 2010). It is important that the children's nurse has a working knowledge of the policies which drive and clarify quality care (see Figure 15.1). Easy access to contemporary evidence should be available and debated by the nursing team. One way of achieving this could be through a journal club by:

- a member of the team being identified to undertake a literature search on a topic
- sharing the literature either on a wall space or in a folder for a given period of time
- the identified member of the team leading a discussion on the topic at an agreed appropriate time, such as the ward meeting.

Ideally, some opportunities for debating the evidence in collaboration with other members of the team, such as physiotherapists, occupational therapists, play specialists and doctors in relation to shared topics of interest should be created.

ACTIVITY 15.4 Journal club ideas for Woodland Ward

Erin has decided that one way of facilitating Rebecca and Louize to reflect on their actions is to undertake a literature review for a journal club. Consider what topic would be appropriate for each of them to consider.

The children's nurse has a duty to listen to the views of the children and young people in their care and involve them as consumers of healthcare (DoH 2001; NMC 2008). Children and young people have a right to be heard and have information presented to them in age or needs appropriate format in accordance with Articles 12 and 13 (UNCRC 1989). There have been a rising number of consultations with children and young people or by joint consultation with them and their parents. To this end, it is not surprising that children and young people have been involved in consultation regarding 'good' and 'not so good' children's nurses.

The Department of Health gave clear indication of service user involvement; therefore, gaining the service user perspective is not a new concept. There has been a political drive to gain the views of service users on healthcare provision (DoH 1999, 2001, 2004). While adult patients are afforded a number of opportunities to have their voices heard, it would seem that engagement with children and young people as consumers of healthcare lagged behind and remains an exceptional occurrence rather than being an embedded concept.

Over time the way in which children and young people have been viewed has changed (see Chapter 4). Childhood is socially constructed and over time children and young people have been placed into the context of adults as 'human beings' and children as 'human becomings' (Qvortrup 1994). Kellett (2010) clarifies that children are citizens in society in the present and should be seen as 'beings' rather 'becomings'. Children and young people

---

RESEARCH NOTE 15.3 Consulting children and young people on what makes a 'good' nurse (Randall and Hill 2012)

The study engaged 11 young people, aged 11 to 15 years, in a consultation to ascertain the views of young people in nurse education. The consultation was over six sessions spread over half an academic term. These young people were very clear in what made a 'good' nurse which has parallels with good nursing practice, understanding patient needs, confidentiality and professionalism. The young people also had clear views on the attributes of a 'not so good' nurse. These attributes have parallels with incompetence, poor attitudes and breaches of confidentiality and lack of professionalism. These attributes are indeed in conflict with the NMC guidance.

Engagement with the process of consulting with children and young people is becoming more frequently reported in the nursing press. Children and young people are being included as service users in giving their views on the performance of children's nurses in practice at Anglia Ruskin University. Meaningful consultations can be an alternative to research with children.

Within the context of school life, there are often recognised opportunities for expressing views through school councils. Randall and Hill (2012) organised their consultation with health and educational partners.

---

have been viewed as 'social actors making interpretations of their world' (James et al. 1998). Political decisions have called for children and young people to be involved as a service user. Children and young people have often been regarded as 'passive participants of healthcare', although since 2003 there has been a political agenda to gain insight into the user's perspective (Darbyshire 1994; DoH 2004).

In recent years there have been research projects involving the 'active participation' of children and young people's views related to their interpretations of healthcare (Maconochie and McNeill

2010). The central foci of these previous projects relate to healthcare services (Doorbar 1995); service development (Lightfoot and Sloper 2004; DoH 2002); user experiences (Sartain et al. 2000); local health services (Curtis et al. 2004); involvement with quality monitoring (Moules 2005); participation in care (Coyne 2006; Gibson et al. 2010); therapeutic relationships (Mottram 2009); and the involvement of children and young people in research to ascertain colour and thematic design preferences for a children's nursing environment (Coad and Coad 2008; Coad et al. 2008).

RESEARCH NOTE 15.4 'They wouldn't know how it feels . . .': characteristics of quality care from young people's perspectives: a participatory research project (Moules 2009)

The researcher identified that children and young people have the potential to make a useful contribution to the clinical audit process and to the quality of care. A participatory research study was conducted to explore whether children and young people could be involved with monitoring the quality of hospital care. The participatory research took place with nine young people as a research team. A further 129 questionnaires were also part of the participatory study. The research identified five characteristics of quality care: 'technical expertise', 'friendly staff', 'respect', 'choices', 'explanations'.

Children clearly identified ideas arising from theorists who potentially published before their grandparents were born. Peplau put forward the idea of 'technical expert' in the 1950s. Although there have been changes in society, nursing and expectations of the NHS, Peplau's research appears to be

relevant to children today. Interestingly, there are similarities with the findings of this research on involvement with quality with the consultation by Randall and Hill where ideas of the characteristics of a children's nurse are identified. 'Friendly staff' notes a characteristic of a 'good nurse'. Explanations are important to the children in this research. In the melee of the workload this part of nursing can be rushed or overlooked and requires children's nurses to consider how they explain ideas and issues to children and young people directly. It was identified that parents have a different evaluative context to their children. Children's views could be systematically fitted into quality systems. Professionals talk in terms of quality but it is not clear what children understand by the term quality. The service user involvement agenda requires children's nurses to include the views of children and young people.

The ethos of children's nursing has always worked in family-centred care and partnership and this coexists with children's rights. Smith and Coleman (2010) clearly identify this change within the phrase 'child- and family-centred healthcare' (Chapter 1). Having considered the young people's perspective on quality through

research, it is important to consider how parents' views can make contributions to the quality of care.

From an idealistic perspective, it may have been useful to have involved service users in the development of an audit tool and audit project. Woodfield (2001) identifies that as 'consumers

PRACTICAL GUIDELINES 15.1

Nurse-facilitated discharge for children and their families into the community can be a straightforward, simple process (accounting for 80% of discharges) or it can be more complex.

Establishing a problem – the senior nursing team and the bed manager identified that a significant number of children were experiencing delayed discharges.

Rationale – to identify the issues associated with delayed discharges so that senior staff could highlight areas for change and improvement.

Developing a tool – no insight into the development of the audit tool was stated. Gibbens (2010) gives insight into the compliments received in connection with the audit project and these would seem to have been from the view of parents. While the general ethos of children's nursing recognises the importance of family-centred care, parents may not always have insight into the views of their children. Seeking the views of both parents and the child or young person would facilitate a more rounded perspective.

Peer review – a steering group was set up with ward nurses, managers and senior nursing team representatives. There was also the support of key members of the multidisciplinary team.

Trust endorsement – there was opportunity for staff to 'opt in' to the audit, undertake training and education to augment their skills. There was opportunity for empowerment through information being available and involvement with the audit process. There were reports from conferences and findings from the literature. There were discharge policies in place and there was the opportunity to consider nurse-facilitated discharge in conjunction with the trust's competency framework. There was also the opportunity to consider practical changes, risk management and accountability as part of the change.

Undertaking the audit – the audit took place over a 3-month busy period.

Data handling – the audit data at 6 months demonstrated that there was a significant increase in nurse-facilitated discharges to include 95% of the total discharges. The remaining 5% was due to changes to medications or procedure which resulted in consulting team reviews.

Sharing of results – there was a central theme of sharing information with staff throughout the project thus facilitating a 'sense of ownership' into the initiative. A series of annual reviews was planned, which included discharge planning and process reviews to ensure the policies continue to meet the aims and objectives. A scheme was developed within the trust for service users to make comments and compliments.

(Gibbens 2010).

---

of healthcare' children and young people can participate in audit processes that may require some thinking related to eliciting their view. Woodfield (2001) recognises that involving children in the audit process can be complex and would require careful consideration. Moules (2005, 2009) suggests that children have the potential to make a significant contribution to clinical audit.

Schemes for receiving service user feedback as suggestion, compliment or complaint are widespread but often these are not brought to the attention of the children or young people themselves to enable them to make their views known (Gibbens 2010). Action planning can be a useful way of guiding improvements or changes to care. These improvements can be from reviewing and refinement of the audit tool, to making substantial changes to the care or systems processes. This may lead to the management of change.

PROFESSIONAL VALUES: CARE MANAGEMENT, THE INDIVIDUAL AND TEAM WORK CARE MANAGEMENT: THE TASK

Caring for children and young people can be rewarding but can also be demanding in terms of balancing time, priorities and resources. This requires a range of skills and competencies which include observing, problem solving, planning and evaluation of clinical actions to ensure the child or young person receives the most appropriate, evidence-based care. To this end, the nursing process has been embedded into practice for over 50 years (Orlando 1961; Casey 2006; see also Chapter 1). Children's nurses have a range of assessment tools to enhance the assessment process that include: AVPU and GSC (see Chapter 8); early warning tools (Monaghan 2006; see Chapter 6); developmental assessment (see Chapter 2) and pain assessment tools (see Chapters 7 and 8) (Wong and Denver, cited in Hockenberry 2005). These assessment tools have been developed in the public, professional and employer contexts (see Figure 15.2).

The Individual Children's Nurse Leadership and Management

Children's nurses work through a range of clinical tasks during the course of a day to facilitate a well-organised holistic approach to care. Through experience a children's nurse will learn from role models, reading and reflection that there are many ways of dealing with particular situations. Each children's nurse will develop her own style or way of dealing with situations. The terms 'leadership' and 'management' are used interchangeably at times but there are key differences (see Table 15.3). There are a range of leadership and management styles and often the children's nurse will develop an 'eclectic' style. Adair's leadership model with be applied to the case study within this section.

Table 15.3 Leadership styles

Leadership styles	
Behavioural styles (Lewin et al. 1939)	Behaviour styles are dependent on the culture of organisation in which the leader is working or the situation the leader is facing These include: **autocratic:** the leader giving clear but behaviour controlling instructions **democratic:** everyone having a say about how a situation is dealt with **laissez-faire:** leader 'takes a back seat' and subordinates 'do their own thing' **bureaucracy:** following rules and instructions to the letter
Theory X and Theory Y (McGregor 1960)	**Theory X:** central principle of Theory X is direction and control through a centralised system of organisation and the exercise of authority. It is assumed that people are lazy and unmotivated, working to survive and must be coerced, controlled and threatened with punishment if the organisation is to achieve its objective. It assumes that the average person avoids responsibility, prefers to be directed, lacks ambition and values security, and that motivation occurs only at the physiological and security levels
	Theory Y: work is seen as natural as play or rest and that people will exercise self-direction and self-control in the service of objectives to which they are committed. Given the right conditions the average worker can learn to accept and to seek responsibility. Work itself is seen as motivating and rewarding and the environment itself key to motivation
Contingency approach (Fiedler 1960)	**Effective leaders:** will adapt their style and behaviour to the environment, the task, the situation and the people
Trait theory of leadership	**Leadership style:** considered that the leader can be chosen for the traits they possess in varying quantities **Emergent traits:** include intelligence and the ability to problem solve; initiative, independence and inventiveness; self-assurance and self-confidence Effectiveness traits include charisma
Situational leadership (Blanchard et al. 1969)	**This style of leadership** supports growth and development of team members. There is no single best fit and the style is defined by followers' needs. There are four styles: **directing**, giving clear instructions **coaching**, giving lessons or teaching them 'on the job' **supporting**, facilitating subordinates to sustain the situation **delegating**, sharing the task required to care for the child or young person
Action-centred leadership (Adair 1993)	**The effective leader** has to: **achieve** the task **develop** the individual **build** and maintain the team Takes account of **variables** Leader-preferred style, follower-preferred style, task and environment

ACTIVITY 15.5 Personal reflection on clinical deterioration

Reflect on a situation where a child or young person was showing signs of clinical deterioration that led to a resuscitation situation with a successful outcome.

Consider:
● Which leadership style was evident?
● What the situation and outcome would be like if a democratic leadership style were used?
● What the situation and outcome would be like if a laissez-faire leadership style were used?
● What the situation and outcome would be like if a bureaucratic leadership style were used?

Action-Centred Leadership

Adair (1990) identifies that there are a number of elements that need to come together in order to move forward as a leader:

● the individual
● the task
● the team.

Applying these concepts to children's nursing provides an 'aide memoire' for thinking about managing care. Combining ideas from the NMC, Adair et al. (1982) and Dimond (2011, 2010) demonstrate how theories are framed differently and are embedded in practice as fused layers. Rebecca, Louize and Erin, as qualified members of staff, will take on different role expectations within their positions on the ward and the care or intervention they are undertaking. At times, they will be planning care or they will be fact finding, problem solving, participating and sharing information (Practical Guidelines 15.2).

In considering Erin's higher authority as matron, she will be adopting a range of 'roles of a nurse', which include, judge, ameliorator, arbitrator and negotiator in trying to diffuse the situation between Rebecca and Louize (see Table 15.4). There is potential for Erin to use her position of authority (power) to apply sanctions as a part of a disciplinary process, if deemed necessary (see Figure 15.6).

Management/Transactional Leadership

Transactional leadership is defined as a leader or manager who functions in a caretaker role and is focused on day-to-day operations. A transactional leader or manager identifies the needs of the followers and provides rewards to meet those needs in exchange for expected performance within the institutional culture. Effort produced and performance obtained is as expected (Huber 2011). Transactional leaders or managers are considered to be a person in a position of employment who is deemed accountable and responsible for achieving the management tasks such as integrating resources, using the functions of planning, organising, supervising, staffing, evaluating, negotiating and representing the organisation who employs them. In sum, the person has been afforded a position in the organisation and has also been given a degree of power, authority and autonomy to enable the work to be undertaken effectively.

Considering unpublished research analysis of a 4 week diary of a Band 7 nurse (Practical Guidelines 15.2), it is possible to see the role expectations of the person or how others perceived

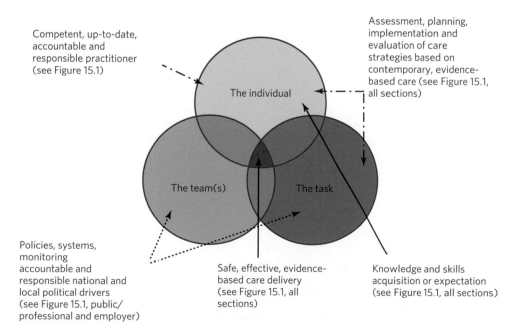

Figure 15.6 Using authority to apply sanctions

Table 15.4 Ideas on power

French and Raven (1959)	Payne (2000)	Related to Woodland Ward case study
Reward power	A thinks B can give rewards	Louize may think that Erin can reward her for bringing Rebecca's mistake to light
Coercive power	Where A thinks B could damage or punish	Rebecca may feel that Louize is a threat to her position on the ward and will 'outshine' her
Referent power	Where A identifies with B	Louize could be identifying with Rebecca recognising how easy it would be to leave the medication at the nurse station yet Rebecca sees her as a threat
Expert power	Where A thinks B is skilful or knows more	Louize may believe that Rebecca is more knowledgeable than she is Likewise, Rebecca may believe she has more knowledge and skills than Louize
Legitimate power (or authority)	Where A accepts a general view in society that B should be able to influence things is correct	Rebecca and Louize respect Erin's position and the power of knowledge and associated expertise

the role. The diary analysis also gives insight into the types of activity that were at the heart of the role and the transactional leadership or management styles that were predominantly used. The diary analysis has also integrated ideas arising in the Woodland Ward case study to enable them to be contextualised.

PRACTICAL GUIDELINES 15.2

Role expectations	Relates to	Recognised leadership styles	Related to the Woodland Ward case study
Planner	Organising Problem solving Decision making		When acting in the 'norming' and 'performing' quadrants Rebecca, Louize and Erin form positive alliances/coalitions to achieve appropriate care for children and young people
Reporter and communication cascade	Information sharing	Directive	
Meeting/conversation convener	Seeking collaborative view		When acting in the 'norming' quadrant collaboration based on knowledge sharing is at an optimum point
Judge	Decision making Difference of opinion		Erin will need to diffuse the 'storming' situation between Rebecca and Louize and bring the situation back to the 'norming' and 'performing' stages
Fact finder	Gaining information Analysis of information Handling information Feedback mechanisms	Facilitative	When acting in the 'norming' and 'performing' quadrants, Rebecca, Louize and Erin form positive alliances/coalitions to achieve appropriate care for children and young people (see Figures 15.1 and 15.7)
Negotiator	Achieving balance emergency/planned admissions and discharges		

Role expectations	Relates to	Recognised leadership styles	Related to the Woodland Ward case study
Colleague	Assisting staff with gaining clinical skills Assisting staff with clinical challenges		
Listener	Advice and support		
Meeting attendee/ 'rounds' attendee	Participation Sharing knowledge, experience and information	Participatory	
Problem solver	Dealing with clinical issues Dealing with staffing issues Exploring options	Directive, facilitative or participatory	Erin was to diffuse the difference of opinion between Rebecca and Louize based on a poor decision to leave medication on the nurses' station and the subsequent conflict arising from it (see Figure. 15.7, 'storming' quadrant)
Ameliorator/arbitrator	Judging situations Difference of opinion Decision making Advising on conflict issues in clinical area Dealing with staff conflict	Facilitative Facilitative or participatory Directive, facilitative	
Communicator	Information sharing	Directive, facilitative or participatory	Rebecca, Louize and Erin working in collaboration to care for children and young people (see Figure 15.7, 'norming' and 'performing' quadrants)

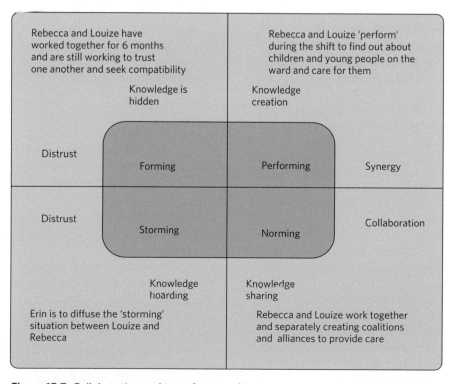

Figure 15.7 Collaboration and team functionality

Source: Goodman and Clemow (2010)

The IntraProfessional Team

The intraprofessional team could be considered as an alternative term for the nursing team that provides care for the child or young person and their parents or carers. Tuckman (1965) developed a model to describe how teams worked together through the 'forming', 'storming', 'norming' and 'performing' stages. Tuckman and Jensen (1977) added the word 'adjourning' to the model as this brings closure to a project, task or team. Payne (2000) identified that team work required competence, communication, cooperation, coordination and collaboration. Improving communication can impact on improved learning and enables team members to develop a sense of belonging that may lead to increased motivation. Teams require a 'settling in' period because they develop over time (Martin 2006). Teams are able to achieve more by working together and sharing the workload. The ultimate aim of teamwork is achieving integrated and seamless care. When teams are functioning or performing well, all team members contribute to the care. Teams value difference and are highly structured. Teams are able to focus on the key problems and set appropriate clear goals, encourage participation and to maintain high standards of care. Well-functioning teams are able to build trust and have external recognition for the work they have undertaken. A well-functioning team will keep clear records and are also able to manage and confront conflict.

After studying the performance of teams, Belbin identified nine key roles required to make any team function well. Belbin's roles are based on enduring personality attributes (Handy 1999; Martin 2006; Goodman and Clemow 2010). These roles are:

- **Plant** who has an idea 'seed' and 'plants' it with the team. It is often someone who has a creative mind, with freedom of thought and an ability to solve problems.
- **Resource investigator** is enthusiastic, is a good communicator and is able to explore opportunities in pursuing contacts and initial ideas. Resource investigators glean ideas from other sources.
- **Coordinator** is able to delegate appropriately, promotes decision making and ensures that all members of the team are acting appropriately according to the decisions made.
- **Shaper** thrives on pressure and ensures that team members are encouraged in their endeavours. The shaper is always sensitive to the emotional feelings of the rest of the team.
- **Monitor evaluator** is able to recognise biases and is often able to explore the options.
- **Teamworker** is able to see more than one side of the argument. The team worker supports the team by listening, encouraging, conflict resolution and harmonising the group to avoid conflicts.
- **Implementer** can turn ideas into practical actions and is a methodical, trustworthy worker. Her actions can lead to team cohesion but she may be slow to respond to changes to plans.
- **Completer/finisher** pays attention to details and ensures that deadlines are met but may not always be the most popular person in the team.
- **Specialist** is a person who provides knowledge and skills that are unique and is passionate about her area of expertise. She may lack interest in other areas and dwell on technicalities.

InterProfessional and Interagency Teams

The interprofessional and interagency teams operate in similar ways to the intraprofessional team. There are differences due to the fact that members of the interprofessional team have different professional backgrounds and values. One of the main considerations may be who will oversee the work and who makes contributions. There have been cases connected to safeguarding that have questioned how interprofessional teams function, particularly after the Victoria Climbié and Peter Connolly cases (Laming 2009) (see Figure 15.7 and Table 15.5).

If teams do not have a leader, then they may not have a solid base and this can give rise to the potential for misunderstanding, miscommunication, decrease in respect for team members and conflict. This could have an impact on decision making within the team which could become vague and reduce the ability to review the team's performance. This could also impact on a lack of objectives, imprecise vision and seeing the strategic view point or even ignore the bigger picture. They may not embrace the interprofessional approach and there may be distrust (Taylor 2007; see Figure 15.x).

Overall, whether it be working in an intraprofessional or an interprofessional team there are distinct advantages or disadvantages that need to be considered and worked through in order to achieve good-quality care that is in the best interests of the child or young person.

Where social policy, effective communication, breaking down of preconceived ideas about other professionals and proactive planning come together, there will be a greater opportunity for successful collaborative working where all members of the team are working in unison.

Manifestation of Power and Influence

Leadership and power are synonymous with one another (Bennis and Nanus 1997). Power can be both a positive and a negative force that can have a direct or indirect impact on the care of children and young people. French and Raven (1959) identified that power is divided into five categories:

- **resource power** (power over resources)
- **information power** (power over/to information)
- **expert power** (specialist knowledge/skill)
- **coercive power** (physical power or punishment-centred approach)
- **position power** (formal position)
- **personal power** (personality/charisma) (see Table 15.x).

Huber (2000) frames power differently and includes coalition/alliances, blocking, ingratiation, exchange, sanctions, assertiveness, upward appeal and rationality (Figure 15.8).

There has been a longstanding acceptance of the importance of interprofessional working at government, professional and interprofessional levels (DoH 2000; NMC 2008; Laming 2009; Ofsted 2010; Munro 2011). There has been an emphasis on interprofessional education from a range of literature sources.

Table 15.5 Interprofessional working

Advantages	Disadvantages
Collective sharing responsibility	Time-consuming consultation
More efficient use of staff (enabling development of specialists)	Increase in admin and communication cost
Effective service provision (overall service planning)	Conflicting and different leadership styles, values and language
Satisfying working environment (more relevant and supportive services)	Reduced independence and autonomy of practitioners
Better risk management, auditing of services and research	Difficult for professionals to make individual decisions
Ease of access for children and families	Inequalities in status
Development of new ideas, roles and ways of working	Minimises the importance of professional differences
Opportunity for shared supervision	Risk of professional collusion
Enhancement of professional skills	Separate educational backgrounds
Avoidance of isolation for practitioners	Blurring roles
Efficient sharing of education and resources	
Promotes professional openness	

Source: Walker and Thurston (2006)

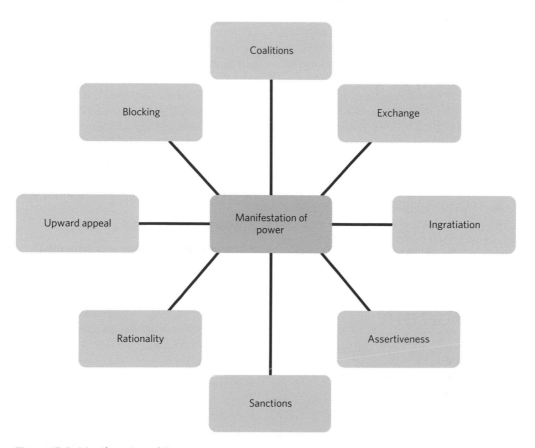

Figure 15.8 Manifestation of Power
Source: Huber (2000)

Coalition and Alliances: Collaboration Working

RESEARCH NOTE 15.5 Role of nurses in interprofessional health and social care teams (Miers and Pollard 2009)

The study built on earlier evaluations of three pre-qualifying courses from midwifery, nursing, occupational therapy, physiotherapy, diagnostic and therapeutic radiography and social work. There were 34 participants of whom 24 participants reported that interprofessional working was rated as good in their areas of practice. Nurses saw themselves as the 'pivot' or 'a cog in a wheel'. It was acknowledged that 'professionals bring a mix of abilities to support interprofessional collaboration, including a relaxed view of role overlap and ambiguity'. Key skills were identified as communication, interpersonal relationship skills, teamwork skills, knowledge of roles, personal qualities and personal attributes. In a further research study, Pollard (2009) reports that hierarchical relationships in the paediatric unit are the 'norm' and that students only spoke when spoken too. Pollard (2009) identified that this is not the case with other students from other disciplines. An implication for children's nursing practice is that nurse managers have a key role in nurturing nurses' collaborative skills and addressing skills deficits.

D'Amour et al. (2005) review 17 articles related to interprofessional working and identified that sharing, partnership, independency and power were key concepts. Taylor (2007) suggests that power is the currency of leadership that determines who has the power, how that power is used and who can access the power bases.

Transformational Leadership

Much has been written and recorded about 'third way' politics and the modernisation agenda for the NHS. Leaders and followers raise one another to higher levels of morality and motivation. Moral leadership has a transforming effect on both and brings out the best in each party. The focus on professional values provides a vision that excites, yet is feasible to achieve and sustain. It provides opportunity for dialogue and actively listening to those working at 'grassroots' level to those responsible for the provision of services. It was this type of strategy that led to the provision of the National Service Framework for children, young people and maternity services. By sharing experiences of practice and establishing an ethos of trust and mutual support, enabled the first Children's Commissioner, this Sir Al Aynsley-Green, to listen to the views of those professionals at grassroots level and to develop a strategy that was concerned with meeting their needs. The views of children, young people and their families were also sought to explore all options to formulate a robust strategy for a 10-year plan.

CONFLICT MANAGEMENT

Conflict can be caused by a range of reasons from personality clashes to clashes related to care management. Communication is potentially a primary cause of conflict. Poor time management of some can also cause conflict with other staff members who manage their time more efficiently. There could be a lack of understanding of why something has occurred a particular way, for example the 'custom and practice' culture rather than an 'evidence-based' culture. It may be that there are incompatible goals (issues becoming polarised). Role conflict can cause conflict, particularly if one person feels 'undermined' or 'usurped'. Conflict can also be caused by situations being left in the hope the problem will disappear, or failure to agree to the issue being passed up the organisation for resolution resulting in 'them and us' situations (see Table 15.6).

Seeking to resolve conflict can be a challenging situation for all parties. There are a number of strategies which can be useful to consider conflict resolution (see Tables 15.6 and 15.7). Adair (1986) suggests one of the first strategies should be to seek to depersonalise the issue and place it into the context of policies and guidelines.

Achieving a resolution to conflict will take time and careful management of the situation. Erin will be seeking to turn this into a successfully resolved situation but it may be that the situation can only be partially addressed in the timeframe (see Tables 15.6, 15.7 and 15.8).

MANAGEMENT OF RESOURCES

Physical Resources

Purchasing equipment can vary from weekly occurrences with the 'everyday consumables' (such as needles, syringes, clinical wipes) to the 'big purchases' (hoists, profiling beds, wheelchairs). The environment and infrastructure play a part when considering physical resources. Consideration of equipment in relation to health and safety issues is important, along with the equipment's suitability for the task.

The National Patient Safety Agency (2005) says:

- All equipment should be fit for purpose and well maintained.
- Mandatory training programmes and record keeping should be implemented.
- Tracking equipment from serial numbers is important.

Table 15.6 Types of conflict

Type	Related to Woodland Ward	
Intra-sender	Conflicting instructions and decisions from a single source	Rebecca's decision-making conflicted with hospital policy and could have had an impact on health and safety factors
Inter-sender	Conflicting instructions and decisions but from 2+ sources	Rebecca's decision making conflicted with her own internal voice of conscience, national and local hospital policy and could have had an impact on health and safety factors Rebecca may also be trying to ingratiate herself to Erin and senior managers by staying late
Inter-role	Having more than one role	It is not clear whether Rebecca was overseeing the care of more than one group of children and young people If Rebecca were overseeing Woodland Ward as well as having a group of patients to care for, there is the greater potential for error
Person–role conflict of organisation	Personal role	Rebecca may find being a leader and manager challenging It is evident from the case study that Rebecca is on duty for longer than she is employed to do so. On the face of this, Rebecca seems to 'distrust' other staff members to deliver appropriate care There is the potential for tiredness or fatigue to impact on conscious and unconscious decision making
Inter-person	Between two managers – for resources	Louize was more junior to Rebecca Louize may believe that her skills match or exceed those of Rebecca and may be seeking more 'power' It could also be that Rebecca perceived that staying late put her in a position of power
Intra-group	Within a group e.g. facing change	Louize was in the early stages of her post, the status quo of the staff had changed It is unknown whether Louize had been a student on Woodland Ward, however, a settling time following reforming may be useful
Inter-group	Between two groups in the organisation	
Role ambiguity	Not having clear guidelines for the role	It may be that Rebecca was not aware of, or had lost sight of the clear guidelines on the administration of medication
Role overload	Too much expected of the individual	Rebecca had responsibility for the ward and could have made a decision to delegate.

Table 15.7 Approaches to conflict resolution

		Related to Woodland Ward
Avoiding	Unassertive and uncooperative	If Erin cannot diffuse the situation then conflict between Rebecca and Louize will continue and there is the potential for avoiding further conflict
Accommodating	Cooperative but unassertive	If a partial resolution is achieved then Rebecca and Louize will work with each other but will not 'stand up' for actions or issues they do not agree with
Compromising	Assertive and cooperative	If Erin resolves the situation between Rebecca and Louize then there is potential for the conflict to be resolved and the 'norming' phase to be re-established in collaborative working together for the benefit of patients or compromising due to priorities in care and working with each other It is important to note that there is a fine line between assertiveness and aggression so both Rebecca and Louize will need to be able to discern between the two
Collaborating	Assertive and cooperative	
Competing	Assertive but uncooperative	If competition remains between Rebecca and Louize they are likely to be uncooperative with each other which can impact on the care of children and young people If the competition remains an issue, then there is the potential for one or the other of them to 'sabotage' the other's actions Erin may need to impose 'sanctions'

Table 15.8 Resolving conflict

Resolution to conflict	Related to Woodland Ward
WIN–WIN	If Erin can diffuse the conflict situation between Rebecca and Louize then the 'norming' and 'performing' stages can be restored
LOSE–WIN	If Erin favours the actions of either Louize or Rebecca
LOSE–LOSE	If a child or young person finds and takes the medication left on the nurses' station then everyone loses as patient care is compromised, the error needs to be escalated and the organisation could be brought into disrepute

There is clear evidence that things go wrong when:

- systems break down
- staff take shortcuts
- communication breaks down
- responsibility is ill-defined
- training systems are poor
- coordination of equipment records, maintenance and repairs is poor.

Financial Resources

Budget control and management play an important part of care within the NHS and while the needs of the individual patients are paramount, the children's nurse should be mindful of the cost of items and of minimising wastage (Wolfe et al. 2011). Budget management can be set at either ward level with the ward manager, or with a group of wards at matron/lead nurse level or at the higher level of the most senior nurse in the directorate/division.

Human Resources

Human resources account for the largest proportion of the NHS budget. Investment in staff development is ever changing and upskilling staff is time consuming. There will be a calculation of the staffing requirements for a particular area which is known as the establishment. The establishment takes into account the skill mix, that is to say the number of particular types of staff and the grades that are required to ensure the safe and effective running of the specific clinical area. This requires strategic planning and is reviewed when there is a change to the specific clinical area. Hurst et al. (2008) identify that nurses can select from a confusing collection of tools that can help calculate the number of nurses required to care for an estimated acuteness of patients within an inpatient setting. Hurst et al. (2008) identified a method which is useful for estimating staffing establishment and short-term planning when a higher number of patients are more dependent on nursing staff. Some of these tools have been based on time and motion studies, some have been based on task and time requirements and others by 'multipliers'. During winter pressures or during unplanned, acute, high dependency admissions the need may arise to adjust the establishment to deal with the immediate planning for unexpected events. Good budgetary management will have contingency provision for this type of situation.

Due to movement of staff, skill mix can change and new priorities will become evident. It is at this point where personal development plans may indicate staff with particular interests for further development. This fits with the notion of lifelong learning and evidence-based practice (NMC 2011). The individual's performance at work can be determined by the extrinsic rewards (external rewards for example salary and status), intrinsic rewards (internal rewards like self-recognition and worthwhileness). If human resources and performance were to be related to Maslow's hierarchy of needs, this could have motivational effects on staff and encourage them to engage with staff development strategies (see Table 15.9).

> ### ACTIVITY 15.6 Staff allocation
>
> Compile a list, with a clear rationale, of what must be considered when deciding on the allocation of staff to an allocation of group of patients.

ORGANISATION OF CARE

Time Management

Time management can have a significant impact on the care and management of children and young people. As children's nurses become more confident in their practice and have higher levels of motivation, their time management skills become more honed. Time is a precious commodity and poor time management has an impact on costs to service delivery (Huber 2010). Care interventions can be planned across the shift pattern rather than condensing it all into a few hours. The children's nurse needs to consider building in time management strategies to deal with any emergency or unplanned situation they are presented with. A few moments checking the functionality of oxygen and suction supplies at the beginning of a shift could save valuable seconds if faced with a resuscitation situation. Routine practice has been debated within the nursing press with supporters and critics. Barton and Semple (2011) point out those routines have a place in the NHS as it facilitates the coordination within organisations and in nursing could provide a positive outcome. Barton and Semple (2011) made comparisons with the airline industry which relies on preflight check lists to ensure no action is omitted. They oppose the use of routine as nursing care is individualised, doing the right thing at the right time to facilitate compassion and dignity. Without advocating the return to a situation where ritualistic nursing practice was the order of the day (Walsh and Ford 1989), it would seem a sensible option that providing the routine practice had an evidence base and a substantial part of the child or young person's care is individualised, the two concepts can work together in contemporary children's nursing.

Decision Making

Decision making is a concept undertaken by everyone as a part of everyday living. When decisions are made a range of options are considered and selected on their perceived appropriateness for the task at hand (see Figure 15.X). Byrnes (2002) highlighted that there was a four-step phase to decision making:

- setting a goal
- compiling options for producing that goal
- rank ordering the options
- selecting the highest ranked alternative.

Table 15.9 Maslow, Hertzberg and work ethic

Physiological (hunger and thirst)	Good salary and conditions
Safety (environment)	Job prospects lead to feelings of security
Love (valued team member)	Need to belong and feel accepted
Esteem (self-respect and achievement)	Status recognition
Self-actualisation	Developing one's own potential through personal development plans, staff development and personal study

Saccomano and Pinto-Zipp (2011) confirm that delegation is an essential skill in the nurse's repertoire as there is a requirement to delegate and remain accountable for the task. Jefferies et al. (2010) add to the conundrum by suggesting that nurses traditionally document patient care at the end of a shift, yet, by implication this means some of the 'audit trail' of decision making in respect of patient care may be become untraceable (see Practical Guidelines 15.3). This would mean that if a child or young person's care become a point of court scrutiny, absent data would not be able to prove or disprove an intervention took place. The NMC (2008) is very clear that a nurse is responsible for actions or omissions to care. On balance, choosing key times to write in the child or young person's notes may improve the quality of the documentation. By the same token, language and meaning changes over time therefore the nurse writing in the child or young person's notes should use plain English language and registrants and students should not be tempted to use 'text speak'. This is simply because the child or young person's notes would become a legal document. In advertisements for nursing posts, words such as 'ward manager', 'ward coordinator' and 'team leader' will convey insight into the organisational culture.

RESEARCH NOTE 15.6 How do children's nurses make clinical decisions? Two preliminary studies (Twycross and Powls 2006)

The research endeavoured to gain an understanding how children's nurses make clinical decisions using the 'think aloud' technique. The participants were presented with clinical scenarios and asked to think aloud. The research analysed verbal protocols to provide insight into how children's nurses made decisions. The research also explored whether there was a difference between the decisions made by experienced nurses and less experienced nurses. All participants appeared to use backward reasoning strategies, which is a non-expert decision-making characteristic and was regardless of their level of expertise. Experienced and less experienced nurses collected similar additional information before planning the nursing interventions, supporting the conjecture that they were functioning at a non-expert level. In relation to decision making, no differences were seen in the information collected by graduate and non-graduate nurses. Several strategies to support nurses' clinical decision making have been proposed but need testing to ascertain their effectiveness. In clinical practice nurses make numerous decisions throughout the course of the shift. Suboptimal decision-making strategies may adversely affect the quality of nursing care provided. It is imperative, therefore, to ascertain how nurses make clinical decisions and the factors that may influence the decision-making strategies used.

Delegation

The NMC (2008) gives clear guidance that in delegating a task a registrant should check that the person to whom the task is delegated understands the instructions and checks that the task has been undertaken to an acceptable standard. The NMC (2008) is also explicit that registrants must supervise and support staff that they are responsible for. Gopee and Galloway (2009) highlight that nurses are responsible for delegating tasks which are achievable by appropriate interprofessional team members, within their professional boundary. There is clear indication that delegation considers a range of factors (Ellis et al. 2004; Zerwekh et al. 2006).

When considering the delegated action of medicines administration, a children's nurse is dealing with a complex and possibly a contentious area (Crawford 2011). Children's nurses should have a working knowledge base of frequently used medications and know the pharmacokinetic (how the body handles the medication over time) and pharmacodynamic actions of them (the effects of the medication on the body) (Blair 2011). Hall (2010) clearly articulates that nursing skills for medicine management should include legal and ethical perspectives, manual dexterity, technical skills and knowledge. Conroy et al. (2012) debate whether there is a case for single or double checking of medicines due to the related complexities. Conroy et al. (2012) clearly emphasise that it is an unacceptable risk for one nurse to read a prescription to another nurse as both should independently check the medication for administration (Table 15.10).

Crawford (2012) reminds children's nurses that there is a set of key principles by which medicine administration takes place and there are legal aspects to this process as well. These include:

- right way
- right child or young person
- right time
- right amount
- right circumstance.

It is equally important to remember that children's nurses are accountable and responsible for any action or omission in the care journey. Documentation is therefore of great importance to record actions. If an adverse reaction arises it is important to report it appropriately. It is extremely important to consider the safety of other patients and supervise the journey of the medication through the entire process:

- right communication
- right supervision.

Table 15.10 Medicines knowledge

Pharmacokinetics (movement of the medication)		Pharmacodynamics (actions of the medication on the body)	
Absorption	Route travelled by medication from the point it enters the body to the blood or lymphatic systems	Idiosyncrasy	A peculiarity of a medication
		Skin reactions	Each medicine may produce a different pharmacodynamic response on the body's systems
Distribution	The transportation of the medication around the body	Blood Gastrointestinal upset	
			Manufacturer information sheets provide insight to these
Metabolism	Chemical converting process to change its form for using and excretion	Central nervous system	
		Photosensitivity	
Excretion	Process by which medications and other substances are removed from the body		
		Tolerance	Acceptable parameters
		Dependence	Reliance

CASE STUDY REVIEW 15.1

Rebecca had delegated responsibility for the administration of medicines and had failed to ensure the medications were securely placed in the clinical environment. It is not clear from the case study whether this was an isolated occurrence of medicines being left at the nurse's station or whether it had become custom and practice as a result of bad habits leading to poor practice. It is in the best interests of the children and young people to follow evidence-based practice at all times and not leave medicines unattended, even for a short time. Rebecca's actions posed a risk for Woodland Ward.

Communication

Communication is central to the caring process and establishing rapport with the child or young person and their family (NMC 2010). Communication is required to establish the factual information about the child or young person to aid the assessment process or clinical interventions. Therapeutic relationships are built on trust, mutual understanding and effective communication (NMC 2010) (see Figure 15.9). Children's nurses are adept at conducting conversations at different levels of understanding in the same timeframe to the child and young person, the parents or carers and maybe other professionals. Conversations can overlap and this gives rise to the potential for confusion, lost meaning or lost data.

The children's nurse may aim direct conversation related to specific questions at the child or the parent and there may be points which could be aimed at either party (see Figure 15.10). The parent may direct responses to the children's nurse and involve the child using statements such as 'that's right, isn't it' or 'you tell the nurse' to augment the quality of the responses. Gibson et al. (2010) confirmed that at times children will want to be in the foreground of the communication and at other times they are happy to be in the background. Although Gibson et al. (2010) undertook the research with children with cancer journey pathways, these can be transferred to the wide population of children and young people in hospital.

The children's nurse also requires skills in appropriate delegation, prioritisation of care, embracing conflict and managing or leading change to ensure care delivery is contemporary and evidenced based (Lewin 1951; Kotter 1996). There are times when the children's nurse uses intuition about particular aspects of care (Kosowski and Roberts 2003).

Professional communication is also crucial when performing specific key tasks as a part of the care and management process. Communication is a vital and continuous component of the management repertoire. In considering communication within children's nursing, it is evident that there are three key areas where

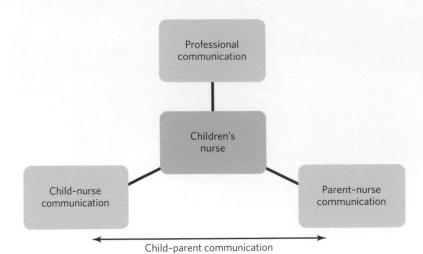

Figure 15.9 Communication networks

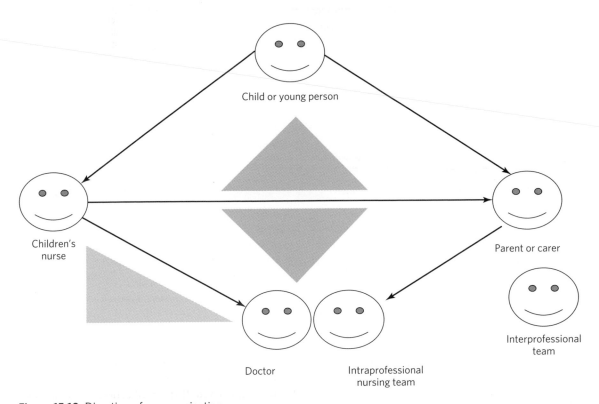

Figure 15.10 Direction of communication

communication needs to be accurate and fully informed to ensure appropriate care is delivered: the handover, ward round and the administration of medications. Each of these events presents the children's nurses with a problem or challenge for which a resolution has to be found. In order to do this, 'fact finding' (seeking information) takes place that, in the event of a handover, prepares staff for taking on responsibility for care at the beginning of a shift or relinquishing care at the end of the shift. Gathering information equips staff to fully understand the needs of the child or young person. The varying options to care can be considered and there should be opportunities for clarification and exploring the options. After considering a range of options, it is then possible

to make an informed decision based on the presenting evidence, knowledge and evidence-based best practice, which leads to a full or partial resolution and then a re-evaluation of the process will take place at a key point in time. Nursing handovers are predominantly uni-professional, whereas the ward round follows a predominantly interprofessional focus (see Practical Guidelines 15.X, 15.X, Figure 15.11 and Table 15.X).

The administration of medications is predominantly a nursing duty, where the nurse takes accountability and responsibility for the administration of medications to children and young people on Woodland Ward. Erin, Rebecca and Louize would all have experienced this activity many times and would have developed expertise

PRACTICAL GUIDELINES 15.3

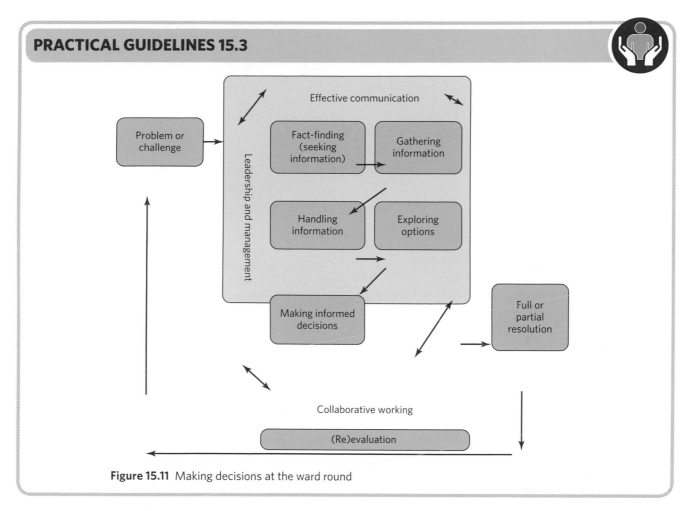

Figure 15.11 Making decisions at the ward round

in the administration of medications. On each occasion where the administration of medications was required a 'fact-finding' (seeking information) period would take place to ensure that the right medication and right dose were legible and appropriately prescribed, according to the child's weight, formulary directions, policies and the 'three whats' formula (Crawford 2012). If an incorrect amount had been administered, it could have disastrous or life-threatening consequences. Merely misreading an LCD or keeping a solar-powered calculator in a pocket can have the potential to give incorrect readings. Correct and careful calculation is essential:

$$\frac{\text{What you want}}{\text{What you have}} \quad \times \quad \text{What is the volume amount in ml}$$

Another way of expressing this may be:

$$\frac{\text{Strength required}}{\text{Stock strength}} \quad \times \quad \text{volume of stock solution}$$

Example: you have a bottle of Ciprofloxacin 500 mg in 5 mls. Prescription is for a dose of 750 mgs. How many mls would you give?

$$\frac{\text{What you want}}{\text{What you have}} \quad = \quad \frac{\text{Ciprofloxacin 750mg}}{\text{Ciprofloxacin 500mg}}$$

$$\times \underline{\text{What is the volume amount in ml}} = 5 \text{ mls}$$

$$\frac{750}{500} \quad = 1.5 \quad \times \quad 5 \text{ mls} = 7.5 \text{ mls}$$

The medication would also need to be given at the right time in order to be effective and retain a therapeutic effect. Randall and Hill (2012) reported that children and young people want their medication when they needed it and this should ideally be considered with the other options. Gathering information equips staff to fully understand the needs of the child or young person and the effectiveness of the medication being administered. If the medication was an antipyretic and there are two common preparations (paracetamol and ibuprofen). There are varying options to the timing of the last dose and whether there were any contraindications for choosing a particular preparation thus Erin, Rebecca and Louize can explore the options and make an informed decision. It may be that changes to the environment such as opening a window or encouraging an improved fluid intake should also be considered to lead to a full or partial resolution and then a re-evaluation of the process will take place at a key point in time. It is crucial that the information is appropriately and accurately recorded to enhance ongoing care and management of high temperature.

The simple action of the administration of paracetamol or ibuprofen requires effective communication between the nurse

ACTIVITY 15.7 Charlie is due his antiepileptic medication

Charlie is 2 years old and is due to have his anti-epileptic medication. Mum says he needs his Epilim. The generic name is sodium valproate and comes as 200 mg in 5 ml doses. The prescription is 150 mg of sodium valproate due at 8 am.

Talk through the procedure of administration of medicines with a colleague or write it down.

Consider the right strategy.

What now? How are you going to approach this?

Problems you may face?

ACTIVITY 15.8 Potential error in the administration of medicines

It is 8.30 am and you have just had handover from the night staff who have gone home. You are in charge of the ward and one of the staff nurses comes to you in a distraught state.

She reports that she has just given an IV antibiotic to a child on the ward while the mother was not in the room. On her return, the child's mother informed staff nurse that the night staff had already given an IV just before they went home.

How do you handle the situation?

and the doctor, with the support of the pharmacy department to check the dosages and the porters to transport the medication to the ward or department: this requires effective collaboration. Rebecca left the medication at the nurses' station so this would imply that the policies and guidelines were not wholly adhered to, leaving the children and young people on the ward exposed to a breach in safety and risk of harm. Rebecca's employers would have systems in place for events such as these through the risk assessment strategies. Louize was potentially advocating for her patients but may not have understood the distinction between aggressive and assertive behaviours.

Management of Change

There are many reasons why change may be required and there are a range of theories as to how change may take place. There are a range of ways in which children's nurses can work to secure quality improvements for children and young people. The first steps are to ensure that the care being delivered is evidence based. By encouraging reflective practice, opportunities will arise for identifying areas for improvement or change. The thoughts and ideas can be followed up by sharing ideas with colleagues at appropriate forums for discussion such as staff or unit meetings. At this point, an exploration of appropriate strategies for improvement to care interventions can be facilitated. From the

discussions a consensus of agreement could be reached to consider the way forward.

Second, by measuring care interventions against contemporary and projected national guidelines there is potential to identify possible discrepancies between best practice and the care interventions being received by the child or young person. The identification of a discrepancy means changing the current state of the care intervention and in order to make changes to care, the children's nurse will need to identify appropriate education strategies and devise appropriate change strategies.

Third, the children's nurse needs to consider the skills and tools required to ensure that the child and young person receive good-quality, consistent care. Good effective communication skills are essential to facilitate appropriate care at the point of delivery. It is important that the children's nurse has a working knowledge of the policies that drive and clarify quality care (see Table 15.X). Easy access to contemporary evidence should be available and debated by the nursing team.

Models of Change

Management of change can be a daunting prospect when facing the change process for the first time. Lewin (1951) put forward a model of change (see Table 15.11).

Table 15.11 Lewin's model of change

Unfreezing	There is problem awareness
	People need to acknowledge that there will be an improvement if changes are made
	Preparations for change made
Moving	Moving towards the change by identifying the problem and setting out the aims and objectives. The change can then be implemented
Refreezing	Stabilisation of the change
	Often people return to the old way of doing things
	Often structural changes are necessary for stabilisation to take place

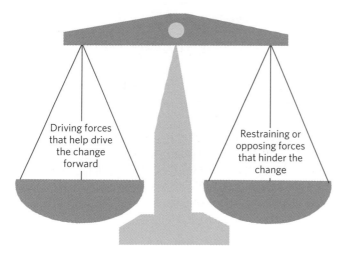

Figure 15.12 Lewin force field analysis

Lewin (1951) also put forward the notion of force field analysis to demonstrate how helping forces can push forward changes and resisting forces can be instrumental in hindering the change (see Figure 15.12).

Other authors have adapted Lewin's ideas and have added their own perspectives. Lippitt and Lippitt (1973) adapted Lewin's ideas on change management to produce a new model.

1 Diagnose the problem.
2 Assess motivation and capacity for change.
3 Assess change agent's resources.
4 Select progressive objectives for change.
5 Define role of change agent.
6 Maintain the change.
7 Terminate the helping relationship.

Managing change in practice may mean that there is a need to engage with changing attitudes of staff involved. This may be a change in cognitive behaviours and coming to terms with new facts, evidence or evaluation of evidence. Engaging with novel opinions or intellectual perspectives are pivotal in presenting both sides of the argument and explicit conclusions. It is important to consider placing strong, positive arguments first. Changes to practice can compel unfamiliar behaviour and can also evoke

ACTIVITY 15.9 Introduction of an isolation policy in paediatric wards

Where and how to care for children with infections, or those requiring protection, is a daily debate in many paediatric settings. The practice of placing patients into single rooms for infection control purposes is well documented but there is little guidance on when to remove patients from isolation rooms. Unless the appropriateness of isolation for each patient is evaluated daily, the availability of cubicles falls, resulting in potentially unnecessary transfers to other hospitals where such facilities are available. A new isolation policy was introduced to improve the availability of isolation rooms on paediatric wards in a large inner city teaching hospital with over 100 paediatric inpatient beds. A change management framework was used that included empowering organisational action and consolidating improvements. A number of strategies were introduced to prompt daily review of children in isolation, including clear criteria for isolation and nursing staff in the emergency department challenging the decision to admit a child into an isolation room. Introduction of the policy and subsequent audits have resulted in improved staff awareness, more effective use of isolation rooms and reduced transfers to other hospitals.

What model do they utilise in their work?

Locate and read Hall et al. (2007).

emotional behaviours because of stress, lack of familiarity with new proposals and being creatures of habit. This requires support and reduction of fear or anxiety. Motivation will be a key factor when emphasising group solidarity. The character of change agent should include respect, fairness and credibility. Understanding the reason for change can serve to reduce fear or anxiety or serve as a motivational force (see Table 15.12).

Dynamics of Change

Change can have a positive or negative effect on practitioners or a team, which can be due to external or internal factors. The

Table 15.12 Reasons why change may be deemed necessary

Achieving excellence in practice	Implementation of national and local policies
Quality assurance	Result of clinical audit
Evidence-based practice	Risk assessment
Financial	Restructuring of workplace
Need for increased efficiency	Technological advances
New services development	Dissatisfaction with the present
Vision for the future	Personal/professional interest

sources of change cannot always be controlled by managers or leaders and may come from external sources such as from political drivers. This change can be radical ('Modernising the NHS' and 'Agenda for change') or subtle (reorganising storage). Some practitioners expect change can be the removal of something (often privileges or pay) or the practitioners believe that more will be expected of them. Reactions to change can vary according to an individual's responses and his flexibility to change. Prior to any planned change it would be important to evaluate the situation and try to anticipate any consequences of change.

For some practitioners there will be the perception of loss or gain as a result of change, which makes them feel threatened, insecure, or be resistant to change, or be complacent. Practitioners may develop inaccurate perceptions related to the change and they may perceive that there will be a loss of power. These practitioners are regarded as 'laggards' (see Figure 15.13).

Other practitioners are more accepting of change and are able to see the need for change, be in agreement with the planned change or wish to support colleagues. This group of practitioners are likely to be feeling valued and secure and will be viewing change as an opportunity, not a threat which may be seen as a criticism of past practices. This group of people are likely to be the 'early adaptors' who can foresee possible rewards for their efforts and have some control of the situation because they have entered the change process at an early stage.

Reasons for Resistance

There are a minority group of practitioners who may either lack understanding of the purpose of the planned change or disagree with the change itself because they lack motivation or deny change is necessary. Some individuals are plainly 'creatures of habit' and simply do not like stepping out of their comfort zone while others will have uncertainty about the future. Other individuals may have a distorted perception of the need for change, or an unrealistic perception of consequences the change may induce, including perceived loss of status, comfort, and pay which may arise from a lack of understanding or trust. Lack of ownership may increase stress and sabotage is seen as a realistic strategy to avoid change (Hall et al. 2007; Marquis and Huston 2012).

Evaluating Change

In order to evaluate the change, it is useful to look at the original objectives that led to change and pushed the change forward. There will be informal and formal evaluations to consider and there would be the opportunity for continuous feedback, providing an opportunity to address any issues as they develop. Once the management of change process has been completed, it will be expected that the results of the change are disseminated to key stakeholders. These results could be disseminated verbally at ward meetings or by presentations or through written reports, sharing information within the team and organisation.

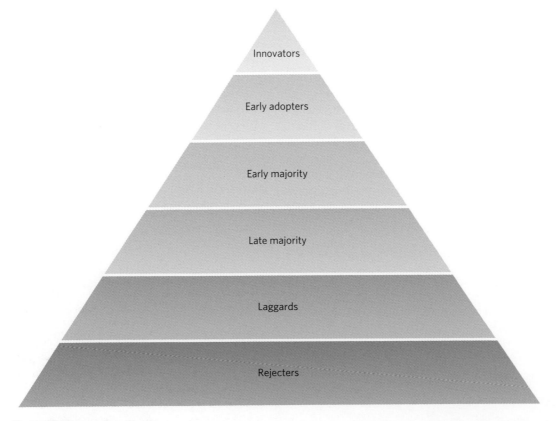

Figure 15.13 Response to Change
Source: Rogers (2003)

Preceptorship

The mission statement of the NMC, 'Protecting patients through standards,' is aimed at preventing harm to patients. Being a children's nurse is about being self-aware and gaining self-development through lifelong learning (NMC 2008). Pearson (2009) identified that joining a team can take time to bond with team members and that it is important to acknowledge personal limitations and seek to acquire new knowledge and skills. One way of doing this may be to write a learning contract or action plan with the named preceptor. Another way may be to produce a SMART action plan (Weir-Hughes 2011):

Specific
Measurable
Attainable
Relevant
Time bound.

A SMART action plan could be used to gain confidence as a newly qualified children's nurse and could be useful in planning out a learning journey (see Table 15.13).

Table 15.13 Assessment tool developed using a SMART Action Plan

Criteria for success in undertaking medicines administration (*indicates minimum grade to achieve a pass grade)	Achieved	Not achieved	Signature of the preceptor
An area for own continuing professional development within the first 6 months of professional registration is identified	*		
Read and understand the trust's drug package	*		
Read and understand all of the legislation, i.e. NMC standards for the safe storage and administration of medication and the Drugs Act	*		
Speak with the pharmacy team to gain an understanding of the indications, doses and contra-indications of the chosen drugs	*		
Learn six of the most common drugs used in your area	*		
Complete the trust drug package	*		
Undertake drug round with preceptor	*		
Undertake drug round with supervision	*		
Undertake drug round with preceptor as assessment of competence	*		
Is aware of all of the resources available, and the hindrances and difficulties that may prevent completion	*		
Preceptor is satisfied with competence and signs off the documentation	*		

Preceptor name ....

Preceptor signature ....

Date ....

Candidate name ....

Candidate signature ....

Date: ....

Ward/department: ....

Acknowledgement to Jan Lovelle (2012, Anglia Ruskin University)

CASE STUDY REVIEW 15.2

Erin has ultimate everyday managerial leadership for staff and by her position as matron in the organisation she holds authority (power and influence) to make the necessary changes for the safe and effective performance of the staff on Woodland Ward.

Rebecca has been in post for a substantial period of time and has established herself as a loyal member of staff who stays on shift later than necessary to 'give extra attention' to children, young people and their families. Although this seems an admirable action that is beyond the call of duty, it could have contributed to fatigue. Fatigue can impair clinical judgements and contribute to the leaving of medications unattended on the children's ward (Peate 2012). Rebecca may be feeling 'threatened' by Louize's enthusiasm for the job and knowledge of contemporary evidence-based practice. Rebecca's knowledge and understanding of contemporary evidence may also pose a threat.

Louize has just finished her period of preceptorship and is still finding her feet. It would be timely for Louize to consider the differences between assertive and aggressive behaviours so that she can be more flexible in her approach to other members of the team. It may also be that Louize is feeling 'over-confident' and has 'staff-nurse-itis', which can impact on the Woodland Ward team. In the exchange of words, in the smallest sense of the word, Louize has become involved in whistleblowing.

Erin is in a position of power and has authority to ensure that evidence-based care is being delivered to a high standard. With Erin at the helm of the meeting between Rebecca and Louize, it should be possible to diffuse the situation, identify the root cause of the problem and begin teambuilding strategies by means of a resolution. It may also mean that Erin has to impose sanctions on either Rebecca or Louize or both of them. It may be prudent for Erin to involve the entire Woodland Ward team in policies and practice guidelines to ensure that Woodland Ward is delivering 'good, evidence-based practice' to children and young people.

The trust in which Woodland Ward is situated will have risk assessment, managing and reporting systems in place for incidents, errors and near-misses to avoid further adverse events. Adverse media reporting would further impact on the trust. Prior to meeting with Rebecca and Louize, Erin would be expected to consider patient safety and redistribution of patient care for the duration of the meeting.

Due to time constraints, it may be that Erin has a brief word with Rebecca and Louize and revisits the situation at a later date and time thus allowing time for personal reflection and stress reduction. Sanctions could result from Rebecca leaving unattended medicines on the nurses' station which could be dealt with either informally through a meeting or formally through disciplinary procedures (power through sanctions). It is evident that Louize's arrival has prompted 'feelings' in Rebecca. Those 'feelings' are compounded when Louize challenges Rebecca's actions and a 'storming' phase occurs. Erin needs a team who can work together as more can be achieved by working collaboratively. Engaging Rebecca and Louize in a shared activity working on a project may prompt 'bonding' and respect. In the long term, it would be prudent for Erin to consider teambuilding activities for Woodland Ward.

SUMMARY OF KEY LEARNING

The management of change can invoke behaviours that are designed to resist or sabotage the change. It can be a helpful strategy to introduce change slowly so that all staff can have an opportunity to ask questions and participate at the initial discussions. By providing full information and allowing time to consider the options and time to try things out, resistant behaviours may reduce. The act of participation and the involvement of all staff in decision making not only provides opportunities for staff development but also facilitates psychological ownership. Identifying the potential advantages and rewards of any change may encourage children's nurses to participate in the planned changes and contribute to the evidence of improvement and success the change brings (Huber 2010; Marquis and Huston 2012).

FURTHER RESOURCES

Nursing quality: **http://www.dh.gov.uk/en/Publicationsandstatistics/Publications/PublicationsPolicyAndGuidance/DH_113450**

NHS Institute for Innovation and Improvement: **http://www.institute.nhs.uk/**

National Patient Safety Agency: **http://www.npsa.nhs.uk/nrls/improvingpatientsafety/patient-safety-tools-and-guidance/risk-assessment-guides/risk-matrix-for-risk-managers/**

Medicines for Children: **http://www.mhra.gov.uk/Howweregulate/Medicines/Medicinesforchildren/index.htm\#l11**

Medicines for Children Research Network: **http://www.mcrn.org.uk/**; **http://www.mcrn.org.uk/networks/grip**

National Audit Office: **http://www.nao.org.uk/**

MONITOR: **http://www.monitor-nhsft.gov.uk/**

Resuscitation: **http://www.resus.org.uk/**

RoSPA: **http://www.rospa.com/about/successstories/default.aspx**

ANSWERS TO ACTIVITIES

ACTIVITY 15.1 NMC Hearings

Access the NMC website and consider how may hearings relate to medicine misuse in nursing and in particular children's nursing.

1 These will vary according to the field of nursing due to the population sizes.

2 The NMC publishes guidelines in relation to the standards of medicines administration.

3 There is guidance within the National Service Framework for children, young people and maternity services.

ACTIVITY 15.2 Evidence-based practice: guiding the care and management of feverish illness in children

Review the NICE Guidance CG47 feverish illness in children **http://guidance.nice.org.uk/CG47**.

What does NICE CG47 say about temperature taking in children 0 to 5 years old?

According to NICE CG47, the oral and rectal routes should not routinely be used to measure the body temperature of children aged 0 to 5 years old.

NICE CG47 also informs us that forehead chemical thermometers are unreliable and should not be used by healthcare professionals.

ACTIVITY 15.3 Personal reflection on clinical deterioration

Reflect back on a situation where a child was showings signs of deterioration which has led to a resuscitation with a successful outcome. Consider:

Q: Which leadership style was evident?

A: It is highly likely that an automatic leadership style would be employed to ensure that

Q: What would the situation and outcome be like if a democratic leadership style was used?

A: Valuable seconds and minutes would be wasted which could have been used for dealing with the needs of the patient.

Q: What would the situation and outcome be like if a laissez-faire leadership was used?

A: A successful outcome for the patient would be in jeopardy.

Q: What would the situation and outcome be like if a bureaucratic leadership style was used?

A: To some extent a bureaucratic leadership style is used when applying the Resuscitation Guidelines to an individual situation. The algorithms act as an aide memoire and guide the resuscitation process.

http://www.resus.org.uk/ last accessed 6 May 2012

ACTIVITY 15.4 Journal club ideas for Woodland Ward

Erin has decided that one way of facilitating Rebecca and Louize to reflect on their actions is to undertake a literature review for a journal club. Consider what topic would be appropriate for each of them to consider.

Rebecca could be asked to undertake a literature review related to the administration of medicines. Louize could be asked to undertake a literature review related to conflict management or both could be asked to undertake a literature review on team working, safeguarding children and young people through quality care.

ACTIVITY 15.5 Personal reflection on clinical deterioration

Reflect on a situation in which a child was showing signs of clinical deterioration that led to a resuscitation situation with a successful outcome.

Consider:

- Which leadership style was evident?
- What the situation and outcome would be like if a democratic leadership style were used?
- What the situation and outcome would be like if a laissez-faire leadership style were used?
- What the situation and outcome would be like if a bureaucratic leadership style were used?

- It is highly likely that an autocratic leadership style would be employed to ensure that.
- Valuable seconds and minutes would be wasted that could have been used for dealing with the needs of the patient.
- A successful outcome for the patient would be in jeopardy.
- To some extent a bureaucratic leadership style is used when applying the resuscitation guidelines to an individual situation. The algorithms act as an aide memoire and guide the resuscitation processes

(http://www.resus.org.uk/.)

ACTIVITY 15.6 Staff allocation

Compile a list, with a clear rationale, of what must be considered when deciding on the allocation of staff to an allocation of patients.

1 May include patients to staff.
2 Patients with higher acuity scores require more interventions and staff should be allocated fewer patients.
3 Allocate staff with an appropriate 'buddy' to care for each other's patients to facilitate breaks and working together for checking medications.

4 The nurse in charge will need to check that all the patients delegated to other staff have received appropriate care and treatment in a timely manner.
5 The patients with the highest acuity scores should be cared for by appropriately qualified staff. As dependency levels change, staff should reform to amend the original allocation of patients.

ACTIVITY 15.7 Charlie is due his antiepileptic medication

Charlie is 2 years old and is due to have his antiepileptic medication. Mum says he needs his Epilim. The generic name is sodium valproate and comes as 200 mg in 5 mls. The prescription is 150 mg of sodium valproate due at 8 am.

$$\frac{\text{What you want}}{\text{What you have}} \times \underline{\text{What the volume amount is in ml}}$$

Another way of expressing this may be:

$$\frac{\text{Strength required}}{\text{Stock strength}} = \frac{150}{200} \times \underline{\text{Volume of stock solution}}$$

$$= 5 \text{ mls}$$

$$\frac{150}{200} \times 5\text{mls} = 3.75\text{mls}$$

Talk through the procedure of administration of medicines with a colleague or write it down:

- liquid or tablet form
- spoon or oral syringe.

Consider the right strategy:

- right drug chart with patient
- right drug – how are you going to check?
- right amount – how are you going to check and calculate?
- right route – orally
- right time – 8 am

What now ? How are you going to approach this?

- tell Mum and Charlie what you are doing, prepare them
- Charlie is 2 years old – how might he take his medication usually?
- consider syringe, spoon or pot
- measure carefully
- oral syringes vs. ordinary syringes? Cost vs. safety?

Problems you may face:

- non-compliance
- safe holding/restraint
- negativity from parents
- refusal
- unavailability
- leaving medication at bedside.

ACTIVITY 15.8 Potential error in the administration of medicines

It is 8.30 am and you have just had handover from the night staff who have gone home. You are in charge of the ward and one of the staff nurses comes to you in a distraught state.

She reports that she has just given an IV antibiotic to a child on the ward while the mother was not in the room. On her return, the child's mother informed staff nurse that the night staff had already given an IV just before they went home.

How do you handle the situation?

- Contact the doctor immediately to report the incident.

- Contact the night staff to check that the medication had been administered.
- Report the incident to the pharmacist for further support and advice.
- Implement instructions from the doctor/pharmacist.
- Report the incident according to trust procedures and clinical governance.
- Talk to the child or young person.
- Monitor child or young person for adverse effects.

ACTIVITY 15.9 Introduction of an isolation policy in paediatric wards

Locate and read Hall et al. (2009). What model do they utilise in their work?

Kotter's eight steps of change leadership:

1 Establish and create a sense of urgency.
2 Create a powerful coalition.
3 Develop both the guiding vision and strategy.

4 Communicate the vision.
5 Empower organisational action.
6 Generate short-term wins.
7 Consolidate improvement.
8 Anchor new vision and strategy in organisational culture.

SELECTED REFERENCES

Adair, J. (1986) *Effective teambuilding: How to make a winning team.* Pan Macmillan: London.

Adair, J. (1990) *Not bosses but leaders*, 2nd edn. Kogan Page: London.

Audit Commission (2001) *A spoonful of sugar.* Medicines Management in NHS Hospitals: London.

Barton, D. and Semple, M. (2011) The pros and cons of routine. *Nursing Management*, 18(5) 11.

Belbin, R.N. (1991) *Management teams: why they succeed or fail.* Heinemann: London.

Bennis, W. and Nanus, B. (1997) *Leaders: strategies for taking charge*, 2nd edn. Harpers Business: New York.

Blair, K. (2011) *Medicines management in children's nursing.* Learning Matters Ltd: Exeter.

Bricher, G. (1999) Paediatric nurses, children and the development of trust. *Journal of Clinical Nursing*, 8, 451–458.

Brookes, J. (2011) Engaging staff in the change process. *Nursing Management*, September, 16–19.

Byrnes, J.P. (2002) The development of decision-making. *Journal of Adolescent Health*, 31, 208–215.

Carlin, J. (2005) *Including me: managing complex health needs in schools and early years settings.* Council for Disabled Children. Department for Education and Skills: London.

Casey, A. (2006) Assessing and planning care in partnership, in A. Glasper and J.A. Richardson (eds) *Textbook of children and young people's nursing.* Churchill Livingstone Elsevier: London.

Coad, J. and Coad, N. (2008) Children and young people's preference of thematic design and colour for their hospital environment. *Journal Child Health Care*, 12, 33–48.

Coad, H., Flay, J., Aspinall, M., Bilverstone, B., Coxhead, E. and Hones, B. (2008) Evaluating the impact of involving young people in developing children's services in an acute hospital trust. *Journal of Clinical Nursing*, 17, 3115–3122.

Collier, S. (2005) An exploration of the children's services co-ordinator/modern matron role, MSc dissertation (unpublished).

Conroy, S., Davar, Z. and Jones, S. (2012) Use of checking systems in medicines administration with children and young people. *Nursing Children and Young People*, 24(3), 20–24.

Cornock, M. (2011a) Legal definitions of responsibility, accountability and liability. *Paediatric Nursing*, 23(3), 25–26.

Cornock, M. (2011b) Whistleblowing: a legal commentary. *Nursing Children and Young People*, 23(8), 20–21.

Cornock, M. (2011c) A legal commentary on negligence. *Paediatric Nursing*, 23(1), 20–21.

Coyne, I. (2006) Consultation with children in hospital: children, parents and nurses' perspectives. *Journal of Clinical Nursing*, 15(1), 61–71.

Crawford, D. (2012) Maintaining good practice in the administration of medicines to children. *Nursing Children and Young People*, 4(4), 29–35.

D'Amour, D., Ferrada,-Videla, M., Rodriguez, L.S.M. and Beaulieu, M. (2005) The conceptual basis for interprofessional collaboration: core concepts and theoretical frameworks. *Journal of Interprofessional Care*, Supplement 1 May, 116–131.

Davis, C. (2011) Touch-screen technology frees nurses to spend more quality time with patients. *Nursing Management*, 18(5), 6–7.

Department of Education (DoE) (2011) *The Munro Review of child protection: final report: a child-centred system.* TSO: Norwich.

Department of Health (DoH) (1998) *The new NHS, modern and dependable, a national framework for assessing performance.* DoH: London.

Department of Health (DoH) (2000) *An organisation with a memory.* DoH: London.

Department of Health (DoH) (2001) *Building a safer NHS for patients: implementing an organisation with a memory.* DoH, London.

Department of Health (DoH) (2003) *Patient and public involvement in health: the evidence for policy implementation, a summary of the results of health in partnership research programme.* DoH: London.

Department of Health (DoH) (2004) National Service Framework for children, young people and maternity services. DoH: London.

Department of Health (DoH) (2010) *Equity and excellence: liberating the NHS.* TSO: Norwich.

Dimond, B. (2011) *Legal aspects of nursing.* Pearson: Harlow.

French, J. and Raven, B. (1959) Power and conflict, in D. Huber (ed.) (2011) *Leadership and nursing management.* 2nd edn. W.B. Saunders: Philadelphia.

Gibbens, C. (2010) Nurse-facilitated discharge for children and their families. *Paediatric Nursing*, 22(1), 14–18.

Gibson, F., Aldiss, S., Horstman, M., Kumpunen, S. and Richardson, A. (2010) Children and young people's experiences of cancer care: a qualitative research study using participatory methods. *International Journal of Nursing Studies*, 47, 1397–1507.

Glebling, H. and Marr, H. (2004) *Quality assurance in nursing.* Nelson Thornes: Cheltenham.

Goodman, B. and Clemow, R. (2010) *Nursing and collaborative practice: a guide to interprofessional learning and working*, 2nd edn. Learning Matters: Exeter.

Gopee, N. and Galloway, J. (2009) *Leadership and management in healthcare.* Sage: London.

Griffith, R. and Tengnah, C. (2008) *Law and professional issues in nursing.* Transforming Nursing Practice Series. Learning Matters: Exeter.

Hall, C. (2010) Medicines administration, in E.A. Glasper, M. Aylott, and C. Battrick (eds) *Developing practical skills for nursing children and young people.* Hodder Arnold: London.

Hall, J., Roopine, S. and McLean, J. (2007) Introduction of an isolation policy in paediatric wards. *Paediatric Nursing*, 19(9), 15–17.

Handy, C. (1999) *Understanding organizations.* Penguin Group: London.

Hockenberry, M.J., Wilson, D., Winkelstein, M.L. (eds) (2004) *Wong's Essentials of Paediatric Nursing*, Elsevier Mosby: St. Louis, MO.

Huber, D. (2000) *Leadership and nursing management*, 2nd edn, W.B. Saunders: Philadelphia.

Huber, D. (2010) *Leadership and nursing care management*. Saunders, Elsevier: Maryland Heights, MO.

Hurst, K., Smith, A., Casey, A., Fenton, K., Scholefield, H. and Smith, S. (2008) Calculating staffing requirements. *Nursing Management*, 15(4).

Kosowski, M.M. and Roberts, V.W. (2003) When protocols are not enough: inuitive decision-making by novice nurse practitioners. *Journal of Holistic Nursing*, 21(1), 52–72.

Kotter, J. (1996) *Leading Change*. Harvard Business School Press: Boston, MA.

Laming, H. (2009) *The protection of children in England: a progress report*. TSO: Norwich.

Langmack, G. (2009) Being qualified, in C. Hall and D. Ritchie, *What is nursing? Exploring theory and practice*. Learning Matters: Exeter.

Laurance, J. (2011) The dangerous power of healing hands, *The Independent*, 26, July: **http://www.independent.co.uk/lifestyle/health-and-families/features/jeremy-laurance-the-dangerous-power-of-healing-hands-2325861.html**

Lightfoot, J. and Sloper, P. (2004) Having a say in health: involving young people with chronic illness or physical disability in local health services development. *Children and Society*, 17, 277–290.

Marquis, B.L. and Huston, C.J. (2012) *Leadership roles and management functions in nursing: theory and application*. Lippincott, Williams & Wilkins, Wolters Kluwer Health: Philadelphia.

Martin, V. (2006a) Learning to lead: part 2. *Nursing Management*, 12(10), 34–37.

Martin, V. (2006b) Leading in teams: part 1. *Nursing Management*, 13(1), 34–37.

Martin, V. (2006c) Leading in teams: part 2. *Nursing Management*, 13(2), 32–35.

Miers, M. and Pollard, K. (2009) The role of nurses in interprofessional health and social care teams. *Nursing Management*, 15(9), 30–35.

Mooney, S. (2010) Unplanned hospital admission: supporting children, young people and their families. *Paediatric Nursing*, 22(10), 20–23.

Mottram, A. (2009) Therapeutic relationships in day surgery: a grounded theory study. *Journal of Clinical Nursing*, 18, 2830–2837.

Moules, T. (2009) They wouldn't know how it feels. . . : characteristics of quality care from young people's perspectives: a participatory research project. *Journal of Child Health Care*, 13, 322.

Nursing and Midwifery Council (NMC) NMC, 2008. The code: Standards of conduct, performance and ethics for nurses and midwives. London, NMC. [online] Available at: http://www.nmc-uk.org/Documents/Standards/The-code-A4-20100406.pdf.

Ofsted (2010) *Learning lessons from serious case review: Ofsted's evaluation of serious case reviews from 1 April 2009 to 31 March 2010*. OFSTED: London.

Orlando, I.J. (1961) *The dynamic nurse–patient relationship: function, process and principles*. G.P. Putnam's Sons: New York.

Payne, M. (2000) *Teamwork in multiprofessional care*. Palgrave: Basingstoke.

Pearson, H. (2009) Transition from nursing student to staff nurse: a personal reflection. *Paediatric Nursing*, 21(3), 30–32.

Peate, I. (2012) Shift working: safety or savings?, editorial, *British Journal of Nursing*, 21(3), 153.

Phillips, A. (2002) *Communication and the manager's job*. Radcliffe Publishing Ltd: London.

Pollard, K. (2009) Student engagement in interprofessional working in practice placement settings. *Journal of Clinical Nursing*, 18, 2846–2856.

Sartain, S.A., Clarke, C.L. and Hayman, R. (2000) Hearing the voices of children with chronic illness. *Journal of Advanced Nursing*, 32(4), 913–921.

Saunders, M. (2003) Audit: the beginning and the end of the change cycle, in S. Pickering and J. Thompson (eds) *Clinical governance and best value: meeting the modernisation agenda*. Churchill Livingstone, Elsevier Science Ltd: London.

Scally, G. and Donaldson, L.J. (1998) Clinical governance and the drive for quality improvement in the new NHS. *British Medical Journal*, 317, 61–65.

Spinks, J. (2010) Developing nurses' power to care. *Paediatric Nursing*, 22(4), 26.

Taylor, V. (2007) Leadership for service improvement: part 3 *Nursing Management*, 15(1), 28–32.

Tozer, J. and Hull, L. (2012) New death at poisoning hospital as police quiz male nurse amid fears fourth patient has become victim: **http://www.dailymail.co.uk/health/article-2082615/Stepping-Hill-hospital-deaths-Male-nurse-arrested-amid-fears-4th-patient-victim.html**

Twycross, A. and Powls, L. (2006) How do children's nurses make clinical decisions? Two preliminary studies. *Journal of Clinical Nursing*, 1, 1324–1335.

United Nations (1989) Convention on the Rights of the Child. **http://www2.ohchr.org/english/law/crc.htm**

Walker, S. and Thurston, C. (2006) *Safeguarding children and young people, a guide to integrated practice*. Russell House Publishing Ltd: Lyme Regis.

Walsh, M. and Ford, P. (1989) *Nursing rituals, research and rational action*. Heinemann Nursing: Oxford.

Weir-Hughes, D. (2011) *Clinical leadership: from A to Z*. Pearson Education: Harlow.

Westwood, C. (2010) Leading by example to aid personal development. *Nursing Management*, 17(2), 32–33.

Wolfe, I., Cass, H., Thompson, M.J., Craft, A., Wiegersma, P.A., Jansom, S., Chambers, T.L. and McKee, M. (2011) How can we improve child health services? *BMJ*, 342, 901–904.

Woodfield, T. (2001) Involving children in clinical audit. *Paediatric Nursing*, 13(3), 12–16.

Zaleznik, A. (1992) Managers and leaders: are they different? *Harvard Business Review*, 70(20), 126–135.

CHAPTER 16
Transferring to Adult Services for Young People with Long-Term Conditions

Chris Thurston

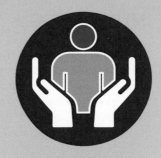
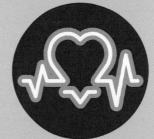
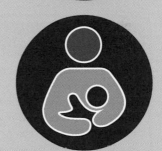

LEARNING OUTCOMES

On completion of this chapter, the reader will be able to:

- Explore transitional processes in relation to young people as they become adults.
- Understand the challenges in the lives of young people with a lifelong or life-limiting illness.
- Critically analyse the issues affecting young people with long-term health conditions.
- Explore the development of services, during and after transferring to adult services.
- Critically evaluate provision for young people with long-term health conditions.

TALKING POINT

'It is time to break the myth that has grown up over the 60 years of the NHS, that health services manage your health for you making it OK to get "hammered" and end up in A&E; or to try a drug and see what happens; or remain ignorant of what is going on inside your body while fretting over glamour and goodies on the outside. Involvement of young people invariably moves into the "too difficult" box, to be dealt with later, but later never comes. Young people are avid learners. They contribute through voluntary activity far more than adults and are deeply committed to and interested in the health services.'

Barbara Hearn, Deputy Chief Executive, National Children's Bureau http://www.bbc.co.uk/news/health-16851926

INTRODUCTION

This chapter will discuss how to improve the practice of health professionals in understanding the transitional experiences of young people with long-term conditions. While the young people have lifelong conditions, they also have commonalities with their peers who are unaffected. Throughout the chapter, the view of the young people within their unique social context and Jenny's as the case study will be considered and professional support offered for young people.

On reading this chapter, you will be able to understand the physical, psychological and social support required when transferring to adult services for a young person with long-term health needs. The changing context of young people's lives and the services they require means that every health practitioner working with young people has to develop the capacity to undertake assessments and interventions in a wide variety of settings.

Such activity needs to be understood in the context of statutory duties, agency requirements, and the needs and wishes of the young people. Young people already feel disempowered by society, and this is before they have any further challenges in their lives. To start the transition into adulthood for Jenny (from the case study in the chapter) with her health needs transferring into adult services, issues may arise as she is required to adapt to adult healthcare. An exploration of the definition of transition and its importance will offer explanations of the journey from child to young adult, when transitioning with a long-term illness. This includes an acknowledgement of the effects of physical and human development on the young person and also the attributes of the young person with long-term illness, including the debilitating effect the condition has on the young person and their body. There will also be a focused exploration of themes related to transition, including youth culture, comparative youth and the biographical perspective of youth.

CASE STUDY 16.1 Jenny, a young person with CF

Jenny is 15 years old and has two older brothers. While her brothers carry the gene, she has cystic fibrosis (CF), which was diagnosed when she was 2 years old. She is in her second year of GCSEs and is worried as she has missed a significant amount of time at school, due to frequent chest infections. Jenny has always had an active social life and spends time with her friends when well. Jenny has found it difficult to maintain her weight and now as well as a port-a-cath for her regular 4-weekly prophylactic intravenous antibiotics, she requires a gastronomy tube for overnight feeding. Another concern Jenny has raised with you on admission to the children's unit with a chest infection is that she is starting the process of transferring to adult services and she is worried that the interventions that she presently receives from children's services both locally and at the tertiary centre are not going to be as readily available.

While the term lifelong illness acknowledges that a young person has a medical condition that will be with them throughout their lives, life limiting goes a stage further by highlighting the life-shortening effect the condition has on their lifespan. By choosing a condition that has this dual aspect, it will enable reflections on both the physical and psychological issues that may occur for these young people as they become young adults and users of adult services. Table 16.1 gives examples of the continuum of illness linked to their severity and risk of a shortened lifespan.

TRANSITION FROM YOUTH TO ADULT

Defining transition from youth to adult within the context of western society for Jenny offers the challenge of acknowledging that it is seen as a generalised longitudinal process, with society's belief that transitioning into adult is equitable in timespan and experience to all individuals. This approach detracts from the young person and their unique life experiences, whether influenced by culture, gender, class or health. Episodes may reveal changes in the young person's stage of physical or psychological development, health status or illness progression and can be seen to be applicable to the transition into adulthood for all young people with or without long-term illness. There may be changes in their sociocultural standing, such as when a young person is able to vote, changes in their circumstance or situation, such as going from college to work, or relationship changes, such as marriage, alongside changes due to critical incidences such as injury or sudden illness and also organisational changes, including changing careers or health service (Kralik et al. 2006; Henderson et al. 2007; Kehily 2007).

Transition can be simply defined as a change for an individual that occurs over time, or change in stage of development, or moving from one environment to another, such as school to college or work (Kralik et al. 2006). This fits well with young people as they move from school and education to work or college studies and, indeed, reflects the young person with long-term illness as they move from the environment of child health services to adult services. However, society does not always judge behaviour consistently and therefore this can lead to young people including Jenny being confused about their responsibilities, especially when it comes to making decisions about their healthcare needs.

Table 16.1 Continuum of illness with examples

Description of life-limiting lifelong conditions	Examples of conditions
Life-threatening conditions for which curative treatment may be feasible but can fail	Cancer Cardiac anomalies Irreversible organ failure
Conditions that may entail long periods of intensive treatment aimed at prolonging life and allowing participation in normal activities, although premature death is still possible or inevitable	Cystic fibrosis Duchenne muscular dystrophy HIV/AIDS Sickle cell Multiple Sclerosis
Progressive conditions without curative treatments, where intervention is exclusively palliative, although it may continue for many years	Batten's disease Mucopolysaccharidosis Creutzfelt Jacob disease
Conditions associated with neurological disability that are not progressive but can entail weakness and susceptibility to health complications leading to premature death	Brain or spinal cord injuries Cerebral palsy
Conditions that have lifelong consequences to health and may lead to a shortened lifespan if a crisis occurs	Diabetes Asthma Epilepsy Eating disorders

Source: adapted from Doug et al. (2009)

ACTIVITY 16.1 Ages of progression to adulthood within UK law

Explore the ages that a young person can undertake these activities:

- heterosexual sex
- homosexual sex
- vote
- able to work full time
- able to drink alcohol
- to babysit a child who is not a relative
- able to smoke
- able to get married
- able to live alone.

What about the age that society believes children and young people need to be to take personal responsibility for their actions:

- gain a criminal conviction
- be sent to an adult jail.

What about the age at which society believes children and young people can make decisions about their healthcare:

- consent for treatment
- consent for contraception
- age sent to an adult ward for treatment
- age sent to an adult mental health unit for treatment.

Independence

Independence in adulthood is often seen as the ideal in western society, where young people strive to move away from home and their parents' control, and begin to work and gain financial independence, leading to a desire for their own family (Morrow and Richards 1996). There are difficulties such as politics, sociolegal issues and financial restrictions which make it more of a challenge for the young person to become completely independent.

It is a commonly held belief in western society that young people become optimally independent in adulthood, as this can be seen to benefit society's requirement for an independent adult workforce not dependent on others for financial or physical support. However, young people, when questioned about the value of independence, did not have a uniform factor that gave them independence: some of the young people felt they gained independence while living at home, while for others the move away and having a career heightened their independence. Holdsworth and Morgan (2005) highlight this in their study.

RESEARCH NOTE 16.1 Transitions out of parental home in Britain, Spain and Norway (Holdsworth and Morgan 2005)

Young people questioned focused on the issues surrounding leaving home, independence and adulthood. They suggested that independence cannot be seen as a purely linear process that occurs with age, but had aspects that related to the young person's relationships with their parents, their gender and whether the young person lived at home or moved out of the home environment; this varied across the young people and the culture in which they lived. It required an acknowledgement of financial stability of the young person alongside the development of adult–partner relationships. Within this context the definition of independence was not seen purely as the ability to function autonomously as an individual although this may be part of the definition for some young people; rather it was seen as being able to balance individual freedom alongside mutual respect, obligation and commitment to others including family, but may also be related to friends, colleagues and the development of adult relationships (Gillies 2001, cited by Robb 2007a).

ACTIVITY 16.2

List the chores that become more relevant to young people as they gain more responsibility in the home.

How may this be different if there are younger siblings or individuals who have a long-term illness?

Independence may be lost when a significant illness occurs, which may lead an individual to feel disempowered and unable to perform all the activities they used to undertake at the time of their choosing, without support or practical help from others, whether family, or professionals (Thurston 2010). With young people such as Jenny, this may lead to feelings of anger and frustration, especially if they have believed they were independent in the past and this has been lost as a result of their illness (this would include cancer as described in Grinyer's (2007) study). However, siblings may also feel frustrated if they are part of the network of support for the young person in terms of practical care, without acknowledgement for the part they play.

Advocacy

An area closely related to independence is advocacy and how young people with long-term illness view the support they are offered by professionals when they require interventions, either for social or physical needs. This can be dependent on the way that youth is constructed in society, either when the transitional process offers incremental opportunities for responsibility or the same level of autonomy to adulthood.

ACTIVITY 16.3

Highlight the nursing or medical interventions you would be happy for a young person with a long-term condition to undertake. List the interventions you would not feel comfortable in their undertaking and why.

Protective Perspective

It could be argued that if the care of young people is seen from a *protective perspective*, the advocacy offered may be passive as the professionals and carers begin by working for the young individual, rather than with them, and initially may reduce the opportunity for the young person's views to be heard (Robb 2007; Boylan and Dalrymple 2009). This adult-focused system fulfils the requirements in a generic way for the adolescent's needs but the power stays with the professional and reduces the likelihood of an individual care package for the young person that incorporates their specific requirements.

Liberationist Perspective

While the protective stance could be seen to offer security for the young person, the *liberationist perspective* offers the young person autonomy in his own right, enabling decisions to be made that are the young person's choice rather than imposed by an adult. This can be seen as controversial, as the young person may be offered the opportunity to work, vote and have financial independence, and also choose the level of treatment he wants to undertake, although there could be a risk of exploitation by individuals who wish to harm him (Corby 2006; Boylan and Dalrymple 2009). While young people may be working towards independence, there needs to be a balance between freedom to make choices and psychological and social support to have the information and knowledge when making those decisions (Thurston and Church 2001).

DEVELOPMENTAL APPROACH TO ENCOURAGING INDEPENDENCE

Professionals may advocate a developmental approach to children and young people who have a life-limiting or chronic illness and this approach can be seen as generic and chronologically based, fitting into already defined developmental stages rather than acknowledging the unique features of the child's or young person's illness, his personality and the dynamics of his family (Eiser 1990). Relating this to Jenny's own characteristics affects how she is viewed, especially coping with daily treatment and level of resilience.

The family's ability to communicate will also shape the way in which Jenny learns to deal with conventional activities such as school and the specific situations with healthcare professionals. This unique situation does not readily fit into the standard adolescent view and starts to dispel the myth that transition is uniform in structure and that every young person experiences this in a similar way; rather, it is socially constructed to fit into the beliefs of the society the young person resides within.

Adolescence

The term or definition of adolescence has a specific focus on the maturity of the body and mind in the context of individual growth and biopsychological development, often used by health and other caring professionals (see Chapter 3) (see Table 16.2). While it could be argued that they endeavour to support and empower the young person, this can be passive due to the distribution of power with the control residing with the professional, especially around decision making including treatment and care (Turney 2007).

ACTIVITY 16.4

Reflect on the young person's physical and psychological attributes that health professionals measure to monitor their increasing growth and development.

- What attributes do professionals measure?
- What do the young people themselves measure?
- Evaluate the similarities and the differences.

During transition to adulthood, Jenny and her peers may – with positive life experiences – further advance feelings around their level of self-worth and identity as an individual, if this has been a consistent feature of their psychological development to the present time, alongside developing further their own personal beliefs and values. While many of the development tasks may seem of value to young people, especially in terms of increasing abilities to problem solve and having insight into how their risk-taking behaviour may affect their health and safety, there has to be some critique of completion of these tasks in relation to the young person with long-term illness. Within the context of a limited life illness it is not uncommon for the individual to have psychological problems (Valentine and Lowes 2007). As Jenny not only has to adapt to the same developmental predicaments as her peers, she has had the challenges to continue her adaptation to the illness, and the added requirements this places on developing her life skills (ACT 2007; Kralik et al. 2006).

While Jenny as a young person is trying to work out her identity, she may be experiencing major physical changes to her body, alongside resolving changing relationships within her family. When discussing psychological development, perhaps shaped to some extent by the genetics received from her parents, her personal identity continues to emerge through late childhood and adulthood and therefore structures how Jenny and her peers learn to function as adults in society (Berk 2006). These are seen as innate characteristics within an individual, which affected their motivation, linked to biological or instinctive features of human behaviour, which may include cognitive ability or personality type from sociable to shy (Bee and Boyd 2006; Berk 2006).

An alternative view would consider social perspectives, focusing on the dynamics of interaction between the young person and their immediate environment. Jenny may be influenced by the environment she is placed within, including the relationship she has with her parents, siblings and peers and her underlying ill health and these progress as they transition through to adulthood (Boyden and Levison 2000; Aldgate et al. 2006; Walker and Thurston 2006).

For Jenny, this adjustment to a variety of environments can highlight further concerns, especially juggling study and home and treatment regime (Valentine and Lowes 2007). The experience of acquiring the skills to adapt and survive in adult society is difficult enough as cultural normalities around language, behaviour and lifestyle seem to shift more quickly than the young person can often comprehend or adjust to (Henderson et al. 2007). This is evidenced by the way in which young people who are not seen to fit into society's ideal of teenage behaviour are labelled as disruptive and excluded from educational or social activities for

Table 16.2 Comparison of the terms adolescence and youth

Adolescence	Youth
Defined in terms of individual bio-psychological growth	A sociological term for the age between 13 and 20 years
Professional term used for comparisons of teenagers' development	Societal concept of the time between transition from child to adult
Related terms: normal adolescence abnormal physiology development tasks	Related terms: youth culture youth comparison youth biography

---

RESEARCH NOTE 16.2 Inventing adulthood: a biographical approach to youth transitions (Henderson et al. 2007)

A study was undertaken over a 10-year period. This was based on 100 young people interviewed from five diverse sites in the UK, including rural and urban, middle class and working class and ran from 1996 to 2006; it highlighted the way that young people examined their lives. The study enabled the balance of themes to occur which could compare and contrast the lives of the young people.

'Young people are often understood in very general terms, with little regard to the diverse pathways and detours that their lives undertake. On the one hand, they are lumped together as a generation – defined historically by the time of their birth and the events, values and opportunities that shape their world... On the other hand, youth is also seen as a phase in the life course that we all experience involving a notion of developmental life stages leading from dependent childhood to independent adult.' (Henderson et al. 2007, page 17).

Because the study used a biographical approach the researchers were able to follow up each individual young person and explore with them their hopes and fears and expectations for the future.

---

behaving rebelliously; this can be seen in the increase in truancy and exclusions from school (Bee and Boyd 2006; Glasper and Richardson 2006; Kehily 2007).

This risk-taking behaviour is most significant when related to family and how Jenny views her place and task within this and also, more broadly, the environment she lives within including the local community, school and peer groups (Walker and Thurston 2006).

ACTIVITY 16.5

List specific risk-taking behaviours the young people you work with undertake; this may include drinking, smoking etc.

- Which of these are seen as typical young people's experiments?
- Do any break the law?
- What risks would you have specific concerns about?

As Jenny had long-term illness, this may become more complex; while teenagers, rebellion around fashion, schooling and leisure may be negotiated within the family. For a young person with long-term illness, treatment regimes, diet and physiotherapy are not so flexible because of the risk of developing further complications of the illness with inconsistent compliance (Valentine and Lowes 2007). Therefore, Jenny may feel hemmed in by her health needs, which could lead to further non-adherence and the potential risk of increased severity of the symptoms of the illness (Kyngas et al. 1998; Foster et al. 2001).

The term 'adolescence' is more focused on the young person as a growing and developing being in a physical or biological sense, rather than as a young person progressing towards independence in society, and so may be seen as a stage of life that was socially constructed for convenience of professionals to assess rates of development and provision of services for the adolescent rather than as a way in which Jenny would view herself (Taylor and Müller 1995; Grinyer 2007; Valentine and Lowes 2007).

Because individuals may learn through their environment, young people may be aware of the changes in their physical and mental health and can recognise that wellness and illness can exist at the same time (Glasper and Richardson 2006; Valentine and Lowes 2007). However, while most young people consider health to be achievable by taking care of oneself and are aware of the internal clues to health including their own role in promoting their own health, this may not be the case for the young individual who has long-term illness. While Jenny can be compliant with her treatment regime, this does not preclude her having further chest infections and admissions to hospital. Therefore she may develop a more cynical approach to health and well-being, which acknowledges the lack of consistency in regards to maintaining health and having a life-limiting condition (Badlan 2006; Williams et al. 2007; Foster et al. 2001).

Jenny could feel different from her peers both in body shape and sexual characteristics and knew from early in her teenage years that she may not be able to have children (Didsbury and Thackray 2009). This awareness of personal difference is not really considered in general development theories regarding adolescent development as the assumption is usually made that individuals can have an adult relationship that leads to production of children. While all young adults may strive and even rebel to gain independence, physically and socially this could be perceived to be more of a challenge for Jenny (Shale 1996; Williams et al. 2007). The challenge of life-limiting conditions also leads to an insight that she often has to rely on others for support in undertaking her treatments and with regular hospital and outpatient attendance which can also feel disempowering if others appeared to be making decisions for her (Huegel 1998; Grinyer 2007).

Youth

In contrast to adolescence, the term youth denotes a sociological approach that enables an exploration of society and transition for Jenny from child to youth and adult within the context of her environment alongside her physical maturation.

McCarthy (2006), in her exploration of knowledge and sociological theories about young people dealing with grief and loss, also viewed the sequence of transition as seen in society as a dual process, related, first, to the physical or biological development of the young person through adolescence and, second, society also constructs transition for young people in terms of emerging from childhood and becoming a young person when seen in the environment of school, work or in society in general. From a sociological perspective McCarthy (2006) commented that:

> The supposed transition between childhood and adulthood is, however argued to have become increasingly multifarious and complex in contemporary western society, with some transitions having become elongated while others have become truncated. (McCarthy 2006, page 23)

The elongation of youth transition can be seen in the extension of school leaving age to encourage young people to continue in further or higher education (Kehily 2007), but cynically could also be seen as a means of delaying the young person's transfer into adult employment. In contrast, truncated or condensed transition can be seen as a reduction in the opportunity for perceived or traditional childhood and youth behaviours and this challenge to behaviour can be observed when society through family, media and peer pressure encourages young people to dress and be seen as a grown up at an increasing earlier age (Wheal 2004; Bee and Boyd 2006). It is suggested that child and adult tastes are merging. In behaviour, language, attitudes and desires it becomes harder to separate youth from adult and can confuse Jennys in her move towards independence and individual identity (Lee 2001; McCarthy 2006). This redistribution of definitions of childhood and youth changes the way in which society constructs the general consensus on when or how a child becomes a young person and a young person becomes an adult (Table 16.3).

These challenges to develop and adjust to changing lives and society's perception of the young person can be more problematic when other influences are involved in Jenny's decision making, including taking chances with her health (Kyngas et al. 1998; Badlan 2006; Walker and Thurston 2006). This

chance taking during the perceived transitional process into adulthood such as carrying out behaviour that may end up in disaster, damage or injury may be linked to a need by Jenny or any young person to walk a fine line between fearfulness and exhilaration, even if only for the thrill of taking chances and not the risk (Walker and Thurston 2006). Difficulties may include responses by Jenny to her developmental responsibilities in regards to maintenance of health or gaining more independence in compliance with treatment regimes. The risk may be related to the need to conform to her peers who are an influence in social activities. This may lead to poor adherence to routines to be included with the social activities of others by reducing or stopping medication, limiting the amount of physiotherapy undertaken or the peer pressure to start to smoke or diet which could have implications on lung capacity or weight loss (Foster et al. 2001; Williams et al. 2007).

Bronfenbrenner (1989, cited by Berk 2006 and Corby 2006) offered explanations of how the complex external factors including friends and peers may affect the young person whether they have a long-term illness or not, starting from their family through to the overarching culture that may influence the individual's development; he focused specifically on how the relationships in the environment may influence the young person. He acknowledged that laws in society could not be free from cultural influences and that the ecological construction within any given society can change the way young people achieve their development during their transition into adulthood due to the society's values, from how the family deal on a daily basis with the requirements for the young person, expanding to the local community and the support offered in the school and society in general. For an individual with long-term illness going through transition both into adulthood and into adult-based services, the support received by the person both within the family and from the community and health service influences how well they adapt to the progressive nature of the illness. While Bronfenbrenner's (1989) model (see Figure 16.1) acknowledges the influences the environment has on the young person's health, intellect and personality it does not offer a detailed explanation of illness transitional. Biological influences are acknowledged, but personal illness is seen

Table 16.3 Society's perceived difference between a young person and an adult

Young person	Adult
School/college	Work
Lives at home	Lives alone or with friends/partner
Relies on family for income	Has own income
Cannot make autonomous decision about healthcare	Can give own consent to healthcare
Unable to vote/not willing	Can vote/will vote
Unmarried	Married/Civil partnership
No dependants	May have dependants

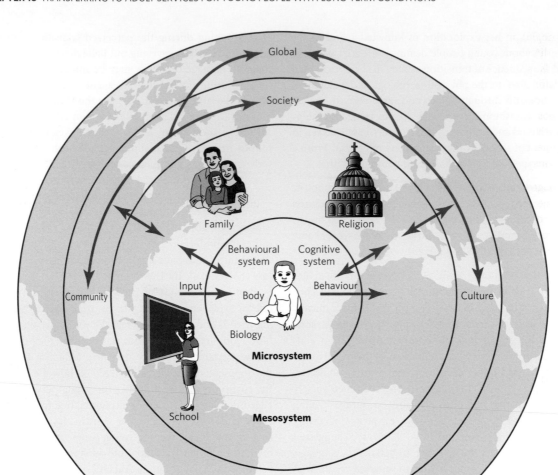

Figure 16.1 Bronfenbrenner's ecological systems theory
Source: Adapted from McLaren and Hawe, 2004, *Ecological perspectives in health research*

only as part of one of many factors rather than as a separate factor (Berk 2006).

Berk (2006) comments that a dynamic system perspective is a more useful approach as it offers explanations that visualise the young person's adaptation as they master new skills:

> A change in any part of it – from brain growth to physical and social surroundings – disrupts the current organism-environment relationship. When this happens, the child actively reorganizes her behaviour so that the components of the system work together again in a more complex effective way. (Berk 2006, page 29)

A holistic and dynamic process for exploring transition needs to consider that for Jenny there may be awareness from a young age that life may be shortened as this could have a variety of consequences related to resilience and adaptation. Jenny could have a perception of life beyond her chronological years, having a wisdom or psychological maturity not often recognised in society for this age group. McCarthy (2006) raises a

point of concern noting it could be seen as pseudo-maturity rather than genuine that the young person appears to develop skills to cope and become independent, especially in a health-care environment when having to make decisions, but in reality was not as emotionally mature as perceived to be.

However, maturity of young people with life-limiting conditions did become apparent in autobiographies from both Lipman (2001) and Pitts (2007) who spoke sensitively and with insight into the daily issues they faced living with long term illness. Also in the reports of joint working parties which have included young people when discussing transferring to adult services. Pownceby et al's (1996) 'Coming of age' project, which worked with young people with long-term illness and explored their experiences of adult services and their needs as they juggled home, school and social life alongside their treatment regime, concluded that services should be tailored to fit their individual needs rather than one size fits all. Also as shown in *Palliative care for young people* (Elston 2001), young people aged 13 years to 24 years showed a depth of knowledge and understanding not only about their life-limiting condition but also a comprehension of the needs of their siblings and family members. What emerged from the findings of both reports was a request to remember the individual was a young person first and that wherever possible they strive to be independent; however, they also wished to have the opportunity of psychological and social support.

From a sociological view of young people:

> The teenage years (can be viewed) as a phase within life course trajectory, as a time of 'transition' between the socially constructed status of child and adult. From this perspective, experiences that individuals may share by virtue of their status as 'teenager' or 'young person' must be primarily understood in terms of different status categories which are relational, based in patterns of power that are underpinned by institutional arrangements and other features of social structure. (McCarthy 2006, page 182)

This highlights the ambiguous nature of change in transitional status, that while a young person has more control over her daily life than a child, within society the indistinctness of youth caused a dichotomy in terms of decision making, for example a young person may get a job or have sex at 16, but may not vote until she is 18. This conceded the mixed messages that young people such as Jenny have had to interpret, that while they are often expected to act responsibly, they felt that they are often treated as a child by family and the wider community, rather than as a young adult (Mayall 2000).

RESEARCH NOTE 16.3   Negotiating childhoods (Mayall 2000)

Research was undertaken for the Economic and Social Research Council (ESRC); the study interviewed children and young people and also undertook group discussions, in inner London. Children and teenagers from school years 5 (139 children) and 7 (67 teenagers) were asked about how they negotiated their typical daily routine, including how they worked out their role and social position in relation to family, friends, adults and other children. The older children and teenagers felt that they were under adult authority and control daily and those adults regarded them as unreliable and disbelieve them, but expect them to carry out other tasks such as school work, household duties and childcare. Also, while predominantly they felt supported and protected, they were not always able to participate fully in expressing their rights.

This study gave insight into the view of negotiation through daily life and could be useful when contemplating the tasks the young person with long-term illness had not only with their mundane daily activities, but also the unique action in managing their long-term illness. The perceived authority that the individual such as Jenny is under can be said to be more pronounced if requirements are made daily for drug and other therapeutic interventions. This requires comprehension of the psychological needs and also the cultural issues which may occur both as a young woman and as a person with a life-limiting illness.

THEORIES OF YOUTH TRANSITION

Cultural Perspective of Youth

The set of socially acceptable behaviours are dependent on the times and challenges for that society and also reflect the status given to young adults as regard to their roles and responsibilities in society. Young people have therefore been viewed differently throughout history and both McCarthy (2006) and Kehily (2007) argued that youth, as with childhood, is a social construct defined by the people, professionals and society around the young person and the environment they inhabit, rather than by the young people. Therefore, the transition into adult society via the experiences of youth is not a fixed reality or time period in all young people's lives; rather a route or life course that was shaped by the time, culture and society.

Young people can often be seen as a challenge to society both productively and economically, not conforming to society's rules and being rebellious, and could be seen to be 'youth as trouble' (Griffin 2004) who need to be controlled and contained. Indeed, some young people may experience failed transitions where they were not able to achieve the society expectation of successful educational results, followed by career, marriage and family (Coles 2004). These examples give rise to societal belief that young people are a menace who endeavour to disrupt society, by nonconformist activities, rather than in a more sympathetic term of 'youth in trouble' who may need help and support as they strive to achieve the goals they set themselves, whether this is to be a young mother or to try to gain qualifications (Griffin 2004). However, young people are also seen as holding hope for the future in terms of potential productivity and are therefore accommodated into the structure of society by being seen as 'going through a phase' usually during their later years in education, as they transferred from the world of the classroom to the world of the adult (Holdsworth and Morgan 2005). Once the young person is perceived as having transitioned through this phase it would be assumed by society that the young person would then have a productive working life. This could, however, lead to potential conflicts for Jenny as society cannot always view individuals with life-limiting conditions as having the ability to pursue productive lives; rather, they were pursuing an illness life course (Barnes et al. 1999). Jenny's illness may offer flexibility in conforming to society's adult behavioural expectations because of the effect of illness on her life course or transition into adulthood and adult responsibility. Society's perception may also restrict Jenny's ability to develop her life further as regard to career and status progression as the illness becomes more debilitating.

> **ACTIVITY 16.6** Reflect on the different groups or subcultures to which you may belong:
>
> - age
> - gender
> - nationality
> - religion (if any)
> - cultural heritage
> - political persuasion
> - single/married/divorced.

Every individual in society including Jenny with long-term illness belongs to a number of groups that may be related to their class, age, religion and gender. However, while some remain fixed throughout the life course such as gender and country of origin, others are transient depending on their age or indeed the person's career, health or lifestyle. Jenny's place in society can be socially constructed as part of the 'youth culture' or between child and adult, for a brief number of years. Kehily (2007) commented that:

> Viewing young people culturally also positions them as active meaning-makers in their own lives through negotiations with the social world and the exercise of agency; young people give shape to their lives and actively ascribe meaning to events. (Kehily 2007, page 12)

Garratt et al. (1997) explored the process of being a young person as more than just a 'problem age' for society; rather, the young people like Jenny may feel oppressed and excluded and not able to challenge the frequently open discrimination received. This may include negating political beliefs or sexual orientation, but is more commonly related to the lack of a voice, as the young person has to struggle to overcome daily matters throughout his teenage life. Roche and Tucker (2003) highlighted this challenge in their comparative study on the life-debilitating illness of ME or when young people care for others with illness. Jenny may feel isolated from her peers and society by her situation and unable to express her feelings to others. This social exclusion not only separates her from society but also restricts her social interaction with her peers, which further alienates her from her local community. This is especially true when the illness that they or their dependants have is seen as 'dirty' or 'embarrassing'.

This is relevant to Jenny who, while being part of the broad culture of youth as perceived by society, can be excluded from fully embracing the experience due to the physical limitation of her body, therefore she may seek reassurance and support from individuals who can empathise with her situation. This mutual support is shown on the CF Trust website (**www.cftrust.org. uk**), where young people can chat openly, and with mutual understanding with peers who also have long-term illness. This can be viewed to be a subculture of life-limiting illness, within the culture of youth and therefore acknowledges the shared narratives of the illness experienced by this rare population of young people.

Comparative Perspective of Youth

This offers an anthropological understanding of the lives of all young people, and the transitional process that is constructed within different culture settings. In exploring culture and youth culture in the context of the global comparisons, it became apparent that young people are viewed differently depending on where they live, including attitudes to chronological age and sexual development and whether there was a perceived 'rite of passage' into adulthood (Montgomery 2007).

While Jenny and every young person with or without long-term illness should be viewed as unique, it is important to acknowledge both the experiences that facilitate those unique characteristics that may enable the young person to adapt to increasing independence and the mutual themes that bring all young adults with long-term illness together.

RESEARCH NOTE 16.4 Extending the social exclusion debate: an exploration of the family lives of young carers and young people with ME (Roche and Tucker 2003)

The issues of isolation from peers and suspicion of professionals are raised by young people with the diagnosis of ME who were interviewed. The young people in the study on exploring social exclusion and the lives of young carers and young people with ME felt at times that professionals did not take their issues seriously enough and they were not always heard and communication was difficult. They felt that the situation would improve if they were able to fully participate in decision making, rather than be seen as part of a family group.

'It appears as if the question of the children's voice is not simply one of practical value (professionals will arrive at better decisions affecting them) but also of symbolic value' (page 453).

The approach suggested by Roche and Tucker (2003) suggests the need to not only give the child or young person the voice he requires, but also views each young person as unique rather than a product of the illness. Social isolation and exclusion did not appear to be a specific burden for all young people with long-term illness and their families. This social construction of long-term illness and the young person makes the individual's ability to conform to socially acceptable behaviours far more difficult, either because the opportunities are not available to him or decision making is taken out of his hands.

Barlow and Ellard (2006) highlighted this psychosocial distress in their systemic examination of six reviews, which explores the well-being of children and young people with chronic illness and their siblings and families. The review concluded that young people are more stressed than their counterparts without a chronic illness and that their siblings are also affected; however, they also commented that the evidence was not systematically researched, and that further evidence-based research was required. This was against the reality that, in 2007, 73 per cent of the adult population with CF, a long-term illness, were employed and could clearly handle the stress of interventions required for long-term illness and a career, until the illness became too debilitating (CF Trust 2009).

Biographical Perspective of Youth

The usefulness of exploring the lives of young people using a biographical approach appreciates that young people, rather than labelled as 'youths', are each unique dependent on their own life experiences rather than purely due to the perceived commonalities that exist due to age, gender or culture. This would appear to be a useful method when exploring transition for Jenny, whether this is related to general life transitions or more directly to transitions from health into ill health (Grinyer 2007; Henderson et al. 2007; Kehily 2007). Thomson (2007) commented that the biographical approach was simply 'the history of the life of the person'. Thomson (2007) links the biographical perspective to individualisation and cites Beck (1992) that the way a person's life develops is not a process that can be taken for granted, and the relationship that an individual has with society changes over time and has been influenced recently by economic and technological processes.

Thomson (2008) uses an example of the increasing use of mobile phones as a way that individuals have changed their relationship with society with the freedom the phone gives, causing disembodiment, as young people, especially young women, have more freedom than was traditionally given. Alongside this is the insecurity and disenchantment due to perceived risk of cancer from overuse of the phones and a new form of bullying via the phone, but finally she surmises the re-embedment occurs when new forms of parenting and social contact are developed due to the ease with which individuals can be contacted (Table 16.4).

This can be translated for young people with long-term illness: traditionally the lack of portable equipment, including oxygen cylinders, meant that once a young person had to rely on oxygen throughout the day, they were restricted in their movements often leaving them housebound and able to spend less time with their peers. Now due to advances in technology the equipment can be easily transported and gives the young person more freedom to carry out the social activities on a par with their peers. The disenchantment that may occur relates to an increasing awareness by the young person with long-term illness that, even with advances in technology, she is still restricted in her movements and activities because of exhaustion and treatment requirements. The reintegration occurs when the young person and family and friends become used to the new technologies and adapt their activities to accommodate a variety of abilities.

When exploring the literature written by young people with long-term illness, it became apparent that wishes and hopes for the future are similar to all young people. They wanted to have careers, partners and families (Lipman 2001; Pitts 2007; Walters 2008). Thomson (2007) argues that young people today have more choice in their life stories than at any time in the past because they have the ability and resources to make things happen, helped by the way their parents view their role in disciplining and supporting their children and their future hopes. There could also be a conflict because Jenny has a life-limiting condition. While parents, teachers and employers offered support in career development, the physical condition may limit her career and life opportunities, depending on the severity of the condition and frequency of acute illness episodes. Jenny therefore has to make decisions that could have both negative and positive consequences; this can be related to her personal circumstance including health and family support.

Table 16.4 Individualisation influenced by economic and technological processes

Disembedding	Disenchantment	Re-embedding
Mobile phones gives more freedom	Risk of cancer/bullying	New forms of parenting and social contact
Advances in medical technology increases mobility due to portability	Still restricted in their activities due to exhaustion	Adaptation of activities to accommodate a variety of abilities

Source: adapted from *Risk society: Towards a new modernity*, Sage Publications (Beck, U. 1992) © 1992 Sage Publications. Reproduced by permission of Sage Publications.

Chumbley (1999) commented on the physical process of transferring to adult services and the challenges of leaving children's services:

> Some people find it very difficult emotionally to leave the children's hospital behind. After all, it's a place where you may have grown up and where you may well have felt very secure... when young adults with CF were asked about their transition to adult care in a survey recently, the major reason for their unhappiness was in-patient treatment in a ward with sick, elderly people. (Chumbley 1999, pages 91–92)

While the practicalities of transfer to adult healthcare are emphasised, it was the emotional aspect highlighting the challenges that the young people and their families faced that was pertinent. Alongside these thoughtful discussions about the social and emotional effects of living with long-term illness were helpful hints on how families can get help and support. This book was a real asset for a family with a child newly diagnosed with CF.

RESEARCH NOTE 16.5 The 'Coming of Age' project (Pownceby et al. 1996)

Another way in which the lives of young people with long-term illness were explored was to investigate the experiences of young people as they transferred to adult services. The study also explored treatment adherence for this group of individuals and utilised 10 specialist centres that offer either child or adult services. Fifty-three subjects were pre-transfer and 51 post-transfer to adult services. The study alongside medical notes used a number of different tools to explore with the young people their family, loneliness and life orientation.

Also during the interview process, information was gathered on their experience of the CF centre they attended, the transitional process to adult services, various elements of treatment and personal health behaviours, and also family and social issues, friends, hobbies and interests. The recommendations were valuable in suggesting greater involvement of the family and a need to view the young person before the condition.

RESEARCH NOTE 16.6 From child to adult: an exploration of shifting family roles and responsibilities in managing physiotherapy for cystic fibrosis (Williams et al. 2007)

This study examined the way in which individuals with CF take increasing responsibility for their treatment as they made the transition from youth to adulthood, especially around physiotherapy requirements. The team explored the changing relationship the young person had with their parents in regards to interventions. The interviews with young people and their families were undertaken using a qualitative approach and appeared to be managed in an ethical and empowering fashion. It was clear that the young people did not always agree with the way their parents wanted to manage their treatment. However, for successful adherence, Williams et al. (2007) suggested for consideration all the factors of wellness, and illness, the ability to undertake treatment successfully and family and daily routine for concordance are needed.

'Concordance advocates a sharing of power in the professional–patient interaction, an acknowledgement of not only health professional expertise and knowledge but also the legitimacy of the patient to determine their desired outcome.' (Williams et al. 2007, page 2143).

The team suggested further that professionals using the approach enabled the parents to move from a paternalistic attitude with the young person to a method that had mutually shared goals and values and focuses on the young person's abilities and skills rather than the parents'. The study explored the bidirectional nature of involvement from parents, predominantly the mother, especially during episodes of illness. Many of the outcomes focused on the shifting roles of the young person and their family geared around therapeutic intervention of physiotherapy and the health belief model.

Insightful accounts build up a picture of the lives of young adults adapting to life-long illness and reflect how normal activities of living are interwoven in the theme of illness. This offers Jenny the added benefit of seeing her peers coping with the condition and to have online chats with them. One concern may be if issues are discussed without professional support, as young people may believe speculation about the condition rather than facts and safe information. Jenny describes in detail through her prose how long-term illness makes her feel especially on bad days, however, she also developed skills and learnt to adapt to the condition.

Andy Lipman (2001), in his autobiography about growing up with CF in the USA, provided a refreshing account highlighting how normal he felt in his worries about his physical development. This was especially true in regards to his physical build as compared to his peers and he discussed his concerns about relationships, family and work. The discussion in his early life focused on his struggle to be seen as the same as his friends and

VOICES 16.1 Chloe's alternative definition of CF

I would say that CF is a condition that affects every aspect of your life. It can affect your lungs, liver, pancreas, joints, sinuses, and even fingernails.

But in real terms, for me this means:

I know I have to wake up the next day facing vitamins, minerals, antibiotics and enzymes, which means over 100 tablets a day. I know I'm going to have to spend hours in my day doing physio and coughing up copious amounts of sputum. I know I'm going to have to spend hours doing nebulisers or puffers to fight infection, thin down mucus and open airways, just so I can breathe. I know I'm going to have to drink high-calorie milkshakes which make me want to throw up, just so my body has some energy to fight with, even though I know no matter how hard I try, I'm always going to need to put more weight on. I know I'm going to

have to inject myself maybe six times to keep my diabetes under control. I don't know whether tomorrow I'll be able to walk because my joints are too painful. I don't know whether my stomach muscles are going to hurt at the end of the day because of all the coughing. I don't know if I'll have enough breath to have a shower, or play with my nephew, or do anything other than sleep. I don't know if tomorrow I'll have to turn down an invite from a friend, because yet again 'I'm sorry, I can't, I'm not well enough.' I don't know if I'll ever be able to have kids or a place of my own. And I don't know if tomorrow I'm going to get a call to have a double lung transplant, which I know I may not wake up from. But I do know that at least it makes you appreciate life, and live it to the full without wasting any time, which is certainly a life worth living (**http://www.pwcf.net/**).

school peers, and also his changing relationship with his family (**http://www.youtube.com/watch?v=_LNQaucfYBk** accessed 15/03/12).

After exploring his struggle for independence and life skills at home, Lipman (2001) went on to describe his transition away from home in his college years and experiences with friends and partners. In his account, areas most prominent were not the illness itself, but rather his journey through denial to adaptation and acceptance of his condition, which was counterbalanced with a passionate will to succeed in all areas of his life.

These accounts hold valuable insights into the world of young adults who have a life-limiting condition and the juggling they have to achieve between health and their burgeoning independence and their illness and the dependency they may have on others. This acknowledges the perceived common experience often constructed by society, where it is assumed that an illness especially a long term condition has similarities for everyone and that is homogeneous in nature. An alternative view is the unique experience of the individual which acknowledges their life course of both their journeying into adulthood and their illness progression.

TRANSITIONAL PROGRESSION FOR LIFE COURSE AND ILLNESS

The investigating of transition of young people across different perspectives has enabled young people to be seen to develop within a specific society or culture. If a young person misses time at school from ill health it could lead to delay in educational development, but may also affect social skills and friendship development. Alternatively, a supportive social network will enable a young person to enhance his social development,

and emotional maturity, regardless of any underlying condition (Sloper et al. 2010).

The transitional experiences of youth for individuals with long-term illness cannot be seen as a linear process but rather a recurring dynamic multifactorial process that changes its nature with the realities of the person, both positively during periods of wellness or emotional stability and negatively during acute escalation of the condition or inadequate professional or family support. An individual grows physically, socially and psychologically, influenced by all their experiences and relationships, and their independence may increase over time from a child to an adult and from an older adult until death (Bee and Boyd 2006; Williams et al. 2007). Independence and dependence need to be acknowledged, for instance when a young person starts working and living independently.

Factors that Influence the Development of Independence

Transition into adulthood is complex and socially constructed within the context of an individual. This is true for any young person such as Jenny because of her own personal and societal experiences (McCarthy 2006). Jenny appears to pursue hopes similar to those of her peers but also has insight into the profound effects a life-limiting condition has on her mind, body and lifestyle (Badlan 2006). This, in turn, is relevant to educational attainment, relationships with family, friends and life partners while times of relative wellness can offer opportunities for activities, including studies, careers and socialising (Pownceby et al. 1996). Jenny therefore has to continuously adapt and strive for autonomy as the illness progresses and as she transitions into adulthood.

The strive for independence during the life course is constantly balanced against the requirements for the interventions for long-term illness, especially when becoming an adult. In my research, this led to the recognition that the mundane and ordinary for young people with long-term illness changes over time, in regards to their lifestyle and illness progression (Thurston 2010).

IMPLICATIONS FOR POLICY AND PRACTICE

The activities that are undertaken by Jenny both as a young person and also because of her long-term illness require professionals in health, education and social care and career services to work alongside her rather than trying to be her advocate, a role that she could be said already to be successfully undertaking (ACT 2007). Adherence to treatment could be argued to be the greatest challenge for her (Foster et al. 2001; Williams et al. 2007; Badlan 2006; Thurston 2010). However, if the context within compliance is explored, including family life, school, college or career obligations, this would offer an opportunity for Jenny to have guidance to develop strategies that gives time for her lifestyle commitments, alongside the requirements of the treatment regime. Mobility both physically and through studying or career can affect her ability to achieve or maintain the balance between lifestyle and treatment regimes.

The Department of Health (2006, 2007) explores ways of supporting young people with complex or long-term conditions as they transferred to adult services, including health, social care and education, with financial allowances. The documentation offered examples of good practice in regards to independent living, housing and transport. Unfortunately, there appeared to be little on the support and resources available for the young person such as Jenny, who is cognitively able to seek a job after her education. While supported employment was mentioned, this was superficial. With the reality that 72 per cent of adults with some long-term illness are working or studying, it would have been useful to have given more detailed information that was user friendly (CF Trust 2009; McNamara 2011).

There is a pivotal role played by families in the support of young people with long-term illness. Whether Jenny is still active or has more underlying symptoms, there appeared to be an inconsistency of service support offered for the family or outside the family. The issues and concerns do not appear to arise for young people during their time in children's services due to the focus of family-centred care (Casey 1993); there is, in fact, a positive element to the care received, which enabled the young people to live as conventional a live as possible (Thurston 2010; McNamara 2011).

Health professionals' utilisation of nursing models when educating individuals and their families about their illness are of paramount importance, especially when the condition has long-term health implications (Casey 1993; Roper et al. 1990; Williams et al. 2006; Holland et al. 2008). However, young adults and their families can also educate the professionals with the knowledge and personal experiences they have gained because of living with the condition. Jenny is unique and therefore transition from specific child services to adult services should be tailored to her specific needs (RCN 2004). When working in partnership with the family, practitioners whether health, education or social care, need to ensure openness to their hopes even if it does not reflect the practitioner's own values and beliefs (Boylan and Dalrymple 2009; Walker and Thurston 2006; Williams et al. 2006).

The developmental and transitional needs into adulthood for Jenny require acknowledgement, alongside the progressive concerns of her condition. Health professionals both at the local hospital and in the tertiary centres sometimes misunderstood basic requirements for safety and reassurance. To rectify this, Hollander (2002) viewed the appropriate practice that enabled young people to feel supported was honest and open communication, which facilitates the voicing of concerns and issues to be shared in a non-critical constructive environment. This would empower Jenny to vocalise her true dilemmas rather than offering a sanitised version of her life, treatment and daily routine.

PRACTICAL GUIDELINES 16.1

● Acknowledge and value the family care especially following increasingly debilitating elements of the condition.

- Offer an atmosphere in which to explore values and beliefs in a safe and confidential manner within and outside the family.
- Offer opportunities for realistic discussions around lifespan.
- Offer Jenny opportunities to discuss having a family.

- Have awareness of potential conflicts with parents.
- Include all family members in planning care.
- Offer support networks for family members.
- Tailor transitional services specifically for Jenny.
- Offer respite care for Jenny and her family when required.

While Jenny may require information and reassurance, in the longer term she will also require practical support from health professionals. Some young people with long term illness are able to go on to further education, others to work, however some may have issues and concerns which may reduce their success in finding a job, or developing adult

relationships (Walters and Warren 2001; Roulstone et al. 2003; CF Trust 2009). If, during transfer, services offered to Jenny are transparent and well resourced with good networking across agencies, then this may ensure that she reaches the potential she strives to achieve, within her own physical capacity (ACT 2007).

PRACTICAL GUIDELINES 16.2

● Accessibility services need to have insight into the progressive nature of Jenny's illness.

● Be aware of up-to-date research in regards to prevention and treatment of infection.
● Respect Jenny regarding commitments outside the remit of the condition including school and work.
● Offer opportunities for peer support (including online).
● Offer opportunities to shape future practice and policies.

● Jenny should be involved in regularly reviewing her care.

PRACTICAL GUIDELINES 16.3

● Offer Jenny flexible programmes of school work.
● Acknowledge her personal abilities and skills to offer a tailor-made service.
● Offer Jenny honest and open communication.
● Give opportunities for interventions in a supportive education environment.
● Specific support to enable the transition into further or higher education.
● Specific support to enable the transition into and maintenance of employment.

● Adaptation of emotional and social support during physical and psychological development.
● Consideration given to Jenny's culture, personal knowledge and cognitive ability.
● Listen without offering judgement, using opportunistic discussion.
● Encourage Jenny to become fully informed and able to make her own choices and decisions.
● Offer Jenny pastoral support.

While nurses and doctors acknowledge the value of progressive services for young adults before they reach adult care, practically, this is much more difficult to plan. The emotional and social support for Jenny needs to change and adapt to her needs as she physically and psychologically grows and develops. The guidelines offered by the CF Trust in their *Standards of care document for children and adults with CF* (2001a) acknowledged this challenging time for the young person both emotionally and physically. The guidelines urged the nurse and other health professionals caring for the young person to be aware and realistic in the issues that may arise, which may include conflict with parents and maintaining and adhering to treatment regimes (Foster et al. 2001; Badlan 2006; Williams et al. 2006).

An associate document to the standards of care from the CF Trust (2001a) is the *The national consensus for nurse management* (2001b). This highlights the roles that the family had to undertake, varying from being the young adult's partner in care, to managing clinical practice and offering advice and education. While this offers clear ideas of the way in which the specialist nurse maintained support, it does not really acknowledge the gap in service for those individuals who are unable to receive the service available due to their geographical location or tertiary centre, although these services are increasing with time and the development of shared clinics (CF Trust 2009; McNamara 2011). It can become an ethical dilemma for health professionals and the individual young people alike, which needs to be addressed if parity of services and resources are to be achieved. Health professionals cannot always gain expertise because they do not have enough new referrals to improve their practice, while Jenny may be unhappy to receive a new service, even if it is local, because the teams of health professionals are not seen as knowledgeable enough in the care and treatment of the individual with long-term illness required.

PRACTICAL GUIDELINES 16.4

● Offer Jenny opportunities for safe and supervised learning/leisure activities.
● Education resources need to be offered to environments of the individual with long-term illness.
● Awareness of the variety of activities that Jenny accesses.

● Support and advice offered to friends and family when requested.
● Support for relationship and family planning.

Implementation of the policies agreed by most specialised centres follow guidelines developed by the CF (2001b, 2002, 2004). While the effective treatment can been seen to be key for Jenny at present with an acute infection and prophylactially to reduce the deterioration in the lungs (Walters and Warren 2001; University of Dundee 2006; CF Trust 2009), this cannot work in isolation; rather professionals in the clinical area need to maintain universal precautions to ensure no undue risks are taken (CF Trust 2001a).

PRACTICAL GUIDELINES 16.5

- Need to work as part of a multiprofessional team.
- Acknowledgement of Jenny as the expert patient.
- Utilisation of resources offered by the CF trust.
- Offer a transparent service with good networking across agencies.
- Uniform approach to care.
- Jenny receives holistic services flexible to her lifestyle.
- Support for the assessment of the financial implications of long-term illness. Support for the family during times of admission.

- Complaints listened to sensitively and constructively dealt with.
- Central sourcing of equipment.
- Spiritual care for frontline staff.
- Support with applying for housing, grants, benefits and equipment.
- Increased levels of education for all professionals on the effects of long-term illness and secondary conditions.
- Offer of specialty clinics acknowledging secondary conditions and pain.

Although specialised services may give Jenny the physical support and interventions required, they do not always take into account the uniqueness of the person and their family. Issues around culture, individual development, personal knowledge and cognitive ability also need to be considered if holistic care is to be offered. Iles and Lowton (2008) explored young people's long-term illness experiences of working with the multi-professional team being offered support and concluded that rather than the team reacting on an informal basis, the young person requested support physically and emotionally as part of the standard package of care. This uniformed approach acknowledged the uncertainty of disease progression, including discussions around transplantation, and palliative care.

PRACTICAL GUIDELINES 16.6

- Key (worker) professional to be the main contact (locally and at the specialist centre).
- Awareness of the tension between dependency and independence.
- Awareness of the context of treatment adherence, including time commitments to school, work and family.
- Openness to Jenny's aims in life.
- Understanding of requirements for safety and reassurance especially around treatment.
- If available, offer a placement when required on an adolescent unit for long-term illness catering for young people within the region.

- Realistic view of issues that may arise in maintaining and adhering to treatment regimes.
- Being Jenny's partner in care.
- Managing clinical practice and offering advice and education.
- Acknowledgement of the uncertainty of disease progression, transplantation, palliative care.
- Working with Jenny to plan terminal care in an appropriate place.

How this would work for Jenny can be seen by the utilisation of the RCN (2004) guidelines for adolescent transition care, which offers a flexible approach that can be tailored for each young person and identified her involvement in each stage of the process from the early stage of transition to the middle and late stage, until she is successfully embedded in adult services.

The framework for each topic gives pointers for discussion, however, other areas may also be highlighted for the young person to pinpoint her own needs.

CASE STUDY REVIEW 16.1

Necessity for independent care with regard to PEG feeding and transfer to adult services

Make sure Jenny understands what resources she needs

By Jenny having information about her option for Percutaneous Endoscopic Gastrostomy (PEG) feeding and transferring to adult services she can then make an informed decision about compliance to treatment both during her stay and following discharge. This will include support from the dietetic team and the transition clinic team.

Discuss any potential problems/barriers

As Jenny is concerned about her transfer to adult services, a discussion of the options will make it easier for her to decide where she would like to go for her inpatient treatment as an adult and who would support her at home. This could be predominantly local or at the tertiary centre (or a mixture of the two) and may be influenced by the relationships with the health professionals involved in her care. Visiting potential hospitals will help this.

Make sure Jenny knows where to get help

Give Jenny contacts of both statutory services such as social services (for financial advice) and NHS (for treatment) alongside voluntary service such as the CF Trust (for peer support and general advice).

Make sure Jenny understands the principles of confidentiality

When Jenny needs to share information, including inconsistency with her compliance of her drug regimen, she needs to feel that the information is discussed only with the professionals directly dealing with her care. This may mean that her parents may have concerns about not being involved in the entire decision making and she and they may require further support about the transitional process.

Actions

Offer Jenny the opportunity to explore the risks and side-effects of the PEG feeding, but also the most appropriate routes and timing of administration.

Evidence

Jenny will then know who is available to support her on a daily basis.

Jenny will be able to identify her preferred feeding regime and discuss likely side-effects.

She will be able to identify which medication and treatments to increase when required.

She also knows how to make urgent appointments and understands the SOS admission to the ward.

She is aware of the confidential nature of the transition programme.

Source: adapted from RCN (2004)

CONCLUSION

While transition into adulthood is socially constructed by society, the definition of transition linked to illness is more complex as there is an acknowledgement of the struggle for independence, but alongside this the use of transition by health professionals endeavours to accommodate the changing nature of the patient's condition and whether it is stable or deteriorating (Kralik et al. 2006). Young people such as Jenny have to negotiate with their family and health professionals to ensure the interventions that they can no longer undertake still occur (Lowton 2002).

SUMMARY OF KEY LEARNING

- Skills are therefore required to support young people as they transfer to adult services and also have continued care.
- Professionals need to listen without offering judgement and use opportunistic discussions to explore issues. Also professionals should offer an atmosphere in which to explore values and beliefs in a safe and confidential manner.
- As adherence to interventions is often seen from the professional rather than the individual's perspective it would be useful not to focus on the trivial elements, rather the important issues respecting the young person's point of view. This is especially true regarding commitments outside the remit of the condition and interventions required.
- Encourage the young person to reflect on their personal experiences and then make their own decisions, offering them further opportunities to develop independence (Walker and Thurston 2006).

FURTHER RESOURCES

Moving into adulthood

This guide highlights the major life changes that young people may experience as a disabled teenager – including choices in education, health and independent living: **http://www.direct.gov .uk/en/YoungPeople/Youngdisabledpeople/DG_10039695**

Transition out of the parental home in Britain, Spain and Norway

http://www.liv.ac.uk/Geography/research/grants/leaving.htm

Ten approaches to help you deliver better outcomes and an enhanced experience of care for people living with long-term conditions. A collaborative resource to support partnership: **http://www.scotland.gov.uk/Resource/ Doc/309257/0097421.pdf**

Rachel's blog about waiting for a lung transplant: **http://lungs-for-life.blogspot.com/**

Asthma support website for young people: **http://www .kickasthma.org.uk/index.html**

Young people with long-term health conditions: **http://www .youtube.com/watch?v=BX5-zRz9zDM**

Diabetes: **http://www.youtube.com/watch?v=b1tiIcHfeMc**

Young people and cancer: **http://www.youtube.com/ watch?v=USkZNNLZatA**

ANSWERS TO ACTIVITIES

ACTIVITY 16.1   Ages of progression to adulthood within UK law

In Great Britain, a person has to be 16 or older to have homosexual (gay) or heterosexual (straight) sex.

To be allowed to vote, you must be 18 years of age or over on polling day, be resident in the UK, be a British citizen, a qualifying Commonwealth citizen or a citizen of the Republic of Ireland and not be subject to any legal incapacity to vote.

There are many rules that control working hours of 14-year-old children, but the basic ones are: during term time, they may only work for 2 hours on weekdays and Sundays, during term time; they may work for up to 5 hours on a week day or a Saturday during a school holiday, they may not work for more than 2 hours on a Sunday and may not work before 7 am or after 7 pm on any day.

While still at school, the rights for 15- and 16-year-olds are almost identical to those of 14-year-olds. However, they are allowed to work for up to 8 hours on Saturdays or during the school holidays.

If no longer at school, 16- or 17-year-olds are referred to by the law as a 'young worker'. Because they are no longer at school, there are fewer restrictions on when they may work and for how long, but there are still some rules. Because they reached school leaving age, they may find that employers may be more willing to offer part-time or full-time employment. They are also not limited to just 'light work', so are allowed to work in places such as a busy shop, restaurant kitchen or as a waiter or waitress (see **http:// www.direct.gov.uk/en/YoungPeople/Workandcareers/ Yourrightsandresponsibilitiesatwork/DG_066272**).

It is against the law to sell alcohol to someone under 18 anywhere, for an adult to buy or attempt to buy alcohol on behalf of someone under 18, for someone under 18 to buy alcohol, attempt to buy alcohol or to be sold alcohol, for someone under 18 to drink alcohol in licensed premises, except where the child is 16 or 17 years old and accompanied by an adult. In this case, it is legal for them to drink, but not buy, beer, wine and cider with a table meal, for an adult to buy alcohol for someone under 18 for consumption on licensed premises, except as just seen and, finally, it is against the law for children under 5 to drink alcohol at home or on private premises unless following a doctor's advice for health reasons.

It is not illegal: for someone over 18 to buy a child over 16 beer, wine or cider if they are eating a table meal together in licensed premises; neither is it illegal for a child aged 5 to 16 to drink alcohol at home or on other private premises (see **http:// www.drinkaware.co.uk/talking-to-under-18s/parents/ the-law?gclid=CKWytu3M96wCFUhrfAod_iuQTA**).

There is no law in England or Wales to prevent anyone of any age from babysitting, but a person under the age of 16 may not be charged with neglect or ill treatment of a child left in her care. Parents remain responsible and can be charged themselves if their child is harmed in any way.

The NSPCC, however, recommends 16 as a minimum age for babysitting (see **www.worcestershire.gov.uk/cms/ PDF/46684%20Babysitting.pdf**).

It is illegal to sell cigarettes, tobacco or cigarette papers to anyone under 18 and smoking is banned in all public places and workplaces, whatever your age (see **http://www. adviceguide.org.uk/index/your_family/family_index_ew/ faq_index_family/faq_family_legal_age_drinking_and_ smoking.htm**).

In the UK, generally speaking, a man and a woman may marry if they are both over 16 and not married to or in a civil partnership with someone else. Individuals aged 16 or 17 in England, Wales and Northern Ireland, however, may only marry if they obtain their parents' consent. Moreover, close blood relatives may not marry – although this does not include first cousins, who may still legally wed one another in the UK.

Lastly, people of the same sex may not marry, but they may register a civil partnership instead (this is currently under review) (see **http://findlaw.co.uk/law/getting_married/index.html**).

At 16, young people have the right to decide where they want to live. Some options include continuing to live at home with their parents or carers, applying for sheltered housing through the council or housing association, moving into private rental accommodation, alone or with friends or applying for a council or housing association house or flat (see **http://www.direct.gov.uk/en/YoungPeople/Youngdisabledpeople/DG_10039695**),

Existing legislation provides for a number of different custodial penalties for 10 to 17 year olds:

- Detention at Her Majesty's pleasure, under section 53(1) of the Children and Young Persons Act 1933 for murder: the sentence may be served in local authority secure accommodation or Prison Service accommodation depending on the age and vulnerability of the offender and the availability of accommodation.
- Long terms of detention, under section 53(2) of the 1933 Act, up to the adult maximum, for other very serious offences such as manslaughter, robbery, domestic burglary and indecent assault: the sentence may be served in local authority secure accommodation or Prison Service accommodation depending on the offender's age and vulnerability and the availability of accommodation.
- Detention of between 2 months and 2 years in a young offender institution for 15 to 17-year-olds convicted of any imprisonable offence.
- A secure training order of between 6 months and 2 years for 12 to 14-year-old persistent offenders to be served in secure training centres (see **http://www.nationalarchives.gov.uk/ERORecords/HO/421/2/nme.htm**, **http://www.archive2.official-documents.co.uk/document/cm57/5778/5778.pdf** and **http://www.direct**

.gov.uk/en/YoungPeople/CrimeAndJustice/Youngpeopleservingyoursentence/DG_10027708).

Once children reach the age of 16, they are presumed in law to be competent. In many respects, they should be treated as adults and may give consent for their own surgical and medical treatment.

The Department of Health recommends that it is, nevertheless, good practice to encourage children of this age to involve their families in decisions about their care, unless it would not be in their interests to do so.

If a competent child requests that confidentiality be maintained, this should be respected unless the doctor considers that failing to disclose information would result in significant harm to the child.

A child aged 16 to 18 may not refuse treatment if it has been agreed by a person with parental responsibility or the court and it is in their best interests. Therefore, they do not have the same status as adults.

The Mental Capacity Act applies to people aged 16 and over in England, Wales and Northern Ireland. In Scotland, the legal framework is set out by the Adults with Incapacity (Scotland) Act 2000.

Children under the age of 16 are deemed not to be automatically legally competent to give consent.

The courts have determined that such children can be legally competent if they have 'sufficient understanding and maturity to enable them to understand fully what is proposed'.

This concept is now known as 'Gillick competency' and initially arose in the case of Gillick vs. West Norfolk and Wisbech Health Authority in 1986. The term 'Fraser competency' is also used in this respect (Lord Fraser was the judge who ruled on the case) (see **http://www.patient.co.uk/doctor/Consent-to-Treatment-in-Children.htm**, **http://www.nhs.uk/NHSEngland/AboutNHSservices/Documents/NSF%20children%20in%20hospitalDH_4067251[1].pdf** and **http://www.gmc-uk.org/static/documents/content/0-18_0510.pdf**).

ACTIVITY 16.2 List the chores that become more relevant to young people as they gain more responsibility in the home.

In Britain, young people tend to help more in the house once they reach their twenties, which may reflect a sense of becoming an adult and taking some responsibility for the household (**http://www.liv.ac.uk/Geography/research/grants/leaving.htm**).

Chores that children aged 10 and older may undertake include: unloading the dishwasher, folding laundry, cleaning the bathroom, washing windows, washing the car, cooking a simple meal with supervision, ironing clothes, doing laundry, babysitting the younger siblings (with adult in the home), mowing the lawn, cleaning the kitchen, cleaning the oven, changing beds and making cookies or cake from a box mix (**http://www.webmd.com/parenting/features/chores-for-children**).

Young carers often take on a level of responsibility that is inappropriate to their age or development. More than half of young carers live in one-parent families and almost one-third care for someone with mental health problems.

The average age of a young carer is 12.

The 2001 census showed that there are 175,000 young carers in the UK, 13,000 of whom care for more than 50 hours a week, 72% cook and clean, over 50% provide general care and 20% help with intimate care such as showering and toileting (**http://www.barnardos.org.uk/what_we_do/turn_around/young_carers_rebecca.htm?gclid=CJna7dTP1KOCFblhtAodshAikw**).

ACTIVITY 16.3 Highlight the nursing or medical interventions you would be happy/unhappy for a young person with a long-term condition to undertake.

Each young person is unique; therefore an acknowledgement of how their long-term condition may affect them is important. Medical interventions performed by one young person on a regular basis such as giving themselves medication via injections or intravenously or undertaking physiotherapy may not be suitable for another (Thurston 2010).

ACTIVITY 16.4 Reflect on the young person's physical and psychological attributes that health professionals measure to monitor their increasing growth and development.

See Chapter 3.

ACTIVITY 16.5 List specific risk-taking behaviours the young people you work with undertake; this may include drinking, smoking etc.

Risk taking is seen as behaviour that may end up in disaster, damage or injury. This can be seen as a need by the young person to walk a fine line between fearfulness and exhilaration, even though the young person may only see the thrill and not the risk.

Examples of risk-taking behaviour include: fighting, joy riding/traffic dodging, drinking alcohol/taking drugs/smoking, vandalism/hooliganism, playing truant, having unprotected sex/having a baby, stealing/burgling, murder, prostitution, becoming homeless, carrying a gun/knife, self-harm/attempting suicide, not complying with treatments for health conditions and playing extreme sports.

The types of risk-taking behaviour can be seen to be on a continuum, from staying out late at night, to getting into fights right through to committing murder or trying to take your own life. A degree of risk taking is thought to be a 'normal' transitional behaviour during adolescence, however, extreme risk taking can lead to self-destructive activities (Visser and Moleko 2005; Walker and Thurston 2006; Chapter 3).

ACTIVITY 16.6 Reflect on the different groups or subcultures to which you may belong:

[Example]
Age: 50
Gender: female
Nationality: British
Religion (if any): agnostic

Cultural heritage: Irish Catholic
Political persuasion: liberal socialist
Single/married/divorced: married

SELECTED REFERENCES

ACT (2007) *The transition care pathway: a framework for the development of integrated multi-agency care pathways for young people with life-threatening and life-limiting conditions.* ACT: Bristol.

Aldgate, J., Jones, D., Rose. W. and Jeffery, C. (eds) (2006) *The developing child.* Jessica Kingsley Publisher: London.

Apel, M.A. (2006) *Cystic fibrosis: the ultimate teen guide*, 4th edn. Scarecrow Press Inc.: Boston, MA.

Badlan, K. (2006) Young people living with cystic fibrosis: an insight into their subjective experience. *Health and Social Care in the Community,* 14(3), 264–270.

Barham, N. (2004) *Disconnected: why our kids are turning their backs on everything we thought we knew.* Random House: London.

Barlow, J.H. and Ellard, D.R. (2006) The psychosocial wellbeing of the child with chronic disease, their parents and siblings: an overview of research evidence base. *Child Care, Health and Development,* 32(1), 19–31.

Barnes, C., Mercer, G. and Shakespeare, T. (1999) *Exploring disability: a sociological introduction.* Polity Press: Cambridge.

Beck, H. (1992) *Risk society: towards a new modernity.* Sage: London.

Bee, H. and Boyd, D. (2006) *The developing child,* 11th edn. Pearson International: New York.

Berk, L.E. (2006) *Child development.* Pearson International Edition: Boston, MA.

Boyden, J. and Levison, D. (2000) *Working paper 2000: 1: children as economic and social actors in the development process,* expert Group On Development Issues, Ministry for Foreign Affairs: Stockholm.

Boylan, J. and Dalrymple, J. (2009) *Understanding advocacy for children and young people.* Open University Press/McGraw-Hill: Maidenhead.

Bury, M. (2005) *Health and illness.* Polity Press: Malden, MA.

Casey, A. (1993) Development and use of the partnership model of nursing care, in G. Glasper and A. Tucker (eds), *Advances in child health nursing.* Scutari Press: London.

Chumbley, J. (1999) *Cystic fibrosis – a family affair*. Sheldon Press: London.

Coles, B. (2004) *Welfare services for young people: better connections?* in J. Roche, S. Tucker, R. Thomson and R. Flynn (eds), *Youth in society*, 2nd edn. Sage: London.

Collins, R. (1994) *Four sociological traditions*. Oxford University Press: Oxford.

Corby, B. (2006) *Child abuse: towards a knowledge base*, 3rd edn. Open University Press: Maidenhead.

Cuckney, P. (1993) *CF rules ok: the story of a life with cystic fibrosis*. Pat Cuckney: Birmingham.

Cystic Fibrosis Trust Clinical Standards and Accreditation Group (2001a) *Standards for the clinical care of children and adults with cystic fibrosis in the UK*. Cystic Fibrosis Trust: Bromley.

Cystic Fibrosis Trust (2001b) *The national consensus for nurse management*. Cystic Fibrosis Trust: Bromley.

Cystic Fibrosis Trust (2002) *Information: clinical guidelines for the physiotherapy management of cystic fibrosis*. Cystic Fibrosis Trust: Bromley.

Cystic Fibrosis Trust (2004) *Annual data report 2004*. Cystic Fibrosis Trust: Bromley.

Cystic Fibrosis Trust (2006) *Factsheet: employment*. Cystic Fibrosis Trust: Bromley.

Cystic Fibrosis Trust (2009) *UK CF registry annual data report 2007*. Cystic Fibrosis Trust: Bromley.

Department of Health (DoH) (2006) *Transition: getting it right for young people: improving the transition of young people with long-term conditions from children's to adult services*. DoH: London.

Department of Health (DoH) (2007) *Transition planning for young people with complex health needs or a disability: a transition guide for all services. Key information for professionals about the transition process for disabled young people*. DoH Publications: London.

Didsbury, J. and Thackray, E. (2009) *Cystic fibrosis and relationships: a collection of real-life experiences, written by people with CF and their partners*. Cystic Fibrosis Trust: Bromley.

Eiser, C. (1990) *Chronic childhood disease: an introduction to psychological theory and research*. Cambridge University Press: Cambridge.

Elston, S. (ed.) (2001) *Palliative care for young people aged 13–24*. National Council for Hospice and Specialist Palliative Care Services, SPA: Bristol.

Foley, P., Roche, J. and Tucker, S. (eds) (2001) *Children in society: contemporary theory, policy and practice*. Open University Press: Basingstoke.

Foster, C. et al. (2001) Treatment demands and differential treatment of patients with cystic fibrosis and their siblings: patient, parent and sibling accounts. *Child Care, Health and Development*, 27(4), 349–364.

Garratt, D. (2004) Youth cultures and sub-cultures, in J. Roche, (eds) S. Tucker, R. Thomson and R. Flynn, *Youth in society*, 2nd edn. Sage: London.

Garratt, D., Roche, J. and Tucker, S. (eds) (1997) *Changing experiences of youth*. Sage Publications/Open University Press: London.

Glasper, A. and Richardson, J. (eds) (2006) *A textbook of children's and young people's nursing*. Churchill Livingstone: Edinburgh.

Griffin, C. (1993) *Representations of youth: the study of youth and adolescence in Britain and America*. Polity Press: Oxford.

Griffin, C. (2004) Representations of the young, in J. Roche and S. Tucker, R. Thomson and R. Flynn, *Youth in society*, 2nd edn. Sage: London.

Grinyer, A. (2007) *Young people living with cancer: implications for policy and practice*. McGraw Hill Education/Open University Press: Maidenhead.

Helman, C.G. (2001) *Culture, health and illness*, 4th edn. Arnold: New York.

Henderson, S. et al. (2007) *Inventing adulthoods: a biographical approach to youth transitions*. Sage: London.

Holdsworth, C. and Morgan, D. (2005) *Transitions in context: leaving home, independence and adulthood*. McGraw Hill Education/Open University Press: Maidenhead.

Holland, K. et al. (2008) *Applying the Roper, Logan and Tierney model in practice*, Elsevier/Churchill Livingstone: New York.

Huegel, K. (1998) *Young people and chronic illness, true stories, help and hope*. Free Spirit Publishing: Minneapolis, MN.

Jenkins, G.W., Kemnitz, C.P. and Tortora, G.J. (2007) *Anatomy and physiology from science to life*. Wiley: Chichester.

Kehily, M.J. (ed.) (2007) *Understanding youth: perspectives, identities and practices*. Sage/Open University Press: London.

Kloep, M. (1999) Love is all you need? Focusing on adolescents' life concerns from an ecological point of view. *Journal Of Adolescence*, 22, 49–63.

Kralik, D., Visentin, K. and Van Loon, A. (eds) (2006) *Transition: a literature review, The Author's Journal Compilation*. Blackwell Publishing Ltd: Chichester.

Law Commission (2008) *Adult social care: a scoping report*. Law Commission: London.

Lee, N. (2001) *Childhood and society. Growing up in an age of uncertainty*. Open University Press: Philadelphia, PA.

Lipman, A. (2001) *Alive at 25*. Longstreet Press: Atlanta, GA.

Lowton, K. (2002) Parents and partners: lay carers' perceptions of their role in the treatment and care of adults with cystic fibrosis. *Journal of Advanced Nursing*, 39(2), 174–181.

Lupton, D. (2003) *Medicine as culture*, 2nd edn. Sage Publications: London.

Marsh. et al. (2009) *Sociology: making sense of society*. Pearson: Harlow.

Mayall, B. (2000) *Negotiating childhoods*. Economic and Social Research Council: London.

McAdams, D. (2001) *The person, an integrated introduction to personality and psychology*, 3rd edn. Harcourt College Publishers: New York.

McCarthy, J. (2006) *Young people's experiences of loss and bereavement*. McGraw Hill Education/Open University Press: Maidenhead.

McNamara, K. (2011) *Transition for young people with life-limiting conditions: the UK picture*. Together for Short Lives: Bristol.

Modrcin-Talbott, M.A. et al. (1998) A study of self-esteem among well adolescents: seeking a new direction. *Issues in Comprehensive Pediatric Nursing*, 21, 229–241.

Montgomery, H. (2007) A comparative perspective, in M.J. Kehily (ed.) *Understanding youth: perspectives, identities and practices*. Sage/Open University Press: Maidenhead.

Morrow, V. and Richards, M. (1996) *Transition to adulthood: a family matter?* Joseph Rowntree Foundation: York.

Penn, H. (2005) *Understanding early childhood: issues and controversies*. Open University Press: Maidenhead.

Pitts, D. (2007) *Living on borrowed time: life with cystic fibrosis*. Authorhouse: Milton Keynes.

Pownceby, J. et al. (1996) *The coming of age project: A study of the translation from paediatric to adult care and treatment adherence amongst young people with cystic fibrosis*, The Cystic Fibrosis Trust: Bromley.

Robb, M. (ed.) (2007a) *Youth in context: frameworks, settings and encounters*. Sage/Open University Press: Milton Keynes.

Robb, M. (2007b) Relating, in M.J. Kehily (ed.) *Understanding youth: perspectives, identities and practices*. Sage/Open University Press: London.

Roche, J. and Tucker, S. (2003) Extending the social exclusion debate: an exploration of the family lives of young carers and young people with ME. *Childhood*, 10, 439–456.

Roche, J., Tucker, S., Thomson, R. and Flynn, R. (eds) (2004) *Youth in society*, 2nd edn. Sage: London.

Roper, N., Logan, W. and Tierney, A. (eds) (1990) *The elements of nursing*, 3rd edn. Churchill Livingstone: London.

Roulstone, A. et al. (2003) Thriving and surviving at work: disabled people's employment strategies. Polity Press: Oxford.

Royal College of Nursing (RCN) (2004) *Adolescent transition care: guidance for nursing staff*. RCN: London.

Schutz, A. (2006) *Stanford encyclopedia of philosophy*. Metaphysics Research Lab, CSLI, Stanford University: Stanford, CA.

Shale, D. (ed.) (1996) *Cystic fibrosis*. BMJ Publishing Group: London.

Silverman, D. (1993) *Interpreting qualitative data: methods for analysing talk, text and interaction*, Sage Publications: London.

Sloper P., Beecham, J., Clarke, S., Franklin, A., Moran, N. and Cusworth, L. (2010) *Models of multi-agency services for transition to adult services for disabled young people and those with complex health needs: impact and costs*. Social Policy Research Unit, University of York: York.

Sparkes, A. (2002) *Telling tales in sport and physical activity: a qualitative journey*. Human Kinetics Press: Champaign, IL.

Sparkes, A.C. and Smith, B. (2008) Men, spinal cord injury, memories and the narrative performance of pain. *Disability and Society*, 23(7), 679–690.

Stokes, H. and Tyler, D. (2001) The multi-dimensional lives of young people: young peoples' perspective of education, work, life and their future. *Scottish Youth Issues Journal*, 3.

Taylor, J. and Müller, D. (1995) *Nursing adolescents: research and psychological perspectives*. Blackwell Science: Oxford.

Taylor, S. and Field, D. (1997) *Sociology of health and health care*, 2nd edn. Blackwell Science: Oxford.

Thomson, A.H. and Harris, A. (2008) *The facts: cystic fibrosis*. Oxford University Press: Oxford.

Thurston, C. (2010) The life and transitional experiences of eight young people with cystic fibrosis (CF). Unpublished thesis in partial fulfilment of the requirement of Anglia Ruskin University for the degree of PhD in social science.

Thurston, C. and Church, J. (2001) Involving children and families in decision making about health, in P. Foley, J. Roche and S. Tucker (eds) *Children in society: contemporary theory, policy and practice*. Open University Press: Basingstoke.

Turney, D. (2007) Practice, in M. Robb (ed.) *Youth in context: frameworks, settings and encounters*, Sage/Open University Press: Milton Keynes.

Valentine, F. and Lowes, L. (eds) (2007) *Nursing care of children and young people with chronic illness*. Blackwell Publishing: Oxford.

Visser, M. and Moleko, A.G. (2005) *High-risk behaviour of primary school learners*: **http://www.sahealthinfo.org/admodule/highrisk.htm**

Wakefield, G. (2002) *Schizophrenia – a mother's story*. Fivepins Publishing Ltd: Salisbury.

Walker, S. and Thurston, C. (2006) *Safeguarding children and young people – a guide to integrated practice*. Russell House Publishing: Lyme Regis.

Walters, S. (2008) *My life with cystic fibrosis*: **http://www.docs-quid.com/mylifecf.htm**

Walters, S. and Warren, R. (2001) *Cystic fibrosis – a millennium survey*, Cystic Fibrosis Trust: Bromley.

Werner, E. (2000) Protective factors and individual resilience, in J.P. Shonkoff (ed.) (2000) *Handbook of early childhood interventions*, 2nd edn. Cambridge University Press: Cambridge.

Wheal, A. (2004) *Adolescence: positive approaches for working with young people*, 2nd edn, Russell House Publishing: Lyme Regis.

Williams, B., Mukhopadhyay, S., Dowell, J. and Coyle, J. (2007) From child to adult: an exploration of shifting family roles and responsibilities in managing physiotherapy for cystic fibrosis. *Social Science and Medicine*, 65, 2135–2146.

CHAPTER 17
Research with Children and Young People

Tina Moules and Darren Sharpe

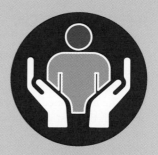
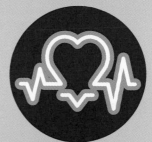
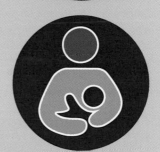

LEARNING OUTCOMES

On completion of this chapter, the reader will be able to:

- Discuss different approaches, techniques and methods for researching with children and young people.
- Search for and interpret information from a variety of sources.
- Understand the ethical issues involved in carrying out research with children and young people.
- Explain the importance of disseminating the findings of research into the practice arena.
- Understand the requirement for developing the capacity for conceptual, critical and independent thinking.

TALKING POINT

'Recognise the implementation of professional ethical guidelines for research with children as desirable and as being premanently irreducible to routine . . . Morally engaged practitioners (researchers) could not hide within professional ethical anaesthesia, but would retain their responsibility for their professional practice and its implications.' (Husband, 1995)

INTRODUCTION

It is said by many authors that Florence Nightingale was the first to identify the importance of research in nursing when she was working in the military hospital in Scutari during the Crimean War. She maintained that practice needed to be up to date and based on the best current research findings available. She was very interested in statistics and was keen on collecting data and was able to use these data to improve conditions in military hospitals. However, not much about research was evident in the literature until the 1950s when a number of developments brought the topic onto the nursing agenda. These included an increase in the number of nurses with advanced academic training, the development of the *Nursing Research* journal, the availability of funding to support nursing research and the formation of the RCN Research Society as a discussion group in 1959.

The late 1960s and 70s saw a number of influential pieces of research undertaken by nurses. These included work by Felicity Stockwell (*The unpopular patient*), Jack Hayward (*Information: a prescription against pain*) and Doreen Norton (*An investigation of geriatric nursing problems in hospital*). In 1993 the *Report of the taskgroup on the strategy for research in nursing, midwifery and health visiting* (DoH 1993) was published and recommended that all nurses should become research literate, an essential skill for knowledge-led nursing practice. Today, the NMC competency framework (Competency 9) states that: 'All nurses must appreciate the value of evidence in practice, be able to understand and appraise research, apply relevant theory and research findings to their work, and identify areas for further investigation'.

If what nurses do is important, then it figures that it needs to be done well. Nurses need to question what they do and how they do it to ensure that the best possible care can be given to the children and young people in their care. Yet research with children and young people is not without its issues, especially the tension between enabling children to take part in research and the responsibility to safeguard them. This chapter starts by giving an overview of how the involvement of children and young people has changed over recent years and the different level at which they can be and are involved. It then goes through the research process, specifically focusing on issues related to doing research with children. The chapter concentrates on non-therapeutic research with children and young people. This type of research aims only to gain new knowledge and so is unlikely to benefit the participants. Therapeutic research, sometimes referred to as clinical research, however, aims to benefit a particular group of patients by improving available treatment. Find out more about this type of research with children and young people in the Case Study 17.1.

CASE STUDY 17.1

Participatory research project

The first phase of the project started with a question – can children and young people be involved in monitoring the quality of care in hospital? This phase used a qualitative approach and recruited nine young people aged between 12 and 16 years, all of whom had been inpatients in hospital. Interviews were used to explore their experiences of hospital.

In phase 2 of the project, the young people became peer researchers with the adult. They took an active part in all stages of the research from deciding the research agenda through to dissemination of the findings.

Source: Moules (2009)

RESEARCH IN CHILDHOOD

Historical Perspectives

The status of children and young people's position in research has changed substantially in recent decades from occupying a marginalised position where they were treated as 'objects of study', to becoming 'study subjects' and now increasingly as 'research participants'. The point of differentiation lay in how researchers conceptualise and work with children and young people to investigate their exterior or interior worlds; the negotiation of 'power' in this trusted relationship; and the navigation of how the meaning of data is represented in research.

Studies that exemplify these changes in attitudes include the 1930s studies by the psychologist Jean Piaget who held the common assumption that children are merely less competent thinkers than adults. He observed his own children – as objects of study – to develop his theory on how children acquire knowledge.

In 1972 the psychologist Walter Mischel began a longitudinal study on deferred gratification with 4-year-olds. He worked with children – as study subjects – and analysed how long each child resisted the temptation of eating a marshmallow. Mischel followed the cohort of children into adulthood to see whether or not patterns of deferred gratification correlated with future success. Clark and Moss (2011) developed the mosaic approach to listening to younger children. Clark and Moss worked with children under 5 – as research participants – at a local day nursery to capture their experiences of the early years educational provision. The mosaic approach presents a framework for listening and treats children as experts and agents in their own lives. These studies demonstrate the gradual shift in how researchers conceptualise and work with children and young people in research.

Taking account of the different ways children and young people have been positioned in research, consider very carefully if the nurse researchers' approach to researching children or young people's experiences are grounded in 'research on', 'research for' or 'research with' young people (Oakley 1994; Darbyshire et al. 2005). To 'research with' young people there is a need to perceive them as active agents, which departs from a 'deficit' model, which views children and young people as unsophisticated or 'silly', as mini or 'incomplete adults'; as 'presocial' and thus incapable of being taken seriously in discussions about their needs (Oakley 1994, page 419) or being unable to articulate a set of coherent political views (Scott 2000; Mayall 2002). This conceptualisation sees childhood and youth as a stage of 'being' as opposed to 'becoming', and engages with the 'new sociology of childhood' (Wyness 2006). This approach to the study of childhood: 'Take(s) it as read that children can be understood as competent social actors [and] as fully constituted social subjects' (Wyness 2006, pages 236–237).

Why Do We Need to Do Research with Children and Young People?

Children and young people's involvement in research is often questioned, marginalised and devalued within public policy and research communities because of misconceptions made about children and young people's capacity and competencies in contributing to the production of robust data that stands up to 'scientific' standards. The public consensus is that children and young people are 'vulnerable', which is attributable to their physical, psychological and emotional development. On this basis, children and young people ought not to bear the burdens of research unless absolutely necessary; yet, if they are to benefit from health-related advances then children must take part in relevant health-related research. At the other end of the spectrum, many people also work under the assumption that 'children and young people-led research' is where the process should be aiming. By definition, it needs to be young person initiated, implemented and focused in its entirety. But the most important question researchers face is the ethical dilemma of how to balance protection and access while giving due recognition to how voices of young people are silenced in research. As researchers there is a need to ensure that a chance is given to all children and young people to get involved in research,

including those who might have limited speech, who are semi-literate, have challenging behaviour, are from different cultural and ethnic backgrounds and who are experiencing highly sensitive and stressful circumstances. There may be times when it is justifiable to use a proxy interviewee, for instance in the case of a baby or toddler or to hear all perspectives on an issue. What is important then is to identify the proxy, whether it be parent or alternative carer (e.g. foster parent). Enabling a child or young person to say 'no' to involvement is also important as non-participation can be just as acceptable as participation. Within a research project the team should consider different spheres where children and young people's voices need to be heard:

- within the research project
- within the organisation/school/youth group
- in the outside world (i.e. policy arena).

Fifteen to 19 year-olds are under-researched and less likely to be involved in clinical studies than other age groups. In the UK 19 per cent of the population are under 16 and 'children's research' (aged 13–16) accounts for only 3 per cent of clinical trials. This is partially because attention towards young people's health-related research has decreased since the 1950s even though people aged 10 to 17 make up 17 per cent of the world population (Fern et al. 2008; Modi 2011). Paradoxically, this is the age range in which adult diseases start to make an appearance and high volumes of young people decide for themselves to opt out of clinical trials.

Against these backdrops, there are important legal as well as moral reasons why children and young people should be involved in doing research. The Local Government and Public Involvement in Health Act (2007) contains reference to the 'duty to involve', requiring that public bodies inform, consult and involve people in decisions on the design and delivery of local services. Table 17.1 gives an indication of some of the other important policies and guidelines underpinning research for and with children and young people. Impetus also came from the UN Convention on the Rights of the Child (UNCRC–adopted in 1989 and ratified by the UK in 1991) in the form of

Table 17.1 Policy and legislation: knowing where to link children and young people's rights and research

UN Convention on the Rights of the Child 1989

Children Act 1989 and Children Act 2004

National Health Service and Health Care Professions Act 2002

Youth Matters 2005

Section 29A of the Education Act 2002

Children's Homes National Minimum Standards 2011

Disability Act 2005

Review of Children's Cases Regulations 1991

Adoption and Children Act 2002

You're Welcome Quality Criteria: Making Health Services Young People Friendly 2007

Local Government and Public Involvement in Health Act 2007

guidelines for the proper conduct of research involving children and young people (Beazley et al. 2009). The UNCRC (1989) is the main driver for increasing children and young people's participation. Children and young people's involvement in research is conceptualised as one way of securing the fulfilment of all rights in the Convention, so positively improving outcomes for children and young people in the UK. This means that adults have to do more than listen. They must give weight to the child's and young person's view taking into account their age and maturity.

VOICES 17.1

'Although they know better medically, they don't know about me personally. They don't know whether I'm more sensitive than normal. Although adults might know in some respects, they might not understand how children feel about that . . . It is good to know that people are researching about the care of young people in hospital because they are getting their voice heard' (young participants cited in Moules 2006).

RESEARCH NOTE 17.1 UNCRC (1989) and links to children's involvement in research

Article 13 gives children and young people the right to receive and give information through speaking, writing, printing, art or any other form. Combined with Article 17, the Convention gives children and young people the right to information, especially information that helps build his or her social, spiritual and moral well-being and physical and mental health. Both Articles (13 and 17) are underpinned by Article 12 of the Convention on the Rights of the Child that gives every child and young person the right to express and have her views given due weight in everything that affects her.

Based on experience, children and young people are keen to participate and/or co-research some of the challenges that they face as they seek to build healthy and liveable lives in the UK. Some of these challenges include poverty, drug and alcohol abuse; HIV/AIDS; gang and gun culture; homelessness; bullying; sex and sexuality; lack of family life and access to good education. As researchers, there is a need to know why to seek to involve children and young people in research and have an open dialogue about this with children and young people. In research discussed by the authors it has been found that sometimes children and young people feel that participation can be a policy agenda or an adult agenda imposed on them. This could work against the overall goals of empowering children and young people to take part in research. From experience it can be seen that research might have different dimensions such as:

- adding quality to the research
- framing young people's voices
- enhancing strengths and competences of young people.

In terms of involvement, research commissioned or undertaken with children and young people will be meaningful, informed, and produce evidence-based contributions that will help to influence and shape policy and practice. Whether the research project originates from the ideas of children and young people or they complete the fieldwork or get involved in the analysis, there is intrinsic value in having them doing research on matters that affect their lived lives. Children and young people know their needs and can best prioritise what is important to them whether as members of society, service users, or consumers.

RESEARCH NOTE 17.2 Young people to have role in shaping health service (AYPH 2012)

In 2012 the Association for Young People's Health (AYPH) was commissioned by the Department of Health's Innovation, Excellence and Strategic Development (IESD) section to set up a project designed to create a bridge between clinical professionals and the youth sector. It is specifically aimed at assisting GPs, clinical commissioning groups and health and well-being boards in their emerging commissioning roles, putting them in contact with community youth projects to meet and improve young people's health needs.

Approaches to Doing Research with Children and Young People

Research projects are seldom child or young person directed and their involvement is often situated – arguably – alongside the lower rungs of Roger Hart's (1997) ladder of participation. Research involving children and young people can be situated on a continuum and may involve young people acting in a wide range of roles from participant, peer researcher through to co-researcher; it may be led by children and young people or by adults working in collaboration with children and young people, or with young people acting as research commissioners.

There are different approaches to doing research all of which can be used with children and young people: exploratory, descriptive and explanatory. The approach taken with children and young people will be influenced by the purpose of the inquiry, the age and will reflect children and young people's competency levels. Much of children and young people's research takes place within services that they use or within their own communities. They are therefore the experts. Consequently, they will be familiar with the geography and risk factors that might limit the scope of the project and ways of working with or involving other children and young people. The approach decided should not determine the research question; rather it should be the other way round. Key points to consider:

- Develop an answerable research question or hypothesis.
- Research methods are selected after the research question is defined and must appropriately address the question.
- Using a combination of different methods (called 'triangulation') will strengthen the research findings by drawing on a number of different sources.

Directly involving children and young people in the research process is an extension of the wider participation agenda in the public health sector that is focused on improving health services for child and youth. Thus, adopting a non-evidence-based practice fails young people in the commitment to ensuring that they have protection, are heard, have choices, are valued, have privacy, enjoy social inclusion and are not discriminated against.

Children and young people's involvement in health-related research often falls under the common descriptor of user-controlled research. User-controlled research is research that is actively controlled, directed and managed by service users and their service user organisations. Service users decide on the issues and questions to be looked at, as well as the way the research is designed, planned and written up. The service users will run the research advisory or steering group and may also decide to carry out the research. Some service users make no distinction between the term user-controlled and user-led research, others feel that user-led research has a different, vaguer meaning. They see user-led research as research that is meant to be led and shaped by service users but is not necessarily controlled by them. Control in user-led research in this case will rest with some other group of non-service users who also have an interest in the research, such as the commissioners of the research, the researchers or people who provide services.

Making change is commonly identified as the central purpose of user-controlled research, although there is also recognition that such change may not always be achieved. User-controlled research can be based on both qualitative and quantitative research methods and is also developing its own research methods. Service users see democratic accountability to service users as a key requirement for good practice in user-controlled research. This might be achieved by the research project itself being democratically constituted or it being located within a democratically constituted service user organisation.

The current emphasis on user-led research is not new, but it has developed considerably in recent years, both in sheer volume and in the scope of its activities. It is a quiet movement, which has been gaining momentum over the last few decades, influencing how public services are designed, delivered and evaluated. User groups have built up their skills, increased their self-confidence and resilience and have developed the ability to campaign and/or lobby behind an authentic and informed voice (see Faulkner 2010). User-led research has also added value to the quality of research 'on', 'for' and 'about' children and young people (see Kellett 2005, 2010; Delgado 2006; Boeck and Sharpe 2009; Sharpe 2009).

ACTIVITY 17.1

Watch this YouTube clip and reflect on the points listed:
http://www.youtube.com/watch?v=sNWIOryWd5I
Changing Our Worlds.

Alternatively, read the report in Faulkner (2010).

This report is intended to increase the understanding and awareness of user-controlled research through exploring, in-depth, seven examples of research in which service users or disabled people controlled the research process. The report provides a description of the seven examples and a summary of the role and value of the user-controlled research.

- **What is user-controlled research?**
- **What challenges do user-controlled research groups encounter?**
- **What changes are created by user-controlled research?**

Ethical Issues

Starting from the premise of ethical symmetry between children, young people and adults this section deals with how the researcher gains voluntary informed consent and acts to guarantee confidentiality in research. Ethics here pertains to principles and guidelines that the researcher can use in order to help make decisions and shape conduct. Various professional research associations in the UK have adopted written codes of standards for research which set out standards and responsibilities. These include the British Sociological Association (2002), the Medical Research Council (2004), the Royal College of Paediatrics, Child

Health: Ethics Advisory Committee (2000) and the Royal College of Nursing (2009). The Mental Capacity Act 2005 is also an important document in considering research ethics in relation to those who are mentally incapacitated. All ethics guidelines can each trace their origins back to the 1947 Nuremberg Code and the 1964 declaration of Helsinki (updated 2008) which gave guidance to research with human subjects, aimed at medics. Usually guidelines are not mandatory or enforceable by law. They do, however, result in the researcher's need to reflect on potential damaging consequences of research and questions of power in research.

Children's nurses will most likely be involving children and young people who seek answers to their own life circumstances that often hinge on moral questions. The children and young people will be coping with some kind of ill health, potentially life-threatening disease or chronic lifelong problems. They might even have had to endure humiliation at the hands of significant adults who should be protecting them. As a result, they do not necessarily come to research ignorant of the consequence of taking part and with nothing to give.

Voluntary Informed Consent

Voluntary informed consent is a process between researcher and child/young person that must contain an information component and a consent component. The *information* component refers to the disclosure of information and comprehension of what is disclosed. (See 'recruitment and selection' for detail about information sheets.) The consent component refers to a *voluntary* decision and agreement to take part in the research study. The voluntary nature of the consent is important and young participants must not be made to feel pressurised into taking part. Coercion is potentially an issue when the research is conducted by teachers in schools, or when parents push for their children to take part in a desire to please staff. It can be potentially difficult for young participants to say 'no'. Consent is also an ongoing process throughout a research project, sometimes referred to as 'process consent'. It acknowledges that participants have the right to withdraw at any stage and that consent is negotiated on an ongoing basis.

The UK law is untested as to legal age of consent for **social research** with minors and it is technically lawful (at the time of publication) to invite under 16-year-olds to choose for themselves without first seeking parental permission or consent (Heath et al. 2007). However normally under 10s should not be approached without parental permission and it may be unwise to accept the consent of a 10- to 16-year-old without parental permission especially if the study addresses sensitive or personal issues. Consent by 16- to 18-year-olds is rather vague but most researchers would acknowledge that young people in this age group are competent to give consent for themselves unless proved otherwise. A key issue is whether the child/young person is competent to understand the information provided and to make up his own mind regarding participation.

RESEARCH NOTE 17.3 Clinical trials

With respect to *clinical trials*, the law is specific in that, in gaining consent for a child's participation:

- the informed consent of the parents or legal representative has been obtained
- the minor has received information according to its capacity of understanding
- the explicit wish of a minor who is capable of forming an opinion and assessing this information to refuse participation or to be withdrawn from the clinical trial at any time is considered.

(See the Medicines for Human Use (Clinical Trials) Regulations 2004 at **http://www.legislation.gov.uk/uksi/2004/1031/contents/made**.

Confidentiality

All research participants are entitled to provide data in the knowledge that what they say will remain confidential; this applies to children and young people as well as adults. There are, however, limitations to this general principle. The NMC Code of conduct (NMC 2002) allows nurses to breach confidentiality when there is concern about a child's safety (e.g. abuse or harm), when they would be obliged to pass on this information to the relevant authority or when it can be justified in the public interest. It is important that parents also realise that they will not be party to information provided by their children; this should be spelt out when permissions are being sought. All data provided must be anonymised and especial care needs to be taken with video and photographic material.

If children and young people are involved as co-researchers it is important for them to take responsibility and make decisions in the formative stages of the research project when everything remains circumspect and time is still available to work through and appreciate the potential risks and challenges that lay ahead. At this stage children and young people can lend their own perspectives to planning for safety in research design, assessing risk in the fieldwork site and strategies for handling risky situations.

SEARCHING AND REVIEWING THE LITERATURE

This section explains the purpose of a literature review and what constitutes literature. It goes on to provide examples of

RESEARCH NOTE 17.4 Project A: impact team (2010): 'The day I told my best mate...', London, Office of Public Management

Participants were young people who were affected by or cared for parents with AIDS or HIV. They feared personal prejudice and hostility (e.g. risk of physical threat or abuse, name calling or isolation) from individuals not sympathetic to people living with AIDS and HIV.

Project B: ethnicity (2009), attitudes to sexual health and services among young people from the BME community, London, Brook. Participants were young people who accessed a sexual health service working predominately with BME teenagers. They were constrained by local politics wishing

to deny the existence of Muslim young people being sexually active.

For both groups of young people, the main concern was with the anonymity of the participants to protect them from the hostility and commendation of the wider community. But both groups felt their stories must be told and devised ethical frameworks to overcome these challenges. Both projects used a teenage sample and obtained consent from each of the participants as well as from the organisations assuming legal responsibility for the groups of young people.

step by step approaches to carrying out a review and reading critically. Starting out on a piece of research can be a daunting task, but it need not be so. Think about it as if the project were going out to buy some new clothes. The process begins by looking in the wardrobe to see what is already there, what is worn out and needs replacing, what new pieces are needed (wanted) and so on – that is basically what a literature search and review is: there is a need to be objective, thorough and critical of relevant available research and non-research literature on the topic. The overall purpose is to identify the body of knowledge associated with a particular topic, critically read it, analyse its strengths and weaknesses, and identify areas for new or further study. It is a really good way of making the argument for new research to be done or of reporting on the current state of knowledge within a given topic area. Doing a literature review will reveal common findings among studies; reveal inconsistencies between studies; and identify methods of investigation, which could be used for further study. A literature review nearly always forms the first part of any research study but may also

be done as part of the work in implementing evidence-based practice (see Table 17.2). For decisions to be made about the implementation of recommendations from research it is important to be able judge the rigour with which the study was carried out and therefore the trustworthiness of the findings. The children's nurse may also carry out a review of literature to develop practice policies, update practice guidelines or as part of an academic assignment.

What is Literature and How Valuable Are the Different Types?

The term 'literature' is used to describe any published material, mostly books, journals, reports, conference proceedings or newspapers. However, other types of literature might be used in different circumstances including film, song, works of art and photographs. The value of each of these depends on what the individual derives from them but practitioners and researchers place more value on some than on others. The value depends

Table 17.2 Main types of literature review

Traditional review	Sometimes called a narrative review. Includes relevant studies but is typically selective with no specific criteria
	An extensive literature review may be carried out to bring the reader up to date with current knowledge. It picks out critical elements of current knowledge
	An example of an extensive literature review can be found in Scott and McSherry (2008) who carried out a review to establish the key concepts associated with evidence-based nursing
Systematic review	A rigorous and defined approach in a specific subject. Used to answer well-focused questions. Specific criteria for selection of papers (see Parahoo 2006) Two types of systematic review: ● meta-analysis – takes a large body of quantitative findings and conducts statistical analysis to integrate the findings and to detect patterns and relationships between the findings ● meta-synthesis – a method used to search, appraise and combine the findings of qualitative studies

Table 17.3 Types of literature and their value

Type of literature	Assessing its value
Research information	Highly valued, is systematic and normally rigorously collected and analysed
Descriptive accounts (e.g. of care)	May contain valuable information but tends to be subjective
Conceptual and theoretical discussions	Need to be structured logically and argued coherently for these to be of high value
Personal opinions	Subjective but can be valuable

on the type and quality of the information contained within the publication and the type of publication itself (Tables 17.3 and 17.4) and on whether it is reported first or second hand:

- primary information – original publications
- secondary information – there is the potential for this type of publication to analyse, discuss, simplify and summarise original ideas or even misinterpret them.

ACTIVITY 17.2   How to evaluate a website

Watch this video on YouTube on how to evaluate a website. **http://www.youtube.com/watch?v=xlqZSg5ER6A**.

Then access the following web page and use the guidelines on the video to evaluate the site **http://www.fairplayforchildren.org/**.

Searching the Literature

Searching is often intuitive but it does help to follow a structure and be methodical. A number of writers suggest a variety of frameworks – have a look on the internet or in textbooks to see which one suits your way of working. One is suggested here that consists of six steps.

> Step 1: Identify the area you are interested in. Read and scan the literature that you have already, books, lecture notes.
> Step 2: Refine and choose a focused and specific research topic.
> Step 3: Identify your search terms/key words and conduct a search for literature.

Select an appropriate search tool. Google Scholar is sometimes a good place to start and some valuable information can be found this way. However, it is best to move on to using bibliographic databases that enable searching for published research across a

Table 17.4 Types of publication and their value

Type of publication	Assessing its value
Books	Good sources of information but by the time they are written, published and read, the information they contain is already out of date
Journals	Academic containing articles of high intellectual quality, or professional, written mainly for practitioners with more emphasis on practice implications
	Most journal papers are subject to 'peer review,' which helps to maintain standards and gives credibility and value as unsuitable papers are rejected
Research reports	Usually written for the sponsors who pay for the research to be done
	More detailed than related journal articles
	Watch out for any bias
Conference proceedings	May be brief but are 'hot off the press'
Web pages	Need to evaluate whether the information is reputable and reliable
Other forms: leaflets, newspapers, letters	All these have limited value, may be biased and subjective

wide range of subjects and sources. As a student, access to a large number of relevant databases is available through the library website. The three most likely to be useful to nurses are MEDLINE, Cumulative Index to Nursing and Allied Health Literature (CINAHL) and Allied and Complementary Medicine (AMED).

Carry out a number of searches using different key terms and set an inclusion and exclusion criteria if appropriate, e.g.

English language only. It is usual to restrict the searches to the past 10 years. Make a note of all the results from every search undertaken. If very little is found there may be a need to broaden the search terms. If this is too much (a very common occurrence), try refining the search terms or limiting by year, type or language.

PRACTICAL GUIDELINES 17.1

It is a good idea to make use of one of the software tools available for online bibliographic management. RefWorks (**www.refworks.com**) is one such tool, which helps you to manage, store and retrieve all types of material. It also helps you to create reference lists and bibliographies.

Another widely available tool is EndNote (**www.endnote.com**).

Have a look to see which tool your university uses first before you look to buy anything.

Step 4: Appraise your results:

- Look through the references briefly; who are the authors, what type of information is it, is it up to date?
- Read the abstract; is it relevant to the level of study, is it central to the topic?
- Refine the search if necessary, revise the search terms if necessary.
- Select the evidence to work with, download or print.

Step 5: Critically read the material: once it is decided that a publication is valuable there is a need to 'critically read' it to make a value judgement about the content. But 'critical reading' is very different from the type of reading when curled up with a favourite novel. Then there is

only interest in what the text is saying. Critical reading is essential to critically analyse and write and requires standing back and gaining some distance from the text being read. So do not read looking only for information but also looking for ways of thinking about the subject matter. First, determine the **central claims** or **purpose** of the text. Then begin to make some judgements about the **context**, distinguish the **kinds of reasoning** the text employs and examine the **evidence** the text employs. Avoid approaching a text by asking 'What information can I get out of it?' Rather ask 'How does this text work? How is it argued? How is the evidence (the facts, examples, etc.) used and interpreted? How does the text reach its conclusions?'

Step 6: Synthesise and write up the review.

PRACTICAL GUIDELINES 17.2

- Find the best place to read in.
- Have a dictionary to hand.
- Use a checklist.

- Always make notes – this is at the heart of critical reading. Use underlining, highlighters, writing in margins.

Using a Checklist for Critical Reading: the PQRS Method (Cohen 1990)

This is another method that might be useful when critically reading. It consists of four steps:

- **Preview:** skim the work, rapid reading is a skill worth learning. Discard articles that are not deemed relevant.
- **Question:** identify questions you want to ask yourself while reading. To do this you will need to determine an article's original purpose so that you can select an appropriate type of checklist to use. Most research textbooks provide tools for critiquing different types of research article and others can be found online (see Further Resources).

- **Read and question:** read without making notes, read actively, take time, concentrate. Look for answers to questions you may have, look up words you do not understand. Question authors' reasoning and the evidence. Note any further questions you want to answer. Be prepared to read papers twice. On the second read, annotate as you read. Note key points and ideas, answers to questions, your own ideas, and highlight arguments.
- **Review your annotations:** have you answered all your questions fully? Summarise each article including key thoughts, comments, strengths and weaknesses of the publication.

ACTIVITY 17.3 Searching Google Scholar

- Try searching Google Scholar using the term 'research with children'. How many results did you get?
- Now do an advanced scholar search to find articles with all of the words 'research with children', with the exact phrase 'voices' and at least one of the words 'hospital'. Now how many results did you get?
- Now try limiting your search to the years '2009–2011'. How many results now?
- Finally, try adding the phrase 'chronic illness' to your search. How many now?

Try this activity with your own search terms.

COLLECTING THE DATA

Before doing any work with the participants there is a need to gain ethical approval. If working with children who are NHS patients, then a submission of an application to the National Research Ethics Service is required (see **http://www.nres.nhs.uk**). In addition, approval is needed to carry out your project with the relevant trust research and development department(s). A letter is also needed of access from the institutional gatekeeper in order to gain ethical approval for the study.

Who will the participants be and how many should there be? This is an important question to answer. The answer will of course depend on the research, and the chosen approach, the cultural background and age group to access. If the approach is quantitative, there needs to be access to a large enough sample so as to make the participants as representative of the chosen population as possible so results can be generalised back to the population.

If the approach is more qualitative, representation is not an issue and the sample size can be quite small. An appropriate sample size for a qualitative study is one that adequately answers the research question. Frequently the sample size becomes apparent when no new information is forthcoming, sometimes called saturation, so a flexible approach is needed and it may not be possible to state your sample size at the beginning of a project. For some studies, the sample might be in single figures when rich descriptive data are required. There are three main approaches to selecting the sample in this type of study; all are non-probability (non-random) techniques that mean that the findings will only apply to the specific population under investigation (Higginbottom 2004).

Three main approaches to selecting the sample are:

- convenience sample – this includes participants who are readily available
- purposeful sample or judgemental sampling – this is the conscious selection of certain participants with specific chacteristics
- theoretical sample (normally associated with grounded theory).

Whichever approach is chosen, you will need to provide a detailed description of how to choose the sample.

CASE STUDY 17.2

In project 1, the participants had to be children who had been hospital inpatients, ideally those who had a chronic health problem as they would have much more experience of being in hospital. Initially, two age groups were chosen with the view to working with children aged 5 to 11 and young people aged 12 to 16. However, as it was difficult to recruit the younger age group only the young people were selected for phase 1 of the project. The sample of nine was a convenient size and was made up of three boys and six girls.

Accessing Participants

Normally, accessing children and young people through institutions such as schools and hospitals can only be done with the agreement of a range of gatekeepers. Gatekeepers are charged with taking responsibility for safeguarding children and young people's welfare (Christensen and Prout 2002). Although this is an important role for gatekeepers in relation to research, they can also exert power over young people, in essence silencing their voices and excluding them from research. In accessing children and young people for research we are faced with a hierarchy of gatekeepers:

- ethics panel
- consultants; head teachers; directors of children's services
- parents/carers/social workers (in the case of looked-after children).

Access may be denied at any one of these levels for a variety of reasons (Figure 17.1). The decisions adults make are often protectionist in nature based on their own realities so it is important to make sure the research is discussed fully so that all gatekeepers are fully informed. However, many gatekeepers are helpful and supportive if provided with full details of the project.

Recruitment and Selection

Once permission is gained to access potential participants, they need to be recruited to the study. There are a number of different ways of recruiting but basically this stage is about giving children and their parents/carers information about the project so enabling them to decide whether or not to participate. Very often information packs are sent to children via the school or

CASE STUDY 17.3

In this study, the ethics panel was the first level of gate-keeper. Ethical approval was sought and gained without too many problems from a local NHS ethics panel. The next level of gatekeeper in the NHS was consultants. Of the 14 consultants contacted, only two were supportive and granted access. Unfortunately, their communications with parents (the third level of gatekeeper) failed to elicit any further interest. The remaining 12 consultants either did not respond or denied the researcher access. In effect, this disempowered young people by preventing their reaching their own decision about taking part. Following a rethink, a head teacher in a local secondary school was approached who was supportive and identified parents and young people on my behalf. Parents are the final level of gatekeeper and, in this study, all but one of the parents agreed to the researcher approaching their sons and daughters.

the hospital ward/department (especially if the researcher does not have access to the contact details of potential participants – see Data Protection Act 1998). If possible, it is hugely valuable for the researcher to go through the information sheet with the child/parent to clear up any confusion. If they are interested in participating they are asked to contact the researcher (often by return of a reply slip giving permission for the researcher to contact them).

Information needs to be clear, concise, age and culturally appropriate, providing details of any benefits or risks and the requirements of participation. Most ethics committees will provide templates for the information that needs to go into an information sheet. These are always a good starting point but you also need to consider using:

- short lines, words, sentences and paragraphs
- one main idea per sentence
- requests rather than commands
- the active rather than passive voice
- a personal rather than an impersonal approach
- specific details rather than vague ones
- appropriate pictures as a useful addition

- a creative mode of presentation, for example taped information can be played to children with reduced vision. (Alderson and Morrow 2004)

Sometimes there may be a need to encourage children and young people to volunteer to take part in research projects other than through institutions. Have a look at this YouTube video, which shows how some researchers in America went about advertising their project with the use of posters (**http://youtube/j14D-I5Vq5k**).

There are a number of ways in which a selection of the sample is chosen depending on the approach undertaken to the research:

1. Select randomly from those who contacted you.
2. Select the first number that is needed e.g. the first 10 who respond positively.
3. Be a little more selective and select in order to get a range of possible participants in relation to, e.g., gender, age, ethnic origin.

Whichever approach is taken, you will need to contact those you do not select explaining why and thanking them for responding.

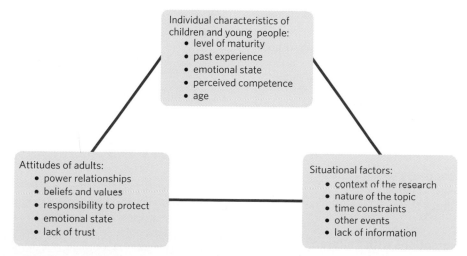

Figure 17.1 Factors at play in decisions made by gatekeepers
Source: Moules (2005)

Methods of Data Collection

Collecting research data from children and young people can be challenging and at the same time very rewarding. Talking with children can open up ways of knowing about their lives and they can provide rich, expressive data if given the right opportunities. The main challenge for researchers in this context is dealing with the power differential between adults and children, finding ways to draw out children's subjective experiences and thoughts. There is no lower age limit on involving children in research providing that the appropriate data collection method is used. However, age is not always synonymous with a child's abilities so a degree of reflexivity is required. While using methods that are sensitive to children's competencies and interests can make for a more trusted atmosphere, the use of methods used with adults need not be ruled out. Most researchers advocate the use of multiple methods (Darbyshire et al. 2005), using traditional 'adult' methods alongside methods considered to be more suitable for use with children and young people. Using this flexible approach respects children's agency as social actors, and gives children an opportunity to choose how they contribute and also helps to generate their engagement and sustain their interest. One specific approach that uses the concept of multiple methods is the mosaic approach (Clark and Moss 2011). This approach was developed as part of a research study specifically to listen to young children's views about early childhood services. It combines the methods of observation and interviewing with participatory techniques to elicit different individual and collective perspectives. Each tool provides one piece of the mosaic. The mosaic approach provides a framework for listening to everyone who has a role to play in the lives of young children within the early childhood setting.

There are many methods of data collection available to researchers but some general principles would be useful to consider, whatever the age of the child/children:

- Be clear about the purpose of the research.
- Pay attention to the time of day; plan to collect data and how long needed.
- Think carefully about the context in which to collect data: it needs to be familiar, and young participants need to know that there are no right or wrong answers.
- Consider the need to carry out the data collection without interference from others, e.g. parents.
- Take time to establish trust and rapport with the child/children.
- Design activities that are fun, enjoyable, varied and accessible. For example, consider the format. Might need different versions for different age groups. Clarity of language is vital.
- Be prepared to involve parents and practitioners as well especially with younger children.
- Always provide feedback to the children who take part.

Interviews or 'Conversations with Children'

Interviews are a common method for collecting data in social research that can be used with children and young people.

Interviewing children in friendship pairs or triads (if the subject is suitable) can help to diffuse the power imbalance when adult researchers are interviewing children (Shaw et al. 2011). However, because children might not be able to express themselves clearly when being interviewed by an adult, it is important to pay attention to the context and approach. Children and young people may not be as inclined to give answers as long as adults would so the use of stimulus materials can help them to expand their views. However, it is important not to be patronising; many young people enjoy straightforward questioning (Punch 2006). A study by Spratling et al. (2010) reviewed qualitative studies that used interviews with children to determine factors that can contribute to the effectiveness of the method. They found six major themes:

Getting to know me: it is really important to establish trust and rapport with a child prior to an interview – this is critical to its success. Beginning the interview with a 'free narrative' can help in this.

Every picture tells a story: the use of journals and drawing, stories, timelines, photographs and pictures before and during interviews can contribute to establishing rapport and enhancing relationships.

Helping with the jitters: decreasing anxiety helps facilitate interviews and this can be helped by group or paired interviews. Choosing a familiar location for the interview also helps to reduce anxiety.

I may be young but I can tell you about me: younger children can participate if the questions are developmentally appropriate.

To be or not to be: the decision as to whether to give parents the option to remain with the child during an interview is an important one as their presence can be both a help and a hindrance.

I don't want to play: children must be allowed to decide for themselves whether to take part in an interview.

VOICES 17.2

'We did it with interviews. If it had been someone else they might not have wanted to talk to an adult. We know how to put things because we've been in care' (Daniel, young researcher).

ACTIVITY 17.4

In the case study project, the initial interviews were carried out in the young person's home. In some cases, parents were either present in the same room or in an adjoining room. List the possible advantages and disadvantages of having a parent present when interviewing a child or young person.

CASE STUDY 17.4

'The purpose of the first stage of the project was to set the context for the young people, to begin to find out their views on the care they had received in hospital and to begin to develop a rapport with them. A semi-structured approach was chosen to encourage a more open response and to enable the young people to take some control over the interview. Using interviews allowed the researcher to treat the young people in the same way as adults and to avoid taking a patronising stance by using "child-friendly" methods. The interviews were designed to explore the types of care received, how care was rated, views on the involvement of young people in monitoring quality and views on participation in research. Two "task-centred" activities were used within the interviews to facilitate discussion. The first activity was a modified brainstorming session using spider diagrams to help the young people remember the various clinical and caring interventions they had experienced. The second activity entailed the use of a prepared chart to rate the care they received. The young people were given the choice of where they wanted to be interviewed. The interviews were semi-structured and each one followed the same format using a topic guide to help shape the interview. Each interview began with the same introduction, rechecking assent, explaining about the tape recorder, explaining about their right to stop at any time and also that there were no right or wrong answers. The interviews took between 45 minutes and one hour. All the interviews were taped using a clip on microphone and then transcribed as soon as possible after completion.'
(*Source*: Moules 2006)

Focus Groups

Focus groups are defined by Powell et al. (1996, page 499) as 'a group of individuals selected and assembled by researchers to discuss and comment on, from personal experience, the topic that is the subject of the research'. Focus groups are different from group interviews in that they aim to encourage interactive conversations between members of the group on a topic supplied by the researcher. They are frequently used in the early exploratory stage of a study either as a data collection method in themselves or as a way of developing further tools. They can also be used towards the end of a study to check out findings or to identify areas for further research. When deciding whether focus groups are an appropriate method to use you need to consider the suitability of the discussion topic. Some topics are too sensitive for group discussions or may be embarrassing for young people to open up about in front of their peers. The size of your focus group is important. Various suggestions exist but most agree that a group of between six to 12 is optimal; the smaller group size should be considered for younger children. These group discussions can engender a safer environment for children and, if facilitated well, can give more control of the discussion over to the young participants. The use of participatory activities in the focus group can stimulate thinking and discussion. A focus group should not last too long, 90 minutes is optimal and ground rules should always be set at the beginning. Starting with an ice breaker can be useful to help participants get to know one another and to settle into the topic to be discussed. When planning focus groups consider the need for:

- Single sex groups: mixed gender groups work well with 9 to 13 year olds. Engaging with mixed-sex groups in discussion in relation to sensitive issues can be challenging.
- Similar age groups: avoid having too large an age gap in the group.

Draw-and-Write Technique

This type of data collection method is popular in health-related research, although it was developed originally for use in schools. Using this method stimulates the child's ability to retrieve information that is encoded more easily than the straightforward semantic stimulus of direct questioning. Driessnack (2006) suggests that the act of drawing becomes the focus for sharing experiences. The technique involves asking a child to draw a picture and then asking the child to talk about it in a semi-structured interview. One of the main advantages of this method is that almost all schoolchildren are familiar with producing drawings. However, not all children find drawing fun and older children may consider it babyish. In addition, it is important to see children's drawings in the context of the wider culture of which they are part. (See Backett-Milbourn and McKie 1999 for a critical appraisal of the draw-and-write technique.)

RESEARCH NOTE 17.5

Children with a diagnosis of cancer were asked to give their views about hospital care. The draw and write technique was one of several methods used and this paper talks about the issues related to using the method.

Brady's study explored the views of hospitalised children about the characteristics of a good nurse. The draw and write technique was used with 22 children. The drawing produced here was by Jason aged 11.

(*continued*)

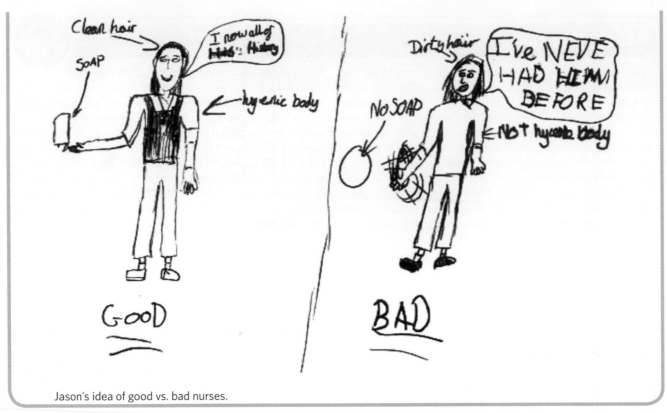

Jason's idea of good vs. bad nurses.

Source: Hospitalized children's views of the good nurse, *Nursing Ethics*, 16, pp. 543–60 (Brady, M. 2009), Sage Journals. © 2009 Sage Publications. Reprinted by permission of Sage Publications.

Questionnaires

While questionnaires tend to be more quantitative in nature they can provide valuable data to support and develop qualitative methods. Questionnaire surveys have been used in a number of studies and if constructed appropriately can have a number of advantages. However, at the same time, the disadvantages must be acknowledged. Self-completion questionnaires can be completed in the privacy of a child's own home. However, it is then impossible to detect who actually completed the questionnaire. The same applies to surveys completed on the internet unless these are completed in school which may itself pose limitations. E-surveys and interviews can be valuable tools for collecting data from children and young people as this is a medium they are familiar with. Questionnaires can be quick to administer and they have the capacity to provide large amounts of data from large samples. On the downside, the response rate is usually low and not all children find it easy to communicate their opinions in writing. The practical design of questionnaires must be flexible and often more than one version may be required. Innovative techniques for example, Likert and visual analogue scales and the use of open questions, can give children more control over how they respond. One example of an innovative approach for use with children can be seen in the British household panel study, which used a prerecorded questionnaire played on a personal stereo which enabled children to answer in a booklet at their own pace (Scott 2000).

RESEARCH NOTE 17.6

Coad and Coad (2008) present the findings from an innovative project that set out to explore children's preferences for the interior design of their new hospital unit. The study was completed in two phases and the second phase was a survey distributed to a sample of 250 children from which 140 responded.

Participatory Techniques

Participatory techniques are being used in many research projects with participants of all ages. They may be used simply as prompts to stimulate discussion or as methods of data collection in themselves. There are a wide range of techniques available and you can be as inventive as you want. Flexibility is the key and techniques can be adjusted to suit different participants and different research questions. Advantages of using these techniques

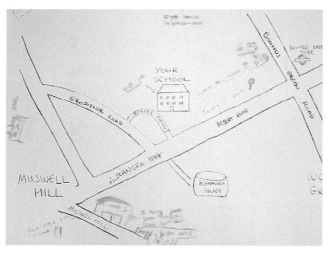

Figure 17.2 A map of places to eat at

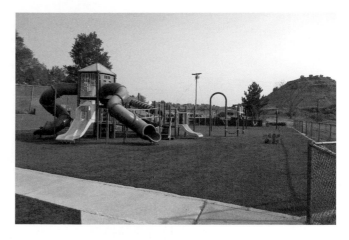

Figure 17.3 Photograph taken of the school playground

RESEARCH NOTE 17.7

This study from Pearce et al. (2009) used mapping (Figure 17.2), photography (Figure 17.3) and focus groups to explore children's perspectives of environmental influences on their eating and physical activity.

---

are that children can choose the degree to which they participate. A few of the more common ones are:

- **Mapping:** this involves the participants simply drawing a map of the area under discussion. For example, you could be discussing the ward environment with a group of children to identify what they see as hazards on the ward. Together they draw a map of the ward and perhaps you give them a red marker pen to identify the unsafe things.

- **Photovoice:** this method entails children being given cameras to take their own photographs. This enables them to feel more autonomous and in control. The children are provided with disposable cameras and are given instructions on what to do. For example, they could be asked to take photographs of things on a ward that they considered dangerous to children. Usually, they would be asked to note why they had taken the photograph or to write a caption for it. This method offers a way of seeing the child's world from a different perspective.

- **Timelines:** a range of methods can be used to enable children to identify chronologies of events, for example their experiences in hospital, or of the trajectory of an illness or track major family events. Timelines can be made on paper, out of different materials e.g. a collage, even using a washing line to peg up events makes for some fun (Figure 17.4)

- **Ranking exercises:** in these types of activity, children are asked to rank items in order of importance. Cards are

often used for this activity but be as creative as you can, for example use photographs taken by children or from magazines. Punch (2002), in a study about young people's problems and coping strategies, gave participants 20 problems written onto cards and simply asked them to put them in three piles of 'big', 'middle' and 'small' worries. One example of ranking is the 'diamond ranking exercise'. This technique is traditionally a thinking skills tool (Rockett and Percival 2002) but has now been used in a variety of research projects. Most commonly nine statements or opinions covering a range of perspectives are set onto cards. Participants usually then work in twos or small groups to sort and rank the statements in a diamond formation in order of significance (could be of interest, importance, value) (see Figure 17.5).

- **Puppetry:** puppet therapy has been used in preparing children for surgery and treatments for over 30 years and has been extremely valuable in helping to explain issues to children. Although the literature on its use in research is limited it can be used to great effect in getting children to talk in the research environment, especially in the case of younger children. Gibson et al. (2010) used 'Tweenie' dolls and other soft toys to talk to children aged 4 and 5 years old about their experiences of cancer care.

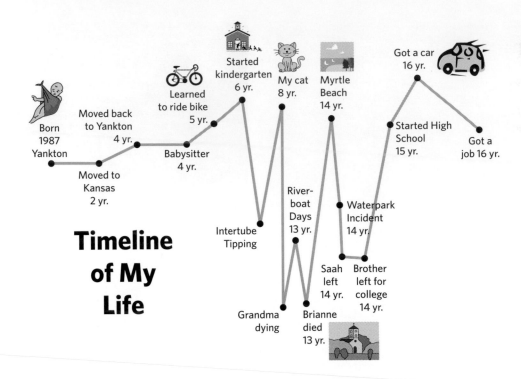

Figure 17.4 Example of a timeline used to identify critical moments in a child's life

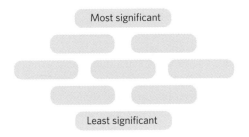

Figure 17.5 Organisation of diamond ranking

ANALYSING DATA

What is Data Analysis?

Data analysis is studying and interpreting the information collected during a research project. It is about making sense of data. The purpose of the analysis is to answer the research question as fully as possible. Just reading or looking at the 'bits of data' (interview transcripts, reflective notes, observation notes) will not give the answer to the research question. Then tease out the meaning during the process of analysis. Sometimes analysis will be done throughout a project, at other times it will be left until the end. However, the approach should be identified at the early stages of the research process before starting the fieldwork and should fit nicely with the method.

Approaches to Analysing Data

Different studies require different types of analysis. For example, surveys will nearly always require some counting and statistical analysis; interviews will require an analysis of the themes or concepts that emerge. There are many different methods of data analysis and a range of excellent textbooks that will help you select the appropriate one for a study (see Further Resources). However, there are two main types of data analysis:

- quantitative analysis
- qualitative analysis.

Quantitative Analysis

This type of analysis involves working with numbers. There are two main approaches to this: the use of descriptive statistics and the use of inferential statistics. This section concentrates on showing how to use the former. (Most of the textbooks about data analysis will have a section on inferential statistics.) Descriptive statistics do what they say – they describe the data collected. If the page is covered with figures the first task is to sort them out and summarise them so that the research and other people will be able to make sense of what is there, to understand the essential features. Descriptive data are ways of representing some important aspect of a dataset by a single number. These can include the sample group's sex, age, ethnicity, faith, number of times he attended a positive activity in a week or the rating he gives to a specific intervention he has experienced.

RESEARCH NOTE 17.8

Thomas (1998) used diamond ranking to explore the thoughts of children in care about decision making. Groups of children were asked to rank in order of importance reasons that other children had given for being involved in decision making (see Figure 17.6). Thomas concluded that what children wanted was to have the chance to take part in discussions with adults about their care.

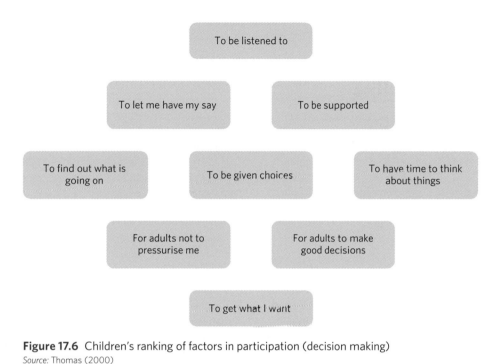

Figure 17.6 Children's ranking of factors in participation (decision making)
Source: Thomas (2000)

CASE STUDY 17.5

In phase 2 of the project, six of the original nine participants joined the researcher as co-researchers. They became the research team with the adult and were actively involved from then on in setting the research agenda and choosing methods of data collection. They chose to use a 'vignette' of a child's experience in hospital made up from their combined experiences and containing examples of positive and negative aspects. The vignette was given to 45 young people aged 13 or 14 in a local secondary school. After reading the vignette, they were asked a number of questions pertaining to the story. The vignette was then turned into a storyboard using a PowerPoint presentation that was shown to 84 children aged 9 to 11 in a local primary school. The same questions were posed after the story had been presented.

ACTIVITY 17.5

What is a vignette?

What might be the advantages and disadvantages of using this method?

The two dimensions most commonly dealt with in this way are:

- The averages (mean, mode, medium): the aim is to find the average number using (one or a combination of) the mean, medium or mode. For instance:
  - the 'mean' is the numeric average, as commonly understood in 'average age' (14 12 10 8 8 8) = 60 ÷ 6 (number of cases) = 10

- the 'medium' is the score below which half the scores lie (14 12 10 [9]8 8 8) = 9
- the 'mode' is the score found most frequently (14 12 10 8 8 8) = 8.
- Rates (disruption): the extent to which the data values in a set of scores are tightly clustered or relatively widely spread

out. The purpose of using rates (100, 1000, 10,000) is chosen depending on how common something is. The purpose of using rates is to make it possible to compare the incidence of something in two or more populations of varying sizes.

PRACTICAL GUIDELINES 17.3

Presentation of descriptive data:

1 Averages and rates are usually presented along with graphs, tables and charts containing all the data. Make sure the layout of tables have accompanying text explaining key figures.
2 The bulk of the graphs and tables can be placed in the appendix.
3 Use clear language – plain English.
4 Always check that titles and scales of tables and graphs are correct.
5 You should draw together your own conclusions, in your own words, from your descriptive data.

6 Conclusions, like the content, should be relevant. They must be consistently related to the questions you set out to answer in the research project.
7 You should indicate how far your interpretations are supported by the data collected and you should identify any deficiencies, such as gaps, inconsistencies and bias, which reduce the value of your data as evidence.
8 Use SPSS or Microsoft data packages to help store and analyse data.

Qualitative Analysis

Qualitative data are collected by a range of methods as discussed earlier. These data most commonly include 'words' either in the form of written words or spoken words but can also be in the form of observed behaviour or all manner of visual material.

There are no 'quick-fix' techniques in qualitative analysis and there are probably as many different ways of analysing qualitative data as there are qualitative researchers doing it. Many would argue that this is the way it should be – qualitative research is an interpretative and subjective exercise and the researcher is intimately involved in the process, not aloof from it (Pope and Mays 2006). However, there are some common processes, no matter which approach is taken. One way of analysis with regard to the analysis of interviews is by following these steps and will achieve a well-organised approach to interpreting and analysing qualitative data. The aim is to build piles of coded data into thematic sets that relate to different dimensions or layers of the big research question:

1 *Transcribe* tape recorded material and interview notes. *Copy* all the data (put original aside and keep securely). Remember to *anonymise* all material.

2 Read all the data from start to finish. Reread until 'sense' of *familiarisation* is achieved.
3 To make sense of the data, find 'paths' through the information. 'Break it up' and rebuild it into thematic categories through a process of focused reading. With the research question in mind, read and note themes that arise, *coding* sections of the transcript using short names or 'tags', ending up with a list of codes and sections of highlighted text. This is *preliminary coding*. Do the same with each transcript.
4 Identify *major themes* that seem to recur bearing in mind the research questions. Put ideas together in broader categories and then *recode* the material. This would be the second round of analysis. This might be done several times over. Remember coding is meant to reduce the amount of data and not increase it.
5 The idea is to arrive at a set of key themes for each research question with sets of codes for each.

PRACTICAL GUIDELINES 17.4

When analysing qualitative data:

- Be organised.
- Use a coding method which can include: the use of computer software e.g. NVivo; cutting and pasting; the use of highlighter pens; a combination of these.

- Keep a record of your thoughts.
- Allow time.

CASE STUDY 17.6

In phase 1 of the study, data were collected through individual interviews with the young people. All the interviews were transcribed. Analysis began by using codes identified from the interview schedule (a priori codes). These were ideas that the researcher wanted to look for and at this stage anything related to care and participation. In coding the care they had received, it was evident that between them they had experienced 29 different aspects of care ranging from technical care through to occupation and hygiene. The transcripts were now reread using the codes (alluding to the quality of care) of 'excellent', 'OK', 'not good enough'. This identified all instances of where the young person had given a view on the quality of care received. A third read used the code 'reasons'. From this five different reasons that accompanied the young people's views about the quality of care were identified. These were: the level of *explanation* given; how well care was actually carried out – *technical* ability; degree of *choice*; *privacy* afforded; and whether the staff were *friendly*.

Doing Analysis with Children and Young People

Sometimes, it may just not be feasible to involve children and young people in this stage of the research process. This is likely when the project is complex and highly technical or when time and resources are limited or constrained. However, leaving children and young people out of the data analysis stage fails to acknowledge that adults and children occupy different cultural worlds and thus may interpret experiences in different ways. So, where possible and appropriate, think about involving young participants in the analysis stage as their experience of health services will help to make sense of the data. Coad and Evans (2008) identify a range of ways in which they may be involved:

- Children may help to verify adult researchers' understandings of data.
- Children may act as a reference or advisory group to consult with and guide the research process and help to interpret the findings.
- Children are actively involved in the data analysis stage, working alongside adult researchers, through strategies such as coding, verification and interpretation.
- Child/young person-led research team plan, collect and undertake data analysis as a group with adults facilitating the process.

Which ever approach is taken, attention must be paid to ensuring sufficient and appropriate training is given and the time and resources are available.

VOICES 17.3

'There's some adults that do this job, they read a book and they think they know it all and they don't. We could step right in to their shoes and do a better job because we know how to relate to a young person. If you get a grip of life before it gets a grip of you you've got a better chance. With a social worker it's by the book' (Anthony, young researcher).

ACTIVITY 17.6 Data analysis

Why are so many chocolate bars named after space?

Pop into your local supermarket and find the confectionery aisle. List all the different chocolate bars that you can see. Once you have produced a list of chocolate bars, start breaking it down into subcategories. For example, by brand name, e.g. Thorntons; by size composition, e.g. double-bar Twix or single-bar Mars and, finally, grouped according to name association. Try this final grouping using the term 'space'. What chocolate bars are named after space? Write down your list.

This is a simplified illustration of how to go about doing the first stages of a thematic analysis.

DISSEMINATING RESEARCH

Dissemination is a key element of all research and is about sharing the findings in an accessible manner. Qualitative research when done well warrants sharing. Dissemination of the findings of research is an essential component of evidence-based nursing as it helps nurses to either verify current practice or development of new ways of caring for children and young people. Following a review of the literature on evidence-based nursing, Scott and McSherry (2008) suggest this definition:

> An ongoing process by which evidence, nursing theory and the practitioners' clinical expertise are critically evaluated and considered, in conjunction with patient involvement, to provide delivery of optimum nursing care for the individual. (page 1089).

In practice, the findings from research studies are often left 'on the shelf', meaning that the potential for impact can be missed. Some of the barriers to using research in nursing practice have been shown to include a lack of knowledge among nurses about the research process and an inability to understand research reports (Rogers 2009). The first priority in any dissemination plan is returning results to study participants. Dissemination to any other stakeholder group must take place following this first step. Planning dissemination should be done at the beginning of a project. Figure 17.7 shows the possible processes involved in dissemination which might be used to draw up the plan.

A dissemination plan should take into account:

- The aim: what are the aims and objectives of the dissemination effort? What impact does it have? What message is wanted to get across?
- The audience: who is affected most by the research? Who would be interested in learning about the study findings? Is this of interest to a broader community?
- The medium: what is the most effective way to reach your audience(s)? What resources does each group typically access?
- The execution: when should each aspect of the dissemination plan occur (e.g. at which points during the study and afterwards)? Who will be responsible for dissemination activities?

Keen and Todres (2006) identify the main features of successful dissemination plans as being the use of a tailored approach, in terms of the content, message and medium to the audience and active discussion of research findings.

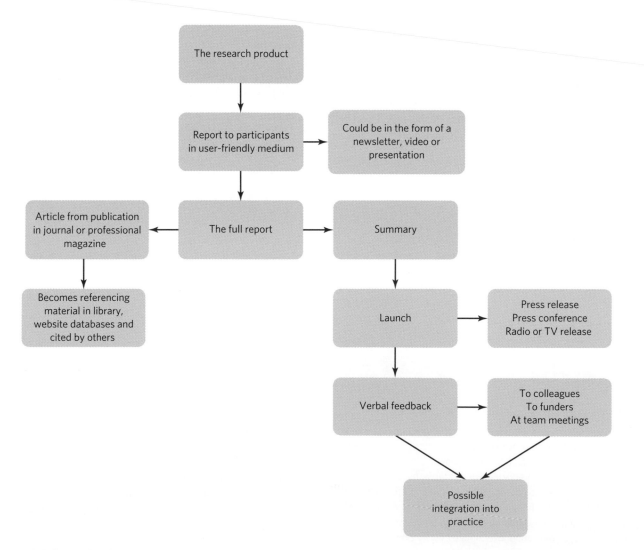

Figure 17.7 Dissemination process

CASE STUDY 17.7

The young researchers decided that they wanted to write an article to publish in a nursing journal. In discussion with the adult researcher, they chose to submit a short article to *Paediatric Nursing* (now called *Nursing Children and Young People* – an RCN publication). They drafted the article together and then asked the adult researcher to finish it off. The young researchers requested that their first names were identified as being the authors of the paper but they did not want their surnames included (Moules 2004).

In addition, the young researchers drafted a leaflet detailing the findings from the project. Copies of the leaflet were given to the local primary and secondary schools and were sent to the head of children's services at the then Department of Health.

The research was also written up for publication in a peer-reviewed journal (Moules 2009) and the findings presented at the RCN International Research Conference.

ACTIVITY 17.7

In the case study project, one of the major findings was that the children and young people identified five characteristics of quality care, which were: technical expertise, friendly staff, respect, choice and explanations. Imagine you were a member of the research team.

Who would you include in your list of possible audiences for the findings?

SUMMARY OF KEY LEARNING

- Involving children in research is vital if we are to hear children's voices in the healthcare system. Deciding how and when to involve them and being sensitive to the ethical issues is part of your role as a children's nurse.
- Being able to search and review the literature is a key element of a nurse's ongoing development. Everything undertaken as nurses is underpinned by knowledge gained by experience and research. Whether reviewing one particular research paper or carrying out an in-depth literature review as part of an assignment, there is a need to be able to develop the skill of critical reading.

- Accessing and recruiting the right children and young people to the study and choosing the most appropriate data collection and analysis method(s) will help to enhance the rigour of any research carried out. An understanding of the research process will enable a more critical approach in appraising of the research.
- The findings of research are of no value and actually a waste of time, if they never reach the correct audiences. Disseminating research is an essential element of evidence-based nursing. But be proactive in searching out the research to underpin practice.

FURTHER RESOURCES

Sampling

Parahoo, K. (2006) *Nursing research. Principles, process and issues*, 2nd edn. Palgrave-Macmillan: Houndmills. Chapter 12: Samples and sampling. A good chapter, which gives guidance on probability and non-probability sampling.

Ethics

Christensen, P. and Prout, A. (2002). Working with ethical symmetry in social research with children. *Childhood*, 9(4), 477–500.

Flewitt, R. (2005) Conducting research with young children: some ethical considerations. *Early Child Development and Care*, 175(6), 553–565.

Alderson, P. and Morrow, V. (2004) *Ethics, social research and consulting children and young people.* Barnardo's: London.

Critical appraisal skills programme: http://www.casp-uk .net/. A valuable resource providing critical appraisal checklist to review all manner of different types of research study including randomised controlled trials and qualitative studies.

Research with children and young people

Shaw, C., Brady, L. and Davey, C. (2011) Guidelines for research with children and young people. NCB: London. **http://www.ncb. org.uk/media/434791/guidelines_for_research_with_cyp.pdf**. Quite a complex publication but does have some valuable resource links and takes you through the whole process of planning and implementing a research project with children and young people.

Christensen, P. and James, A. (2008) *Research with children: per-spectives and practices.* Falmer Press: London. Discusses various aspects of childhood research and includes a chapter by Alderson on children as researchers.

Fraser, S., Lewis, V., Ding, S., Kellett, M. and Robinson, C. (eds) (2004) *Doing research with children and young people.* Sage: London. An excellent introduction to the whole topic, with a chapter on involving children and young people.

Greig, A, Taylor, J and Mackay, T. (2007) *Doing research with children*, 2nd edn. Sage: London. Provides a comprehensive practical introduction to undertaking a research project with children. The book looks at research with children as both the objects of the research and as co-researchers.

Kellett, M. (2010) *Rethinking children and research.* Continuum: London. Takes a more philosophical approach and from a per-spective of participation, but is a broader overview of childhood research in society.

Therapeutic research

Caldwell, P., Murphy, S. B., Butow, P. N. and Craig, J. C. (2004) Clinical trials in children. *The Lancet*, 364, 803–811. This paper explores issues relating to participation by children in clinical trials including consent issues and the factors that influence participation.

Davidson, A.J. and O'Brien, M. (2009) Ethics and medical research in children. *Pediatric Anesthesia*, 19(10), 994–1004. This paper discusses the ethical issues of doing medical research with children, including a discussion about consent, the issue of risk, the potential for children to be disadvantaged by not being involved in this type of research.

The following two articles are from studies that both used interviews as a data collection method but with two different age groups: Kyronlampi-Kylmanen, T. and Maatta, K. (2010) Using children as research subjects: how to interview a child aged 5–7 years. *Educational Research and Reviews*, 6(1), 87–93.

Punch, S. (2006) Interviewing strategies with young people: the 'secret box', Stimulus material and task based activities. *Child & Society*, 16, 45–56.

Gibson, F. (2007) Conducting focus groups with children and young people: strategies for success. *Journal of Research in Nursing*, 12(5), 473–483. This paper gives a description of focus groups and discusses the main methodological and practical issues asso-ciated with running them as a data collection method with chil-dren and young people.

Epstein, I., Stevens, B., McKeever, P., Baruchel, S. and Jones, H. (2008) Using puppetry to elicit children's talk for research. *Nursing Inquiry*, 15(1), 49–56.

Data collection methods

The VideoVoice Collective (**http://video-voice.org/**) is a health advocacy, research and evaluation team that gives cameras to the people who know their communities best. This link (**http://www.youtube.com/user/VideoVoiceCollective**) will take you to clips from a number of videos taken by members of marginalised communities in the USA and around the world. Look for one called 'Living at Bernal Dwellings'. The Healthy Redevelopment Video Project is a public health research project that put video cam-eras in the hands of teens to find out what a healthy community looks like to them. In this video, teen resident Marteka shows the strength, resilience and concerns of residents of Bernal Dwell-ings in San Francisco. She touches on themes such as the health impact of public housing conditions, safety, social programmes and social cohesion.

Deacon, S. (2000) Creativity within qualitative research on fami-lies: new ideas for old methods. *Qualitative Report*, 4, (3 & 4): **http://www.nova.edu/ssss/QR/QR4-3/deacon.html**. This is an interesting paper that discusses some of the creative and active methods researchers can use to involve their participants in the research process. The methods discussed include sculpt-ing, photography and videography, art and drawing, role playing, writing exercises, metaphors and timelines.

The Data Protection Act 1998: **http://www.dh.gov.uk/en/Managingyourorganisation/Informationpolicy/Recordsman-agement/DH_4000489**. This is a useful page which gives information about the application of the Data Protection Act to Research in the NHS.

Access

Stalker, K., Carpenter, J., Connors, C. and Phillips, R. (2004) Ethical issues in social research: difficulties encountered gaining access to children in hospital for research. *Child Care, Health and Development*, 30(4), 377–383. This paper describes some of the difficulties encountered in gaining access to children in hospital in a study that sought to explore the experiences of children with complex health needs.

Gardner, H. and Randall, D. (2012) The effects of the presence or absence of parents on interviews with children. *Nurse Researcher*, 19(2), 6–10.

Data analysis

Polit, D.F. (2010) *Statistics and data analysis for nursing research*, 2nd edn. Humanalysis, Inc.: Saratoga Springs, NY. This book uses a conversational style to teach students how to use statistical methods and procedures to analyse research findings. Students are guided through the complete analysis process from per-forming a statistical analysis to the rationale behind doing so. In addition, management of data, including how and why to recode variables for analysis, how to 'clean' data and how to work around missing data is discussed.

Raingruber, B. (2009) Assigning poetry reading as a way of intro-ducing students to qualitative data analysis. *Journal of Advanced Nursing*, 65(8), 1753–1761. Does what it says on the tin.

Hancock, B. (2002) *Trent focus for research and development in primary health care. An introduction to qualitative research:* **http://faculty.cbu.ca/pmacintyre/course_pages/MBA603/**

MBA603_files/IntroQualitativeResearch.pdf. This is a valuable resource that takes the reader through the process of analysing qualitative data, giving a number of exercises to carry out.

Useful centres

In January 2004 the Open University established a children's research centre: **http://childrens-research-centre.open.ac.uk**.

the Young Researcher Network at the National Youth Agency: **www.nya.org.uk/youngresearchernetwork**

INVOLVE does an excellent guide on involving children and young people in health research: **www.invo.org.uk**

International Childhood and Youth Research Network: **http:// www.icyrnet.net/**

ANSWERS TO ACTIVITIES

ACTIVITY 17.1

What is user-controlled research?
At its simplest user-controlled research is about users being in control of the research question.
What are the challenges encountered?

- funding
- negotiation of the power imbalance of the user–researcher and professional researcher in the direction of the study.

What are the changes resulting from user-controlled research?

- Making a difference in how services are designed and delivered.
- Training and empowerment of service users to be change makers.
- Positive impact on the individual (e.g. self-esteem and confidence) and wider community (e.g. new or enhanced treatments and services).

ACTIVITY 17.2 How to evaluate a website

How did you find the web page? Well, we gave it to you but we found it via Google search.
Who is responsible for the content? It is difficult to find out just who the 'we' is on this site. However it is a registered charity, and was a founder member of the multiagency group Children's Play Council; its national secretary is Jan Cosgrove who is on the governing body of the Children's Rights Alliance for England (CRAE). The organisation has a group of directors and a management council.
What is the website? It basically promotes the child's right to play and it contains resources, carries out research (although there is no explicit link to any of its research on the site), and

provides some training. There are no adverts (except for donation and its online shop) or pop-ups. There are many publications available, which suggest a balanced view.
When was it last updated? No update date given at bottom of pages. Documents dated 2011 have been uploaded but none found dated 2012.
Where is it? This is clearly a UK page. Contact details are in the UK.
The URL? Denotes this is a not-for-profit organisation. There could be potential bias, then, in the fact that one of the main purposes of its website is to raise funds.
Overall? This could be useful for resources but would not be suitable for referencing an academic essay.

ACTIVITY 17.3 Searching Google Scholar

On 7 June 2012:

- there were 3,050,000 results when using the term 'research with children'. Obviously, far too many to look through!
- down to 238,000 – still far too many

- now down to 16,500 – better but still too many
- after adding 'chronic illness', the number of results went down to 5150.

This shows how by refining your search terms, you can reduce the number of results to a manageable list.

ACTIVITY 17.4

Advantages of having parents present:

- Parents can complement children's contributions positively.
- Parents can prompt children's recall of events.
- Insights can be gained about the parent–child relationship.

- Children may feel more at ease if a parent is present.

Disadvantages of having parents present:

- Opinions of children may differ from those gained if interviewed alone.

- Children might withhold information.
- Parents may limit how children are able to express their views.
- Children may assume parents' views are more important than theirs.

- Parents may answer for their children.
- May prevent development of trusting relationship between child and researcher.

ACTIVITY 17.5

You may have found one of the following definitions: Finch (1987, page 105) describes them as 'short stories about hypothetical characters in specified circumstances, to whose situation the interviewee is invited to respond'. While Hill (1977, page 177) says they are 'short scenarios in written or pictorial form, intended to elicit responses to typical scenarios'.

Advantages:

- Vignettes can be useful in exploring potentially sensitive topics that participants might otherwise find difficult to

discuss, as commenting on a story is less personal than talking about direct experience.
- Vignettes also offer the possibility of examining different groups' interpretations of a 'uniform' situation.

Disadvantage:

- The relationship between beliefs and actions is the biggest problem in using this technique in isolation – what people say they will do in a made up context is not always what they would do in a real life situation.

ACTIVITY 17.6

You may have the following in your list:
  Mars Bar
  Galaxy

Milky Way
Aero.

ACTIVITY 17.7

- fellow nurses
- other medical staff, e.g. physiotherapists, doctors
- ward sister/charge nurse

- managers
- policymakers
- Royal College of Nursing specialist group.

SELECTED REFERENCES

Alderson, P. and Morrow, V. (2004) *Ethics, social research and consulting children and young people.* Barnardo's: London.

Backett-Milbourn, K. and McKie, L. (1999) A critical appraisal of the draw and write technique. *Health Education Research*, 14(3), 387–398.

Barker, J. and Weller, S. (2003) 'Is it fun?' Developing children centred research methods. *International Journal of Sociology and Social Policy*, 23(1), 33–58.

Beazley, H., Bessell, S., Ennew, J. and Waterson, R. (2009) The twentieth anniversary of the UNCRC: reflections on the rights-based approach for research with children and young people in the south. *Children's Geographies: Advancing interdisciplinary understanding of younger people's lives*, Issue No. 4. London: Routledge.

Boeck, T. and Sharpe, D. (2009) *An exploration of participatory research with young people, in Coyote, Strasbourg.* The Council of Europe and the European Commision, No. 14.

Brady, M. (2009) Hospitalized children's views of the good nurse. *Nursing Ethics*, 16, 543–560.

British Sociological Association (BSA) (2002) Statement of Ethical Practice for the British Sociological Association: **http://www.britsoc.co.uk/about/equality/statement-of-ethical-practice.aspx**

Clark, A. and Moss, P. (2011) *Listening to young children. The mosaic approach*, 2nd edn. National Children's Bureau: London.

Coad, J. and Coad, N. (2008) Children and young people's preference of thematic design and colour for their hospital environment. *Journal of Child Health Care*, 12(1), 33–48.

Coad, J. and Evans, R. (2008) *Reflections on practical approaches to involving children and young people in the data analysis process.* Children & Society, 22(1), 41–52.

Darbyshire, P., MacDougall, C. and Schiller, W. (2005) Multiple methods in qualitative research with children: more insight or just more? *Qualitative Research*, 5(4), 417–436.

Delgado, M. (2006) *Designs and methods for youth-led research.* Sage: London.

Faulkner, A. (2010) *Changing our worlds: examples of user-controlled research in action.* INVOLVE: Eastleigh.

Fern, L., Davies, S., Eden, T., Feltbower, R., Grant, R., Hawkins, M., Lewis, I., Loucaides, E., Rowntree, C., Stenning, S., and Whelan, J. (2008) Rates of inclusion of teenagers and young adults in England into National Cancer Research Network clinical trials: report from the National Cancer Research Institute (NCRI) teenage and young adult clinical studies development group. *British Journal of Cancer*, 12, 1967–1974.

Finch, J. (1987) The vignette technique in survey research. *Sociology*, 21, 105–14.

Gibson, F., Aldiss, S., Horstman, F., Kumpunen, S. and Richardson, A. (2010) Children and young people's experiences of cancer care: a qualitative research study using participatory methods. *International Journal of Nursing Studies*, 47(11), 1397–1407.

Hart, R. (1997) *Children's participation: the theory and practice of involving young citizens in community development and environmental care*. Earthscan: London.

Heath, S., Charles, V., Crow, G. and Wiles, R. (2007) Informed consent, gatekeepers and go-betweens in child- and youth-orientated institutions. *British Educational Journal*, 33(3): 403–417.

Higginbottom, G. (2004) Sampling issues in qualitative research. *Nurse Researcher*, 12(1) 7–15.

Hill, M. (1997) Research review: participatory research with children. *Child and Family Social Work*, 2, 171–183.

Horstman, M., Aldiss, S., Richardson, A. and Gibson, F. (2008) Methodological issues when using draw and write technique with children aged 6–12 years. *Qualitative Health Research*, 18, 1001–1011.

Husband, C. (1995 The morally active practitioner and the ethics of anti-racist social work, in R. Hugman, and D. Smith, (eds) *Ethical Issues in Social Work*. London: Routledge.

Keen, S. and Todres, L. (2006) *Communicating qualitative research findings: an annotated bibliographic review of non-traditional dissemination strategies*. Institute of Health and Community Studies, Bournemouth University: Bournemouth.

Mayall, B. (2002) *Towards a sociology for childhood: thinking from children's lives*. Open University Press: Buckingham.

Medical Research Council (2004, rev. 2007) Medical research involving children: **http://www.mrc.ac.uk/Utilities/Documentrecord/index.htm?d=MRC002430**

Mischel, W., Ebbe, B., Ebbesen, A. and Zeiss, R. (1972) Cognitive and attentional mechanisms in delay of gratification. *Journal of Personality and Social Psychology* 21(2): 204–218.

Modi, N. (2011) 'Turning the tide': increasing and strengthening child health research. *Arch Dis Child*, 96, 988.

Moules, T. (ed.) (2004) Whose quality is it? *Paediatric Nursing*, 16(6), 30–31.

Moules, T. (2006) Whose quality is it? Children and young people's participation in monitoring the quality of care in hospital: a participatory research study. Unpublished thesis, Anglia Ruskin University.

Moules, T. (2009) 'They wouldn't know how it feels . . . ': characteristics of quality care from young people's perspectives: a participatory research project. *Journal of Child Health Care*, 13(4), 322–332.

Pearce, et al. (2009) Gaining children's perspectives: a multiple method approach to explore environmental influences on healthy eating and physical activity. *Health & Place*, 15(2), 614–621.

Piaget, J. (1932) *The moral judgment of the child*. Kegan Paul, Trench, Trübner & Co.: London.

Polit, D.F., Beck, C.T. and Hungler, B.P. (2010) *Essentials of nursing research: methods appraisal and utilization*, 7th edn. Wolters Kluwer/Lippincott Williams & Wilkins: London.

Pope, C. and Mays, N. (2006) *Qualitative research in health care*, 3rd edn. Wiley-Blackwell: Chichester.

Punch, S. (2002) Interviewing strategies with young people: the 'secret box', stimulus material and task-based activities. *Child & Society*, 16, 45–56.

Rockett, M. and Percival, S. (2002) *Thinking for learning*. Network Educational Press: Stafford.

Rogers, J.L. (2009) Transferring research into practice. An integrative review. *Clinical Nurse Specialist*, 23(4), 192–199.

Royal College of Nursing (RCN) (2009) Research ethics. RCN guidance for nurses. **http://www.rcn.org.uk/__data/assets/pdf_file/0007/388591/003138.pdf**

Royal College of Paediatrics, Child Health: Ethics Advisory Committee (2000) Guidelines for the ethical conduct of medical research involving children. *Arch Dis Child*, 82, 177–182.

Scott, J. (2000) Children as respondents: the challenge for quantitative research, in P. Christensen, and A. James, (eds) *Research with children: perspectives and practices*. Falmer Press: London.

Scott, K. and McSherry, R. (2008) Evidence-based nursing: clarifying the concepts for nurses in practice. *Journal of Clinical Nursing*, 18, 1085–1095.

Sharpe, D. (2009) The value of young people doing research: where do young people's voices count? *Research, Policy and Planning: The Journal of the Social Services Research Group*, 27(2), 97–106.

Spratling, R., Coke, S. and Minick, P. (2010) Qualitative data collection with children. *Applied Nursing Research*, 25, 47–53.

Thomas, C. and O'Kane, C. (1998) The ethics of participatory research with children. *Children and Society*, 12, 336–348.

Tisdall, E.K. and Liebel, M. (2008) Children's participation in decision-making: exploring theory, policy and practice across Europe. European Science Foundation Seminar: Berlin. **http://www.childhoodstudies.ed.ac.uk/research/Tisdall+Liebel%20Overview%20Paper.pdf**

Wyness, M. (2006) *Childhood and society: an introduction to the sociology of childhood*. Macmillan: Basingstoke.

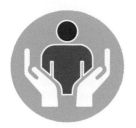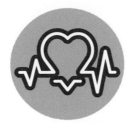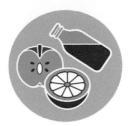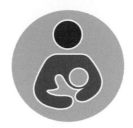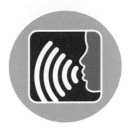

GLOSSARY

Abortion Medical or surgical termination of a pregnancy.

Absolute poverty A standard that is the same in all countries and does not change over time.

Accountability Liable to call to account.

Acetylcholine A neurotransmitter involved with sending messages between the motor nerves and muscles.

Acuity Dependency needs of patients measured to predict staffing requirements.

Adolescence Maturity of the body and mind in the context of individual growth and biopsychological development often used by health and other caring professionals.

Advocate Someone either professional or lay who intercedes for and acts on behalf of a client or young person.

Aetiology The cause or origin of a disease, condition or mixture of symptoms or signs, as determined by medical diagnosis.

Aggression Physical or verbal behaviour that is hostile and enacted to intimidate others.

Ambu bag Ventilating bag.

Amenorrhoea An absence of menstrual bleeding.

Analgesics Medication used for specific purpose of reducing and alleviating pain (although may also have anti-inflammatory properties as well as antipyretic properties).

Anthropology The study of the development of mankind especially of origins, customs and beliefs.

Antipyretics Medication that has the potential to reduce fever.

Approved Mental Health Professionals (AMHPs) are trained to implement coercive elements of the Mental Health Act 1983, as amended by the Mental Health Act 2007, in conjunction with medical practitioners. They have received specific training relating to the application of the Mental Health Act.

Aseptic technique Set of specific practices and procedures performed under carefully controlled conditions with the goal of minimizing contamination by pathogens.

Asymptomatic virus shedding Shedding particles of herpes virus when not suffering any symptoms of the disease.

Atopic eczema An inflammatory condition that is a result of an allergen, known or unknown in origin.

ATP Adenosine triphosphate, which supplies large amounts of energy to cells for various biochemical processes, including muscle contraction and sugar metabolism.

Bibliographic database An organised collection of machine-readable records that describe books, journal articles, reports or other primary sources of information.

Bilevel positive airway pressure (BiPAP) This can be utilised in spontaneous or timed mode. Sensing the changes in flow thus triggers the ventilator and this can be adversely affected by leak at the mask.

Biographical perspective This approach appreciates that individuals are each unique dependent on their own life experiences rather than purely due to the perceived commonalities that exist due to age, gender or culture.

Blood gases Any of the gases that become dissolved in blood plasma, including oxygen, nitrogen and carbon dioxide.

Body mass index (BMI) Measure of the weight for height of the individual. It is calculated as the weight in kilograms divided by the height squared in metres (kg/m^2).

BPD (bronchopulmonary dysplasia) Respiratory problem caused by mechanical ventilation.

Bradykinin A very powerful vasodilator, which increases capillary permeability; in addition, it constricts smooth muscle and stimulates pain receptors.

Bronchoscopy Examination of the bronchi through a scope.

Brown adipose tissue (BAT) Brown fat is one of two types of fat or adipose tissue.

CAF Common assessment framework: the universal starting point for information gathering and referral process used as a common form within and between all agencies involved in safeguarding vulnerable children.

Calcineurin inhibitors In treatment of eczema, calcineurin inhibitors in cream and ointment form (e.g. Tacrolimous) can be used when topical steroids are not effective. These creams appear to have less detrimental effect on the immune system (Hultsch, Kapp and Spergel 2005).

Caps Reusable contraceptive device designed to be placed over the cervix by the user prior to intercourse.

Care of the dying Care of the patient and family in the last hours and days of life. It incorporates four key domains of care: physical, psychological, social and spiritual, and supports the family at that time and into bereavement.

Catecholamine Adrenaline and noradrenaline that are produced in the medulla of the adrenal gland. They function as neurotransmitters in the sympathetic nervous system. The inflation of the lungs during the first inflation breaths.

Cerazette™ Tradename for a newer progesterone-only pill containing desogestrel.

Cervical canal Route through the cervix (bottom portion of uterus) by which sperm enter the womb through the vagina.

Cervix Bottom third of the uterus which projects into the top of the vagina.

Child or adolescent antisocial behaviour This category can be used when the focus of clinical attention is antisocial behaviour in a child or adolescent that is not due to a mental disorder.

Children's hospice services Provide palliative care for children and young people with life-limiting conditions and their families.

Children's palliative care An active and total approach to care from the point of diagnosis or recognition, embracing physical, emotional, social and spiritual elements through to death and beyond.

Chlamydia A sexually transmitted infection.

Clinical network Connections across disciplines, which provide integrated care across institutional and professional boundaries, raising clinical quality and improving the patient experience.

Clinical trial A particular type of clinical research that compares one treatment with another. It may involve patients or healthy people or both.

Coil An intrauterine device (see later) sometimes referred to as a copper coil.

Collaboration Working together to produce, collate or manage something.

Combined hormonal patch A contraceptive patch worn on the skin (like a nicotine patch). It contains both oestrogen and progesterone (combined). It is highly effective. The presence of oestrogen means it has the same benefits, risks and contraindications as a combined oral contraceptive pill. Each patch is worn for a week and then replaced.

Combined oral contraceptive pill (COCP) A contraceptive pill containing two hormones, usually a combination of oestrogen and progesterone. The presence of oestrogen makes the pill very effective at preventing pregnancy and controlling menstrual bleeding, but also increases the side-effects and risks associated with using a contraceptive pill.

Comparative perspective An anthropological understanding of the lives of individuals in the context of global comparisons, depending on where people live, including attitudes to age and development.

Concept An abstract idea representing an object or phenomenon.

Condoms (male) Latex or non-latex contraceptive barrier devices designed to be placed over the penis to collect sperm.

Conjunctivitis Infection of the eye.

Connector Outside edge of the tracheostomy tube that connects to equipment.

Consumption An old name for pulmonary tuberculosis.

Contact tracing *See* **partner notification**.

Contraceptive implant A contraceptive device that is inserted under the skin of the upper arm. It contains only progesterone. It is highly effective. The Nexplanon implant (available in the UK) lasts for 3 years. It is therefore an LARC.

Contraceptive injection A depot injection of synthetic progesterone that is given into the buttock. It is highly effective. Each injection lasts for 12 weeks. It is therefore an LARC.

Copper intrauterine device Contraceptive device consisting of a plastic core surrounded by copper which is placed in the womb (uterus). *See also* **coil**, **IUD**.

CPAP Continuous positive airway pressure. Assisted ventilation that supports the infant's own respiratory efforts. The ability to provide continuous positive airway pressure during spontaneous breaths in ventilated patients has been demonstrated to benefit some patients. Currently a new generation of ventilators is being marketed for the home setting. These have flow generators and variable flow triggers that can provide pressure support as an alternative mode.

CPR Cardiopulmonary resuscitation. A method for getting someone to breathe again once they have stopped.

Culture The set of socially constructed acceptable behaviours are dependent on the times and challenges for that society.

Cystic fibrosis (CF) The most common genetic disorder with around one in every 2500 live births in the UK. Due to a gene dysfunction, individuals with CF have problems with a number of body systems: breathing because of the thick mucus in their lungs, digestion due to lack of pancreatic enzyme, reproductive function both in males and females and heat control due to levels of sodium chloride in the person's sweat.

Data Information (which can be numerical or descriptive) that are analysed and used as the basis for making decisions in research.

Depo Contraceptive injection (see earlier).

Developmental milestones Pointers in the normal development of a child, such as walking.

Diagnostic overshadowing The tendency of clinicians to overlook symptoms of mental or physical health problems and attribute them to being part of 'having a learning disability'.

Diaphragm Reusable contraceptive device made of latex on a compressible frame. Designed to be inserted high into the vagina by the user prior to intercourse.

Direct payments Cash payments given to service users in lieu of community care services they have been assessed as needing and are intended to give users greater choice in their care. Direct payments and personal budgets are a central part of the personalisation agenda to give service users choice and control over their care and support.

Disability The Disability Discrimination Act defines disability as 'a physical or mental impairment which has a substantial and long-term adverse effect on a person's ability to carry out normal day-to-day activities. People who have a disability, and those who have had a disability and no longer have one, are covered by the Act.'

DoH Department of Health. Lead government department for children's services and safeguarding policy and legislation.

Double discrimination Where two issues rather than one are discriminated against, for example a woman with a disability may face discrimination because of gender as well as disability.

'Double Dutch' Using condoms to prevent STIs and another more effective method of contraception to prevent pregnancy.

Duty of care A legal obligation imposed on a children's nurse to provide care.

DVT Deep venous thrombosis. A potentially serious condition where blood clots in the veins of the legs.

Easy read format Created to help people with learning disabilities understand information easily. People with learning disabilities need access to all information, not just disability-specific information but also about their health, voting, work and gaining skills. Easy read uses pictures to support the meaning of text. It can be used by a carer to talk through a communication with someone with learning difficulties so that they can understand it.

Effectiveness Ability of contraceptive device to prevent pregnancy. Usually expressed in percentages (e.g. 96%). This can be thought of as equivalent to the number of women who would remain not pregnant if 100 women used the device for a year.

Efficacy The result of which achieves the desired goal and effect.

Elective surgery Performed when surgical intervention is the preferred treatment for a condition that is not imminently life threatening or to improve the client's life.

ellaOne™ Tradename for a non-hormonal emergency contraceptive pill containing ulipristal.

Emergency contraception (EC) Contraceptive method that is used after intercourse, as an emergency measure.

Emergency surgery Performed immediately to preserve function or the life of the patient.

Emollients Creams that have a softening, soothing and moistening property.

End of life The end-of-life phase begins when a judgement is made that death is imminent. It may be the judgement of the health/social care professional or team responsible for the care of the patient, but it is often the child/young person or family who first recognises its beginning.

End-of-life care Care that helps all those with advanced, progressive, incurable illness to live as well as possible until they die. It focuses on preparing for an anticipated death and managing the end stage of a terminal medical condition.

End-of-life care services Services to support those with advanced, progressive, incurable illness to live as well as possible until they die. These are services that enable the supportive and end-of-life care needs of both child/young person and the family to be identified and met throughout the last phase of life and into bereavement. It includes management of pain and other symptoms and provision of psychological, social, spiritual and practical support.

Enzyme-inducing drugs Drugs such as rifampicin, which speed up the metabolism of other drugs in the liver. This can cause some hormonal contraceptives to become less effective.

Epididymo-orchitis Infection of the testis and epidydimus.

Ethics Code of conduct for researchers. Researchers will have responsibilities and obligations to encourage participation and protection of those involved in the research. Ethics are dependent on particular circumstances of the research project.

Failure rates Inverse of the effectiveness of a device. It expresses the number of pregnancies (i.e. failures of contraception) that are expected when the device is used. It is usually expressed in percentages (e.g. 4%). This can be thought of as equivalent to the number of women who would become pregnant if 100 women used the device for a year.

Family Includes parents, other family members involved in the care of the young person or other carers who are acting in the role of parents. Family includes informal carers and all those who matter to the child/young person.

Family focus Characterised by a collaborative approach to care-giving and decision making. Each party respects the knowledge, skills and experience that the other brings to healthcare encounters. The family and healthcare team collaboratively assess the needs and development of the treatment plan.

Family therapy Psychotherapeutic treatment of the family as a unit to clarify and modify the ways they relate together and communicate.

Female sterilisation Permanent division, destruction or blockage of the ovarian tubes, leading to irreversible infertility.

Femidom™ Tradename for a female condom.

Framework A basic structure underlying a system, concept or text.

Gangsta A sociopathic member of the inner-city underclass, known primarily for being antisocial and uneducated.

Gatekeepers Those people who attempt to safeguard the interests of others.

Gene Basic unit of human heredity, contained within the chromosome.

General anaesthetic Acts by blocking awareness centres in the brain so that amnesia (loss of memory), analgesia (insensibility to pain), hypnosis (artificial sleep) and relaxation (rendering a part of the body less tense) occur.

Genital herpes A sexually transmitted infection.

Glaserian grounded theory Systematic generation of theory from data that contain both inductive and deductive thinking.

Global developmental delay (GDD) General term used to describe a condition that occurs during the developmental period of a child between birth and 18 years. It is usually defined by the child being diagnosed with having a lower intellectual functioning than what is perceived as 'normal'. It is usually accompanied by having significant limitations in communication.

Glycogen A substance deposited in bodily tissues as a store of carbohydrates.

Glycogenesis Conversion of glucose to glycogen for storage in the liver.

Gonorrhoea A sexually transmitted infection.

Grunting Noise produced due to forced expiration and a sign of respiratory distress.

Habituate To cause physiological or psychological habituation.

Herpes simplex virus Virus responsible for genital herpes and cold sores.

Histamine Released in allergic inflammatory reactions.

HIV Human immunodeficiency virus. The virus that attacks the human immune system and can lead to AIDS.

HME Heat and moisture exchanger. A filter device that fits onto the end of the tracheostomy tube and warms and moistens the air the child breathes.

Holism Relates to the notion that all individuals are made up of many parts that are interlinked. When caring for children and young people, our care must address mind, body and spirit.

Hospice at home Term commonly used to describe a service that brings skilled, practical children's palliative care into the home environment. Hospice at home works in partnership with parents, families and other carers.

Human papilloma virus (HPV) The family of viruses responsible for genital warts and most cases of cervical cancer.

Humidity Moisture in the air.

Hyaline membrane disease A disease causing respiratory distress usually in premature newborns in which hyaline, a glassy, eosinophilic material, is seen in the alveoli. Also known as respiratory distress syndrome.

Hypoglycaemia Low level of glucose concentration in the blood (low blood sugars).

Hypovolaemia Low volume of circulating blood.

Hypoxia Reduction and insufficient oxygen supply to cell, tissue or organ.

Implantation Process whereby a fertilised egg becomes incorporated into the lining of the womb, allowing a pregnancy to be established. Usually occurs about 5 days after fertilisation.

In vitro fertilisation Refers to fertilisation of the ovum (egg) outside the body. It is a technique often used by couples when there have been difficulties in conception in the conventional way.

Independence in adulthood Seen not purely as the ability to function autonomously as an individual; rather, it is the balance of individual freedom alongside mutual respect, obligation and commitment to others including family.

Individualisation The consequence of social changes in which individuals are increasingly required to construct their own lives.

Insensible loss Water/fluid loss that is uncontrolled coming from skin, lungs, bowel and digestive tract.

Interagency Representing or working taking place between government bodies.

Intergenerational cultural dissonance (ICD) A clash between parents and children over cultural values – occurs so commonly among immigrant families that it is regarded as a normative experience.

Intermenstrual bleeding Endometrial bleeding outside the time of the usual menstrual 'period'.

Intermittent bleeding Endometrial bleeding that occurs outside the usual time of menstrual 'period'.

Interprofessional Interprofessional working between two or more professional groups to deliver quality evidence-based care.

Intraprofessional Intraprofessional working is one profession group to deliver quality evidence-based practice.

Intrauterine system (IUS) Plastic contraceptive device placed in the womb, with a collar that releases progesterone.

Intravenous cannula A device used to access the venous system in order to deliver intravenous fluids. It is usually an indwelling device designed to remain in situ for duration of treatment.

IUD Intrauterine device. By convention refers to a copper intrauterine device (see earlier).

Key working Or care coordination. A service involving two or more agencies that provides disabled children and young people and their families with a system whereby services from different agencies are coordinated.

Labia Part of the female perineum, which forms the entrance to the vagina.

Learning difficulty (LD) A condition often affecting children of normal or above-average intelligence, characterised by difficulty in learning such fundamental procedures as reading, writing and numeric calculation. The condition may result from psychological or organic causes and is usually related to slow development of perceptual motor skills. Conditions include attention deficit disorder, dysgraphia, dyslexia and dyspraxia.

Levonelle™ Tradename for a hormonal emergency contraceptive pill.

Levonorgestrel A synthetic form of progesterone.

Liability Being responsible for a decision, action or aspect of care.

Life-limiting conditions Those for which there is no reasonable hope of cure and from which children or young people will die. Some of these conditions cause progressive deterioration rendering the child increasingly dependent on parents and carers.

Life-limiting lifelong conditions Conditions that may entail long periods of intensive treatment aimed at prolonging life and allowing participation in normal activities, although premature death is still possible or inevitable.

Long-acting reversible contraceptives (LARCs) Contraceptive methods that can be left in place for longer than a month without being replaced or renewed. They are usually more effective than short-acting reversible contraceptives because they reduce the chances of user error. This means that 'typical use' failure rates are nearly the same as 'perfect use'.

Long-term ventilation (LTV) Required by any child who, when medically stable, continues to use a mechanical aid for breathing, after an acknowledged failure to wean, or a slow wean, 3 months after the institution of ventilation.

Maintenance fluids Intravenous fluids administered to a level that will sustain homeostasis of the circulation.

Medical/clinical stability A period of 2 weeks with no change in treatment plan with regard to the ventilator settings or oxygen supplementation. Over this time the child should have demonstrated adequate growth on the present feeding regimen without life-threatening episodes of aspiration and stable acid-base and metabolic status without changes in medications such as diuretics. Once these patients are clinically stable, they can be transferred from a PICU to a separate area within an acute care hospital or a freestanding rehabilitation centre. The child must have either a secure airway or be able to tolerate non-invasive ventilation.

Medical model Presented as viewing disability as a problem of the person, directly caused by disease, trauma or other health condition that therefore requires sustained medical care provided in the form of individual treatment by professionals. In the medical model, management of the disability is aimed at a 'cure', or the individual's adjustment and behavioural change that would lead to an 'almost-cure' or effective cure. In the medical model, medical care is viewed as the main issue.

Medically stable Generally implies: the presence of a stable airway; stable oxygen requirements (if required) usually less than 40%; arterial carbon dioxide tensions can be maintained within safe limits on ventilatory equipment that can be operated by the family or carers at home; nutritional intake is adequate to maintain expected growth and development; all other medical conditions are well controlled.

Meiosis The production of gametes (sex cells).

Meme A term used by Richard Dawkins to describe the basic unit of cultural heredity.

Mental illness Physical, cognitive, affective, behavioural and social patterns that interact dysfunctionally with the environment.

Metabolic alkalosis A pH imbalance in which the body has accumulated too much of an alkaline substance, such as bicarbonate, and does not have enough acid to effectively neutralise the effects of the alkali.

Migraine headaches with aura An aura is a disturbance of vision that occurs before the onset of the headache. It usually involves loss of a C-shaped area of vision with scintillation, i.e. zigzag lines, at the edges.

Mirena™ Tradename for IUS in the UK.

Mitosis Replication of all cells in the body apart from gametes.

Model Structure that allows the issues to be examined in two or three dimensions before being applied to the real situation.

Mucus plug Thick mucus that blocks the passage of sperm through the cervical canal.

National Institute for Health and Clinical Excellence (NICE) Provides independent, authoritative and evidence-based guidance to healthcare professionals and others working in areas where healthcare is delivered. Their role is to enhance the provision of the most effective ways to prevent, diagnose and treat disease and ill health, reducing inequalities and variation.

Needs led Term used to describe how services should be provided on the basis of the needs of the patient and family and not as a result of assessing the resources that are available. To deliver a needs-led service, it is important to assess and thoroughly understand the needs of the children, young people and families first.

Negligence Failure to take reasonable care, which results in damage, error or an untoward incident.

Neutral thermal environment The environmental temperature at which an infant can maintain his rectal temperature at 37°C with minimal oxygen consumption.

Non-invasive positive pressure ventilation Although less cumbersome, the interface between the patient and ventilator is critical to its success. Most frequently this is accomplished with a nasal or facemask though mouthpieces have also been used. Fit and comfort are essential and this can present a hurdle in infants or patients with facial malformations. Continuous positive airway pressure is maintained in the CPAP mode by increasing inspiratory flow. This effectively holds the airway open and maintains lung volume. When the ventilator is set on spontaneous mode, the patient triggers each breath spontaneously, whereas in a timed mode the ventilator is set to deliver a mandatory breath at a fixed rate.

NSPCC National Society for the Prevention of Cruelty to Children. One of the leading charitable organisations and a pioneer in promoting the welfare of vulnerable children.

O_2 Saturation Oxygen saturation value is the amount of oxygen that has passed into the blood and is being carried by the haemoglobin. One haemoglobin molecule carries four molecules of oxygen. If all the sites available on the circulating haemoglobin are full then it will measure 99% oxygen saturation.

Obturator The semi-rigid stick you put into the tracheostomy tube to help guide it into the opening in the neck.

Oestrogen A sex hormone used in combined hormonal contraceptive preparations.

Off-label Products not licensed for use in children; however, there may have been approval for use in adults or animals.

Orthopaedic surgery Concerned with conditions involving the musculoskeletal system. Surgeons use both surgical and non-surgical means to treat trauma, sports injuries, degenerative diseases, infections, tumours and congenital disorders.

Ovulation Production of an egg from the ovary of a woman.

Parents Term used to mean any carer for a child whether that be a married or unmarried couple, a single parent, guardian or foster parent.

Partial pressure of carbon dioxide (PCO_2) Quantifies the amount of carbon dioxide that is dissolved in the plasma. Carbon dioxide values are maintained by alterations in the respirations by the rate of respirations and the depth of respirations. The partial pressure of carbon dioxide assesses the ability of the lungs to rid the body of CO_2. An increased partial pressure of CO_2 can indicate either the blood supply to the lungs is reduced and there is vasoconstriction or the CO_2 is unable to diffuse from the blood to the lungs through the alveolar membranes. There is decreased air movement out of the lungs to expire the CO_2. There is depressed activity of the respiratory centre. A decreased partial pressure of CO_2 is associated with increased respiration and expiration resulting in hyperventilation.

Partial pressure of oxygen (PO_2) The amount of oxygen that has passed from the alveolus of the lungs and is being transported by the blood to the tissues and cells. An increased PO_2 means there is increased oxygen in inspired air. A decreased PO_2 means there is reduced oxygen passing into blood.

Participatory research Carried out *with* people, rather than *on* people. Those being researched take an active role in the research project.

Partner notification Tracing and contacting of sexual partners of a person diagnosed with an STI, with a view to treating those partners.

Patency Refers to a pathway being free from obstruction.

Peer research Carried out by people who share the same set of circumstances as those being researched. For example, people of the same age group or who live in the area under study. In many cases, young researchers who research other young people are carrying out peer research.

Peer review Evaluation of creative work by other people in the same field in order to maintain or enhance the quality of the work in that field.

PEG A feeding tube that passes through the abdominal wall directly into the stomach, so that nutrition can be provided without swallowing or, in some cases, to supplement ordinary food. The PEG tube can be connected to a 'giving set' to provide feeds continuously or a syringe can be used to receive feeds at intervals.

Pelvic inflammatory disease (PID) Severe infection of the uterus and ovaries, which can lead to secondary loss of fertility.

Perfect use Refers to the situation in which a contraceptive device is used perfectly for every act of intercourse. Failure rates for perfect use are usually lower than for typical use, but the rate does not reflect what can be expected in a 'real-life' situation for most populations.

Perfusion Refers to the action of oxygen as it 'pours through' the circulatory system and perfuses the end organs and tissues of the body.

Peri-hepatitis Infection of the capsule of the liver.

Person-centred Activities that are based on what is important to the person from her own perspective and that contribute to her full inclusion in society. Person-centred approaches design and deliver services and support based on what is important to a person. Hence person-centred planning can promote person-centred approaches.

Personal budgets Allocation of funding given to users after an assessment that should be sufficient to meet their assessed needs. Users can either take their personal budget as a direct payment or – while still choosing how their care needs are met and by whom – leave councils with the responsibility to commission the services. Or they can have a combination of the two.

Personalisation Putting individuals firmly in the driving seat of building a system of care and support that is designed with their full involvement and tailored to meet their own unique needs.

Pessary Bullet-shaped preparation designed for delivery of medication via the vagina.

Phlebitis Inflammation of the vein, which can manifest with swelling, redness and pain.

Phobia Described as a strong fear of an event, object or animal.

PICU Pediatric intensive care unit.

Postcode lottery Term used when healthcare provision is determined by location rather than need.

Preceptor Someone who is on the same part of the register as the preceptee and who can provide support, guidance, help and advice when 'internalising' learning from a pre-registration nursing programme.

Primary care Care services that occur at the initial point of contact and usually in a community environment.

Proctitis Infection of the rectum.

Progesterone-only pill (POP) A contraceptive pill containing only progesterone. The absence of oestrogen in a POP removes many of the contraindications and risks of a COCP. However, control of menstrual bleeding is less and intermittent bleeding can be a problem.

Progesterone A sex hormone used in contraceptive preparations.

Prostatitis Infection of the prostate gland.

Psychoanalysis An approach to treating mental health disorders based on the theories and teachings of Sigmund Freud.

Pulse oximeter Machine that monitors the oxygen saturation of the blood using an infrared detector placed across a capillary bed such as a digit or ear.

Qualitative research Often described as in-depth research, using words or imagery rather than numbers (quantitative research). It concentrates on understanding *why* and *how* things happen and how they are *understood*. Common methods include interviews, focus groups and observations.

Quantitative research This type of research has an emphasis on counting and numbers; it is often used to find out *what* happened or *how much*. Common methods include surveys and using statistical information.

Reactive arthritis (Reiter's syndrome) Inflammatory condition of the joints secondary to an STI.

Reality Orientation (RO) is a programme designed to improve cognitive and psychomotor function in persons who are confused or disoriented. Aids such as calendars and clocks and sensory stimuli such as distinctive sights, sounds, and smells are used to improve sensory awareness.

Reasonable adjustments Equality law recognises that bringing about equality for disabled people may mean changing the way in which environments are structured, such as the removal of physical barriers and/or providing extra support for a disabled person. This is the duty to make reasonable adjustments. The duty to make reasonable adjustments aims to make sure that, as far as is reasonable, a disabled person has the same access to everything that is involved in doing and keeping a job/accesses services as a non-disabled person.

Relative poverty The poverty threshold, or poverty line, is the minimum level of income deemed necessary to achieve an adequate standard of living that differs between countries.

Research Asking questions, exploring issues and reflecting on findings. It is concerned with extending knowledge, pursuing 'truth' and must always be ethical.

Respiratory acidosis Condition in which a build-up of carbon dioxide in the blood produces a shift in the body's pH balance and causes the body's system to become more acidic.

Respiratory alkalosis Condition in which the amount of carbon dioxide found in the blood drops to a level below normal range.

Responsibility A person, thing or event a children's nurse is responsible for.

Risk management Covers all the processes involved in identifying, assessing and judging risks, assigning ownership, taking actions to mitigate or anticipate them and monitoring and reviewing progress.

SALT (speech and language therapist) Person trained to help with speaking and swallowing problems.

Screen Test for disease or condition in an asymptomatic population.

Secondary care Care services that occur in an acute hospital setting.

Self harm a way of expressing very deep distress. Often, people don't know why they self-harm. It's a means of communicating what can't be put into words or even into thoughts and has been described as an inner scream. Afterwards, people feel better able to cope with life again, for a while.

Sexually transmitted infection (STI) Infection contracted from another person through sexual activity.

Short breaks Short breaks may offer the whole family an opportunity to be together and to be supported in the care of their child or it may offer care solely for the child or young person, to provide opportunities for siblings to have fun and receive support in their own right.

Skin prick allergy testing Commonly used skin test to identify allergens. The test is usually performed on the inner arm and a tiny amount of each allergen is introduced into the skin with the tip of a lancet, which is not painful. A positive result is recorded if a wheal develops during the following 15 minutes. There is a recording of the test available.

Smog Smokey fog.

Social model of disability Sees the issue of 'disability' as a socially created problem and a matter of the full integration of individuals into society. In this model, disability is not an attribute of an individual, but rather a complex collection of conditions, many of which are created by the social environment. Hence, the management of the problem requires social action and it is the collective responsibility of society at large to make the environmental modifications necessary for the full participation of people with disabilities in all areas of social life.

Speaking valve A one-way valve that lets air come in through the tracheostomy tube, but then sends it out past the vocal cords and mouth to make talking possible.

Spermicide Chemical presented as gel, foam, film or pessary that has the effect of killing sperm.

Stoma Hole or opening in the neck into which you insert the tracheostomy tube.

Stridor Description of the sound of breathing when the upper airway is obstructed.

Suctioning Vacuuming up mucus in the tracheostomy tube.

Supervision An emerging concept in nursing prompted by the Children's Workforce Development Council, not to be confused with line management or operational procedures. A reflective, non-judgemental discussion to aid practice development.

Surgery Any procedure performed on the human body that uses instruments to alter tissue or organ integrity.

Sweat test A rudimentary test that relies on measurement of the amount of salt released from the sweat glands following a stimulus of a small electrical charge; the test is still effective and with further physical and symptomatic assessments, it can still be used as one of the tools for diagnosis, combined with more advanced genetic testing.

Swedish nose *See* **HME**

Symptom management Management of common symptoms associated with life-limiting conditions. It is often used to refer to symptoms that are primarily physical, but in palliative care symptom management also includes attention to psychosocial and spiritual aspects of symptoms where appropriate.

Systematic Carrying an action out in an organised manner.

Systemic treatment Treatment that addresses the problem through the whole body system, rather than just addressing part of the problem.

Tertiary care A care service that delivers specialised care and is generally accessed through referral from primary or secondary centres.

Thermal humidifying filter *See* **HME**

Thermogenesis Production of heat.

Thermovent T *See* **HME**

Tracheostomy Opening into the trachea.

Tracheotomy A medical procedure creating an opening in the trachea.

Transition A change for an individual that may occur over time or in stages of development or by physically moving from one environment to another, such as school to college, work.

Typical use Refers to the situation in which a device is used in a typical population, under usual conditions. The failure rates of a contraceptive device during typical use are higher than during perfect use, because it reflects the numbers of people who may forget to use the device, use it imperfectly and so on.

Ulipristal Active ingredient in emergency contraceptive pill ellaOne™.

Unlicensed These products have a specific legal status. The manufacturer may not have any liability for the drug and liability could rest with the prescriber, dispenser and administrator of the medicine. Prescribing under the remit of a licence is desirable.

Unprotected intercourse Intercourse carrying a risk of pregnancy or sexually transmitted infection because no contraceptive or barrier method is used.

Urethra Tube leading from the bladder to the outside, through which urine is voided.

Urethral discharge Pus or mucous coming from the urethra in a man or woman.

Urgent surgery Necessary for client's health to prevent additional problem from developing; not necessarily an emergency.

User-controlled research Research that is actively controlled, directed and managed by service users and their service user organisations.

Vaginal contraceptive ring A contraceptive ring, containing oestrogen and progesterone which is worn high in the vagina. It is highly effective. The presence of oestrogen means it has the same benefits, risks and contraindications as a combined oral contraceptive pill. Each ring is worn for three weeks before being removed for a week and then replaced with a new ring

Vaginal discharge Pus or mucous coming from the vagina.

Vaginal mucosa Membrane lining the inside of the vagina.

Venepuncture The introduction of a sharps device (needle or cannula) to obtain a blood sample or give access for intravenous therapy.

Ventilator A machine that helps a person breathe.

Whistleblowing An informant who exposes wrong doing.

Young person The term young person describes a person from their 13th – 19th birthday.

Youth A sociological term which enables an exploration of transition for the young person from child to youth and adult within the context of their environment.

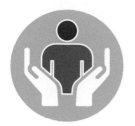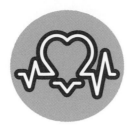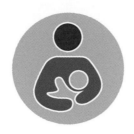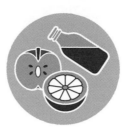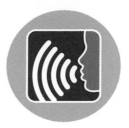

INDEX